We believe that illustrations can more effectively convey some informat
words, and since illustrations today can be so readily incorporated into boc
modern publishing techniques, we used them when we felt that they would
effective than words alone.

Such is the breadth of medical disorders involving the immune system that
inevitably there are omissions in some areas, and unintended brevity, or overem-
phasis in other areas. We hope however, that this text will serve as a starting point
for trainees in clinical immunology, general physicians, other clinical specialists
and advanced medical students seeking a syllabus for this fascinating discipline.

We wish to record our thanks to all who have made this book possible, contribu-
tors and colleagues; students and trainees both past and present, and especially to
our wives and families for being so tolerant of the time and effort consumed.

February 1997   J. B
Australia   J. McC.

Preface

Clinical immunology has become recognized as a fascinating and evolving speciality with very flexible boundaries. It has contributed substantially to our understanding of many human diseases and also in the development of new diagnostic techniques and therapeutic interventions. The past decade has seen the introduction of fruits of the molecular era to this area with diagnostic use and therapeutic administration of monoclonal antibodies and recombinant products. Whereas clinical immunology has developed into a clinical and laboratory discipline in Australia, in other parts of the world it has remained mainly a laboratory discipline, or it has been identified exclusively with the clinical treatment of allergic disorders. In Australia, the clinical areas directly associated with this speciality include allergy, rheumatology, renal medicine and HIV/AIDS, and other infectious diseases. For more than twenty years in Australia specialists in clinical immunology have trained as specialists in internal medicine (physicians), in pathology, or both (pathologists/physicians). One purpose of this book was therefore to demonstrate what we consider to be the area of practice for the clinical immunologist.

This book aims to define the more specialized aspects of immunological medical practice. There have been many books on the laboratory aspects of clinical immunology and the area has been well covered. However, the clinical area has been more difficult to clearly define. This is because increasingly, immunology is seen to be a basic underlying science for understanding many disease processes relevant to many clinical specialities. An aspiring specialist in clinical immunology may not need to be quite as familiar with these areas as the specialist renal physician, endocrinologist, or neurologist. However, it is important that there should be a sophisticated understanding of the role of immunological involvement across clinical medical practice if there is to be appropriate advice to clinical colleagues on the role of investigation in diagnosis, and on the possibility of manipulation of immune responses in their management.

We have therefore relied on our own experience as clinical and laboratory specialists; as supervisors of trainees; and as examiners in this speciality to decide what should be included in this book. In addition over the past few years there has been an expansion of knowledge about the molecular side of this speciality. While there are already books in this area we believe that there is place for one which gives greater emphasis to the clinical and molecular sides of the speciality.

Practitioners of clinical immunology need to understand the immunopathogenesis of human diseases; be masters of the immunological diagnostic tests used to aid diagnosis and management of disease; be authoritative advisers on the ordering of diagnostic tests and therapy of the disease; and be good clinical practitioners. There should be many opportunities for the clinical immunologist who is orientated to preventing the progression of diseases in the future. More effective and focused therapy with the use of cytokines, monoclonal antibodies, peptides, immunosuppressants, together with immunoreconstitution, and transplantation of tissues are areas where the specialist in immunology will increasingly be effective because of the core scientific base knowledge of the discipline.

Nothing is more important in a textbook than being up-to-date. For this reason, it is noteworthy that all the authors are working leaders in their subject, and that quite a few could still be classified as young! Most of the authors confront their clinical problems on a daily basis and have that uniquely urgent spur to keep them at the cutting edge. The editors are to be congratulated on their choices. As a result of the collective labour of a large number of creative people, we now have a textbook which admirably fills a real need – and in one of the most exciting branches of modern medicine.

Foreword

G. J. V. Nossal

The Walter and Eliza Hall Institute of Medical Research, Melbourne, Australia

The unique nature of immune recognition leads to deep consequences. In most recognition systems in biology (enzyme–substrate, ligand–receptor, transcription factor–DNA motif), eons of evolution have shaped the reaction to have a particular, appropriate affinity. In immune recognition, the problem is that the T- and B-cell repertoire does not know what it will be asked to recognize next! This is why we needed extraordinary somatic minigene shuffling events to create random sets of T-cell and immunoglobulin receptors, and adjunct mechanisms, different for T and B cells, to raise the strength of binding between lymphocytes and introduced antigen. Nowhere else in nature is there a million-fold range in binding affinities for a given type of recognition. This leads to a system which is intrinsically difficult to regulate.

In the main, clinical immunology deals with situations (like autoimmunity or allergy) where immunoregulation has gone wrong; or with situations (like transplantation or non-sterilizing immunity in certain infections) where we would like to interfere therapeutically with immunoregulatory mechanisms. Taking autoimmunity as an example, it is clear that the immune system has good mechanisms of getting rid of some of the most dangerous 'anti-self' lymphocytes but needs elaborate control mechanisms for some others. Fortunately, our knowledge of immunoregulation has expanded greatly in recent years, as has understanding of congenital and acquired immunodeficiencies.

What makes this timely and authoritative volume on clinical immunology so particularly useful is the way in which the authors have managed to underpin their descriptions of immunopathological states, and their analyses of diagnosis and treatment, with an orderly and not unduly onerous presentation of the basic immunological facts underlying each disease group. This has been achieved *inter alia* through the use of appealing figures and tables. As immunology has this curious capacity to infiltrate itself into virtually every nook and cranny of medicine, clinical immunology has become quite a compendious discipline. Despite this, the editors have managed to cover the subject in a volume of reasonable size. This is important, because immunology has another peculiarity: it is hard to understand one pat of it without some knowledge of all of it. You cannot define an antigen without reference to antibody, tolerance without immunity, B-cell function without reference to T cells, immunodeficiency without a good working knowledge of primary and secondary lymphoid organs. So it is with clinical immunology: it is hard to be an allergist without knowing all that transplantation has taught us about T cells and cytokines, and so forth. To have a reference work that is not unconscionably detailed yet embraces all the main subheadings of clinical immunology does a favour not only to advanced trainees reading their way into the subject for the first time since undergraduate days, but also to experts in the various subspecialties needing, as they all do, a genuine overview.

Oxford University Press, Walton Street, Oxford OX2 6DP
Oxford   New York
Athens   Auckland   Bangkok   Bombay
Calcutta   Cape Town   Dar es Salaam   Delhi
Florence   Hong Kong   Istanbul   Karachi
Kuala Lumpur   Madras   Madrid   Melbourne
Mexico City   Nairobi   Paris   Singapore
Taipei   Tokyo   Toronto
and associated companies in
Berlin   Ibadan

Oxford is a trade mark of Oxford University Press

Published in the United States
by Oxford University Press Inc., New York

A catalogue record for this book is available from the British Library

Library of Congress Cataloging in Publication Data
Clinical immunology / edited by John Bradley and Jim McCluskey.
(Oxford medical publications)
Includes index.
1. Clinical immunology.   I. Bradley, John.   II. McCluskey, James.
III. Series
[DNLM: 1. Immunologic Diseases—immunology.   2. Transplantation
Immunology.   WD 300 C64145 1997]
RC582.C548   1997   616.07′9—dc20   96–30986

ISBN 0 19 2625187

Typeset by EXPO Holdings, Malaysia
Printed in Hong Kong

Clinical Immunology

Edited by

John Bradley

Sandoz Professor and Head of Department
of Clinical Immunology, Flinders University
and Flinders Medical Centre, Adelaide, Australia

and

James McCluskey

Professor and Director, Clinical Immunology
Flinders University and Medical Centre, and
Transplant Services, Blood Transfusion Service
Adelaide, Australia

Oxford   New York   Melbourne
Oxford University Press
1997

OXFORD MEDICAL PUBLICATIONS

Clinical Immunology

Contents

Contributors

John ALPERS
Associate Professor, Head of Respiratory Medicine, Acting Head Dept of Medicine, Flinders University and Medical Centre, Adelaide, Australia

Anthony J. d'APICE
Director of Department of Clinical Immunology, St Vincents Hospital Melbourne, Australia

Ross St Clair BARNETSON
Professor of Dermatology, University of Sydney, Royal Prince Alfred Hospital, Sydney, Australia

Peter BRADDING
Faculty of Medicine, University of Southampton, Southampton General Hospital, UK

John BRADLEY
Professor and Head Department of Clinical Immunology, Flinders University and Medical Centre, Adelaide, Australia

Sam BREIT
Centre for Immunology, St Vincent's Hospital, Sydney, Australia

WARWICK J. BRITTON
Associate Professor, Department of Clinical Immunology, Royal Prince Alfred Hospital, University of Sydney, Australia

Eric J. BROWN
Professor, Division of Infectious Diseases Washington University School of Medicine, St Louis, Missouri, USA

Michael J. BROWNING
Department of Microbiology and Immunology, University of Leicester, Leicester, UK

Kevin CHENEY
Associate Professor and Director, Australian Red Cross Blood Transfusion Service, Adelaide, Australia

Frank CHRISTIANSEN
Associate Professor and Clinical Immunologist, Institute for Molecular Immunology and Instrumentation, Royal Perth Hospital, Perth, Australia

Keryn CHRISTIANSEN
Department of Microbiology, Royal Perth Hospital, Perth, Australia

A. G. CUMMINS
Senior Consultant, Department of Gastro-enterology, Queen Elizabeth Hospital Adelaide, Australia

Angus G. DALGLEISH
Professor, Division of Oncology, St George's Hospital Medical School, London, UK

Ian van DRIEL
Senior Lecturer, Department of Pathology and Immunology, Monash Medical School, Melbourne, Australia

Roger L. DAWKINS
Professor and Head, Institute of Molecular Immunology and Instrumentation, University of Western Australia, Royal Perth Hospital, Perth, Australia

John FINLAY-JONES
Associate Professor, Department of Microbiology and Infectious Diseases, Flinders University and Medical Centre, Adelaide, Australia

Kevin FORSYTH MD
Professor and Head, Department of Pediatrics and Child Health, Flinders University and Medical Centre, Adelaide, Australia

Anthony FREW
Faculty of Medicine, University of Southampton, Southampton General Hospital, Southampton, UK

Roger GARSIA
Senior Lecturer Department of Clinical Immunology, Royal Prince Alfred Hospital, University of Sydney, Sydney, Australia

Reem GHALIB
Department of Medicine, Washington School of Medicine, St Louis, Missouri, USA

Paul GLEESON
Reader, Department of Pathology and Immunology, Monash Medical School, Commercial Road Prahran, Melbourne, Australia

Michael GOOD
Professor and Head Molecular Immunology, Director CRC for Vaccine Technology, Queensland Institute of Medical Research, The Bancroft Centre, Brisbane, Australia

Tom GORDON
Associate Professor, Department of Clinical Immunology, Flinders University and Medical Centre, Adelaide, Australia

Amanda GRAMP
Dermatopathologist and Director, Gramps Skin Pathology Adelaide, Australia

Len HARRISON
Professor, and Director of Burnet Clinical Research Unit, The Walter and Eliza Hall Institute, Royal Melbourne Hospital, Australia

Robert HEDDLE
Senior Lecturer, Department of Clinical Immunology, Flinders Medical Centre, South Australia

A. M. HEITZ
Department of Clinical Immunology, Royal Perth Hospital, Perth, Australia

Stephen T. HOLGATE
MRC Clinical Professor of Immunopharmacology, University of Southampton Faculty of Medicine, Southampton General Hospital, UK

Peter HOLLINGSWORTH
Director, Department of Clinical Immunology, Sir Charles Gairdner Hospital, Perth, Australia

Margot HONEYMAN
Burnet Clinical Research Unit, The Walter and Eliza Hall Institute, Royal Melbourne Hospital, Melbourne, Australia

D. B. JONES
Tenovus Research Institute, University of Southampton, UK

Christine KINNON
Reader of Molecular Immunology, Institute of Child Health, University of London, UK

Ann KUPA
Senior Lecturer, Department of Clinical Immunology, Flinders Medical Centre, Adelaide, Australia

Kevin J. LAFFERTY
Professor and Research Director of John Curtin School of Medical Research Australian National University, Canberra, Australia

Robert LECHLER
Professor of Molecular Immunology and Honorary Consultant in Medicine, Department of Immunology, Royal Postgraduate Med. School, London, UK

Marc LeMIRE
Department of Microbiology and Infectious Diseases, Flinders University and Medical Centre, Adelaide, Australia

Roland J. LEVINSKY
Dean and Professor, Institute of Child Health, University of London, London, UK

Susan LIGHTMAN
Professor and Director, Clinical Ophthalmology, Moorfields Eye Hospital London, UK

Christopher Martin LOCKWOOD
Wellcome Reader, School of Clinical Medicine, Addenbrooke's Hospital, Cambridge, UK

Ravindar N. MAINI
Professor and Director, The Mathilda and Terence Kennedy Institute of Rheumatology, London, UK

Nick MANIOLIS
Senior Lecturer, Department of Rheumatology, Royal North Shore Hospital, Sydney, Australia

Philip D. MASON
Department of Medicine and Immunology, Royal Postgraduate Medical School, London, UK

James McCLUSKEY
Professor and Director Transplant Immunology, Flinders University and Medical Centre, Adelaide, Australia

P. McCLUSKEY
University of New South Wales, Sydney, Australia

Ronald PENNY
Professor and Director, Centre for Immunology, St Vincent's Hospital, Sydney, Australia

Marion PETERS
Associate Professor, Department of Medicine, Washington School of Medicine, St Louis, Missouri, USA

N. PETROVSKY
Burnet Clinical Research Unit, The Walter and Eliza Hall Institute, Royal
Melbourne Hospital, Melbourne, Australia

David POWER
Department of Clinical Immunology, St Vincents Hospital Melbourne,
Australia

Morris REICHLIN
Professor of Medicine, Chief Arthritis/Immunology Section, Oklahoma Medical
Research Foundation Oklahoma, USA

Donal ROBERTON
Professor and Chairman of Department of Paediatrics, Womens and Childrens
Hospital, King William Road, Adelaide, Australia

Ian ROBERTS-THOMSON
Director, Department of Gastroenterology, Queen Elizabeth Hospital, Adelaide,
Australia

Peter ROBERTS-THOMSON
Associate Professor and Head of Rheumatology Unit, Department of Clinical
Immunology, Flinders University and Medical Centre Adelaide, Australia

Leslie SCHRIEBER
Associate Professor, Department of Rheumatology, Royal North Shore Hospital,
NSW, Australia

R. S. SCHMIDLI
Burnet Clinical Research Unit, The Walter and Eliza Hall Institute, Royal
Melbourne Hospital, Melbourne, Australia

David SCHULTZ
Neurology Department, Queens Hospital University of Nottingham, Nottingham,
UK

Jonathan SEDGWICK
Wellcome Trust Senior Research Fellow, Centenary Institute of Cancer Medicine
and Cell Biology, Australia

Charmaine J. SIMEONOVIC
Fellow, Division of Molecular Medicine, John Curtin School of Medical Research,
Australia National University, Canberra, Australia

Michael STEEL
Professor of Biomedical Science, School of Biological and Medical Sciences,
St Andrews, Scotland, UK

George STEVENSON
Institute Director and Professor, Tenovus Research Institute, General Hospital,
Southampton, UK

Ban Hock TOH
Professor and Head Department of Pathology and Immunology, Monash Medical
School, Melbourne, Australia

Denis WAKEFIELD
Associate Professor of Pathology, Director of Immunology and Immunopathology,
Prince of Wales Hospital, Sydney, Australia

Steven L. WESSELINGH
Staff Specialist, Department of Micirobiology and Infectious Diseases, Flinders University and Medical Centre, Adelaide, Australia

Keryn WILLIAMS
Fellow, Department of Ophthalmology, Flinders Medical Centre, Adelaide, Australia

Section I

Immunodeficiencies

1 Congenital immunodeficiencies

K. Forsyth, C. Kinnon, and R. J. Levinsky

Introduction

The congenital immunodeficiencies are a group of disorders characterized by an enhanced susceptibility to infection. Throughout history infection has been a major cause of death for the human race and still remains so for people in poorly developed countries. With the introduction of improved housing and nutrition, combined with the availability of antibiotics earlier in the twentieth century, it became apparent that there were groups of individuals uniquely susceptible to infection in spite of appropriate antimicrobials. In the 1920s and 1930s some of the phenotypes of diseases which we now recognize as congenital immunodeficiencies were first described. However, it was not until 1952 with Bruton's description of congenital agammaglobulinaemia that the first specific and characterized congenital immunodeficiency was described. Since that time there has been a considerable increase in the number of congenital immunodeficiency disorders that have been identified. This increased ability to discern immunological abnormalities parallels our increasing understanding of basic immune mechanisms.

The hallmark of congenital immunodeficiency is infection presenting during childhood. Many of the children presenting with congenital immunodeficiency disorders have been reviewed by paediatric immunologists. The cooperation between clinical paediatric immunologists and basic scientists working in the laboratory have led to an explosion of understanding and knowledge in these disorders. Before the advent of molecular biology techniques, the immunodeficiencies were characterized according to clinical and immunological phenotype. Such classification systems have many faults. As the genetic basis for the immunodeficiencies have been better understood and molecular biology techniques enabled isolation and characterization of specific gene and protein disorders, the congenital immunodeficiencies have been characterized with much more precision.

Throughout this chapter the disorders will therefore be described, where possible, according to both the phenotype and the genotype. Increasingly, the congenital immunodeficiencies are being well characterized at the molecular level. It is anticipated that there will be an explosion in molecular understanding of other immunodeficiencies over the next few years.

Classification

Immunodeficiencies can be classified as primary (*i.e.* congenital) or secondary. The secondary immunodeficiencies, which will not be discussed in this section, may be due to immaturity or other illnesses, drugs, medical intervention, etc.

The congenital immunodeficiencies can be classified as: (i) antibody deficiency syndromes; (ii) T-cell deficiencies; (iii) combined B- and T-cell immunodeficiencies; (iv) complement deficiencies; and (v) defects in natural killer (NK) cells and phagocytic cells.

Incidence

The overall incidence of primary immunodeficiency, excluding immunoglobulin A (IgA) deficiency, is about 1 per 10 000 live births. IgA deficiency is the most common immunodeficiency with an incidence of about 20 per 10 000 live births or about 1 in 500–1500 adults.

Clinical phenotype

The hallmark of congenital immunodeficiency is increased susceptibility to infection. This may be characterized by recurrent infections, an unusually severe infection or infection with an unusual or atypical organism, or atypical recovery from an infection.

The definition of recurrent infection in childhood may be problematic given that throughout the first few years of life it is common for children to have multiple infections. Studies suggest that children who have 10 or fewer infections per year have a normal immune profile. Children who have more than 10 infections per year or who have severe or persistent infections or infections with organisms generally considered non-pathogenic should be referred for analysis of their immune function. Additional clues which may suggest an immunodeficiency in childhood are failure to thrive, recurrent candida infection, diarrhoea and malabsorption, recurrent sinusitis or pneumonia/bronchiectasis, absent lymphoid or tonsillar tissue, and evidence of autoimmune or haematological abnormalities.

Laboratory diagnosis of immunodeficiency

Considerable numbers of otherwise normal children will fulfil the criteria for suspected immunodeficiency. It is therefore important to have screening tests which are cheap and have a high sensitivity to enable adequate screening to be performed. A full blood count should always be performed. Screening for antibody disorders is most easily accomplished by the measurement of IgG, IgA, and IgM in serum. Screening for T-cell disorders is best accomplished by using a delayed-type hypersensitivity skin test such as the CMI Multitest™ together with lymphocyte subset enumeration and functional studies. Age-related reference ranges for these tests are available. As one of the more common immunodeficiencies is human immunodeficiency virus (HIV) infection, the laboratory examination for a child with suspected immunodeficiency should include HIV antibody or antigen testing. It is important to note that transplacental transmission of maternal HIV antibodies makes HIV antibody testing unreliable in the first 18 months of life. Additionally, the reference ranges for lymphocyte subset numbers are much higher in infancy than in adults. A standard blood film and blood counts would also assist in screening for immunodeficiency. Phagocytic defects are best screened for by the nitro blue tetrazolium dye reduction test and complement abnormalities by the estimation of C3 and C4 levels in serum along with a functional test of complement such as a CH50 activity measure.

Genetics of immunodeficiency

Table 1.1 summarizes the major congenital immunodeficiencies, dividing them into X-linked and autosomal recessive patterns of inheritance. The defective genes and their chromosomal locations, where known, are indicated. The chromosomal localization information has been important for the identification of the genes in many cases. Such information is essential for the successful deployment of the positional cloning strategy.

Positional gene cloning strategy has been particularly important in the elucidation of the X-linked genes, with the first successful use of this strategy resulting in the identification of the gp91-*phox* gene as being responsible for X-linked chronic granulomatous disease (CGD). More recently, the positional cloning approach was successfully employed to isolate the *Btk* gene, identified as causing X-linked agammaglobulinaemia (XLA). At the same time, the equivalent murine gene was isolated independently and suggested to be a candidate for the XLA gene based on its chromosomal localization. Similarly, the CD40 ligand (CD40L) and the common γ chain of the interleukin (IL) 2 and additional cytokine receptors were suggested as being candidates for XLA with hyper-IgM (HIGMI) and X-linked severe combined immunodeficiency (SCIDXI), respectively.

In some cases the genes for the autosomal recessive disorders have been identified, most notably, for the autosomal recessive forms of CGD and increasingly for the various forms of severe combined immunodeficiency (SCID), but in many cases they have yet to be elucidated. Problems hindering their characterization are that affected families are much rarer than are those with X-linked conditions and the autosomes are less well mapped than the X chromosome. Perhaps elucidation of the defective genes for the remaining disorders will rely more heavily on candidate genes being suggested.

The precise mapping of the genes causing the various immunodeficiency diseases has provided opportunities for the prevention of these diseases. Most often this has been through the identification of carrier females in affected families and first trimester prenatal diagnosis. This approach has been particularly successful for the X-linked immunodeficiencies where it has been possible to use assays based on X-inactivation analysis and gene tracking.

X-inactivation analysis relies on the determination of unilateral patterns of X-inactivation in particular cell lineages, and particularly those where the expression of an X-linked gene is essential for the development of that cell type. This has been most useful in cases of mothers of single affected males where there has been no previous family history of the disease. Gene tracking is dependent on the use of closely linked polymorphic probes.

Where the genes are now identified it is possible to diagnose the diseases and assess carrier status unambiguously for 'at-risk' females by direct mutation analysis or through the use of intragenic polymorphisms. The identification of the causative genes should lead to an improved understanding of the nature of these disorders and, in time, to improved management and treatment. The currently available treatments remain far from adequate and, in many cases, these diseases are still fatal. Perhaps the most exciting prospect in this area is treatment by somatic gene therapy.

▮ **Table 1.1** Inherited immunodeficiencies

Disease and pattern of inheritance	Gene defect	Chromosomal location
X-linked disorders		
Severe combined immunodeficiency	γ chain of IL-2R and other cytokine receptors	Xq 13.1
Chronic granulomatous disease	gp91-*phox*	Xp 21.1
X-linked agammaglobulinaemia	*Btk*	Xq 22
X-linked agammaglobulinaemia with hyper IgM	CD40 ligand	Xq 26
Properdin deficiency	Properdin	Xq 11.23–21.1
X-linked lymphoproliferative syndrome	?	Xq 25
Wiskott–Aldrich syndrome	*WASP*	Xp 11
Autosomal recessive disorders		
Severe combined immunodeficiency		
	Adenosine deaminase	20q 13.11
	Purine nucleoside phosphorylase	14q 11.2
	Zap 70?	2q 12
	CD3ε and γ	11q 23
Major histocompatibility complex	RFX5	?
class II deficiency	CIITA	?
Chronic granulomatous disease	p47-*phox*	7q 11.23
	p67-*phox*	1q 25
	p22-*phox*	16q 24
Leucocyte adhesion deficiency	CD18	21q 22.3
Immunoglobulin heavy chain deficiency	Immunoglobulin heavy chain constant regions	14q 23
Immunoglobulin light (kappa) chain deficiency	Immunoglobulin kappa light chain	2p 11 ?
IgA deficiency	?	6p 21
Common variable immunodeficiency	?	6p 21
Ataxia telangiectasia	ATM	11q 23
Di-George syndrome	?	22q 11
Chediak–Higashi syndrome	LYST	?
Mannose binding protein deficiency		

Congenital antibody deficiency syndromes

Antibody deficiency syndromes are primarily associated with B-cell defects. However, as T cells interact with B cells and are frequently required to provide 'help' to B cells for antibody production, some antibody deficiency disorders are due to deficient T-cell help.

Sex (X)-linked agammaglobulinaemia

XLA is an X-linked humoral immunodeficiency characterized by severe pyogenic infections. In early infancy transplacentally acquired maternal antibody gives protection to affected boys. Symptoms therefore generally present during the latter part of the first year of life. Upper respiratory tract (sinuses and ears) and lower respiratory tract infections are the usual presenting complaints. Affected boys may also present with gastroenteritis, pyoderma, aseptic arthritis, septicaemia, or meningitis/encephalitis.

There is frequently a delay in diagnosis of this condition with the mean age of diagnosis in unaffected families of 3.5 years. The majority of the sinopulmonary infections are due to *Haemophilus influenzae*, *Streptococcus pneumoniae*, and *Staphylococcus aureus*. Diarrhoeal symptoms may be due to bacterial overgrowth in the bowel or bowel infection with *Giardia lamblia*.

In general boys with XLA have normal immunity to viral infections. An exception to this are the neurotropic viruses such as ECHO 19 which can cause a persistent meningo-encephalitis. Additionally, XLA subjects are at risk of becoming prolonged excretors after oral polio vaccination from vaccine with the possibility of the virus regaining virulence.

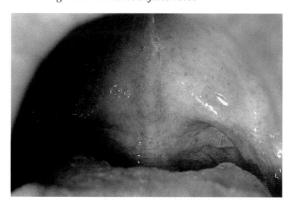

∎ **Fig. 1.1** Congenital sex-linked hypogammaglobuli-naemia demonstrating absence of tonsils.

Clinical findings

Clinical findings in XLA are generally those due to recurrent respiratory tract infections. There is likely to be evidence of recurrent and persistent pneumonia with or without sinus or middle ear infections. Associated with the persistent lower respiratory tract infections may be growth failure, finger clubbing, and chest wall shape abnormality. There may be evidence of skin infections. Arthritis due to bacterial or chlamydial infections may be a presenting feature in older children. Giardia may colonize the gut and be a cause

of growth failure without overt diarrhoea. Neutropenia may be a problem but this is usually readily corrected upon treatment with intravenous immunoglobulin.

Hypoplasia of lymph nodes and tonsils is present, and on histological examination germinal centres and plasma cells are not seen.

Laboratory findings

Serum levels of IgM and IgA are generally undetectable. IgG is generally present at very low levels (40–100 mg/dl). B-cell numbers in blood are markedly decreased or absent. However, pre-B cells with cytoplasmic μ are present in normal numbers in the bone marrow. Tests for antibodies to blood group substances and to antigens given by immunization (e.g. diphtheria, tetanus toxoid) are useful diagnostic aids.

In most patients the number of T-cells is normal or increased, and T-cell function is normal. The thymus is normal histologically.

Molecular defect

The primary defect in XLA is a failure of pre-B cells to mature into antibody producing cells. It is caused by defects in a single gene which has been localized to Xq22. Two research groups simultaneously identified a previously unknown B-cell-specific protein tyrosine kinase (called *Btk* for Bruton's agammaglobulinaemia *tyrosine kinase*). This enzyme is analogous to members of the *Src*-related non-receptor tyrosine kinase family

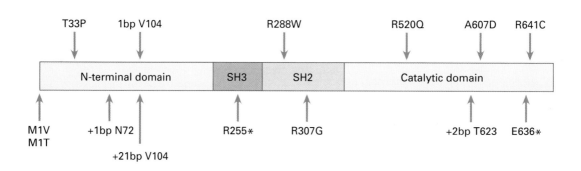

∎ **Fig. 1.2** Mutations of all varieties have been described affecting all domains of the *btk* gene. This figure illustrates a few of these. Depending upon the mutation the phenotype of the disease may differ slightly; for instance the two mutations in the SH₂ domains have incomplete and classical phenotypes, respectively. Deletions of the whole or part of the gene is found in <10% of patients.

of proteins, many of which are involved in signal transduction in haematopoietic cells.

Deletions within the *Btk* gene in XLA patients suggested that XLA is caused by loss of function of the protein encoded for by this gene. *Btk* expression is reduced or absent in cell lines derived from patients with XLA, but not from normal individuals.

A number of distinct point mutations covering all the major domains of the protein have now been identified in *Btk* and continued mutation analysis of both classical and atypical XLA patients will allow greater characterization of the functionally important residues in the protein. There is now evidence that *Btk* may play some part in signal transduction in mature B cells, as increased autophosphorylation may be shown upon B-cell receptor cross-linking. However, its precise role in pre-B-cell maturation is still to be discerned.

Previously, the Xid mouse was not thought to be an animal model of XLA. Recently, it has been shown that the same gene is involved in the Xid mouse, although the phenotype is quite different. The mouse has B cells of a predominant CD5 subset and can produce immunoglobulins, although antibodies to carbohydrate antigens are deficient. A number of Btk knockout mice have now been described, all with the xid phenotype. Clearly, the differentiation pathways for B cells in humans and mouse are different.

Treatment

Current treatment is by intravenous immunoglobulin given three to four weekly to achieve trough IgG levels above the lower range of normal for that particular age group. Trials have shown that such treatment may prevent progressive pulmonary disease. The volume of injection required to achieve similar levels by the intramuscular route make this impractical, although slow subcutaneous infusion may be an alternative to intravenous IgG. Management should also include regular pulmonary function testing.

Identification of the gene defect in XLA opens the way for antenatal testing and specific targeted gene therapy. However, before the latter treatment can be considered, it will be important to investigate the effects of over-expression of *Btk*, as it is possible that it might have a potential for oncogenesis. XLA results from loss of function of *Btk*, in contrast to diseases where constitutive activation of the kinase domain is associated with an oncogenic potential (e.g. the oncogenes v-src and BCR-abl associated with haematological malignancies). If such a treatment can be achieved safely, it should be a much more effective therapy than intravenous immunoglobulin.

X-linked agammaglobulinemia with hyper-IgM syndrome

This is a rare syndrome characterized by recurrent bacterial infections. There is also susceptibility to opportunistic infections including *Pneumocystis carinii*. There may be lymphadenopathy with splenomegaly. Most cases are found in males with an X-linked pattern of inheritance. An identical phenotype with an autosomal recessive inheritance has been described, and it may also occur post-congenital rubella.

Laboratory findings

IgG, IgA, and IgE are either very low or undetectable in serum. There are normal to increased levels of serum IgM and IgD. Serum IgM levels may be very high. The IgM is polyclonal but may be monomeric. Plasma cells can be found in lymphoid tissue. There are no germinal centres.

Molecular defect

Clinically, there are indications that there may be a T-cell deficiency in these patients in that they are prone to infections more typical of T-cell deficiencies, for example *P. carinii* and cryptosporidial diarrhoea. Additionally, it is noted that a supernatant from a T-cell line obtained from a patient with Sezáry syndrome was able to induce IgG and IgE production by a patient's B cells when incubated in co-culture. The gene defect was mapped to Xq26. The CD40 ligand (CD40L, found on activated T cells and which binds CD40 on B cells) became a candidate gene as it also mapped to this region. Activation of CD40 on B cells induces IgE secretion, and cross-linking of CD40 with antibodies has been shown to rescue cells from apoptosis. It is also known that the CD40L when binding to CD40 on B cells is able to induce immunoglobulin heavy chain switching, all these features being deficient in HIGMI.

It therefore became very likely that CD40 or the CD40 ligand were abnormal in this syndrome. Mutations in the CD40L gene in males with this disorder have now been identified. Therefore, the defect in XHIgM is failure of activated T cells to provide appropriate B-cell help through the CD40L, with failure of immunoglobulin isotype switching or failure of rescue from apoptosis.

Treatment.

As levels of IgG are very low in this disorder, treatment consists of regular infusions of immunoglobulin in a manner analogous to that required in XLA. Given the recent improvements in

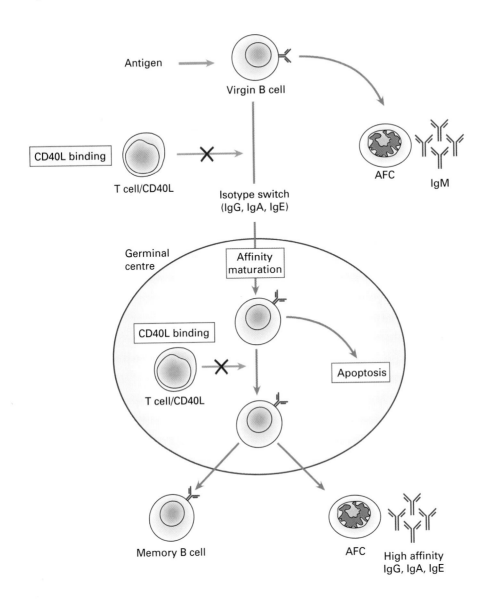

▎ Fig. 1.3 CD40 ligand is expressed on activated T cells and this interacts with CD40 on B cells as one particular signal in T/B cooperation for antibody production. Absence of CD40 ligand binding as found in XHIgM results in failure of isotype switching from IgM to IgG, IgA, and IgE. AFC — antibody-forming cell.

understanding the molecular defects in this condition, it may be possible to envisage a strategy for treating XHIgM by somatic gene therapy techniques. This would perhaps be best achieved by expressing CD40L under the control of endogenous promoter/control elements in bone marrow stem cells or mature T cells.

Common variable immunodeficiency

Common variable immunodeficiency (CVID) is characterized by recurrent bacterial infections. The syndrome may present during infancy and childhood or in early adulthood. The clinical presentation is generally with sinopulmonary infections. The pulmonary infections may have progressed to bronchiectasis before the diagnosis becomes apparent. As in XLA, these patients may have gastrointestinal symptoms, particularly diarrhoea with steatorrhoea and malabsorption. Infection with *G. lamblia* is quite common in such individuals.

Although the symptoms and signs resemble those of XLA the differences are:

(i) the later age of onset; (ii) an equal sex incidence; (iii) a tendency for T-cell function to become compromised; (iv) a tendency to develop autoimmune disease; (v) greatly increased incidence of lymphoma; and (vi) recurrence of herpes zoster and *Pneumocystis* infection.

Laboratory findings

Serum levels of IgG and IgA are low. In about half of the patients levels of IgM are low or absent. B-cell numbers may be normal or low. There is a weak antibody response to immunization and often poor switching from IgM to IgG. T-cell numbers are generally normal, although in a subset of patients there may be low numbers of T cells and poor delayed-type hypersensitivity skin tests.

Molecular defect

The genetic basis of common variable immunodeficiency is not known. As the common variable immunodeficiency phenotype is heterogeneous, it has been suggested that it is a multigenic disorder. Many of the common variable immunodeficiency patients share a common major histocompatibility complex (MHC) haplotype with IgA-deficient patients. This makes it likely that both disorders share at least one gene, which is suggested to lie in the class III region of the MHC. Exogenous factors in genetically susceptible individuals will determine the outcome.

Treatment

Symptomatic therapy with antimicrobials may be required. Intravenous immunoglobulin (*vide supra*) should be given for hypogammaglobulinaemia.

Immunoglobulin A deficiency

IgA deficiency is defined as markedly diminished serum IgA levels but normal or near normal levels of other immunoglobulins. This is the most common primary immunodeficiency with a prevalence of 1:500 to 1:1500. Associated with IgA deficiency may be other autoimmune disorders or other abnormalities of IgG subclasses. There may also be abnormalities of T cells.

Clinical characteristics

Given that many of the normal population have a selective IgA deficiency, there may be no clinically apparent symptoms in this disorder, about 50% having no symptoms. As IgA is particularly expressed at mucosal surfaces, including the upper respiratory tract, it is not surprising that many of the symptoms of IgA deficiency relate to recurrent upper respiratory tract infection. In patients with allergy there is an increased incidence of selective IgA deficiency.

There have been some reports suggesting that in childhood, IgA deficiency may be categorized into two groups. In the group with no detectable IgA in serum, the IgA deficiency appears permanent and symptoms are more prevalent. Transfusion reactions may occur in this group due to development of antibodies to IgA. In the other group, IgA is present in serum but at levels below the reference range for age. In this group the IgA deficiency is frequently transient, levels returning to within the reference range within 2 years and patients becoming asymptomatic.

Laboratory findings

Serum IgA is low (~33%) or absent (~67%) levels. Some patients may develop transfusion reactions due to development of anti-IgA after exposure to IgA. Selective deficiency of IgA2 is associated with more clinical complications than IgA1 deficiency.

Molecular defect

No single defect at the molecular level has been characterized in IgA deficiency, although there are many similarities in this condition with common variable immunodeficiency. Given the heterogeneous nature of this disorder, the variable phenotype of the association in some patients with autoimmunity, it is likely that this condition represents abnormalities in the interrelationships between T and B cells.

Treatment

If clinically warranted treatment is directed at the primary symptoms, generally recurrent upper respiratory tract infections using antibiotics as required. There is no place for infusion of immunoglobulins. Immunoglobulin preparations, although low in IgA, may sensitize the recipients.

Selective immunoglobulin M deficiency

This rare poorly characterized condition consists of recurrent or severe bacterial infections associated with low levels of serum IgM but normal levels of the other immunoglobulins. It is likely that this condition is caused by abnormalities in T-cell help, as in HIGMI.

Immunoglobulin G subclass deficiencies

Antibodies to protein antigens are generally IgG1 or IgG3, whereas those to polysaccharide antigens, e.g. of pneumococcus and *H. influenza*, are predominantly IgG2. The clinical phenotype of IgG subclass deficiency is as variable as that for IgA deficiency. In this heterogeneous condition total levels of IgG may be normal despite markedly reduced levels of one or more IgG subclasses. Indeed IgG2 deficiency can be associated with deficiencies of IgA and IgG4. Clinically normal individuals with a deficiency of IgG subclasses have been reported, as have those with symptoms of recurrent infection. This would suggest that IgG subclass deficiencies are heterogeneous in aetiology, some being isolated and others involving other arms of the immune system. In a few families deletions of the immunoglobulin constant region genes on chromosome 14 have been described. These deletions can be detected by Southern blotting using immunoglobulin probes and are of varying extents. The deletions generally do not span the entire locus, but they can encompass one or more constant region gene segments. Although the serum of affected individuals lacks immunoglobulin of the relevant isotypes and subclasses most individuals do not have a history of recurrent infections. However, some have presented with recurrent pyogenic infections.

Kappa light chain deficiency

Two families have been described who fail to make κ light chains. Only λ light chains are expressed by the affected individual. Circulating B-cell numbers are normal and antibodies may be normal or reduced. In one family a point mutation in the gene coding for the κ chain at chromosome 2p11 has been reported.

Treatment

For symptomatic patients in whom conservative medical management is ineffective, intravenous immunoglobulin has been shown to be effective.

Antibody deficiency with normal immunoglobulins

There are a group of patients who have recurrent bacterial infections and normal levels of immunoglobulins. If these subjects are selectively immunized with agents such as tetanus toxoid, pneumococcal polysaccharide vaccine, or diphtheria toxoid, it is possible to demonstrate a lack of antibody response to a particular antigen. It is likely that these subjects have poorly characterized abnormalities of B-cell function. If symptomatic, treatment consists of infusion of immunoglobulin.

Transient hypogammaglobulinaemia of infancy

Transplacental transmission of maternal antibodies gives the newborn an immunological advantage with respect to antibody. However, by 3 months of age serum antibody levels have reached a nadir. There follows a gradual increase in serum IgG levels towards adult levels later in childhood. In some infants there is a prolonged trough in antibody levels because of a delay in the onset of immunoglobulin synthesis. In affected subjects antibody production becomes apparent generally by 18–36 months of age. The failure to switch on antibody production may be due to delayed maturation of helper T-cell function. If the affected individuals are asymptomatic no therapy is required. However, if there are severe or recurrent bacterial infections, a brief period of parenteral immunoglobulin administration may be appropriate.

Primary T-cell immunodeficiencies

It is important to recognize these early, and to avoid immunization with live vaccines and orthodox blood transfusion because of the risk of graft-versus-host disease.

Severe combined immunodeficiencies

These deficiencies are characterized by complete absence of all immune responses. Children with SCID present within the first 6 months of life. Their major presenting problems are infection and failure to thrive. The infective episodes are fungal (particularly candida), bacteria, and viral infections. Pulmonary infection is common with bacterial or viral agents. Many of the children present with *P. carinii* pneumonia. Patients are likely to have gastrointestinal symptoms which may be an infective diarrhoea due for example to *Rotavirus* or

Campylobacter or *G. lamblia*. They may also have an infective hepatitis.

Laboratory findings

There are variable degrees of lymphopenia. Lymphocyte subset enumeration will reveal varying degrees of T-cell abnormality. Lymphocyte proliferation to specific antigens or in a mixed lymphocyte reaction is absent. Immunoglobulin levels are generally very low. There may be absence of a thymic shadow on chest X-ray.

Molecular defects

Approximately 60% of cases of SCID are due to the X-linked form, the rest being autosomal. At least 25% of cases of autosomal recessive SCID are caused by defects in enzymes involved in purine metabolism, the more common (<15% of total SCIDs) being adenosine deaminase (ADA), and purine nucleoside phosphorylase (PNP) being exceptionally rare (<2% of total SCIDs). There are additional rare autosomal recessive forms of SCID which can involve defects in various components of the T-cell receptor (TCR), and T-cell activation pathways and which are becoming increasingly well understood. However, in many cases the precise abnormalities in autosomal recessive SCID remain to be elucidated.

X-linked severe combined immunodeficiency

Phenotypically these patients have markedly decreased numbers of T cells but normal or elevated B-cell numbers. The thymus shows lymphocyte depletion with precursor thymocytes not detectable. There are in addition very low levels of all classes of immunoglobulin.

Molecular defect

Mutations in the gene encoding the interleukin 2 receptor γ chain (IL-2RG) have been found to cause the X-linked form of SCID. IL-2RG maps to Xq13, as does the SCIDXI locus. Originally identified as a component of the high and intermediate affinity IL-2R that is required to achieve full ligand-binding affinity and internalization, the γ chain is constitutively expressed in haematolymphoid cells and is now known to be a component of additional cytokine receptors, including the IL-4, IL-7, IL-9, IL-15, and also possibly IL-13 receptors. It is postulated that in each of these receptors the unique chain recognizes the specific cytokine, and thus confers the signalling specificity, while the common γ chain transduces the signal via its cytoplasmic domain. All these receptors are involved at different stages of T- and B-cell growth and maturation and the combined effect of disrupting their expression may augment the immune defect. The humoral

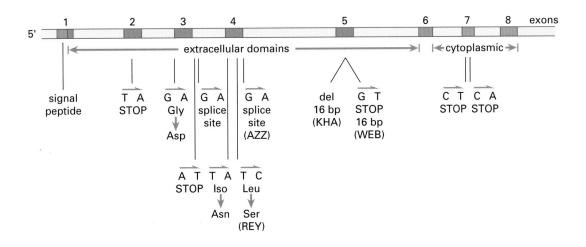

∎ **Fig. 1.4** Mutations of different varieties shown for the IL-2γ chain gene in patients with SCIDXI.

immunodeficiency observed in SCIDXI may be due to poor T-cell help. However, it is more likely that abnormalities of the γ chain also suppress B-cell function in these patients. B cells from SCIDXI patients respond to IL-4 and IL-13 in a similar way to those from unaffected children in assays for B-cell activation, proliferation and IgE secretion, but do not respond to IL-2 or IL-15. Bone marrow progenitor cells (CD34+CD7+) from normals, but not from SCIDXI patients, will differentiate along the T-cell lineage when cultured with stem cell factor plus IL-7 suggesting that lack of responses to IL-7 are crucial in this disease.

Treatment

The treatment of choice is bone marrow transplantation with an human leucocyte antigen (HLA)-matched donor, matched for both maternal and paternal chromosomes. In haploidentical bone marrow transplants, if immunosuppressive therapy is utilized at the time of transplantation, B and T cells from the donor are likely to engraft with full immunological reconstitution. With an HLA identical donor 95% survival with full immune function may be expected but this drops to 50–60% survival with varying degrees of haemopoietic reconstitution even in haploidentical transplants. If immunosuppression is not used in haploidentical transplants, a chimeric state with only donor T-cell engraftment is likely to occur. The residual B cells lacking the γ chain will be poor antibody producers and humoral immunodeficiency will persist.

Adenosine deaminase severe combined immunodeficiency

This immunodeficiency is characterized by progressive accumulation of deoxyadenosine in lymphocytes, which leads to gradual immune paresis. Clinical presentation occurs generally by 2–3 months of age with diarrhoea, respiratory tract infections, and failure to thrive. Although most cases of ADA deficiency present within the first 2–3 months of life, there may be milder forms of the disease with some residual enzymic function. There appears therefore to be a spectrum of abnormalities which present with the ADA SCID phenotype.

Laboratory findings

Both B and T cells are absent, as are immunoglobulins; however, there may be functional NK cells present. ADA deficiency is established by the presence of ADA in patient's erythrocytes or lymphocytes. In

about half of the patients there are characteristic X-ray findings with flaring and cupping of the rib ends.

Molecular defect

Despite the relative rarity of this disorder, a number of different mutations have now been identified throughout the ADA gene, most of which are point mutations. The resulting accumulation of toxic metabolites in developing and mature T cells is thought to inhibit their function.

Treatment

The treatment of choice is bone marrow transplantation with an HLA-matched donor. However, when no matched donor is available there are now other options and bovine ADA coupled to polyethylene glycol (PEG-ADA) to increase stability and half-life and decrease immunogenicity, given by three times weekly injection may restore immune function for several years until somatic gene therapy techniques are perfected. However, efficacy may be reduced under long-term treatment conditions because of problems of immunogenicity.

Severe combined immunodeficiency due to T-cell receptor — CD3 abnormalities

Defective expression and function of the TCR–CD3 complex of T cells can occur as a result of rare mutations in the ζ or ε genes of the CD3 complex. The phenotype of this disease varies from full-blown SCID to mild respiratory symptoms or no apparent effects.

Severe combined immunodeficiency due to ZAP 70 defects

Rare mutations of ZAP 70, a TCR-associated protein tyrosine kinase that is associated with the ζ chains of the TCR–CD3 complex, produce a distinctive form of SCID. This is characterized by profound immunodeficiency, absence of CD8+ and abundance of CD4+ peripheral T cells. The CD4+ T cells, however, fail to proliferate following TCR stimulation. It is thought that absence of ZAP 70 protein function results in an inability to couple the TCR to more downstream signalling events. Lack of ZAP 70 expression intrathymically apparently results in a differential production of peripheral T cells, with immature CD8+ cells being more refractory to ZAP 70 absence than CD4+ cells.

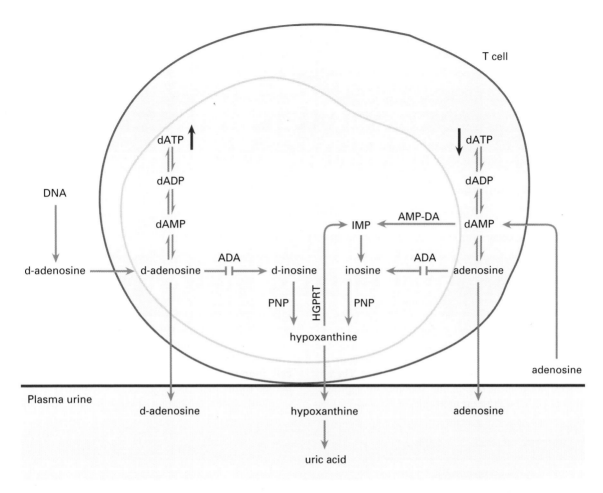

▌ Fig. 1.5 Metabolic pathways of purine metabolism. The absence of the enzyme ADA diverts the metabolism of d-adenosine and leads to metabolic build up of deoxyATP which at high concentrations is toxic to lymphocytes, especially T cells.

Severe combined immunodeficiency due to recombination activating genes (RAG1 and RAG2) defects

It has recently been reported that perhaps as many as 20% of autosomal recessive SCID patients are affected by mutations in the RAG1 and/or RAG2 genes. These proteins are involved in the process of VDJ rearrangement which is essential for production of functional immunoglobulin and TCR proteins. The phenotype of these patients is very variable, with absence of B cells and absent or low numbers of T cells. When T cells are present they are either as a result of maternal-fetal engraftment or a less severe mutation giving a 'leaky' phenotype.

Severe combined immunodeficiency due to major histocompatibility complex class II deficiency

MHC class II deficiency is characterized by the presence of normal levels of T and B cells, but these cells have apparently little functional activity as they fail to make cellular or humoral responses to foreign antigens. In these respects the resulting syndrome behaves much like other forms of SCID. This condition has also been called the 'bare lymphocyte syndrome'.

Clinical characteristics

The presentation is generally similar to that seen in severe immunodeficiency. There may be gastrointestinal, respiratory tract infections, *P. carinii* pneumonitis, or overwhelming septicaemia. This condition also demonstrates considerable clinical heterogeneity. Some people without evidence of immunodeficiency but with absence of MHC class II have been described.

Laboratory findings

All bone marrow-derived cells in affected individuals fail to express HLA class II antigens (DR, DQ, and DP), and this feature forms the basis of the diagnosis of the disease.

Molecular defect

This lack of expression of MHC class II antigens is the consequence of a failure to synthesize the α and β chain proteins. The defect is not in the class II genes themselves and does not appear to be located within the MHC locus. Instead the defect appears to be in the regulation of expression of the class II genes. There is a specific abnormality in the binding of a protein factor, RFX5 a dimeric molecule of 36 and 75 kDa

chains, to the highly conserved X box of the HLA class II promoter in some of these patients. In another group of patients which do not display this defect, mutations have been found in another protein, CIITA, which acts as an MHC gene transactivator. This novel regulatory gene is essential for the constitutive expression of all MHC class II genes in B lymphocytes. Thus, three types of HLA class II regulatory mutants can now be distinguished at the molecular level which involve different sets of patients. The RFX5 and CIITA genes have now been cloned and transfection experiments have demonstrated full complementation of the deficiencies in MHC class II expression in cell lines from the relevant groups of patients. This raises the possibility of treating at least some patients with this disease by somatic gene therapy in the future.

Di George syndrome

This clinical syndrome of congenital immunodeficiency is characterized by recurrent or severe infection, unusual facies, hypocalcaemic tetany, and congenital heart disease.

There is considerable heterogeneity in Di George syndrome. In the complete form there is absence of T-cell immunity and abnormal B-cell immunity. In partial forms there may be normal or partial T-cell immunity with normal or partial B-cell immuno-

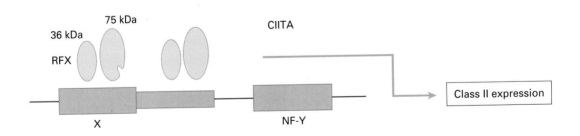

3 Complementation groups

A: mutations in CIITA - a general regulator of MHC class expression mediated by IFN γ

B: mutations in 36 kDa chain of RFX heterodimer

C: mutations in 75 kDa chain of RFX heterodimer

∎ **Fig. 1.6** The three different defects resulting in the human leucocyte antigen class II deficiency syndrome are illustrated. To date these are the only known genetic defects due to transactivating factors. MHC, major histocompatibility complex.

deficiency. The cardiovascular abnormalities are likely to be right sided aortic arch, right ventricular infundibular stenosis, aberrant left subclavian artery, ventricular septal defect, atrial septal defect, tetralogy of Fallot, pulmonary artery atresia, or hypoplastic pulmonary artery. The hypocalcaemia is likely to be symptomatic within the first 1–2 days of life. Infection develops over the subsequent few months.

Laboratory findings

The presence of congenital heart disease along with congenital hypoparathroidism in association with variable levels of T or B cells and immunoglobulins will lead to the diagnosis. There will be an absent thymus on chest X-ray.

Molecular defect

Di George syndrome is a component of the congenital malformation syndrome CATCH 22 (**C**ardiac defect, **A**bnormal facies, **T**hymic hypoplasia, **C**left Palate, **H**ypocalcaemia, **22**q11 deletions), all caused by hemizygosity of chromosome 22q11. Di George syndrome has extensive phenotypic overlap with Shprintzen or velocardiofacial syndrome and it is likely that these disorders are aetiologically related. Candidate genes from the region have now been isolated and one called Tuple 1 is expressed in the correct branchial arch region of the early developing mouse embryo. Further research in a knockout mouse model is required to establish whether this is indeed the gene involved.

Cartilage hair hypoplasia — short limbed dwarfism with immunodeficiency

These patients are short with metaphyseal or spondyloepipyseal dysplasia. Hair is fine and lightly coloured. Infection in the middle childhood years, particularly with varicella has been noted. Some subjects have severe infection in infancy.

Laboratory findings

Decreased lymphocyte numbers and poor T-cell function. Generally, humoral immunity is normal.

Molecular defect

This is unknown.

Treatment

For milder forms of the condition, appropriate antimicrobials and varicella prophylaxis following exposure is recommended. Bone marrow transplantation may be required for the severe form.

Sex (X)-linked lymphoproliferative syndrome

This condition is characterized by severe abnormalities associated with Epstein–Barr virus (EBV) infection.

Following primary infection with EBV, affected boys may develop severe hepatic failure, progressive systemic disease and death. In those who survive the acute infection hypogammaglobulinaemia or subsequent lymphoma sometimes develops.

Laboratory findings

After EBV infection there may be decreased lymphocyte numbers, decreased antibody responses with pan-hypogammaglobulinemia, and inflammatory cell infiltrates into lymph nodes, spleen, liver, and the central nervous system.

Molecular defect

The molecular defect in this condition has not been characterized. The gene has been mapped to a 2 Mb region of chromosome Xq25. There is evidence to suggest that T-lymphocyte proliferation and NK cell activity are reduced in these subjects, or that generation of uncontrolled NK cells occur.

Treatment

Acyclovir may be tried for the EBV infection but is not usually effective in fulminant infections. The hypogammaglobulinaemia can be treated with intravenous immunoglobulins.

Ataxia telangiectasia

Ataxia often develops at the age of 2–4 months and telangiectasia on the nose, ears, and conjuctivae later. Survival is reduced due to development of malignancy. There is considerable heterogeneity in the phenotype of ataxia telangectasia (AT). Some patients have the characteristic oculocutaneous telangiectasias with progressive cerebellar ataxia and immunodeficiency.

Laboratory findings

There are reduced levels of IgA, IgE, and IgG2. T-lymphocyte numbers may also be reduced.

Molecular defect

AT is characterized by DNA fragility. The DNA is particularly sensitive to ionizing radiation. All forms of the disease have been found to have mutation in the *ATM* gene which encodes a protein that appears to be similar to several yeast and mammalian phosphatidyli-nositol-3' kinases that are involved in mitogenic signal

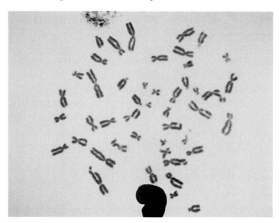

▮ **Fig. 1.7** A chromosome spread after low-dose ionizing radiation from a patient with ataxia telangiectasia showing the typical gaps and breaks (illustrated by the arrows). In the absence of the molecular basis for the disease, diagnosis is based upon the demonstration of chromosomal fragility as an index of failure of DNA repair.

transduction, meiotic recombination and cell cycle control.

Wiskott–Aldrich syndrome (WAS)

This is a combined cellular and humoral X-linked immunodeficiency which is characterized by the triad of thrombocytopenia, eczema, and recurrent infection.

Laboratory findings

There is thrombocytopenia in which characteristically platelets are small in size, and variably low levels of immunoglobulins, particularly IgM, with elevated levels of IgE. T-cell numbers may be variable with either increased or decreased numbers of CD4 and CD8 cells.

Molecular defect

WAS maps to chromosome Xp11. WAS is associated with abnormalities of CD43 with either reduced amounts of CD43 on lymphocytes or abnormal glycosylation of the protein causing interference in T-cell function. CD23 expression has been reported to be reduced along with a blunted response to antibody cross-linking on B cells. Recently, the gene has been isolated (named *WASP*) and has been found to code for a proline rich protein of about 65 kD, which is expressed in lymphocytes, spleen, and thymocytes. The gene does not share any homology with any known gene families and the function has not yet been determined. Point mutations have been described in many patients confirming that this was indeed the gene involved in the disease.

Treatment

Symptomatic treatment with antimicrobials may be required in milder cases. In more severe cases bone marrow transplantation is indicated. Splenectomy is sometimes indicated if thrombocytopenia is a major problem.

Phagocytic cell disorders

Chronic granulomatous disease

Clinical and laboratory findings

CGD consists of a group of several disorders characterized by defective phagocyte function. Phagocytic cells in children with CGD ingest organisms normally but fail to kill them as a result of defects in the superoxide-producing pathway. This results in recurrent and chronic bacterial and fungal infections in affected individuals.

Treatment

Treatment with prophylactic antibiotics, especially trimethoprim and sulphamethoxazole, may partially control the frequency of infections. There is now evidence that treatment with gamma interferon (INFγ) improves patient phagocyte function. In a recent trial after treatment with IFNγ 70% CGD patients remained free of severe infections for a year compared with 30% receiving placebo. In addition, in a small number of cases bone marrow transplantation using HLA-matched donors has been successful in curing the disease.

Molecular defects

All forms of the disease affect the various components of the nicotinamide adenine dinucleotide phosphate (NADPH) oxidase system of phagocytic cells. The NADPH oxidase is now known to consist of four specific components, two of which are cytosolic: p47-*phox* and p67-*phox*, and two are the membrane bound flavocytochrome *b*558 components: gp91-*phox* and p22-*phox*. Defects in any of these components give rise to CGD, with over 90% of all cases caused by defects in p47-*phox* and gp91-*phox*.

Leucocyte adhesion deficiency

Clinical and laboratory findings

Leucocyte adhesion deficiency (LAD) is a rare autosomal recessive disorder that leads to delayed detach-

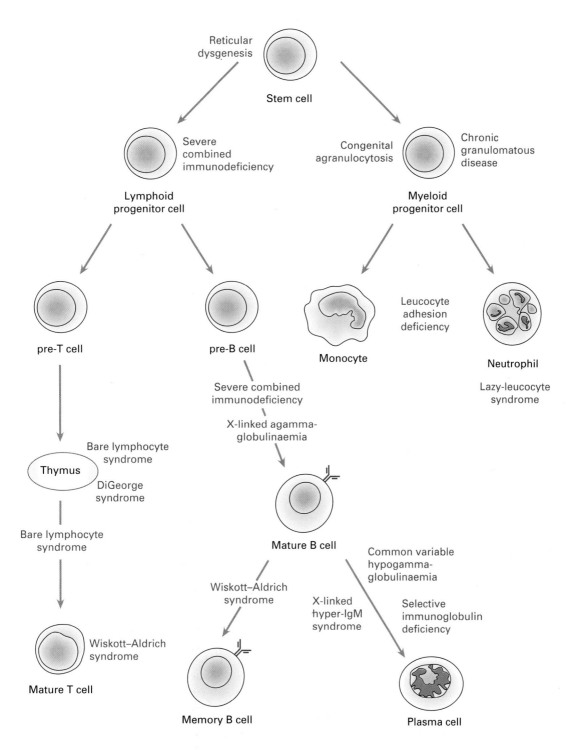

∎ **Fig. 1.8** Sites of the congenital immunodeficiencies on the differentiation pathways of cells from the precursor stem cells.

ment of the umbilical cord and to recurrent severe infections due to impaired leucocyte function. The disease leads to an inability of phagocytic cells to adhere to endothelial cells and subsequently to migrate to sites of infection.

Molecular defects

The disorder is caused by defects in the β chain (CD18) of the adhesion molecules LFA-1, Mac-1 (CR3), and p150,95, which results in their reduced or absent expression. Each of these molecules is a heterodimer consisting of a different α chain (CD11a, CD11b, or CD11c) and a shared common β chain (CD18). The CD18 gene has been cloned and heterogeneous mutations described which alter the expression and/or structure of this component. The severity of the disease seems to correlate with the level of expression of these molecules. Biochemical and genetic studies have defined five different types of LAD, including severe and moderate phenotypes.

Chediak–Higashi syndrome

The Chediak–Higashi syndrome is caused by an abnormality of neutrophil function, resulting in recurrent bacterial and fungal infections. Neutrophils from affected individuals contain large cytoplasmic inclusions. On the basis of similarity with the mutant beige mice, a gene, *LYST*, has recently been isolated and a mutation found in this gene in one patient so far.

Mannose-binding protein deficiency

Mannose-binding protein (MBP) is a major acute phase protein. MBP circulates in the blood in a wide range of concentrations (0.1–50 mg/ml). Structural analysis shows that it resembles C1q by binding to ligands which activates a serine protease and can then form a C3 convertase.

During the past few years it has become a prime suspect for unexplained immunodeficiency. In 1976 Soothill found that the blood of 11 of 43 children with a history of recurrent infection had an inability to phagocytose yeast cells properly. This was subsequently found to be due to lack of a protein that bound to mannan, a MBP, which was absent or present in very low concentration in the blood of those with this impairment of phagocytosis.

Yeast, bacteria, and some viruses carry mannose which is recognized by MBP, and the complement pathway is activated by this 'innate immunity'. After cloning of the gene in 1989 it was possible to identify the genetic cause of low MBP levels in affected individuals. Mutations in the MBP gene have been identified as replacements: at position 54 glycine by aspartate; at 57 glycine by glutamic acid; and a less common one at 52 of arginine by cysteine. These mutations apparently prevent MBP from polymerizing and performing its function.

However, the existence of mutation in MBP, in 17% of Caucasians, is more frequent than the problems of immunodeficiency, and why this should be so has yet to be explained.

Complement defects

Inherited defects have been described for most components of the complement system (see Chapter 2). These are very rare, giving rise to susceptibility to autoimmune disorders for the early component deficiencies (C2 and C4), and susceptibility to bacterial infections such as *Neisseria meningitidis* for the later components (C5–9). Of the alternative pathway components, X-linked properdin deficiencies have been described with defined mutations in three or four families worldwide.

C1 esterase deficiency is the most common defect, presenting as angioedema, and/or abdominal pain. Three discrete mutations of the MBP gene have been described. This protein, which has structural similarities to bovine conglutinin, is involved in the classical pathway, and is probably a non-specific activator of complement. More details of these complement deficiencies are provided in the chapter on complement deficiencies.

Future prospects: gene therapy for immunodeficiency

The inherited immunodeficiencies make particularly good candidate disorders for treatment by somatic gene therapy; they are caused by single gene defects and the genes in many cases are now cloned (Table 1.1). In many cases expression of the relevant genes is restricted to cells of the haematopoietic lineage. This provides a relatively accessible target organ for treatment, the peripheral blood or bone marrow. In many cases these disorders are already treatable by bone marrow transplantation. Correction of the defect and reconstitution of a functioning immune system may only require low levels of expression of the relevant protein in some of these situations. This means that, although the techniques available at present are far from perfect, it may still be acceptable to attempt this type of treatment in cases where the genetically modified cells may have a selective advantage over the unmodified cells and where there is often no satisfactory alternative treatment.

Although other treatments, such as administration of intravenous PEG conjugated bovine ADA can be used to treat ADA-deficient SCID, this disorder has become the prime target immunodeficiency disorder for treatment by somatic gene therapy techniques. So far this is the only inherited immunodeficiency for which clinical trials have been undertaken using these techniques.

From patient studies it is clear that only low levels of enzyme expression are sufficient to reconstitute normal immune function. There is no requirement for the regulated expression of the gene as it is expressed in all cells of the body but only appears to be critical for the normal function of T cells.

Several ADA-deficient SCID patients have now been treated at different centres in the USA and Europe with retroviruses containing a functional ADA gene. The aim is to correct their defects by reconstituting expression in peripheral T cells. This has been attempted directly by introducing the gene into peripheral blood T cells expanded with IL-2 *in vitro* — the first clinical application of somatic gene therapy for ADA–SCID was for the retrovirus-mediated transduction of IL-2 expanded T cells, and a second protocol involved transduction of both T cells and T-cell depleted bone marrow. In more recent protocols 'stem' cell or progenitor cell populations have been used, derived from either the peripheral blood or bone marrow. The advantages of using precursor cells is that they should provide a renewable long-term source of mature T cells. The approach using more mature cells is technically easier but does not effect a long-term cure, requiring the treatment to be repeated at regular intervals and only generating a limited repertoire. Although the stem cell approach is more difficult, success will mean that there is lifelong correction of the defect. So far, the results of these trials have not been published, but anecdotal evidence suggests cautious optimism as the gene has been shown to be present in bone marrow cells many months post-transduction, but expression of the gene product remains inadequate for immunological correction.

Gene therapy experimentation to date in the area of primary immunodeficiencies has made extensive use of retroviral vectors to introduce DNA sequences into the target cells. Increasingly, attempts are being made to transduce purified stem cell populations derived from bone marrow and peripheral blood. However, these populations are still rather heterogeneous in nature. It is likely that stem cell purification procedures must be improved to give higher yields of stem cells, rather than the presently obtained mixture of progenitors and stem cells, before this approach can be completely successful.

A major disadvantage affecting the use of retroviral vectors is that they have a very low efficiency of integration in cells not actively in cycle, including stem cells. One particularly attractive gene transduction system for potential use in clinical protocols is based on adeno-associated virus (AAV). AAV is an endogenous human virus with many properties which suggests it could be utilized as a safe vector for stem cell transduction. Perhaps most significantly, cell division is thought not to be a prerequisite for AAV infection.

The experiments in ADA deficiency have resulted in substantial progress in establishing somatic gene therapy as a viable treatment and potential cure for many of the inherited immunodeficiencies. However, in the majority of these diseases tight regulation of the expression of the gene in question will be required and knowledge of tissue-specific promotor and enhancer elements for successful gene correction will be needed. Future prospects are exciting and the next few years should see the development and refinement of the techniques necessary for successful treatment of a wide range of these diseases by gene therapy.

Further reading

Allen, R. C., Armitage, R. J., Conley, M. E., *et al.* (1993). CD40 ligand gene defects responsible for X-linked hyper IgM syndrome. *Science*, 259, 990–3.

Arnaiz-Villena, A., Timón, M., Rodriguez-Gallego, C., *et al.* (1992). Human T-cell activation deficiencies. *Immunology Today*, **13**, 259–65.

Arpaia, E., Shahar, M., Dadi, H., Cohen, A., and Roifman, C. M. (1994). Defective T cell receptor signaling and CD8+ thymic selection in humans lacking Zap-70 kinase. *Cell*, **76**, 947–58.

Barbosa, D. F. S., Nguyen, Q. A., Tchernev, V. T., *et al.* (1996). Identification of the homologous beige and Chediak–Higashi syndrome genes. *Nature*, **382**, 262–5.

Blaese, M. (1993). Development of gene therapy for immunodeficiency: Adenosine deaminase deficiency. *Paediatric Research*, **33**, 549–55.

Bordignon, C. (1993). Progress toward the clinical application of somatic gene therapy. *Current Opinion in Hematology*, ,246–51.

Cournoyer, D. and Caskey, C. T. (1993). Gene therapy of the immune system. *Annual Review of Immunology*, **11**, 297–329.

Derry, J. M. J., Ochs, H. D., and Francke, U. (1994). Isolation of a novel gene mutated in Wiskott–Aldrich syndrome. *Cell*, **78**, 635–44.

DiSanto, J. P., Bonnefoy, J. Y., Gauchat, J. F., *et al.* (1993). CD40 ligand mutations in X-linked immunodeficiency with hyper IgM. *Nature*, **361**, 541–3.

Fischer, A. and Lisowska-Grospierre, B. (1988). Leukocyte adhesion deficiency: Molecular basis and functional consequences. *Immunodeficiency Reviews*, **1**, 39–54.

Hirschhorn, R. (1990). Adenosine deaminase deficiency. *Immunodeficiency Reviews*, **2**, 175–98.

Kinnon, C., Hinshelwood, S., Levinsky, R. J., and Lovering, R. C. (1993). X-linked agammaglobulinemia — gene cloning and future prospects. *Immunology Today*, **14**, 554–8.

Kroczek, R. A., graf, D, Brugnoni, D, *et al.* (1994). Defective expression of CD40 ligand on T cells causes "X-linked immunodeficiency with hyper-IgM (HIGMI)". *Immunological Reviews*, **138**, 39–59.

Leonard, W. J. (1994). The defective gene in X-linked severe combined immunodeficiency encodes a shared interleukin receptor subunit: implications for cytokine pleiotropy and redundancy. *Current Opinion in Immunology*, **6**, 631–5.

Macchi, P, Villa, A, Frattini, *et al.* (1995). Mutations of Jak-3 gene in patients with autosomal severe combined immune deficiency (SCID). *Nature*, **337**, 65–8.

Mach, B., Steimle, V., and Reith, W. (1994). MHC Class II-deficient combined immunodeficiency: A disease of gene regulation. *Immunological Reviews*, **138**, 207–21.

Markert, M. L. (1991). Purine nucleoside phosphorylase deficiency. *Immunodeficiency Reviews*, **3**, 45–81.

Noguchi, M., Nakamura, Y., Russell, S. M., *et al.* (1993a). Interleukin-2 receptor γ chain: A functional component of the interleukin-7 receptor. *Science*, **262**, 1877–80.

Noguchi, M., Yi, H., Rosenblatt, H. M., *et al.* (1993b). Interleukin-2 receptor γ chain mutation results in X-linked severe combined immunodeficiency. *Cell*, **73**, 147–57.

Padayachee, M., Feighery, C., Finn, A. *et al.* (1992). Mapping of the X-linked form of hyper IgM syndrome(HIGM1) to Xq26 by close linkage to HPRT. *Genomics*, **14**, 551–3.

Pelham, A., O'Reilly, M-A., Malcolm, S., *et al.* (1990). RFLP and deletion analysis for X-linked chronic granulomatous disease using the cDNA probe: Potential for improved prenatal diagnosis and carrier determination. *Blood*, **76**, 820–4.

Perlmutter, R. M. (1994). Zapping T-cell respons. *Nature*, **370**, 370, 249–50.

Philip, R., Brunette, E., Kilinski, L., *et al.* (1994) Efficient and sustained gene expression in primary T lymphocytes and primary and cultured tumor cells mediated by adeno-associated virus plasmid DNA complexed to cationic liposomes. *Molecular and Cellular Biology*, **14**, 2411–18.

Porter, C. D., Parkar, M. H., Levinsky, R. J., Collins M. K., and Kinnon, C. (1993). X-linked chronic granulomatous disease: Correction of NADPH oxidase defect by retrovirus-mediated expression of gp91-*phox*. *Blood*, **82**, 2196–202.

Puck, J. M., Deschênes, S. M., Porter, J. C., *et al.* (1993). The interleukin-2 receptor γ chain maps to Xq13.1 and is mutated in X-linked severe combined immunodeficiency, SCIDX1. *Human Molecular Genetics*, **2**, 1099–104.

Ramesh, N., Fuleihan, R., Ramesh, V., *et al.* (1993). Deletions in the ligand for CD40 in X-linked immunoglobulin deficiency with normal or elevated IgM (HIGMX-1). *International Immunology*, **5**, 769–73.

Remold-O'Donnell, E, Rosen, F. S., and Kenney, D. M. (1996). Defects in Wiskott–Aldrich syndrome blood cells. *Blood*, **87**, 2621–31.

Roos, D, de Boer, M, Kuribayashi, F, *et al.* (1996). Mutations in the X-linked and autosomal recessive forms of chronic granulomatous disease. *Blood*, **87**, 1663–81.

Russell, S. M., Keegan, A. D., Harada, N., *et al.* (1993). Interleukin-2 receptor γ chain: A functional component of the interleukin-4 receptor. *Science*, **262**, 1818.

Savitsky, K, Bar-Shira, A, Gilad, *et al.* (1995). A single ataxia telangiectasia gene with a product similar to PI-3 kinase. *Science*, **268**, 1749–53.

Seger, R. A. and Ezekowitz, R. A. B. (1994). Treatment of chronic granulomatous disease. *Immunodeficiency*, **5**, 113–30.

Sekhsaria, S., Gallin, J. I., Linton, G. F., *et al.* (1993). Peripheral blood progenitors as a target for genetic correction of p47phox-deficient chronic granulomatous disease. *Proceedings of the National Academy of Sciences USA*, **90**, 7446–50.

Steimle, V., Otten, L. A., Zufferey, M., and Mach, B. (1993). Complementation of an MHC class II transactivator mutated in hereditary MHC class II deficiency (or bare lymphocyte syndrome). *Cell*, **75**, 135–46.

Sugamura, K., Asao, H., Kondo, M., *et al.* (1996). Interleukin-2 receptor gamma chain: its role in multiple cytokine receptor complexes and T cell development in XSCID. *Annual Review of Immunology*, **14**, 179–207.

Thompson, C. (1995). Protein proves to be a key link in innate immunity. *Science*, **269**, 301–2.

Thrasher, A., Cheety, M., Casimir, C., and Segal, A. W. (1992). Restoration of superoxide generation to a chronic granulomatous disease-derived B-cell line by retrovirus mediated gene transfer. *Blood*, **80**, 1125–9.

Tsukada, S., Saffron, D. C., Rawlings, D. J., *et al.* (1993). Deficient expression of a B cell cytoplasmic tyrosine kinase in a human X-linked agammaglobulinemia. *Cell*, **72**, 279–90.

van Beusechem, V. W., Kukler, A., Heidt, P. J., and Valerio, D. (1992). Long-term expression of human adenosine deaminase in rhesus monkeys transplanted with retrovirus-infected bone marrow cells. *Proceedings of the National Academy of Sciences USA*, **89**, 7640–4.

Vetrie, D., Vorechovsky, I., Sideras, P., *et al.* (1993). The gene involved in X-linked agammaglobulinaemia is a member of the src family of protein-tyrosine kinases. *Nature*, **361**, 202–3, and **363**, 590.

Villa, A., Notarangelo, L. D., DiSanto, J. P., *et al.* (1994). Organization of the human CD40L gene: Implications for molecular defects in X chromosome-linked hyper-IgM syndrome and prenatal diagnosis. *Proceedings of the National Academy of Sciences USA*, **91**, 2110–14.

2 Complement deficiencies

E. J. Brown

Introduction

Complement deficiencies are rare, generally hereditary, disorders of the complement system. The proteins of the complement system are listed in Table 2.1.

These components can be divided into the proteins of the classical pathway of activation (C1, C4, and C2); the alternative pathway of activation (factor D, factor P [properdin], and factor B; C3, which is at the intersection of the two activation pathways; the late components (C5-C9); and the control proteins (C1EI; C4bp; 1H [factor H]; C3INA; vitronectin [S protein]). The classical pathway of activation is most often triggered by immune complexes; activation of the alternative pathway is accelerated by bacterial surfaces (Fig. 2.1). In addition, there are multiple host cell-associated proteins which regulate complement activation and deposition. These include CR1 (CD35); CR2 (CD21); CR3 (CD11b/CD18); CR4 (CD11c/CD18); decay accelerating factor (DAF, CD55); homologous restriction factor (HRF, CD59), and membrane cofactor protein (MCP).

Most complement components are encoded on autosomes, so almost all deficiency states are autosomal recessive traits (Table 2.2). Because of this, homozygous deficiency states are quite rare. An interesting exception is C1 esterase inhibitor (C1INH) deficiency, in which the heterozygous state is associated with a symptomatic phenotype known as hereditary angioedema. Another exception to strict autosomal inheritance of deficiency is for the classical pathway component C4. Because there are two active C4 genes, total C4 deficiency is extremely rare, with fewer than 25 reported cases. However, the products of the two C4 genes differ subtly in their ability to bind to immunoglobulin (Ig) G and the C4A gene makes a protein which is particularly important for detoxifying immune complexes. Perhaps for this reason, C4A deficiency has been epidemiologically associated with

systemic lupus erythematosus (SLE), even in the heterozygous state. However, the C4 genes, like factor B and C2, are encoded in the major histocompatibility gene complex. The C4A^{null} genotype is in linkage disequilibrium with other human leucocyte antigen genes, and it is not yet clear which of these is most strongly associated with autoimmunity.

This section will be a brief review of the clinical syndromes associated with complement deficiency states. In general, the early classical component deficiencies are associated with autoimmune diseases. C3 deficiency is associated with increased susceptibility to pyogenic infections, as are deficiencies of factors H and I, which result in enhanced consumption of C3 and secondary C3 deficiency. Deficiencies of the other alternative pathway components and the proteins of the membrane attack complex are associated with a unique susceptibility to *Neisseria* spp. infections. Interestingly, C9 deficiency seems not to be associated with disease.

Deficiencies of specific complement components

Classical pathway

C1 deficiency

C1 is composed of three subunits: C1q, C1r, and C1s. C1q binding to immunoglobulin or other activating surfaces leads to a conformational change within the C1 molecules, with autoactivation of C1r and C1s which have latent serine protease activity. Patients with C1q deficiency have been described. These patients have autoimmune disease which resembles SLE. Human C1r deficiency has also been described and these patients show a similar propensity to autoimmune disease. The pathophysiological mechanism for

∎ **Table 2.1**   The complement system

	$M_r \times 10^3$)	(Serum) g/ml	Chains	Chain function
Classical pathway				
C1q	410	70	6×3	Binds to Fc of IgG and IgM
C1r	190	34	2	Serine protease; activates C1s
C1s	85	31	2	Serine protease; activates C4 + 2
C2	117	25	1	Serine protease; C2b binds to C4b; activates C3
C4	206	600	3	C4 binds C2a; C4a is an anaphylotoxin
Alternate pathway				
Factor D	25	1	1	Serine protease; activates B
Factor B	95	225	1	Serine protease; Bb binds C3b to act as convertase for C3 and C5
Factor P (Properdin)	190	25	4	Stabilizes C3b Bb
Factor H	300	500	2	Blocks formation of C3b Bb
Factor I	90	35	2	Cleaves C4b or C3b using a co-factor
C3	200	1000–2000	2	C3b binds to C3b.Bb or C4b2a; C3a is an anaphylotoxin
Membrane attack component (MAC)				
C5	180	85	2	C5b part of MAC; C5a- anaphylotoxin
C6	128	60	1	Part of MAC
C7	120	55	1	Part of MAC
C8	150	55	3	Part of MAC
79	60	1		Polymerizes; forms MAC
Plasma control proteins				
C1INH	105	180	1	Serine protease inhibitor
C4. BP	560	8		Blocks C3 convertase C4b 2a
Vitronectin	75	500	1	
Membrane proteins				
CR1 (CD35)	160–240		1	On RBC, neutrophil; monocytes; B cells, some T cells
CR2 (CD21)	140		1	B cells; some T cells
CR3 (CD11b/CD18)	165, 95		2	Monocytes; neutrophil; natural killer; some T cells
DAF (CD55)	70		1	
CD59 (HRF)	18		1	Binds C5b,6,7,8; block C9 binding
MCP	40–70		1	Blocks C3 convertase in both classical and alternate paths

development of disease is not known, but is suspected to be failure to detoxify and clear immune complexes by normal routes.

C4 deficiency

Complete human C4 deficiency is a rare condition which has been associated with severe SLE. There are two C4 genes in humans located in the class III region of the major histocompatibility complex (MHC) locus which encode slightly different proteins. The product of the C4A gene is more capable of forming ester bonds from its internal thioester upon activation; the C4B product is more capable of forming amide bonds. In addition to complete C4 deficiency, C4A deficiency has been associated with SLE. Although C4A deficient serum has less activity for detoxifying immune complexes, it is not clear whether this is the defect which leads to autoimmune susceptibility or whether there are other loci within the extended haplotype which contribute to this phenotype rather than, or in addition to, C4A[null].

A complete deficiency of C4 in the guinea-pig has been known for over 20 years. These animals have a

∎ **Table 2.2** Complement deficiencies

Deficiency state	Acquisition	Clinical association
C1q	AR	SLE with GN
C1r[a]	Unknown	SLE
C4	AR	SLE[b]
C2	AR	SLE, AI[c]
C3	AR 2° other C deficiencies	AI, pyogenic infections, GN
Factor D	Unknown	Neisseria infection
Factor P	X-linked	?Neisseria infection
Factor H	AR	2° to C3 deficiency
Factor I	AR	2° to C3 deficiency
C5	AR	Neisseria infection
C6	AR	Neisseria infection
C7	AR	Neisseria infection
C8	AR	Neisseria infection
C9	AR	Probably none
C1.INH	AD	Hereditary angioedema
DAF	Acquired[d]	Hemolysis
CD59 (HRF)	Acquired[d]	Hemolysis
CR3	Autosomal recessive	Pyogenic infections

AD = Autosomal dominant
AI = autoimmune phenomena
AR = Autosomal recessive
GN = glomerulonephritis
SLE = systemic lupus erythematosus

[a] Associated with partial C1s deficiency
[b] Discoid and systemic lupus erythematosus associated with both complete C4 deficiency and C4A deficiency. This is part of an extended haplotype involving MHC Class I, II and III alleles
[c] About half of people with C2 deficiency are clinically normal. AI = autoimmune phenomena, including GN, vasculitis, polymyositis
[d] These are PIG-linked proteins deficient in paroxysmal nocturnal hemoglobinuria

decreased ability to clear some infections, an inability to switch from IgM to IgG production upon intravenous secondary immunization with $\varphi \times 174$, and hampered clearance of model immune complexes. The lifespans of C4-deficient guinea-pigs are normal, and these animals do not appear to develop autoimmune diseases spontaneously.

C2 deficiency

C2 deficiency is the most common human complement deficiency, with a frequency for the C2^{null} allele of about 1 in 200. About half of patients with complete C2 deficiency are asymptomatic; the other half have autoimmune diseases ranging from very mild (discoid lupus erythematosus) to more severe. As C2, like C4 is encoded within the class III region MHC, it is possible that the more severe phenotypes are associated with other abnormal genes within the MHC. In particular, some of these patients have low levels of Factor B, which may contribute to disease susceptibility. The most common form of C2 deficiency results from a 28 bp deletion at the 3' end of exon 6 which results in loss of a splice donor site.

Guinea-pigs with complete C2 deficiency have been described. These animals, like C4D guinea-pigs, are unable to switch from IgM to IgG production after repeated intravenous immunization. These animals have no other striking abnormalities.

C3 deficiency

Human C3 deficiency is associated with increased susceptibility to pyogenic infection and with autoimmune nephritis. The autoimmune disease may occur because of immune complex deposition during chronic antigenic stimulation from subclinical infection. There are multiple genetic bases for C3 deficiency described, including deletions of 60–700 bases, with serum C3 levels ranging from none detectable to 1% of normal C3 levels.

Guinea-pigs with C3 deficiency have been described. These animals appear to synthesize about 2% of normal levels of C3. This may occur because macrophages from these animals are able to synthesize C3, while hepatocytes, the main source of C3, are not. The molecular basis of C3 deficiency in the guinea-pig is unknown, as C3 mRNA is made and apparently encodes a protein identical to that synthesized by normal animals.

Alternative pathway

Patients with factor B, properdin, and factor D deficiency have been described. They seem to have a host defence defect similar to patients with C3 deficiency. This makes sense, as these components are required for C3 activation by the alternative pathway and for amplification of C3 activation when complement activation initiates via the classical pathway.

Membrane attack complex

C5–C8 deficiencies

Patients with late complement component deficiencies are susceptible to infection with *Neisseria* species, but apparently do not have a broader host defence defect. The reason for the special sensitivity to this one genus of micro-organism is unknown.

Murine C5 deficiency is rather common in inbred mouse strains. The basis for the deficiency is a 2 bp (TA) deletion in the C5 gene near the beginning of the protein coding region. This leads to mRNA encoding a truncated non-functional and rapidly degraded protein. C5 deficient mice are about 10-fold more susceptible to pneumococcal infection than their C5-sufficient litter mates. Rabbits with C6 deficiency have also been described. These rabbits breed poorly, and have been studied only minimally.

C9 deficiency

Complete C9 deficiency is apparently common in Japan, with a frequency among Japanese blood donors of 0.035–0.095%. No systematic studies from other large populations have been reported. There is no phenotype known to be associated with C9 deficiency, although there are a few case reports of association with recurrent *Neisseria meningitis*. The apparent health of these C9 deficient individuals prompted a search for other late complement component deficiencies among Japanese blood donors. C5, C6, C7, and C8 deficiencies were found, at a rate about 10% that of C9 deficiency. These individuals were also without obvious disease. Thus, it may be that there are other

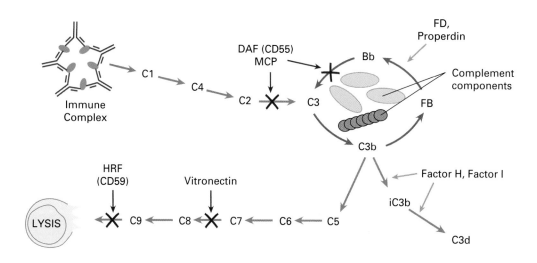

∎ **Fig. 2.1** Pathways of complement activation.

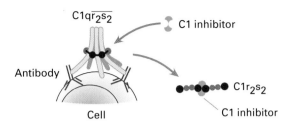

C1 inhibitor dissociates C1r/C1s
from the active $C1qr_2s_2$ complex

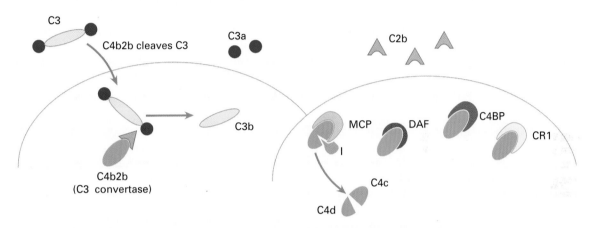

C4BP, DAF, MCP and CR1 displace C2b from the C4b2b complex.
When bound by C4BP, MCP or CR1, C4b is cleaved by a
soluble protease I to its inactive components C4c and C4d

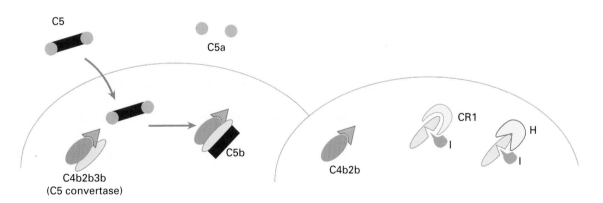

The C4b2b3b complex cleaves C5 to C5a and C5b.
CR1 and H are able to displace C3b and act as cofactors
in the subsequent cleavage of C3b by I

▌**Fig. 2.2**   Factors controlling or inhibiting complement activation.
C4BP: C4 binding protein
DAF : decay accelerating factor
MCP : mannose binding protein
R : Receptor
I : Factor I

factors in addition to late complement deficiency required for increased susceptibility to *Neisseria* infection. As many of the patients with late complement deficiencies and overwhelming *Neisseria* infections have high titre antibody against their infecting organism, antibody cannot overcome the host defence defect. Possibly, the late complement components play an as yet undiscovered part in the intracellular killing of phagocytosed *Neisseria*.

Control proteins

Factors H and I deficiency

Patients with factors I and H deficiencies have been described. Factor H is the alternative pathway equivalent to C4BP. It accelerates the decay of C3 convertase, and acts as a co-factor for cleavage of C3b by Factor I. These patients have low levels of C3 secondary to inadequate control of spontaneous C3 activation via the alternative pathway. Thus, these patients have a syndrome very similar to C3 deficiency, with increased propensity to infections and manifestations of chronic immune complex disease.

C1INH deficiency, hereditary angioedema

Perhaps the most common control protein deficiency is C1 inhibitor deficiency, a syndrome known as hereditary angioedema. The factor which causes the vascular dilatation and leak is probably bradykinin, as C1INH also inactivates the kallikrein-mediated conversion of kininogen to bradykinin as well as activated C1r and C1s. Interestingly, hereditary angioedema has an autosomal dominant inheritance pattern, even though it is a deficiency disease that results from a number of distinct genetic abnormalities which lead to failure of protein synthesis or synthesis of non-functional protein. Apparently, this is because synthetic function of two normal C1 inhibitor genes is required for a normal phenotype, so that it is the heterozygous state which is associated with hereditary angioedema.

This syndrome is characterized by episodic swelling in the extremities, in the gastrointestinal tract, and in the face and larynx. Episodes of swelling, frequently subcutaneous, facial, or oral can be induced by trauma, but may also be spontaneous, without an apparent inciting cause. Oedema can be severe, leading to acute abdominal symptoms of pain and swelling, pharyngeal and laryngeal swelling, stridor, or even death.

Therapy for acute attacks of swelling in hereditary angioedema involve supportive care and infusions of C1 inhibitor have been used. Chronic therapy usually involves treatment with androgenic steroids, which increase protein synthesis from the C1 inhibitor gene (see Chapter X on urticatia).

Cellular control proteins

The most common deficiency of plasma membrane proteins which control complement activation is paroxysmal nocturnal haemoglobinuria, an acquired

■ **Table 2.3** Distribution of complement components

Form	Complement components		
	Activation	**Regulatory**	**Receptors**
In serum	C1q,C1r,C1s; C4; C2; C3; MBP; MASP; B; D C5; C6; C7; C8; C9.	C1inh; C4BP; H; I; P; S protein C3a/C5a inact.	
In membrane		CR1, DAF, MCP HRF, CD59	C1qR, C5aR CR1, CR2, CR3

C1 inh = C1 inhibitor
C3a/C5a inact = C3a/C5a inactivator
C4BP = C4 binding protein
DAF = decay accelerating factor
HRF = homologous restriction factor
MASP = mannose binding protein associated serine proteinase
MBP = mannose binding protein
MCP = membrane cofactor protein
R = receptor

clonal defect of bone marrow stem cells which results in failure of expression of all membrane proteins with a phosphoinositol glycan (glycosyl phosphatidylinositol) anchor. There is absence of two complement control proteins, DAF and HRF (CD59), which leads to abnormal complement activation, deposition on, and enhanced sensitivity to lysis of these erythrocytes. The disease is characterized by increased complement consumption primarily by the alternative pathway, on the surfaces of these abnormal bone marrow derived cells. Lysis of erythrocytes leads to the primary clinical manifestation, severe haemolytic anaemia.

There are at least five distinct biochemical defects which can result in paroxysmal nocturnal haemoglobinuria.

Further reading

Colten, H. R., and Rosen, F. S. (1992). Complement deficiencies. *Annual Review of Immunology*, **10**, 809–34.

Kolble, K. and Reid, K. B. (1993). Genetic deficiencies of the complement system and association with disease: early components. *International Review of Immunology*, **10**, 17–36.

Liszewski, M. K. and Atkinson, J. P. (1993). The complement system. In *Fundamental immunology*, 3rd edn (ed. W. E. Paul), pp. 917–40. Raven, New York.

Mathieson, P. W. and Peters, D. K. (1993). Deficiency and depletion of complement in the pathogenesis of nephritis and vasculitis. *Kidney International*, **42**, S13–18.

Morgan, B. P. and Walport, M. J. (1991). Complement deficiency and disease. *Immunology Today*, **12**, 301–6.

Volanakis, J. E. (1995). Transcriptional regulation of complement genes. *Annual Review of Immunology*, **13**, 277–305.

Wurzner, R., Orren, A., and Lachmann, P. J. (1992). Inherited deficiencies of the terminal components of human complement. *Immunodeficiency Reviews*, **3**, 123–47.

3 Human immunodeficiency virus infection and acquired immunodeficiency syndrome

A. Carr and R. Penny

Definition

The Centers for Disease Control and Prevention (CDC) first defined acquired immune deficiency syndrome (AIDS) on clinical criteria in the absence of a known cause. When AIDS was subsequently found to be viral in origin, the classification was altered to incorporate known seropositivity for human immunodeficiency virus (HIV) and was separated into four groups separated on clinical grounds. These four groups were:

(i) primary HIV infection (group 1); (ii) asymptomatic infection (group 2); (iii) persistent generalized lymphadenopathy (PGL) (group 3); and (iv) symptomatic disease (group 4).

AIDS was defined as one or more clinical illnesses associated with opportunistic infection, malignancy or neurological dysfunction in the presence of seropositivity for antibodies to HIV. In 1993, the classification was further modified primarily also to stratify patients by CD4+ lymphocyte counts in recognition of the strong link between HIV-induced immunodeficiency and disease outcome (Tables 3.1 and 3.9). In the USA, AIDS is also defined by a CD4+ lymphocyte count

less than $200/\mu$l, regardless of the clinical status, although this recommendation has not been widely adopted in other countries.

Introduction

Epidemiology

The first reports of AIDS were in 1981, when a cluster of cases of *Pneumocystis carinii* pneumonia and Kaposi's sarcoma were identified in previously healthy homosexual men in the USA. This syndrome of acquired T-lymphocyte immunodeficiency with opportunistic infections was reported soon after in industrialized nations and in Africa. Although AIDS appears to have arisen in large numbers simultaneously between continents, there is good evidence that AIDS first arose in sub-Saharan Africa and subsequently in North America, Europe, Australia, South America, and more recently Asia. Current World Health Organization estimates suggest that there are 10–13 million cases of AIDS worldwide and that this number could grow to between 20 and 100 million by

▮ **Table 3.1** Summary of the 1993 Centres for Disease Control (CDC) Classification of HIV infection

CD4+ T-cell categories	Clinical categories		
	(A) Primary infection asymptomatic or persistent generalized lymphadenopathy	**(B)** Symptomatic (not A or C conditions)	**(C)** AIDS-defining illness
(1) CD4 > 500	A1	B1	C1
(2) CD4 200–499	A2	B2	C2
(3) CD4 < 200	A3	B3	C3

the year 2000. The vast majority of new cases of AIDS appear to be in sub-Saharan Africa and Asia, particularly South-east Asia and India.

AIDS is caused by infection with HIV. The average time to the development of AIDS appears to be approximately 10 years from infection, although this varies from a period of months to a period in excess of 15 years. Most of this period prior to developing AIDS is asymptomatic, with the mean survival time after developing AIDS being 1–2 years. Whether or not all people infected with HIV will eventually develop AIDS is unknown. What characteristics determine whether a person has rapid progression to AIDS, or is a long-term survivor without evidence of disease or immunodeficiency, are not well understood (see below).

Transmission

Globally, HIV infection is a heterosexual disease, particularly in Africa and Asia, with almost half of all new infections occurring in women. However, the mode of transmission varies between different countries and continents. For example, in the Americas, northern Europe, and Australia the predominant mode of transmission is by homosexual sex, whereas in the Mediterranean and some regions of Asia a more common mode of transmission is injecting drug use. The other modes of transmission include transfusion of infected blood and blood products, maternal–fetal transmission, via breast milk, occupational exposure, and from patient to patient during surgical procedures.

The relative risk of HIV transmission varies significantly according to the mode of transmission,

▌ **Table 3.2** Relative risks for HIV transmission according to mode of transmission

Route of transmission	Relative risk (%)
Sexually	
Male to male	1
Male to female	0.1
Female to female	0.05
Maternal–fetal transmission	10–30
No breast feeding	15–20
With breast feeding	30–40
Blood product	100
Solid organ transplantation	100
Sharing needles	?
Artificial insemination	?
Occupational, e.g. needle stick injury	0.03–0.05

with the greatest risk occurring after transfusion with an infected blood product (Table 3.2). However, the risk of transmission is not solely dependent upon the route of transmission nor even the size of the inoculum. For example, sexual transmission is more likely where there is mucosal disruption, either by trauma or by ulceration (e.g. concomitant sexually transmitted disease). Also, maternal–fetal transmission is more common from women with more advanced HIV disease, but is substantially reduced by zidovudine therapy and perhaps also by Caesarean section. There are some individuals who appear to be less susceptible to infection in the absence of safe sexual practices, suggesting that host immune responses may protect some individuals from infection, at least with some strains. Similarly, despite exposure to multiple viral quasi-species from an HIV-infected individual, there is evidence that only one quasi-species of HIV is usually transmitted, suggesting that particular viral strains are associated with the greatest risk of transmission. The characteristics that define such transmissible strains of HIV are not understood, but may relate to specific HIV envelope sequences. Importantly, it is not known whether an HIV-1-infected individual can be superinfected with a separate HIV-1 strain or strains, although dual infection with HIV-1 and HIV-2 may occur.

Human immunodeficiency virus

HIV receptors and cellular distribution

HIV has been demonstrated in a wide range of tissues. These include CD4+ T lymphocytes, dendritic cells, Langerhans cells, monocytes, macrophages, and thymocytes. These cells all share in common the presence of the CD4+ molecule on the cell surface which acts as the principle ligand for HIV. There is low density CD4+ expression also on some glial, cervical, endothelial, and trophoblastic cells. However, surface CD4+ alone appears insufficient to allow entry of HIV into cells; a recently defined surface protein called fusin appears to be a key co-receptor for HIV infection of CD4+ cells. In contrast macrophage trophic HIV-1 isolates appear to require another fusion co-factor which is the receptor for the c-c-chemokines RANTES, MIP-1α and MIP-β. Both fusin and cc CKr5 are heterodimeric GTP-binding proteins (G proteins). Accordingly elevated levels of β chemokines may play a role in controlling viral load and replication.

HIV can also infect cells that do not express CD4+ such as neuronal, endothelial, fibroblast, and

∎ **Table 3.3** *In vitro* cellular host range of HIV

Blood-derived cells
  CD4+ lymphocytes
  HTLV-I transformed CD8+ lymphocytes
  HHV-6 infected CD3+CD4-CD8+ lymphocytes
  B lymphocytes
  Monocytes/macrophages
  Bone marrow CD34+ precursor cells
  Promyelocytes
  Dendritic cells
  Langerhans cells

Nervous system derived cells
  Microglia
  Macrophages
  Astrocytes
  Fetal neuronal cells
  Neuroblastoma cells

Bowel-derived cells
  Colorectal carcinoma cell lines (e.g. SW620, HT29, SW480, SW1463)

Other cells
  Kupffer cells
  Hepatocellular carcinoma
  Fibroblastoid cell lines (e.g. Hos, RD, HuF)
  Rhabdomyosarcoma
  Trophoblast derived cell line
  Primary chondrocyte cells
  Synovial cells

natural killer (NK) cells, Epstein–Barr virus (EBV)-transformed B cells and some bone marrow progenitor cells. However, *in vivo* HIV infection of B cells or CD8+ lymphocytes has not been detected. Probably the most important of the CD4– target cells are microglial cells. The receptor on microglial and endothelial cells is galactosyl ceramide.

HIV has been detected in virtually all bodily fluids. However, transmission from fluids such as tears, saliva, or urine has not been demonstrated.

Structure of HIV

HIV is a retrovirus and has two major subtypes, designated HIV-1 and HIV-2, which have similar structures and demonstrate the same cell tropism. The nucleotide sequence homology between HIV-1 and HIV-2 is 42%, but nevertheless the clinical consequences of infection with either form of HIV are similar.

The HIV virion is a 90–130 nm diameter, icosahedral structure with a lipid bilayer envelope expressing viral glycoproteins as well as host cell class I and class II major histocompatibility antigens (Fig. 3.1). The two major viral surface proteins of HIV-1 are gp41 and gp120, which insert into and protrude through the envelope, respectively. The equivalent proteins for HIV-2 are gp36 and gp104, respectively. Within the virion is a nucleocapsid containing HIV RNA and various replicative enzymes.

The genome of HIV-1 is composed of diploid, single-stranded positive-sense RNA. Three genes

∎ **Table 3.4** Functions of HIV-1 structural and regulatory genes

Gene	Protein	Function(s)
env	gp120	Ligand for CD4 and galactosyl ceramide
	gp41	Internalization of HIV into target cell
gag	p24	Core protein
	p17	Core matrix protein
	p9	
	p7	
pol	p66	Reverse transcriptase — creates single-stranded DNA copy from HIV RNA
	p31	Integrase — incorporation of HIV DNA into target cell genome
	p10	Protease — splicing of HIV precursor proteins to mature forms and subsequent viral packaging
tat	p14	Accelerates initiation of HIV transcription, increases stability, transport or translation of mRNA
rev	p19	? Stabilizes mRNA and facilitates its transport to cytoplasm essential for expression of env proteins, inhibits mRNA translation of rev, tat, and nef
nef	p27	Shown to both up and downregulate HIV replication
vif	p23	Increases release of HIV from infected cells perhaps by maturation of env proteins
vpu	p16	? Enhances viral budding (not essential for survival)
vpr	p15	controls expression of vpu
		? Weak positive effect on replication
vpx	p16	Unknown

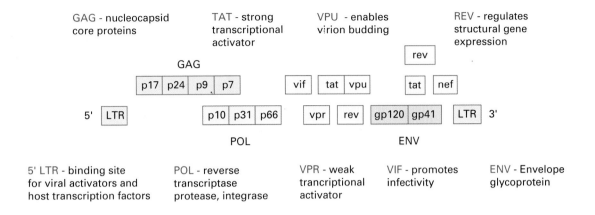

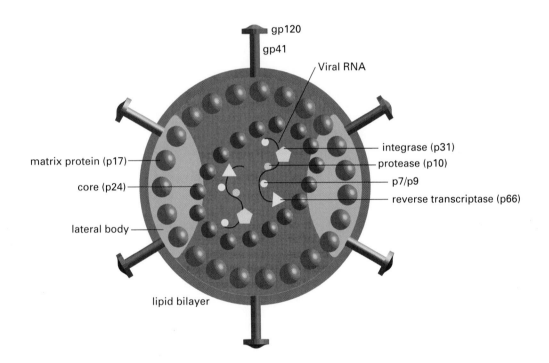

∎ **Fig. 3.1** Structure and genome of HIV-1.

encode for the structural proteins of the mature virion (*gag, pol, env*) while at least six genes encode for proteins involved in the regulation of viral expression (*tat, rev, vif, vpu, vpr, nef*). The gag and pol proteins are derived by cleavage of a common *gag–pol* precursor by HIV-encoded protease. The *gag* genes are transcribed to produce a 55 kDa (p55) precursor protein, which is cleaved by the HIV-encoded protease to produce 24 kDa (p24), 17 kDa (p17), 15 kDa (p15), 9 kDa (p9), and 7 kDa (p7) proteins. The major constituent of the virus core is the p24 protein. The enzymes of HIV-1, namely reverse transcriptase (p66), integrase (p31), and protease (p10), are encoded by the *pol* gene. The *env* gene encodes a glycosylated precursor protein (gp160), which is cleaved to produce the non-covalently linked external 120 kDa (gp120) and transmembrane 41 kDa (gp41) proteins.

Two variants of HIV deserve mention because of their clinical relevance, which is discussed below. Syncytium-inducing (SI) variants of HIV are those which cause the MT-2 T cell line to form non-functional, giant cells *in vitro*. SI variants appear to arise from mutations in hypervariable regions of gp120, in particular its V3 loop, although other regions are involved. The other principal variants are those arising after exposure to antiretroviral agents, especially zidovudine. These are due to mutations in the antiretroviral drug target, and are discussed below.

Life cycle of HIV

The CD4+ molecule, at amino acids 42–55 of its first immunoglobulin-like domain, acts as the principal ligand for the gp120 envelope protein of HIV-1. Once bound to CD4+, HIV is internalized in a process involving the V3 loop of gp120, a hydrophobic region of gp41 and perhaps fusin on the target cell surface. HIV may enter the cell by other means, perhaps as an HIV–anti-HIV antibody complex via an Fc or complement receptor, by direct binding of HIV-1 to neuronal and epithelial cells via the glycolipid galactosyl ceramide and by fusion of infected with uninfected cells.

As with other retroviruses, the outer proteins are removed as the virus enters the cell, exposing the viral capsid, including its RNA and reverse transcriptase. Reverse transcription results in a DNA copy of the RNA, which together form a DNA–RNA hybrid. The reverse transcriptase enzyme has a high error rate of approximately 1 nucleotide in 103 bp, a critical factor in determining the genomic diversity that is characteristic of HIV. Ribonuclease H, a 51 kDa fragment of reverse transcriptase, degrades the viral RNA strand of the RNA–DNA hybrid, so that the DNA strand can act as a template for synthesis of a complementary DNA strand. Double-stranded viral DNA then enters the nucleus and, via the action of viral integrase, is incorporated into host DNA. Once integrated, viral DNA remains part of the genome until cell death and is passed on to progeny should cell division occur.

HIV is often latent for a variable period within cells due to impairment of RNA reverse transcription or of integrated viral DNA transcription. Transcription of viral DNA is usually triggered by host cell activation by antigen, mitogens, cytokines, or gene products of other viruses such as EBV, *cytomegalovirus* (CMV), *human T-lymphotropic virus type I, hepatitis B virus*, and *human herpesvirus type 6* (HHV-6). These triggers upregulate host regulatory proteins, a notable example being the induction of nuclear factor kappa B (NF-κB)

by interleukin-1 (IL-1), interleukin-6 (IL-6), and tumour necrosis factor-alpha (TNFα), as well as by NF–κB itself. NF-κB binds to regulatory sequences in host DNA to activate transcription of various genes; in an HIV-infected cell, NF-κB also binds to regulatory sequences in the 5′ long terminal repeat of the viral DNA and upregulates viral transcription.

Other cytokines which upregulate the replication of HIV include IL-2, IL-3, IL-4, TNFβ, macrophage colony-stimulating factor, and granulocyte–macrophage colony-stimulating factor. In contrast, interferon-alpha (IFNα) and interferon-beta (IFNβ) downregulate HIV expression. Interferon-gamma (IFNγ) and transforming growth factor-beta (TGFβ) have variable effects on HIV replication. The dependence of HIV upon activation signals for effective transcription is underlined by the observation that cyclosporin A and FK-506, which are inhibitors of interleukin-2 (IL-2) production, decrease HIV replication and pathogenicity *in vitro*. The production of long transcripts of viral RNA is assured by the combined actions of the tat and rev proteins. Packaging of viral proteins is regulated by protease. As it buds through the cell surface, HIV becomes enclosed by an envelope of host cell membrane, completing both virion and life cycle.

Pathology

Host response to HIV infection

Primary HIV-1 infection is characterized by high levels of infectious HIV-1 in plasma and peripheral blood mononuclear cells (PBMC) during the first few weeks of infection; in one study levels of 1000–10 000 tissue-culture-infective doses per millilitre of plasma and 100–10 000 infective doses per million PBMC were found. The short and intense period of viral replication is followed in the ensuing weeks by a rapid decline in peripheral blood viral load (at least 100-fold) and concurrent resolution of the acute illness.

Viral clearance might be due either to a progressive lack of susceptible target cells or, more likely, to the emergence of an effective host mechanism for viral clearance. The mechanisms of this partial viral clearance during primary HIV-1 infection are not fully delineated, but humoral, cellular, and cytokine responses all apparently play a part. Nevertheless, clearance during primary infection is the most effective response to HIV, and is certainly far greater and more sustained than that produced by current antiretroviral agents.

Neutralizing antibodies to gp41 and gp120 may contribute to viral clearance, although a direct correlation between decline in viral load and development of

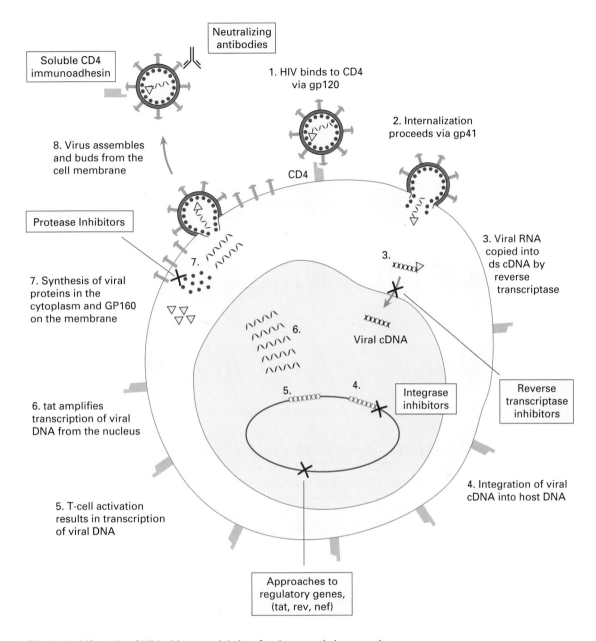

Soluble CD4
immunoadhesin

Neutralizing
antibodies

1. HIV binds to CD4
via gp120

2. Internalization
proceeds via gp41

8. Virus assembles
and buds from the
cell membrane

CD4

Protease Inhibitors

7. Synthesis of viral
proteins in the
cytoplasm and GP160
on the membrane

3. Viral RNA
copied into
ds cDNA by
reverse
transcriptase

Viral cDNA

6. tat amplifies
transcription of viral
DNA from the nucleus

Integrase
inhibitors

Reverse
transcriptase
inhibitors

5. T-cell activation
results in transcription
of viral DNA

4. Integration of viral
cDNA into host DNA

Approaches to
regulatory genes,
(tat, rev, nef)

∎ **Fig. 3.2**   Life cycle of HIV with potential sites for therapeutic intervention

neutralizing antibody has not yet been demonstrated. These antibodies tend to develop after resolution of primary infection, suggesting that they are not the main mechanism of viral control. Neutralizing antibodies directed against the initial infecting quasispecies tend to persist for years, but do not evolve to subsequent variants, a possible factor in disease progression. Antibodies that inhibit syncytium formation

and antibodies that mediate antibody-dependent cellular cytotoxicity (ADCC) against virally infected cells also develop soon after infection. Their *in vivo* significance is unclear. Antibodies develop to all major HIV proteins, although with disease progression, antibodies to p24 tend to reduce in titre.

An appreciable CD8+ lymphocytosis occurs during primary HIV-1 infection, generally beginning in the

(a)

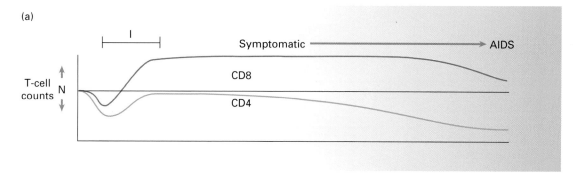

(b)

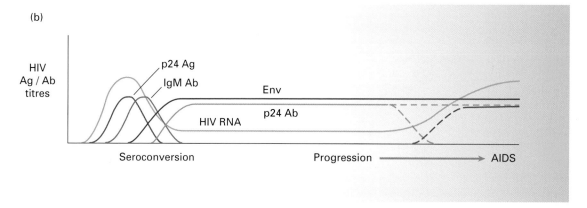

▌ **Fig. 3.3** Time course of serum HIV-specific p24 and gp 41 antibodies (IgM and IgG), p24 antigen, plasma viral load, CD4+ and CD8+ lymphocyte counts.

second week after onset of illness. Unlike the development of neutralizing antibodies, the increase in the number of CD8+ cells during primary HIV-1 infection occurs concomitant with resolution of clinical symptoms and a decrease in the detectable levels of serum p24 antigen, suggesting that the CD8+ cell response to primary HIV-1 infection has a part in controlling viral replication *in vivo* as it has been shown to have *in vitro*. These CD8+ cells represent HLA-restricted, HIV-specific cytotoxic T cells, and the HIV epitopes are gradually being characterized. Autologous CD8+ cells have been found to inhibit HIV replication *in vitro* by both cell–cell contact and by secretion of cytokines. However, it is possible that some cytotoxic T lymphocytes (CTLs) are detrimental to the host, as they could recognize and attack an uninfected cell presenting HIV antigens such as gp120 on its surface. Recently, it has been shown that restricted usage of T-cell receptor Vβ genes at the time of primary infection may correlate with a poor outcome as opposed to those subjects who generate a greater response using several Vβ genes. As HIV infection becomes chronic the CD8+ CTL response can become pauciclonal and directed towards a few immunodominant epitopes.

Variants of the dominant HIV epitopes expressed by quasi-species within the infected host can specifically antagonize recognition of the parental epitope thwarting the ability of HIV-specific CTL to control the infection.

Increased levels of IFNα, IL-1, IL-6, and TNFα have been detected in blood and cerebrospinal fluid (CSF) during primary HIV-1 infection and in more advanced disease, reflecting activation of the cellular immune system. High circulating levels of these cytokines may cause some of the clinical manifestations of HIV-1 infection (e.g. fevers, chills, myalgia, headache, fatigue, leucopenia, and weight loss). Such early rises in cytokine levels occur before the development of HIV-specific antibodies and before the rise in CD8+ cells, suggesting that it is a first line of defence against HIV-1 infection; the precise source of each of these cytokines is unclear.

The cytokine profile secreted by activated immune cells with progressive HIV disease may change. *In vitro*, T cells from patients with early stage disease may secrete a Th1 pattern of cytokines (i.e. IL-2, TNF, IFNγ), whereas those with more advanced disease secrete a Th2 profile of cytokines (i.e. IL-4, IL-5,

IL-10), although not all data support this hypothesis. This change may determine whether the primary response to HIV is cellular or antibody in nature. However, as cellular responses appear to be the more important, this Th1–Th2 switch may be detrimental to the patient; the reasons for such a switch are unclear.

Following initial clearance of circulating virus, there is a clinical state of symptomless infection during which HIV can often not be isolated from the circulation and which may last from only a few months to over 10 years. However, during this period of relative clinical latency, HIV accumulates and replicates in lymphoid tissue despite a low viral burden in peripheral blood. Because of its high replicative and mutative capacity, with time a multitude of quasi-species appears in a given individual. HIV appears to be retained within lymphoid tissue by follicular dendritic cells which may present HIV to local immune cells. Concurrently, there is a gradual reappearance of HIV in blood as well as in non-lymphoid tissue coupled with a reduced load in lymphoid tissue. Dissemination of HIV may be a result of the immune system failing to develop effective immunological responses to these new quasi-species of HIV, although the response to the initial infecting strain may be well preserved.

Recent research suggests that HIV undergoes rapid replication after the initial infection, and destroys many T cells but that it is met with a vigorous response by the immune system, and the viral load drops after the primary illness. However, over time the immune system often, but not always, fails to keep the virus under control, and HIV becomes ascendant in the struggle, the immune system fails, and full blown AIDS develops. Nowak and McMichael (1995) put forward the suggestion that the HIV virus continually evolves and in doing so produces such a plethora of new epitopes that the immune system loses its way and fails to keep up with the new targets. However if the initial immune response to conserved epitopes is strong the immune system defence will not be influenced by mutation in other epitopes, and the body should control the virus indefinitely. If the response is directed more to non-conserved epitopes the HIV levels should rise as there is the emergence of mutants that escape recognition and because of increased diversity of viral epitopes.

Pathogenesis of the immune deficiency

Infection with HIV produces a wide range of qualitative and quantitative immunological changes, including defects in T-cell, NK cell, monocyte, and B-cell function. Prominent among these changes are those that affect the CD4+ T lymphocyte. Normally, the CD4+ T cell provides regulatory factors that enhance the function of many other cell types. It is believed that many of the defects in function seen in HIV disease in these other cells are linked to changes in CD4+ T-lymphocyte number and function.

Effects on T lymphocytes

Depletion

There is a characteristic and progressive fall in the peripheral blood CD4+ T-cell number that closely parallels the clinical deterioration in patients with HIV infection. How HIV produces this effect remains unclear, although a number of mechanisms have been proposed. Which mechanism is most important *in vivo* remains unknown, although the loss of CD4+ T-cell numbers and function is likely to be multifactorial.

Recent studies have demonstrated that HIV has a very short plasma half-life (about 12–24 h), with greater than 10^9 virions being produced daily, even in those with asymptomatic disease and relatively well preserved immune function. Mathematical modelling suggests that most T cell turnover is the result of death soon after acute infection of T cells, and that relatively normal CD4+ T cells numbers are maintained by a correspondingly high rate of new T cell production.

HIV protein and DNA accumulation in the host cell cytoplasm may be directly cytopathic to CD4+ T cells. The budding of HIV from the cell surface has been proposed to disrupt cellular integrity, and an intracellular interaction between gp120 and CD4+ may occur, interfering with normal cellular metabolism. These studies have demonstrated a direct correlation between viral burden and depletion of CD4+ T cells, suggesting that indeed HIV may be directly involved in destruction of CD4+ T cells. In keeping with these data, HIV DNA has been found in 1–13.5% of CD4+ T cells in patients with AIDS versus 0.01–1% of CD4+ T cells in asymptomatic patients.

A second hypothesis states that infected CD4+ T cells which express gp120 on their cell surface may bind to uninfected CD4+ T cells via the interaction of gp120 with CD4+. Large syncytia can form rendering the targeted cells non-functional and susceptible to lysis. This phenomenon, although well documented *in vitro*, has not been clearly demonstrated *in vivo* except in brain. However, patients infected with an SI strain have a more rapid progression to AIDS and significantly shorter life expectancy than patients with non-SI (NSI) strains. Patients with SI strains appear to have minimal, if any, response to antiretroviral therapy with AZT. Although the frequency of SI phenotype increases as CD4+ cell count decline, perhaps only

∎ **Table 3.5**   Possible mechanisms of HIV-induced immunodeficiency

---

CD4+ T lymphocytes
  Directly cytopathic
  Intracellular interaction between gp120 and CD4
  Syncytium formation by cells expressing gp120 on their cell surface may
  Binding to uninfected CD4+ T cells
  Free gp120 may make CD4+ cells targets for antibody-dependent cellular cytotoxicity or cell-mediated
    cytotoxicity
  Superantigens expressed by HIV may lead to selective depletion of T cells bearing
  Specific T-cell receptor Vβ sequences at the thymic level
  Induction of apoptosis by stimulation by antigens
  Impaired IL-2 production
  Impaired antigen and mitogen responses
  Altered surface expression of IL-2R, T-cell receptor and CD4
  gp120 or gp41 can impair binding of CD4 to MHC II
  Glutathione deficiency resulting in unopposed tumour necrosis factor activation of HIV replication

Macrophages
  Reduced chemotaxis
  Reduced monocyte-dependent CD4 T-cell proliferation
  Reduced Fc receptor function
  Reduced C3-mediated immune complex clearance
  Reduced MHC II expression leads to reduced antigen presentation
  Impaired antigen presentation
  Reduced intracellular killing

CD8+ lymphocytes
  Reduced IL-2, IL-2R, and IFNγ production
  Reduced cytotoxic activity

Natural killer cells
  Reduced cytokine production
  Reduced cytotoxic activity

B lymphocytes
  Polyclonal activation by HIV (via follicular dendritic cells), Epstein–Barr virus, and cytomegalovirus
  Increased IgG1, IgG3, IgA, and IgE
  Reduced IgG2 and IgG4
  Reduced neoantigen responses

Other
  Infection of bone marrow precursors
  Infection of thymocyte precursors

MHC, major histocompatibility complex

50% of patients with CD4+ cell counts less than 50/μl have an SI virus. Once an SI strain develops, NSI strains have not been shown to re-emerge.

Autoimmune phenomena could also be responsible for CD4+ T-lymphocyte depletion. Free gp120 may bind to CD4+ T lymphocytes making such cells targets for ADCC or cell-mediated cytotoxicity after processing and presentation of viral protein. HIV infection of CD4+ thymocytes could contribute to CD+ T-cell depletion by preventing replenishment of the CD4+ T cells. HIV preferentially infects memory CD4+ T cells and could selectively deplete these cells which mediate recall antigen responses.

Putative superantigens that might be expressed by HIV have been implicated in T-lymphocyte depletion at the thymic level, as selective depletion of T cells bearing specific T-cell receptor Vβ sequences has been found, by some but not all investigators. In addition, cells bearing such sequences have been found to be more susceptible to productive HIV infection. Lastly, stimulation of CD4+ T cells by mitogens and super-antigens from asymptomatic HIV-infected individuals results in rapid apoptosis of these cells, a phenomenon that may be dependent upon interactions between the CD28 receptor on T cells and its B7 (CD80) ligand on HIV-infected dendritic cells, and be accelerated by the HIV-associated IL-2 deficiency.

Dysfunction

CD4+ T-cell dysfunction, as well as depletion, contributes to the immune deficit. CD4+ T cells from HIV-infected patients are defective in their ability to proliferate in response to soluble antigen and to induce immunoglobulin production from B cells, although their responses to mitogens are relatively preserved and decline later in disease. IL-2 production has been shown to be defective in both antigen- and mitogen-stimulated CD4+ T cells. IL-2 has some homology with gp120; it is possible that an interaction between gp120 and the IL-2 receptor (IL-2R) may interfere with IL-2 action. Defects in major histocompatibility complex (MHC) class I-restricted cytotoxicity have also been demonstrated which are reversible with the addition of IL-2, reinforcing the suggestion that defects in the function of CD4+ T cells may partially explain changes in the function of other cell types. HIV infection also alters the expression of a number of important CD4+ T-cell surface molecules, including the IL-2R, the T-cell antigen receptor and CD4+. Exposure of CD4+ T cells to HIV proteins such as gp120 or gp41 can impair binding of CD4+ to its physiological ligand (the constant region of MHC II molecules), disrupting antigen-presenting cell/T-cell interactions and potentially disturbing post-receptor signal transduction pathways. The selective infection of memory CD4+ lymphocytes may also explain the reduced responses of CD4+ T cells to soluble antigen seen well before CD4+ T-cell numbers are depleted.

Following primary infection, there is a characteristic CD8+ lymphocytosis that persists until very late-stage disease; some of these CD8+ cells are HIV-specific cytotoxic T cells as well as non-specific NK cells. This response is thought to be responsible, at least in part, for suppression of HIV replication, resulting in resolution of primary infection and maintenance of the asymptomatic phase. The late-stage decline in CD8+ cell numbers suggests that CD4+ lymphocytes have a part in maintenance of CD8+ cell numbers and function, perhaps via secretion of IL-2 and other cytokines.

Lastly, it has been found that plasma and leucocyte levels of glutathione are decreased in some patients with both asymptomatic and moderately advanced HIV disease. Glutathione and *N*-acetyl cysteine (used for synthesis of glutathione) inhibit the *in vitro* expression of HIV in acutely and chronically infected CD4+ lymphocytes and monocytes by downregulation of NF-κB and inhibition of TNFα. Glutathione also enhances lymphocyte activation and proliferation by mitogens. Consequently, glutathione has been suggested as an immunomodulatory agent in the treatment of HIV disease. The cause of this glutathione deficiency is unknown, but has been hypothesized to be a depletion arising from chronic inhibition of TNFα induced by HIV.

Effects on monocyte/macrophage lineage cells

In contrast to infection of CD4+ T cells, HIV infection of cells of the monocyte/macrophage lineage does not result in significant cell death. Rather, persistent infection with the potential for sustained viral production is the rule. Also, there is variation in the tropism of HIV isolates, with some showing greater tropism for monocytes/macrophages than for CD4+ T cells. Thus, monocyte–macrophage lineage cells may act as an important reservoir of HIV.

Some functions of monocyte/macrophage lineage cells, such as superoxide anion release, intracellular antimicrobicidal activity and response to IFNγ, are unaltered by HIV infection. Infection of these cells, however, has a number of important functional consequences, including reductions in monocyte chemotaxis, monocyte-dependent CD4+ T-cell proliferation, Fc receptor function, and C3-mediated immune complex clearance. In addition, HIV infection causes a decline in the accessory cell function of monocyte cell lines, perhaps due to a reduction in MHC class II antigen expression on infected cells, although this finding has been disputed.

Production of cytokines, monokines, and their receptors is significantly altered in HIV-infected patients. *In vitro*, the expression of transforming growth factor β, IL-1, IL-6, IL-2R, IFNα, TNFα and IL-1β are increased in monocyte/macrophage lineage cells. Increased serum IFNα, IFNγ, TNFα, and TNFβ levels probably reflect macrophage and CD8+ T-cell production of these factors. Such changes may contribute to cachexia, constitutional symptoms, and bone marrow impairment, as well as activate HIV replication in infected cells. They may also contribute to the B-cell changes discussed below.

Effects on B lymphocytes

Polyclonal B-cell activation is characteristic of HIV infection and is marked by hyperimmunoglobulinaemia and persistent generalized lymphadenopathy. The immunoglobulin may show restricted mobility on routine electrophoresis, suggesting a limited idiotypic specificity. Much of the immunoglobulin is directed against HIV epitopes, although neutralizing antibody to HIV is frequently not produced. The immunoglobulin is mainly IgG and IgA, with IgG1 the dominant subtype. Some patients with advanced HIV disease have elevation of total serum IgE which has been postulated to be due to various microbial antigens, including HIV itself, as well as to relative IFNγ deficiency. Serum IgA and IgE levels have been found to have prognostic significance, although it is not known whether either has value above and beyond more established prognostic markers such as serum p24 antigen, neopterin, β_2-microglobulin, and SI phenotype (see below). Nodal and peripheral blood B cells from HIV-infected patients spontaneously produce immunoglobulin and express surface activation markers, implying they are in an activated state. Despite this substantial immunoglobulin production, antigen-specific responses are impaired and antibody production distorted, as typified by the diminished responses to vaccination against hepatitis B, *Streptococcus pneumoniae*, and *Haemophilus influenzae*. Lastly, abnormal antibody production can result in thrombocytopenic purpura, haemolytic anaemia, and systemic vasculitis, perhaps a result of immune complex deposition.

How HIV infection produces these B-cell changes is unclear, although peripheral blood and nodal B cells do not appear to harbour HIV. However, nodal follicular dendritic cells contain large amounts of HIV, and may be responsible for ongoing B cell activation. Direct B-cell stimulation by HIV proteins has been clearly demonstrated *in vitro*. The *tat* gene product can be taken up by B cells, leading to transactivation of the cell and immunoglobulin production. However, B-cell activation and immunoglobulin production often subside in late AIDS, despite an abundance of viral proteins. This has suggested that a cytokine-driven B-cell proliferation occurs in response to HIV antigens. Freshly isolated peripheral blood and nodal B cells spontaneously proliferate and produce immunoglobulin and this phenomenon is IL-6 dependent, as it is blocked by anti-IL-6 antibodies. IL-6 levels are known to be elevated in HIV-infected patients; the IL-6 probably derives from monocyte/macrophage lineage and endothelial cells. IL-1 and TNFα can promote B-cell proliferation and the serum levels of these cytokines are elevated in HIV-infected patients, mainly in those with advanced disease. The production of such 'helper' cytokines by B cells, endothelial cells, and monocyte/macrophage

lineage cells may allow for the persistence of B-cell activation despite the severe effects of HIV on CD4+ T-cell number and helper function. Indeed, the antibody secretion of B cells isolated from PGL nodes is diminished by monocyte, but not CD4+ T-cell removal *in vitro*. It is only as the CD4+ T-cell defect becomes extreme that B-cell proliferation declines and the lymphadenopathy involutes.

B-cell activation is also driven by EBV, a virus often associated with polyclonal B-cell activation. The EBV genome has been demonstrated in the benign and malignant B-cell proliferations of transplant recipients, of patients with hereditary B- and T-cell deficiencies and of those with HIV disease. EBV has almost universal prevalence, potential immunosuppressive effects, lymphotropism, and transforming capacity, making it a good candidate for the polyclonal B-cell activation seen in HIV-infected patients. Immune regulation of EBV infection is inadequate in HIV-infected patients, as demonstrated by the increased number of B cells that harbour EBV and the defective regulation of EBV-transformed B cells by CD8+ T cells isolated from HIV-infected patients.

CMV infection also is extremely prevalent in patients with HIV disease. As with EBV, CMV infection has been associated with B-cell activation (although CMV does not infect B cells), and regulation of latent CMV infection is impaired in HIV-infected subjects. Patients who are seropositive for CMV have a more rapid progression to AIDS than seronegative subjects, and this progression is independent of CD4+ cell count. CMV may accelerate HIV disease by increasing the secretion of cytokines by immune cells, and/or by the induction of Fc receptors on cells which become more susceptible to HIV infection.

Diagnosis

The diagnosis of HIV disease is a serological one and is made by the detection of HIV-specific IgG in peripheral blood by enzyme-linked immunosorbent assay (ELISA). Current available ELISAs are highly sensitive and are in fact designed for maximum sensitivity at the expense, to a small degree, of specificity, it being more acceptable for such assays to generate false positive than false negative results. More rapid agglutination assays which do not require laboratories or highly skilled technicians have also been developed, mostly for use in developing countries.

A positive HIV antibody result in isolation is not diagnostic of HIV infection. Immunoblotting, detection of viral DNA, or viral isolation is required to distinguish biological false positives from true infection. Immunoblotting identifies various banding patterns,

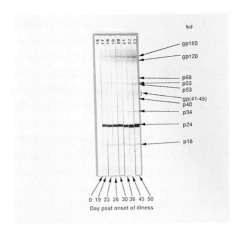

▌Fig. 3.4 Immunoblots of HIV infected patient seroconverting

which have distinct clinical significance. There are no universally accepted consensus criteria for diagnosis of HIV infection by immunoblotting. However, the simultaneous presence of a glycoprotein band and several non-glycoprotein bands is virtually diagnostic of HIV infection. Rarely, a glycoprotein band in the absence of other bands may represent a false positive, but this pattern is more commonly seen in HIV seroconversion or in late-stage disease. A p24 band in isolation either represents a biological false positive or early seroconversion. Biological false positives are more common in multiparous women and intravenous drug users, although the causes for these false positives, which are often transient, are not known. These entities may, of course, be distinguished on clinical grounds, the results of T-cell subset enumeration, presence of serum p24 antigen, and occasionally by virus isolation or detection of HIV-specific DNA.

Serum p24 antigen is especially of diagnostic value in the setting of HIV-1 seroconversion and is often positive when antibody results are negative or indeterminate. However, p24 antigenaemia is transient in seroconversion and so a negative result does not exclude the diagnosis. Assaying for HIV-specific IgM alone is rarely performed because of problems with both sensitivity (IgM is only present for about 3 months after seroconversion) and specificity and has been superseded by more sensitive IgG-based assays.

The polymerase chain reaction (PCR) has been used to detect HIV-specific sequences. There was suggestion from some studies that PCR positivity might proceed detection of specific IgG by months or even years (so-called seronegative HIV infection), but more recent work has suggested this is rarely if ever the case. PCR-based assays may be of benefit in the

setting of seroconversion or the presence of indeterminate serology and/or immunoblotting. They remain a research assay only at this stage, although commercial diagnostic assays are in the late stages of development.

A negative antibody result does not exclude HIV infection, particularly if seroconversion is suspected. In this setting, serology and immunoblotting should be repeated at regular and frequent intervals.

HIV quantitation

Until recently, the only assay which gave information regarding the amount of viral burden in an individual was the HIV-1 p24 antigen assay. This assay, like all other blood-based assays, only gives information on the amount of circulating virus and not on virus resident within tissues. Nevertheless, there is a good correlation between the level of p24 antigenaemia and circulating viral burden as measured by more sensitive assays. Immune complex dissociation pretreatment of serum increases the sensitivity of p24 assays, which can as a result measure both free p24 antigen and p24 antigen conjugated to circulating p24 antibodies.

Molecular biology has been applied to HIV RNA quantitation using both quantitative PCR and branch-chain DNA-based assays, each with an assay range of about 500–1 000 000 copies/ml plasma. The level of RNA correlates strongly with prognosis, and is a marker for disease progression independent of the CD4+ T cell count. Changes in RNA levels of greater than 0.5 log are likely to be clinically relevant in terms of progression or in response to anti-retroviral therapy.

Quantitative plasma and intracellular viraemia assays have also been developed using cocultivation, with HIV-uninfected PBMC, but these are expensive, time-consuming, not standardized, and to date are performed by few laboratories.

Surrogate markers

Because of the great variation in latency of HIV infection, it is important to have markers that identify individuals at greatest risk of disease progression. The most useful such surrogate marker is the CD4+ lymphocyte count and in particular trends in CD4+ cell counts over time. Patients with CD4+ lymphocyte counts less than 500/μl (i.e. below the generally accepted lower limit of normal) are at increased risk of progression to AIDS. Once the CD4+ count falls below 200/μl, there is a greatly increased risk of opportunistic infections, neurological disease, and malignancy. The CD4+ cell count is best performed at regular intervals to guide decisions such as initiation or changes to antiretroviral therapy. However, other variables such as intercurrent illness and diurnal variation

	IMMUNE DEPLETION:	EARLY (CD4 > 500)	INTERMEDIATE (500>CD4>200)	ADVANCED (CD4<200)
General	Fever, pharyngitis, lymphadenopathy arthralgia			
Skin	Erythematous macular rash, urticaria, desquamation	Tinea, Seborrhoeic dermatitis	Molluscum contagiosum, herpes zoster, oral candida, Kaposi's sarcoma, warts	Kaposi's sarcoma
CNS	Headache, meningoencephalitis., Guillain–Barré	Acute or chronic demyelinating neuropathy Polymyositis Bells palsy		AIDS dementia, CNS Lymphoma, Neuropathy
GI	Mucocutaneous ulcer, candidiasis, diarrhoea	Sjögrens syndrome, Bacterial gastroenteritis, Oral hairy leucoplakia	Gastrointestinal candidiasis, non-Hodgkin's lymphoma	Oesphageal candidiasis, persistent HSV, cryptosporidiosis, CMV enteritis
Eye		Reiters Sicca syndrome	HIV microvasculopathy, HSV keratitis, Optic neuritis	CMV retinitis (<200), Toxoplasmosis
Infection			Tuberculosis (200–400), candida *Pneumocystis carinii* (<200)	Toxoplasmosis, cryptosporidiosis, cryptococcus (<100) CMV *Mycobacterium avium* (<50)
Haema-tology	'Atypical lymphocytes'	Persistent generalized lymphadenopathy	Lymphoma	Thrombocytopenia Anaemia

10 WEEKS   5 YEARS   10 YEARS

∎ **Fig. 3.5** CD4+ lymphocyte counts in relation to HIV clinical conditions. CMV, cytomegalovirus; HSV, herpes simplex virus.

▌ **Table 3.6**   Surrogate markers and prognostic variables of HIV disease

Surrogate markers
  CD4+ lymphocyte count
  CD4 percentage
  HIV RNA Load
  β_2-microglobulin
  Neopterin
  Viral phenotype (i.e. synctium-inducing or non-synctium-inducing strain of HIV)
  Delayed-type hypersensitivity (DTH) skin testing
  High-grade zidovudine resistance
  p24 antigenaemia

Adverse prognostic variables
  Coinfection with cytomegalovirus, mycoplasma, and HHV-6
  Infants and the elderly
  Various human leucocyte antigen haplotypes
  Primary HIV infection
    illness lasting longer than 14 days
    acquisition of HIV from an index case with late-stage HIV-1 disease
    infection with SI viral strain
    low p24 antibody titres
    high gp120 antibody titres
    higher HIV RNA load after resolution of illness (i.e. high 'set point')
    level of total plasma IgM before the appearance of specific antibodies
    presence of specific anti-HIV-1 IgM and IgA after infection
    immunodeficiency at time of infection

may cause fluctuations in CD4+ cell counts; therefore, changes in CD4+ counts should be confirmed if alteration to clinical management is possible. The CD4+ percentage may be a more reliable marker as it demonstrates less intrinsic fluctuation over time.

Other surrogate markers which have independent prognostic value include levels of serum β_2-microglobulin and neopterin, viral phenotype (i.e. the presence of SI or NSI strain of HIV), delayed-type hypersensitivity (DTH) skin testing, and lastly the presence of high-grade zidovudine resistance. β_2-microglobulin is the invariant component non-covalently associated with cell surface MHC I proteins. Neopterin is a metabolic end-product of the synthesis of guanosine triphosphate (GTP). Increased levels of β_2-microglobulin and neopterin represent increased cellular activation and turnover. Patients who are anergic to recall antigens on DTH testing are also at increased risk of disease progression, although the sensitivity and specificity of DTH testing depend in part on the prevalence of antigen exposure in the patient population. Therefore, DTH test results are best compared with previous results of a given patient. SI strains of HIV are detected by their ability *in vitro* to cause syncytia of target cells (usually the MT-2 T cell line) in culture. Switching in an individual from a NSI to an SI phenotype usually precedes a rapid decline in CD4+ cell count and a poor subsequent response to therapy. AZT resistance is discussed below. Serum p24 antigenaemia has not been shown to have independent prognostic value in all populations, although it remains a valuable tool for evaluating therapy and disease progression especially in later stage disease. Of the above markers, the CD4+ lymphocyte count, p24 antigen, β_2-microglobulin, and neopterin are all in clinical use and a combination of two or three of these variables is commonly used for monitoring patient disease progress.

There is now increasing evidence that the quantity of HIV RNA in plasma correlates with prognosis, although it is not clear whether this will supplant the CD4+ count as the best single surrogate marker.

Prognostic variables

Apart from the above-mentioned surrogate markers, other clinical and laboratory variables also have prognostic significance. Coinfection with organisms such as CMV, mycoplasma, and HHV-6 may be associated with accelerated HIV disease progression. There does not appear to be a great variation in disease progression between various adult risk groups who are infected with HIV. Nevertheless, both infants and the elderly infected with HIV have a more rapid disease progression which may be dependent upon their less evolved or preserved immune responses. Similarly, various HLA haplotypes have been associated with rapid progression including the common Caucasian haplotype HLA B8 DR3 DQ2. It is not clear, however, whether this association is due to the various HLA types themselves or to other linked inherited genes such as various alleles of TNF.

Variables at the time of primary infection may be useful in predicting the subsequent course of disease. Symptomatic primary HIV-1 infection (versus 'asymptomatic' seroconversion), a primary illness lasting longer than 14 days, acquisition of HIV from an index case with late-stage HIV-1 disease, infection with SI viral strains at seroconversion, low p24 antibody titres and high gp120 antibody titres at seroconversion, higher quantities of infecting virus, the level of total plasma IgM before the appearance of specific antibodies, and the presence of specific anti-HIV-1 IgM and IgA after infection have all been found to predict rapid disease progression. Persisting low CD4+ counts or p24 antigenaemia are also indicate a relatively poor prognosis.

Clinical manifestations of HIV disease

Primary HIV infection

An acute clinical illness associated with HIV-1 seroconversion occurs in about 50–90% of cases. The time from exposure to HIV-1 to the onset of this illness is typically 2–4 weeks, although incubation periods range from 6 days to 6 weeks. The illness has a median duration of 2 weeks. The illness can be associated with an appreciable degree of morbidity, and patients may require hospitalization. Most clinical manifestations of primary HIV-1 infection are self-limited, although in a few cases mild to moderate symptoms may persist.

The main clinical symptoms and signs of primary HIV-1 infection are fever (97%), night sweats, fatigue, generalized lymphadenopathy (77%), pharyngitis (73%), rash (70%), and myalgia or arthralgia (58%). Lymphadenopathy may persist after the acute illness but tends to decrease with time.

The most common dermatological feature is an erythematous, non-pruritic, maculopapular rash (Fig. 3.6a). This rash is generally symmetric, with lesions 5–10 mm in diameter, and affects the face or trunk, but it can also affect the extremities, including the palms and soles, or can be generalized. Desquamation and alopecia typically occur in the second month following onset of primary HIV-1 infection, after resolution of

❚ **Table 3.7** Clinical manifestations of primary HIV-1 infection

General
Fever
Pharyngitis
Lymphadenopathy
Arthralgia/myalgia
Lethargy/malaise
Anorexia/weight loss

Neuropathic
Headache/retro-orbital pain
Meningoencephalitis
Peripheral neuropathy
Radiculopathy
Brachial neuritis
Guillain–Barré syndrome
Cognitive/affective impairment

Dermatological
Erythematous maculopapular rash
Roseola-like rash
Diffuse urticaria
Desquamation
Alopecia
Mucocutaneous ulceration

Gastrointestinal
Oral/oropharyngeal candidiasis
Nausea/vomiting
Diarrhoea

Respiratory
Cough

other symptoms. Mucocutaneous ulceration may involve the buccal mucosa, gingiva, palate, oesophagus, anus, and penis.

Although described in the CDC classification of HIV disease as a 'mononucleosis-like' syndrome, primary HIV infection clearly differs from primary EBV infection by its acute onset and the prominence of rash, non-suppurative pharyngitis, and diarrhoea.

Asymptomatic primary infection may also occur. It is not clear what factors influence the development or lack of symptoms during primary infection. Possible viral factors include the inoculum, tropism, or virulence of the infecting HIV strain. Symptomatic primary infection appears more common in those infected by persons with late-stage disease than those infected by persons at an earlier disease stage.

Following an initial and transient lymphopenia, during which the level of CD4+ cells may be as low as

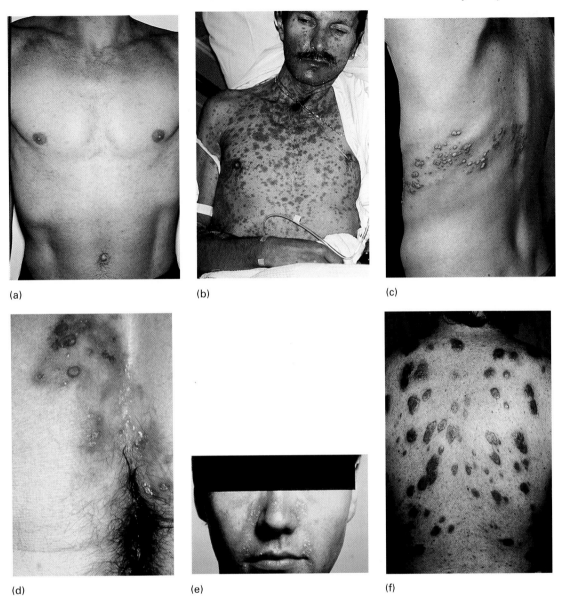

▮ **Fig. 3.6** Cutaneous manifestations of HIV infection: (a) rash of primary HIV infection; (b) morbilliform rash of drug hypersensitivity; (c) herpes zoster; (d) peri-anal herpes simplex type 2; (e) seborrhoeic dermatitis; (f) Kaposi's sarcoma.

that of patients with advanced HIV-1 disease, a CD8+ lymphocytosis develops, generally in the second to third week of infection. The most marked increase in CD8+ cells is observed in those with the most pronounced clinical signs of primary infection. Atypical lymphocytosis is detected in less than 50% of patients and may be profound. Severe lymphocytic hyporesponsiveness to both mitogens and antigens and

impairment of B-cell function occurs and persists after resolution of the acute illness.

Specific HIV-1 antibodies are usually detectable within the first few weeks of onset of the acute illness. IgM antibodies are followed by HIV-specific IgG usually 2–6 weeks after the onset of illness. Immunoblotting usually first detects antibody to p24, p55, gp41, or gp120. Assay for serum p24 antigen is important as p24 antigen can be detected before *gag* and *env* seroconversion and has been detected in serum as early as 24 h after the onset of acute illness. The level of p24 antigen typically decreases as viral burden decreases and p24 antibodies develop.

There is preliminary evidence that prophylactic zidovudine manotherapy will prevent primary HIV-1 infection reducing the risk of occupational HIV transmission fivefold. However, cases have been reported in which AZT clearly failed to prevent HIV-1 infection even when administered within 1 h following inoculation. Antiretroviral intervention could also lessen the initial viral load and subsequently improve long-term prognosis. Primary infection with AZT-resistant HIV-1 has now been reported; the presence of a AZT-resistant isolate in a seroconvertor would make other antiretroviral drugs attractive.

Constitutional disease

Following primary infection, there is an asymptomatic phase during which there may be fluctuating degrees of generalized lymphadenopathy, although this gradually declines with time. Numerous illnesses related to progressive immunodeficiency may occur during this time, and include recurrent herpes zoster, oropharyngeal candidiasis, and oral hairy leucoplakia (Figs 3.5 and 3.7) and thrombocytopenia. Non-specific features are common and include persistent fevers, unexplained weight loss, and fatigue. The mechanisms of these latter manifestation are unclear, although the peripheral blood viral load appears directly related to the frequency and severity of these symptoms.

Infections

Pneumocystis carinii pneumonia (PCP)

P. carinii was long considered a parasite because of its microscopic appearance but recent RNA studies have suggested that it may be a fungus. It has a life cycle of three stages, namely cysts, sporozoites (smaller bodies found within cysts), and trophozoites (extracystic, possibly intermediate forms). *P. carinii* has not being cultured *in vitro* which has hampered efforts to identify subtypes, in particular drug-resistant variants and variants of high pathogenicity.

In industrialized nations there is a high seroprevalence to *P. carinii* approaching 95% by the age of 5 years. In Africa the rate of seroprevalence appears to be substantially lower. Therefore, PCP appears to be a reactivated latent infection and, as for most opportunistic infections in AIDS, reactivation is most dependent upon depletion of CD4+ lymphocytes, although CD8+ lymphocytes and specific antibodies also appear to play a part. The risk of PCP increases substantially

in patients with a CD4+ cell count less than $200/\mu l$ or a CD4+ per cent less than 20%. Primary PCP developed within 6 months in 0.5% of those with a CD4+ count between 200 and $350/\mu l$ versus 8.4% within 6 months if the CD4+ count was less than $200/\mu l$. Because PCP tends to occur at higher CD4+ cell counts than other major opportunistic infections, it remains the most common AIDS-defining condition in industrialized nations.

The cardinal symptoms of PCP are fever, nonproductive cough, and dyspnoea. The onset tends to be more gradual than in HIV-uninfected patients with immunosuppression. These features may be particularly subtle or slow in onset in those who are receiving PCP prophylaxis, especially with aerosolized pentamidine. Auscultation of the chest is often unremarkable, but fine crepitations may be heard. Chest radiography typically demonstrates bilateral, interstitial infiltrates (Fig. 3.7a), although mass lesions, lobar consolidation, or pneumothorax may occur. Pleural effusion is rare. In patients receiving aerosolized pentamidine, the infiltrates may be confined to the upper lobes. This may be due to reduced deposition of pentamidine in the upper lobes due to their relatively reduced ventilation as compared with the lower lobes.

Diagnosis of PCP is made definitively by demonstration of *P. carinii* in sputum or lung tissue. Sputum is induced by inhalation of a 3% saline solution and best stained with methenamine silver, toluidine blue, and fluoresceinated monoclonal antibody stains for detection. Use of PCP prophylaxis reduces the sensitivity of sputum induction. For those patients with a negative-induced sputum result, bronchoalveolar lavage with transbronchial biopsy increases the sensitivity, although the latter carries the risk of pneumothorax. The use of PCR-based diagnostic methods may further increase the sensitivity.

Extrapulmonary pneumocystosis has been documented in the skin, external auditory canal, lymph nodes, heart, pleural space, liver, spleen, meninges, eye, and intestine. Such episodes appear to occur mainly in those who are receiving either no PCP prophylaxis or aerosolized pentamidine. Diagnosis requires histological identification of *P. carinii*.

Therapy consists of at least 21 days therapy with either trimethoprim–sulphamethoxazole (TMP-SMX) or intravenous pentamidine; pentamidine and TMP act by inhibition of dihydrofolate reductase and SMX by inhibition of dihydropteroate synthetase.

For patients with arterial oxygen less than 70 mmHg, a 3 week course of corticosteroid therapy is added to the regimen at the commencement of antimicrobial therapy, as this reduces morbidity, hospital stay, and mortality. Early in the HIV epidemic, mortal-

∎ **Table 3.8**   CDC classification of AIDS indicator diseases (1993 revision)

Category A
 Asymptomatic: no symptoms at the time of HIV infection
 Acute Infection: see Table 3.7
 Persistent generalized lymphadenopathy: lymph node enlargement persisting for 3 or months with no evidence of infection

Category B
 Bacillary angiomatosis
 Candidiasis, oropharyngeal (thrush)
 Candidiasis, vulvovaginal; persistent, frequent, or poorly responsive to therapy
 Cervical dysplasia (moderate or severe)/cervical carcinoma *in situ*
 Constitutional symptoms, such as fever (38.5) or diarrhoea lasting >1 month
 Hairy leucoplakia, oral
 Herpes zoster (shingles) involving at least two distinct episodes, or more than one dermatome
 Idiopathic thrombocytopenic purpura
 Listeriosis
 Pelvic inflammatory disease, particularly if complicated by tubo-ovarian abscess
 Peripheral neuropathy

Category C
 Candidiasis of bronchi, trachea, or lungs
 Candidiasis, oesophageal
 Cervical cancer, invasive[a]
 Coccidioidomycosis, disseminated or extrapulmonary
 Cryptococcosis, extra-pulmonary
 Cryptosporidiosis, chronic intestinal (>1 month's duration)
 Cytomegalovirus disease (other than liver, spleen, or nodes)
 Cytomegalovirus retinitis (with loss of vision)
 Encephalopathy, HIV-related
 Herpes simplex: chronic ulcer(s) (>1 month's duration); or bronchitis, pneumonitis, or oesophagitis
 Histoplasmosis, disseminated or extrapulmonary
 Isosporiasis, chronic intestinal (>1 month's duration)
 Kaposi's sarcoma
 Lymphoma, Burkitt's (or equivalent term)
 Lymphoma, immunoblastic (or equivalent term)
 Lymphoma, primary, of brain
 Mycobacterium avium complex or *M. kansasii*, disseminated or extrapulmonary
 Mycobacterium tuberculosis, any site (pulmonary[*] or extra-pulmonary)
 Mycobacterium, other species or unidentified species, disseminated or extrapulmonary
 Pneumocystis carinii pneumonia
 Pneumonia, recurrent[a] (≥ 2 episodes in 1 year)
 Progressive multifocal leukoencephalopathy
 Salmonella septicaemia, recurrent
 Toxoplasmosis of brain
 Wasting syndrome due to HIV

[a]added to revised definition 1993

ity rates as high as 25% per episode were reported, although with improved therapy mortality is now 5–8%.

PCP prophylaxis is indicated for all HIV-infected patients who have not had PCP and who have an absolute CD4+ lymphocyte count less than 200/μl (or CD4+ percentage less than 20%) and for all patients with prior PCP, regardless of CD4+ cell count. Low-dose TMP-SMX is the most effective form. Aerosolized or intravenous pentamidine or dapsone +/– pyrimethamine or TMP are alternatives for intolerant patients.

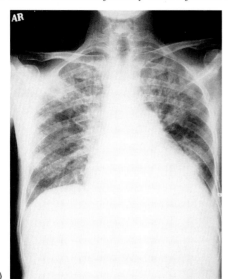

(a)

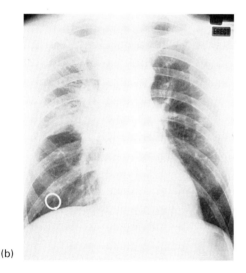

(b)

■ **Fig. 3.7** Chest radiographs: (a) *Pneumocystis carinii* pneumonia (diffuse, bilateral pulmonary interstitial infiltrates); (b) tuberculosis (right upper lobe infiltrate with hilar lymphadenopathy).

Toxoplasmosis

Toxoplasmosis in HIV-infected patients is a reactivated latent infection with *Toxoplasma gondii*, an obligate intracellular protozoan found principally in the cat, although livestock and humans may be an incidental host. Seroprevalence for *T. gondii* is greatest in central Europe and sub-Saharan Africa where consumption of less well cooked meat or less purified water is commonplace. Worldwide, the rate of seroprevalence varies between 8 and 90%.

Most cases of infection result in focal encephalitis, the principal features of which are fever, headache, altered mental state, focal neurological deficit, and seizures. Forty to 50% of patients will have residual neurological impairment and up to 15% of patients die from toxoplasmosis. Infection less commonly involves the retina, lung, heart, and rarely the gut.

Diagnosis of toxoplasmic encephalitis is made definitively by identification of *T. gondii* by light microscopy of infected brain tissue. As brain biopsy is not widely available, however, the diagnosis is made presumptively by appropriate clinical and radiological features in the presence of *T. gondii*-specific IgG in the blood (greater than 97% of patients). Computerized tomography (CT) classically shows multiple space-occupying lesions in the basal ganglia and corticomedullary junctions, often with surrounding oedema (Fig. 3.8a). However, none of these diagnostic features is completely sensitive or specific for the diagnosis. In particular, cerebral lymphoma may have similar findings. Magnetic resonance imaging (MRI) may be more sensitive than CT scanning, but a greater specificity has not been demonstrated. Other less well defined diagnostic techniques include isolation of *T. gondii* from blood or of *T. gondii*-specific DNA from CSF using PCR. Given the above, a response to at least 14 days antimicrobial therapy is also a presumptive diagnostic criterion.

The most important antimicrobial therapy is pyrimethamine, an inhibitor of dihydrofolate reductase in combination with sulphadiazine or clindamycin. Other agents with less well defined efficacy include atovaquone, azithromycin, clarithromycin, dapsone as well as tetracyclines, and TMP-SMX. IFNγ has activity against *T. gondii in vitro* and is being studied in humans.

Lifelong secondary prophylaxis with pyrimethamine and either sulphadiazine or clindamycin is mandatory to prevent relapse. Primary prophylaxis is being increasingly adopted, given the morbidity and mortality due to toxoplasmosis and the fact that patients seropositive for *T. gondii* have a 30–50% risk of developing toxoplasmosis over time.

Cytomegalovirus infection

Most patients with HIV have latent CMV infection with a prevalence of almost 100% in homosexual men. CMV viremia and viruria is common at all stages of infection, although neither appear to be predict the risk of CMV disease. In contrast, CMV–DNA levels in the blood may be predictive for disease onset. CMV disease is a common manifestation of late-stage HIV infection, usually in patients with CD4+ cell counts less than 50/μl, and characteristically affects the

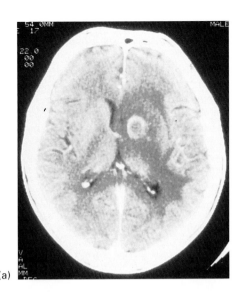

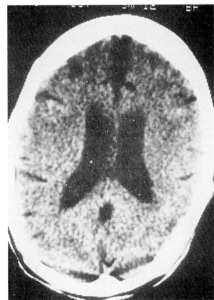

(a)

(b)

▌ **Fig. 3.8** Computerized tomography: (a) cerebral toxoplasmosis (contrast-enhancing lesion in right basal ganglia with surrounding oedema and mass effect); (b) AIDS dementia complex (loss of white matter with dilatation of ventricles and sulci; no focal lesion).

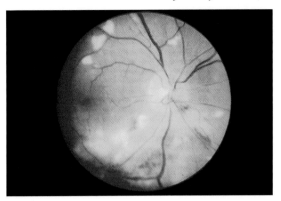

▌ **Fig. 3.9** Cytomegalovirus retinitis (superior retina) with cotton wool spots (inferior retina).

retina, the gastrointestinal tract, and the nervous system.

Cytomegalovirus retinitis

The pathogenesis of CMV retinitis is unclear as it is a rare finding in other immunocompromised patients with CMV infection. It may be a sequelae of HIV-induced microvascular damage to the eye with subsequent seeding of the retina by circulating CMV.

CMV retinitis has a subacute or acute onset of blurred vision and visual floaters. More profound losses are associated with secondary retinal detachment. The degree of symptoms is dependent upon the site of infection, with even mild macular involvement or retinal detachment resulting in substantial symptoms. Fundoscopy demonstrates exudates, increased vascularity, and haemorrhage (Fig. 3.9). There may be associated vitreal inflammation or retinal detachment. Disease is bilateral in about 25% of patients.

Therapy is in the form of intravenous ganciclovir or foscarnet. Induction therapy with either drug should be for 2–3 weeks. Each drug appears to have similar efficacy, although foscarnet may be associated with greater patient survival, perhaps on account of its anti-HIV activity. Nevertheless, ganciclovir is usually the drug of first choice because it does not require central venous access with concomitant risks of line infection. Ganciclovir may cause cytopenias and zidovudine therapy is usually contra-indicated in patients receiving ganciclovir. Apart from the risk of catheter infection, foscarnet may also induce interstitial nephropathy with secondary hypocalcaemia and hypomagnesaemia; haematological toxicity is uncommon. Penile ulceration may develop, which is probably due to direct local toxicity of foscarnet in the urine. Intravitreal ganciclovir and foscarnet are useful for subjects who are intolerant of or appear to be failing intravenous therapy, as the local concentrations achieved of either drug is greater than with intravenous administration.

Indefinite secondary CMV prophylaxis is essential. Despite this, the average time to relapse on either drug is approximately 2–3 months, whereupon reinduction and secondary prophylaxis with the alternate agent is usually required. Oral ganciclovir is slightly less effective as secondary prophylaxis but it allows for out-patient therapy and causes less haematological toxicity. Sodofavir is a nucleoside analogue being developed for treatment of CMV disease; although nephrotoxic, it has the advantage of once weekly administration. Primary prophylaxis with oral ganciclovir or valaciclovir is effective, reducing the incidence of CMV disease by ~50%.

Cytomegalovirus and the gastrointestinal tract

CMV may cause oesophagitis, gastritis, duodenitis, cholangitis, and colitis. In the oesophagus, it is commonly associated with distal ulceration, in the stomach and colon with diffuse but patchy inflammation often with ulceration, and in the biliary tree with sclerosing cholangitis and biliary obstruction. Clinical manifestations are obviously related to the affected organ and tend to be of subacute onset, but pain is often prominent. Diagnosis is by identification of CMV inclusions with or without positive immunoperoxidase staining at sites of inflammation. The significance of CMV inclusions in the absence of inflammation is unknown and is sometimes not treated.

Ganciclovir and foscarnet are useful therapies. Maintenance therapy may not be essential after a first episode as relapse may not occur for many months and maintenance therapy may incur substantial morbidity. Sucralphate may be more useful than H_2 antagonists as adjunctive therapy for oesophagitis as most patients with advanced HIV disease are achlorhydric.

Cytomegalovirus encephalitis

CMV encephalitis develops over days to weeks with a picture of progressive obtundation, fever, seizures, and impaired higher functions. CMV organ involvement elsewhere is not always present. However, there are no clinical or radiological features specific for the diagnosis which makes diagnosis difficult. Examination of CSF may demonstrate a polymorphonuclear pleocytosis which is highly suggestive of CMV infection in the absence of bacterial or tuberculous meningitis. Detection of CMV-specific DNA by PCR may also be a sensitive, specific, and rapid means of diagnosis. Therapy with ganciclovir and/or foscarnet may be beneficial but no objective data are available.

Cytomegalovirus radiculomyelopathy

This disease has a subacute presentation of bilateral, ascending leg numbness associated with weakness, back pain, and occasionally bowel and bladder dysfunction. Generally, there is distal sensory loss in the legs with areflexia and weakness. Involvement of the upper limbs is unusual. The disorder affects approximately 2% of HIV-infected patients with CMV disease elsewhere, although it may be a first manifestation of

CMV disease. CT scanning or MRI may be useful to exclude a compressive spinal lesion. However, CSF analysis is more useful and yields results as seen for CMV encephalitis.

Ganciclovir or foscarnet may be useful, although disease may develop in patients receiving ganciclovir or foscarnet therapy, in which case the alternative drug may be tried. The appropriate dose and duration of induction therapy are unclear. Indefinite maintenance therapy is required. Nevertheless, patients frequently relapse despite such secondary prophylaxis.

Cytomegalovirus at other sites

There is considerable controversy regarding the significance of CMV isolation at other sites, particularly the lungs. CMV has been associated with cholangitis, but the degree to which it causes disease in the absence of bacterial or parasitic superinfection is unknown. CMV pneumonitis in the absence of other pathology that responds to specific CMV therapy appears rare. Likewise, adrenalitis at autopsy may be associated with CMV inclusions, but this has not been well correlated with hypoadrenalism during life. In particular, it is not known whether CMV therapy will reverse HIV-associated hypoadrenalism.

Other herpetic infections

Infections with herpes simplex and herpes zoster are both common problems in HIV disease, and are more likely to be recurrent and more aggressive (Fig. 3.5). Both perioral and genital herpes simplex are common but may be effectively treated with acyclovir which is also an effective prophylaxis. Rarely, HSV may cause oesophageal ulceration or encephalitis, either of which should be suspected in a patient with acute disease, no history of CMV disease, and concurrent mucocutaneous HSV.

Treatment and secondary prophylaxis with acyclovir is usually effective. Acyclovir-resistant HSV strains occasionally develop; such strains can usually be effectively treated with foscarnet.

Herpes zoster is more likely to be recurrent, multidermatomal, or aggressive in patients with HIV disease. High-dose acyclovir or famciclovir is effective therapy and prophylaxis is rarely indicated. Encephalitis due to herpes zoster is also a rare phenomenon and can be treated with intravenous acyclovir or ganciclovir.

Mycobacterium avium complex (MAC)

Infection with atypical mycobacteria and in particular *Mycobacterium avium* is an increasingly prevalent complication of late-stage HIV infection, mostly in patients with CD4+ cell counts less than 50/μl. Other species such as *M. intracellulare* are occasionally seen. The pathogenesis of the infection is unclear. *M. avium* may on occasion be isolated from the gut or the respiratory tract prior to the onset of systemic illness and identification in the blood, suggesting that one or both of these organs are the ports of entry. Nevertheless, it is unclear whether infection is a primary infection or a reactivated latent infection.

The clinical presentation is of gradual onset fever, night sweats, weight loss, pancytopenia, and on occasions symptomatology localized to the gut or the respiratory tract such as intermittent diarrhoea or non-productive cough. Diagnosis may be made by the growth of the organism from blood or by identification of atypical acid-fast bacilli in stools, gut biopsy, respiratory secretions, or bone marrow aspirates.

Combination therapy including clarithromycin or azithromycin is essential as monotherapy is either ineffective or results in rapid development of drug resistance. Without therapy, the average prognosis of MAC is 3–4 months.

Tuberculosis

Infection with *Mycobacterium tuberculosis* is an increasingly prevalent manifestation of HIV infection and is the commonest AIDS-defining illness in Africa, Asia, and economically disadvantaged groups in industrialized nations, and also a major cause of death. Infection may be a reactivation or a primary infection, with recurrences representing relapse in perhaps 70% of patients, and new infections in the remainder.

Symptoms and signs are manifold in that the disease may have an acute and/or chronic onset and may affect any organ. The typical findings seen in HIV-uninfected individuals are often blurred by the lack of immunological response as well as coinfection. In addition, extra-pulmonary infection is more common as is miliary disease. Clinical and radiological features tend to be more atypical in patients with advanced immunodeficiency, with less cavitation and lymphadenopathy (Fig. 3.7b).

The predominant features are fever, weight loss, constitutional symptoms, a non-productive cough, and symptoms related to extrapulmonary sites of infection. The ideal therapy is not known but should include at least one of isoniazid and rifampicin and either two or three other drugs at onset for at least a 2 month period. The duration of maintenance therapy is unclear with recommendations of a minimum of 9 months through to lifelong, especially in those with more advanced HIV disease. Other effective agents include pyrazinamide, streptomycin, ethambutol and in less developed countries, thiacetazone, although this last drug is a frequent cause of severe hypersensitivity reactions.

Diagnosis is made with identification of acid-fast bacilli with staining such as Ziehl–Nielsen in appropriate tissue. Microscopic identification, however, may be negative and so diagnosis may rely upon tissue culture which can take up to 6 weeks. Molecular diagnostics such as PCR are being evaluated with a view to more rapid diagnosis. Likewise, given the problem of drug sensitivity, a rapid sensitivity assay based on the capacity of luciferase to chemiluminesce in the presence of adenosine triphosphate (ATP) produced by viable mycobacteria has been developed.

Outbreaks of multidrug resistance to tuberculosis, including several nosocomial outbreaks, have been reported, particularly in areas of poor drug compliance or inadequate medical supervision. In such areas, at least four drugs should be used until sensitivity results are available as the mortality of multidrug resistant tuberculosis exceeds 50%. Several cases of multidrug resistant tuberculosis in health care workers highlight the significance of the problem.

Prevention of tuberculosis requires adequate public health resources, access to and supervision of therapy, and perhaps the use of DTH testing early in disease, with tuberculin-positive patients being offered isoniazid prophylaxis for at least 1 year.

Cryptococcosis

Infection with *Cryptococcosis neoformans* affects perhaps 10% of patients with HIV infection usually with CD4+ cell counts of less than 150/mm^3. Whether cryptococcosis is a reactivated or primary infection is unknown, with only occasional clear-cut environmental exposure (to pigeons) being related to clinical episodes. The two most common sites of infection are the meninges and the lungs. The clinical features of meningitis are rapid onset fevers and headaches; in early cases, the only early clinical abnormality may be meningism, but with late presentation there may be obtundation, seizures, and even focal deficits.

Analysis of CSF may show cryptococci on India ink staining and positive cryptococcal antigen, although the titre of antigen is a poor guide to clinical severity, prognosis, and response to therapy. Serum cryptococcal antigen may be positive, occasionally in the absence of CSF antigen.

Lung involvement usually manifests as a fever and non-productive cough with a variety of air space, interstitial or nodular abnormalities on radiography.

Therapy is generally with fluconazole or amphotericin B. Although fluconazole is less effective than amphotericin B, fluconazole is substantially less toxic and is absorbed orally. However, patients with a depressed level of consciousness, evidence of raised intracranial pressure, or a high organism load in the

CSF, should receive amphotericin B as they have a poor prognosis.

Candidiasis

Oropharyngeal or vaginal infection with *Candida albicans* is a frequent occurrence in patients with mild to moderately advanced immunosuppression (Fig. 3.8). The presence of oral candidiasis is an independent prognostic factor for progression to AIDS, although it may develop or be exacerbated by the use of broad-spectrum antibiotics.

Candidiasis appears as erythema of the tongue, buccal mucosa, pharynx, and oesophagus, with or without plaques or ulceration. Diagnosis of oral infection is clinical. With advancing disease oesophageal candidiasis may present with dysphagia, odynophagia, and concurrent oral candidiasis. The oesophageal lesion, however, should be biopsied to exclude herpetic infection, lymphoma, reflux oesophagitis, or idiopathic oesophagitis. Systemic candidiasis is rare, presumably because of relatively spared neutrophil function in patients with even advanced HIV disease. Systemic infection with other candida species such as *C. kruzei*, which is intrinsically resistant to azole agents, has been noted in patients receiving long-term azole therapy.

Therapy for less severe disease is with topical amphotericin B or nystatin. Ketaconazole and fluconazole are effective therapies for more advanced disease; daily maintenance therapy may, however, increase the likelihood of eventual azole drug resistance. Intravenous amphotericin B, often on an intermittent basis, is effective for severe or persistent disease. As is the case with cryptococcosis, both ketaconazole and fluconazole are effective primary prophylaxis but their use may also result in azole resistance, drug interactions, hepatoxicity, hypersensitivity, and is expensive.

Histoplasmosis

Infection with *Histoplasma capsulatum* is most common in areas of endemic infection such as southern and central USA and South America. The fungus grows best in moist surface soils, particularly when enriched by droppings of certain birds and bats. Disease in HIV-infected patients is a reactivation of a previous primary healed focus. It has an acute or subacute onset with fever, constitutional symptoms, and on occasion pneumonia, splenomegaly, cytopenias, and ulceration of the upper respiratory tract. Chest radiography may show pneumonitis, nodules, or a miliary pattern. Serological assays are largely unhelpful and diagnosis is made by culture or histology of sputum, bone marrow, or other biopsy specimens.

Amphotericin B is the therapy of choice, although itraconazole may also be effective. Indefinite secondary prophylaxis is mandatory.

Penicilliosis

Infection with *Penicillium marneffei* has been found to be a major complication of advanced HIV infection in South-east Asia. This infection typically presents with constitutional symptoms, anaemia, papular skin lesions with central umbilication, and hepatomegaly. Diagnosis is by staining of involved tissue, which demonstrates intra- and extracellular polymorphic yeast-like organisms. Amphotericin B and itraconazole appear to be effective, but the optimal therapy is unknown. Secondary prophylaxis appears to be required.

Bacterial respiratory tract infections

Bacterial respiratory tract infections with community acquired pathogens such as *Streptococcus pneumoniae* and *Haemophilus influenzae* are frequent in patients with moderate to advanced HIV disease. The presence of two episodes of pneumonia within a 12 month period in an HIV-infected patient with no prior predisposition is now an AIDS-defining illness, recognizing the substantial morbidity associated with these infections.

Therapy with conventional antibiotics is often effective but may be confounded by poor drug absorption, drug interaction, poor patient tolerance, and poor host immunity. These features may necessitate prolonged oral therapy or intravenous therapy.

Cryptosporidiosis

Cryptosporidium parvum is a protozoan which infects the microvillus border of the intestinal epithelium. It is a common infection of relatively late-stage HIV disease. It may infect any region within the gastrointestinal tract, but most commonly the small intestine. Infection manifests with frequent watery diarrhoea, weight loss, and abdominal pain. Dissemination to the biliary tree may result in progressive biliary obstruction and recurrent bacterial superinfection due to sclerosing cholangitis. Diagnosis is by identification of typical basophilic structures in stool, biliary secretions, or intestinal biopsy. Light microscopy of the small bowel shows mild to moderate villous atrophy, crypt enlargement, and a mononuclear cell infiltrate of the lamina propria, all of which of course are quite nonspecific for this infection. The pathophysiology of the associated diarrhoea is not clear, but may be due to an enterotoxin.

There is no proven, effective therapy for cryptosporodiosis. Agents such as paramomycin and azithromycin may be effective, although paramomycin is not absorbed and therefore will have no action in the biliary tree. Nutritional support is very important as for all gastrointestinal infectious complications of HIV disease. Gut infection may also compromise other systemic illnesses by impairing drug absorption. Any treatment found to be effective in an individual should probably be continued indefinitely because of the likelihood of relapse.

Other gastrointestinal infections

Microporidiosis is a more recently identified parasitic infection of the small bowel and biliary tree. There are two causative agents, *Enterozoon bienusi* and *Septata intestinalis*. The pathogenesis of the disease is unclear, and effective treatment for *E. bienusi* is unknown, although albendazole may be effective for *Septata intestinalis*. Infections due to microsporidia were previously labelled as HIV-associated enteropathy, and it is unclear whether HIV itself has direct effects on the gut and so be a cause of wasting syndrome. Other intestinal pathogens are often related to the underlying host (e.g. poor sanitation in developing countries, pathogens associated with homosexual sex), and include *Salmonella*, *Shigella*, *Campylobacter jejuni*, *Giardia lamblia*, and *Clostridium difficile*. Infection by multiple pathogens is common, and should always be suspected in those who fail to respond to appropriate therapy.

Malignancies

Kaposi's sarcoma

Kaposi's sarcoma is a proliferation of endothelial cell origin, although it is not clear whether it represents a true malignancy. Kaposi's sarcoma appears to be due to an infection of endothelial cells by a new herpes virus, called KSHV (Kaposi's sarcoma-associated Herpes virus). How KSHV induces KS is unclear. It is more common in homosexual men with HIV infection than in HIV-infected patients from other risk groups. The prevalence of Kaposi's sarcoma is declining in HIV-infected patients, although it still affects approximately 15% of patients; and Kaposi's sarcoma has been seen, rarely, in homosexual men and immunosuppressed patients without HIV infection. Growth of Kaposi's sarcoma appears dependent upon the HIV tat protein, IL-1, IL-6, TNFα, oncostatin, and other cytokines, some of which are in part synthesized by the abnormal proliferating endothelial cell.

Kaposi's sarcoma may affect virtually any organ with the exception of the brain. It most commonly involves the skin (Fig. 3.6f), although the hands and scalp are not commonly involved. Mucosal involvement of the gastrointestinal and respiratory tracts is not infrequent, particularly of the oropharynx (Fig. 3.10e). Lymph nodes, lung, gut, and liver may also be involved. Gut involvement usually presents with pain and occasionally bleeding or obstruction. Pulmonary disease may present with slow-onset cough, dyspnoea, haemoptysis and interstitial infiltrates indistinguishable from those due to PCP, although a bronchoscopy will usually show visible submucosal lesions. Diagnosis of cutaneous Kaposi's sarcoma is usually clinical but may be confused with bacillary angiomatosis.

Many patients with Kaposi's sarcoma require no therapy. Cutaneous disease may require treatment for cosmetic reasons, or because of local pain, ulceration, or compression of surrounding structures with complications such as peripheral oedema or secondary infection. Localized disease responds well to radiotherapy and sometimes to intralesional chemotherapy, cryotherapy or topical retinoids. More generalized cutaneous or visceral disease usually requires systemic combination chemotherapy, most commonly with bleomycin and vincristine or vinblastine. This chemotherapy is usually well tolerated, although vincristine may exacerbate peripheral neuropathy and vinblastine may cause cytopenias. Doxorubicin is also effective; its toxicity may be reduced by use in a liposomal formulation. IFNα at relatively high doses (9–36 million units daily) is effective, but mainly in those patients with CD4+ cell counts greater than 200/μl. When given in combination with zidovudine, IFNα may also be effective in those with lower CD4+ cell counts.

Non-Hodgkin's lymphoma

Non-Hodgkin's lymphoma (NHL) is an increasingly prevalent problem and manifestation of HIV disease with increasing survival and better opportunistic infection prophylaxis. The lymphomas are of high grade, being of immunoblastic, small non-cleaved (Burkitt's), or diffuse large cell subtypes. They are invariably of B-cell origin. About 50% of peripheral NHL and 100% of cerebral NHL have evidence of EBV infection of the malignant cells, suggesting a part for EBV in the pathogenesis of NHL.

NHL is uncommonly an AIDS-defining condition. The presentation tends to be atypical as compared with HIV-uninfected patients, particularly in patients with advanced disease, in that constitutional symptoms are less prominent and extra-nodal disease is more frequent. Although nodal presentation is still most common, primary cerebral lymphoma is also common, with involvement of the gut, lungs, skin, and bone marrow relatively less frequent. Diagnosis of peripheral NHL is by histological typing and to a lesser extent, clinical and radiological staging. Primary cerebral NHL has a clinical and radiological presentation often indistinguishable from that of cerebral toxoplasmosis, although imaging procedures usually demonstrate only one mass lesion. However, patients will not respond to toxoplasmosis therapy. Demonstration of EBV-specific DNA in the CSF may be specific for the diagnosis.

Regardless of the location and histological type, the treatment and outcome of HIV-related NHL is determined largely by the stage of HIV disease. Patients with only modest immunosuppression and no other AIDS-defining illnesses have a reasonable prognosis as they generally tolerate chemotherapy well and their management is less complicated by the presence of other diseases. Conventional chemotherapy with cyclophosphamide, vincristine, epirubicin, and prednisolone in such patients often leads to a significant response and occasionally prolonged complete response. Patients with more advanced disease are often intolerant of maximal doses of therapy and so for many such patients any treatment is palliative. Agents such as G-CSF may be useful for the treatment of neutropenia, although it is not proven to reduce the incidence of serious infections when used prophylactically.

Primary cerebral NHL is treated with local radiotherapy. Responses to radiotherapy are usually transient and incomplete, and the overall prognosis is poor. Dexamethasone is of use for symptoms associated with cerebral oedema.

Other malignancies

Other malignancies more prevalent in patients with HIV disease include Hodgkin's disease and squamous cell carcinomas of the cervix and rectum related to human papilloma virus infection. Such diseases also tend to behave in a more aggressive fashion. Indeed, the aggressive nature of invasive cervical neoplasia led to its being classified as an AIDS-defining condition, and Pap smears every 6 months are recommended for infected women. Other malignancies such as melanoma tend to have a more aggressive course, perhaps because the normal control of melanoma is in part dependent upon an intact host immune response.

Neurological complications

AIDS–dementia complex

AIDS–dementia complex (ADC) is a subcortical dementia as the usual cortical features of aphasia, alexia, and agraphia that characterize Alzheimier's disease are absent. Symptoms and signs of ADC can be grouped into three series of abnormality, these being cognition (poor concentration, disturbed short-term memory, slowing of thought processes), motor function (incoordination, poor handwriting, and

unsteadiness of gait), and behaviour (social apathy and withdrawal). These features generally develop over a period of weeks to months, although a more rapid onset may occur. On examination, the mini-mental state is usually normal and generally signs are subtle such as slowing and inaccuracy of saccadic and pursuit eye movements and fine finger movements. With more progressive disease there is impaired insight, global dementia, mutism, paraparesis, and incontinence of urine and faeces. ADC generally occurs with advanced immunosuppression with most patients having a CD4+ cell count of less than $200/\mu l$. Prevalence varies widely but is thought to be approximately 7% per year in patients with symptomatic HIV disease.

There are no investigations diagnostic of ADC. CT scanning usually demonstrates cerebral atrophy and MRI scanning may reveal T2 weighted periventricular abnormalities that are either patchy or diffuse. However, neither of these investigations are specific for ADC and their chief utility is for the exclusion of focal CNS disease. CSF analysis may yield detectable p24 antigen and elevated concentrations of β_2-microglobulin, neopterin, quinolinic acid, TNF, and interleukins, but these are non-specific findings. The main value of CSF analysis is for the exclusion of alternative diagnoses such as CMV encephalitis, cryptococcal meningitis, and tertiary syphilis. Neuropsychological testing may demonstrate impaired attention and slowing of intellectual processes, but these features also are not specific for ADC.

The most common histopathological finding is HIV leucoencephalopathy (diffuse but especially subcortical damage to white matter, reactive astrocytosis, and multinucleated giant cells with minimal or no inflammatory infiltrates). There may be reactive astrogliosis, microglial activation and atrophy of grey matter, a perivascular inflammatory infiltrate or vacuolation of white matter, and rarely cerebral vasculitis.

It is unclear as to whether ADC is a direct result of viral infection of the central nervous system. Alternatively, it may represent a toxic response to either productive HIV infection of microglial cells with release of neurotoxins from these cells or be a bystander phenomenon due to toxins secreted locally by reactive inflammatory cells. Nevertheless, it is clear that ADC is related to immune activation during a time of advanced immunodeficiency, that the clinical deficit is disproportionately greater than the amount of HIV in the brain and that the neural cells which support HIV infection are not the ones that die, all of which suggest an indirect pathogenesis.

ADC is best treated with the highest tolerated dose of zidovudine. Responses are generally seen after 8 weeks of therapy in about 50% of patients. Rarely, intrathecal zidovudine has been used for some intolerant patients.

The efficacy of other antiretroviral agents is not clear. Didanosine has demonstrated variable efficacy and zalcitabine does not penetrate the blood–brain barrier. Utility of other agents such as non-nucleoside reverse transcriptase inhibitors is unproven. There are no surrogate markers which have proven benefit in following response.

Zidovudine is also beneficial as primary prophylaxis of ADC in a dose-dependent fashion. This benefit appears to persist even where there is loss of immunological response to zidovudine. Consequently, there is an argument of continuing zidovudine therapy even when additional antiretroviral therapy is commenced for more general indications. The minimum effective prophylactic dose of zidovudine is unclear.

Progressive multifocal leucoencephalopathy (PML)

PML affects approximately 4% of HIV-infected patients, usually with advanced disease. The causative agent is the JC virus. The clinical picture is of a focal neurological deficit which develops gradually over several weeks, but is often not multifocal. Fever and headache are uncommon, and the level of consciousness is preserved. CT scanning or MRI reveals one or more areas of hypodensity in white matter without mass effect or contrast enhancement (Fig. 3.8b). The disease may also be diagnosed by histology of affected tissue or detection of Creuzfeldt–Jakob virus-specific DNA in the CSF by PCR.

There are anecdotal reports of the efficacy of cytosine arabinoside with or without IFNα for PML; neverthless the prognosis remains poor. Therapy is usually given intravenously, although intrathecal therapy has been rarely used. The optimal dose and duration of therapy are not known.

Other central nervous system manifestations

An aseptic meningitis, usually of acute onset, may occur in patients with mild to moderate immunodeficiency or as part of primary infection, occasionally in combination with cranial neuropathy. There may be a CSF pleocytosis, although such a pleocytosis may occur in asymptomatic HIV-infected patients. Low doses of amitryptiline are usually effective.

Seizures may occur as a result of underlying infection, lymphoma, PML, or electrolyte imbalance. Investigation and management should be primarily directed towards exclusion of an underlying treatable condition. However, many seizures remain idiopathic and are presumably due to HIV itself. More than 70% of patients with a first seizure will suffer subsequent seizures and therefore anticonvulsant therapy is indicated. Both phenytoin and carbamazepine frequently cause hypersensitivity and clonazepam is a useful alternative.

Transient neurological deficits may occur in the absence of an underlying cause. Some of these events may have a vascular nature and at autopsy 20% of patients have small infarctions of the basal ganglia. Rarely, herpes zoster may cause cerebral vasculitis that may sometimes be confirmed by PCR of CSF. Treatment is generally as for the HIV-uninfected patient with consideration of anticoagulation or occasionally of high-dose acyclovir.

Neurosyphilis tends to have similar manifestations as that in HIV-uninfected patients. It may occur in the presence of adequate therapy for primary syphilis and may behave more aggressively than in HIV-uninfected patients. CSF serology is usually adequate for diagnosis and in the absence of prior therapy a positive result mandates therapy. Treatment is as for HIV-uninfected subjects.

Vacuolar myelopathy

The main features of this disorder are a mild spastic paraparesis without a definite sensory level. Posterior column loss of diminished proprioception and vibration sense may occur. All features are largely confined to the legs and the onset is over a period of weeks to months. Progression to severe impairment is uncommon.

The aetiology and therapy of vacuolar myelopathy are unknown. Histopathology shows multiple vacuoles of the white matter of the posterior and lateral columns of the thoracic spinal cord, occasional lipid-laden macrophages and separation of the myelin sheaths. There are no useful diagnostic imaging procedures and CSF analysis is done to exclude other pathology. The condition does not appear to respond to zidovudine or other antiretroviral agents.

Peripheral neuropathy

HIV-related peripheral neuropathy most commonly manifests as a distal symmetrical polyneuropathy and occurs in approximately 45% of patients with AIDS. There is diminished pain and temperature sensation with absent or depressed ankle jerks, even in the absence of symptoms. Subsequently, patients develop paraesthesia or numbness in the feet which may progress to the knees. The hands are rarely involved and weakness is uncommon. The condition may be exacerbated by administration of agents such as didanosine, zalcitabine, or vinka alkaloids. Treatment with capsaicin cream, low-dose amitryptyline, sodium valproate or clonazepam may be beneficial.

Narcotic analgesia may be required for some patients. The pathogenesis is unknown and no specific therapy is available.

Autonomic neuropathy may occur in advanced HIV disease and is characterized by postural hypotension, diarrhoea, and occasionally cardiac arrhythmias. Autonomic neuropathy usually occurs in conjunction with peripheral sensory neuropathy and may have the same aetiology. Fludrocortisone may be used to treat symptomatic hypotension but is often unsuccessful.

Other forms of peripheral neuropathy include mononeuritis multiplex and inflammatory demyelinating polyneuropathy. Both usually occur in those with less advanced HIV disease and occasionally may require immunosuppression. Treatment is the same as for HIV-uninfected patients (i.e. plasmapheresis or immunosuppression) and responses appears to be similar.

Other manifestations

Drug hypersensitivity

Drug hypersensitivity is far more common in HIV-infected patients than in immunocompetent or HIV-uninfected immunodeficient subjects. The most common causes are sulphonamides, but β-lactams and anticonvulsants are also frequent causes. The reactions generally comprise a maculopapular rash after about 10 days therapy, often with fever and constitutional symptoms (Fig. 3.6b). Hepatitis, nephritis, and Stevens–Johnson syndrome occur less commonly. Hypersensitivity reactions adversely impact on therapy by necessitating drug withdrawal and institution of alternative therapy, that may have less efficacy or incur other toxicities.

Hypersensitivity in HIV-infected patients has been postulated to be either allergic (i.e. immune-mediated) or toxic in nature but its aetiology is unknown. The development of true drug allergy in HIV-infected patients appears paradoxical, considering the profound anergy that develops in these patients to other immune stimuli; this paradox has yet to be explained. Risk factors, at least for TMP-SMX, appear to be a slow acetylator phenotype, glutathione deficiency, a higher cumulative dose, and perhaps a CD4+ cell count between about 20 and $200/\mu l$. The reactions may be generated by reactive drug metabolites and be mediated by CD8+ lymphocytes, perhaps with the assistance of CD4+ cells, via cytokine release. Overall, hypersensitivity appears to have a multifactorial pathogenesis, which remains to be fully elucidated. Treatment with desensitization has been found to be of benefit.

Other mucocutaneous diseases

Cutaneous involvement is common at all stages of HIV infection. As mentioned, rashes associated with primary HIV infection and drug hypersensitivity are frequent. Non-AIDS-defining cutaneous manifestations of HIV disease include seborrhoeic dermatitis, cutaneous mycoses, generalized eczema, folliculitis, and scabies, as well as herpetic infections and Kaposi's sarcoma which are discussed above.

Seborrhoeic dermatitis is common in early symptomatic disease in patients with only modest immunodeficiency. Its cause is as yet unknown but has been linked to fungal infections. It has a classical distribution involving the nasolabial folds, forehead, scalp, ears, and central chest, although other areas may be affected. Treatment with topical hydrocortisone is often effective, but both topical and oral ketaconazole have also been reported to be of benefit.

Folliculitis is a common disorder in early disease and has been linked to multiple pathogens including fungi, but is in many case idiopathic. Treatment is largely empirical and includes antihistamines for pruritus, topical antisepsis with agents such as clindamycin or erythromycin, and systemic antimicrobials such as erythromycin, flucloxacillin, and doxycycline. The most effective acute and maintenance therapy is unknown.

Aphthous ulceration may occur in the oropharynx or oesophagus (Fig. 3.10d). In the oesophagus they should only be diagnosed after exclusion of other causes such as CMV, HSV, lymphoma, tuberculosis, or locally irritating drugs such as zidovudine. Treatment with thalidomide is effective, perhaps by its anti-TNF activity. Short courses of corticosteroids also appear to be safe and effective.

Autoimmune disease

The most common autoimmune manifestation of HIV infection is thrombocytopenia, a phenomenon of predominantly early symptomatic HIV disease. Although platelet antibodies have been detected, their role in disease is unclear, and bone marrow dysfunction may also contribute to the pathogenesis. Diagnosis requires the exclusion clinically of other causes, a bone marrow aspirate showing plentiful megakaryocytes and often a therapeutic trial of zidovudine (to which the disorder is often responsive) or platelet transfusion (which is ineffective). Bone marrow examination is necessary to exclude disorders such as mycobacteriosis and lymphoma. Apart from zidovudine, other effective therapies include intravenous immunoglobulin, corticosteroids (although long-term corticosteroids are contra-indicated) and splenectomy. Other antiretroviral agents do not appear beneficial, and zidovudine

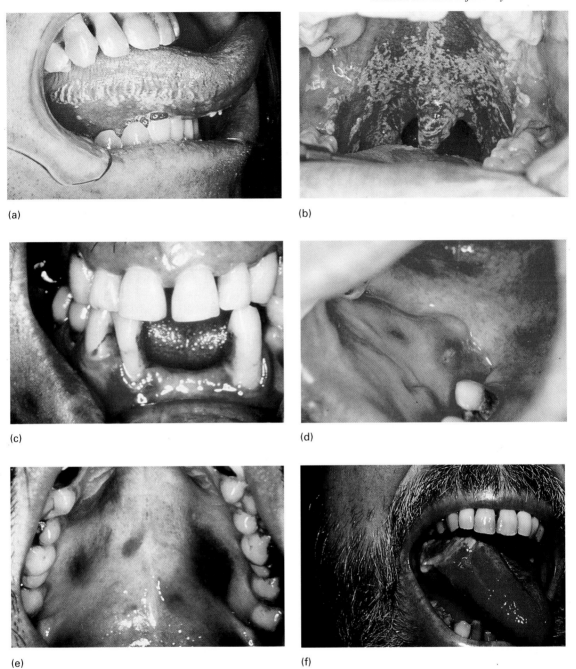

▌**Fig. 3.10** Oral manifestations of HIV infection: (a) oral hairy leucoplakia; (b) candidiasis; (c) gingivitis; (d) aphthous ulceration; (e) Kaposi's sarcoma; (f) lymphoma.

may be effective even the face of high-level zidovudine resistance. Intravenous immunoglobulin often has only transient benefit but is useful, particularly preoperatively. Splenectomy is usually reserved only for patients with otherwise asymptomatic HIV disease with symptomatic thrombocytopenia.

Another common manifestation is sicca syndrome, which may be due to a CD8+ + lymphocytic infiltration of the salivary glands in response to infection of salivary epithelium by EBV and perhaps hepatitis C virus. Autoantibodies against extractable nuclear antigens such as SS-A and SS-B may rarely be seen.

There is an appreciable frequency of IgG and IgM phospholipid antibodies in HIV-infected patients. It is unclear, however, whether these are causally related to the hypercoagulable syndrome comprising deep venous thrombosis, pulmonary embolism, and/or cerebrovascular ischaemia that is an increasingly prevalent manifestation of HIV disease.

The main rheumatological complication of HIV disease is spondyloarthropathy which may be related to enteric or genitourinary pathogens, but also may be idiopathic. A classical clinical and radiological pattern of sacro-iliitis, with or without involvement of peripheral joints, is usual. After exclusion of underlying infections, treatment with non-steroidal anti-inflammatory agents is often adequate. Additional therapy with agents such as salazopyrine may be required and is of benefit. Spondyloarthropathy tends to decline in severity with advancing immunosuppression.

Treatment of HIV infection

Treatment of HIV infection currently revolves around antiretroviral therapy and specifically the use of nucleoside analogues and protease inhibitors. However, as shown in Fig. 3.2, there are numerous potential targets for the antiviral treatment of HIV infection from the moment of HIV attachment to an uninfected cell to the point of release of a new virion from an infected cell. The other major, as yet undeveloped, approach is for improving the underlying immunological deficit.

Antiviral therapy

The ideal antiretroviral therapy would be active against cell-associated and cell-free virus, against both latent and productive stages of HIV, against all strains of HIV in all body sites including the brain, would be non-toxic, cheap, orally available and have indefinite action. No agent currently available possesses these qualities, and so therapy is not commenced immediately after diagnosis.

The currently licensed antiretroviral nucleoside, analogues are zidovudine, didanosine, zalcitabine, stavudine, lamivudine. Of these, zidovudine is the most effective as monotherapy, and will delay progression to AIDS in patients with CD4+ counts less than $500/\mu l$ and delay death in those with more advanced disease. It is also effective therapy and prophylaxis for ADC and thrombocytopenia, and greatly reduces the risk of maternofetal transmission when used in pregnancy and the peripartum period. The best time to ini-

tiate monotherapy is unclear, but probably with a CD4+ cell count between 200 and $500/\mu l$ depending upon clinical symptoms, surrogate markers, and patient preference.

Zidovudine therapy invariably fails, usually after 6–18 months. Failure is probably a result of mutations in reverse transcriptase resulting in phenotypic resistance, and perhaps also altered drug metabolism and patient tolerance for an active dose. Zidovudine in combination with lamivudine didanosine or zalcitabine is more effective than monotherapy or alternating monotherapies, leading to more pronounced and sustained immunological responses and greater reduction in circulating viral load and greater and more sustained clinical responses.

Toxicities due to zidovudine include anaemia, headaches, nausea, and a mitochondrial myopathy, the last usually occurring after 9 months of therapy. Didanosine is an effective alternative, particularly for those patients on long-term zidovudine therapy likely to have high-level zidovudine-resistant strains of HIV. In such circumstances, zalcitabine monotherapy appears to have equivalent efficacy to didanosine. Toxicities of didanosine include peripheral neuropathy and pancreatitis, whereas zalcitabine may cause peripheral neuropathy, mouth ulcers, and mild cytopenias. The only significant toxicity of stavudine is peripheral neuropathy. There is no specific toxicity of lamivudine.

Non-nucleoside reverse transcriptase inhibitors are agents which bind to the non-active site of reverse transcriptase and are more active *in vitro* than the nucleoside analogues. They are active against zidovudine-resistant HIV, but are inactive against HIV-2. Their use as monotherapy is limited by the rapid evolution of resistant HIV strains, as well as a relatively high frequency of drug hypersensitivity, both of which usually occur within 8 weeks of commencing monotherapy. A combination of a non-nucleoside reversed transcriptase inhibitor with a nucleoside analogue such as zidovudine appears to prevent the early development of resistance, allows for synergy between the two drugs and can reverse the high-level zidovudine resistance phenotype associated with the codon 215 mutation in reverse transcriptase.

Three proteinase inhibitors, saquhavit, ritonavir, and indinavit, have been licensed for the treatment of HIV infection. Their toxicities do not generally conflict with reverse transcriptase inhibitors with which they exhibit synergy *in vitro* and *in vivo*. Although potent HIV inhibitors resistance does develop *in vivo* particularly when used as monotherapy. Triple combination regimens incorporating a protease inhibitor have resulted in eradication of HIV from the peripheral blood in excess for in excess of one year, but not in complete reconstitution.

Tat inhibitors, although a promising *in vitro* class of agents, are no longer undergoing clinical evaluation because of their lack of efficacy in clinical trials. No integrase inhibitor has been developed.

Foscarnet has anti-HIV activity in addition to its benefit against CMV. Its toxicity, however, precludes its use as an anti-HIV agent, but its use for CMV disease over the long term may incur a small survival advantage. IFNα has direct antiviral activity against HIV but its expense and toxicity complicate its modest antiviral activity and it is not undergoing widespread evaluation.

Co-therapy is a concept that refers to the treatment of underlying factors such as other infections which may accelerate the progression of HIV disease. For example, use of acyclovir may inhibit the growth of EBV, CMV, and HHV-6 and its use in moderate to high doses in relatively late-stage HIV disease has been associated with reduction in mortality despite lack of any evidence of CD4+ cell count response. Similarly, the use of heat-treated and purified factor VIII concentrates may be associated with slower immunological decline in haemophiliacs than factor VIII concentrates in general.

Convergent therapy is a concept that describes the capacity of HIV to become non-replicative and non-infectious when it mutates in the presence of multiple concurrent antiviral agents. A report of such an outcome with *in vitro* triple therapy of zidovudine, didanosine, and nevirapine has since been discredited. Nevertheless, convergent therapy remains an interesting concept.

Other potential agents for use as antiviral agents include antisense oligonucleotides and ribosomes targeted to one or more conserved sequences of the HIV genome.

Immunotherapy

Several generalized specific immunomodulators are being evaluated at various stages of HIV disease. In addition to IFNα, other therapies such as immunoglobulin, HIV-specific immunoglobulin, HIV-specific therapeutic vaccines, recombinant soluble CD4, cytokines such as IL-2, TNF inhibitors such as

▌ **Table 3.9**   Prophylaxis of opportunistic infections and AIDS dementia complex

Illness	Primary prophylaxis	Secondary prophylaxis
Pneumocystis carinii pneumonia	**Trimethoprim-sulphamethoxazole** Dapsone Pentamidine — aerosolized Pentamidine — IVI	**Trimethoprim-sulphamethoxazole** Dapsone Aerosolized pentamidine Intravenous pentamidine
Toxoplasmosis	**Trimethoprim-sulphamethoxazole** Dapsone/Pyrimethamine Pyrimethamine	**Sulphadiazine/Pyrimethamine** Clindamycin/Pyrimethamine
Cytomegalovirus	Ganciclovir-oral	Ganciclovir — IV Foscarnet Ganciclovir — oral
Tuberculosis	Isoniazid ? combination	Isoniazid + rifampicin + ? other drugs
Mycobacterium avium complex	Rifabutin **Clarithromycin** **Azithromycin**	At least three drugs including: **clarithromycin** ethambutol rifabutin/ clofazamine
Candidiasis	Ketoconazole **Fluconazole**	Ketoconazole **Fluconazole**
Cryptococcosis	Fluconazole ? ketoconazole	**Fluconazole** Amphotericin B
AIDS dementia complex	Zidovudine	Zidovudine

Bold font denotes most effective agent where more than one option is available.

pentoxyfiline and thalidomide, glutathione, and cellular therapies are all currently undergoing evaluation.

Intravenous immunoglobulin is effective in reducing the prevalence of bacterial infections in children and perhaps in adults. Whether this confers a survival advantage is not known. Recombinant soluble CD4+ was active against laboratory isolated but inactive against clinical isolates.

Cytokine therapy has been explored for many years. It is clear that IL-2 can increase CD4+ cell counts, but whether IL-2 plus antiretrovirals result in greater suppression of HIV viral load than use of antiretrovirals alone is not known. The clinical efficacy of IL-2 is currently under evaluation. Pentoxyfiline and thalidomide are specific inhibitors of TNF, which has been associated with the cachexia and constitutional symptoms seen with progressive disease, as well as being a potent HIV growth factor. However, these agents appear to have minimal activity when used at doses that are well tolerated.

Adoptive cellular transfer of autologous CD8+ lymphocytes is currently being evaluated. In some instances, the cells are being 'vaccinated' *ex vivo* with various HIV strains as well as being expanded prior to storage, with the aim of protecting the host against new autologous quasi-species that appear not to induce an effective immune response and which may antagonize the CTL response to the parent strain. However, no consistent benefit on CD4+ counts or viral burden has been demonstrated by these manipulations.

The ideal doses, routes of administration, and combinations of these therapies with antiretrovirals is unknown.

The ideal HIV vaccine, either therapeutic or preventative, should be active against all strains of HIV, all roots of exposure, all inoculum sizes and in the case of therapeutic vaccination would work at all stages of disease; but at present vaccination strategies for treatment and prevention of HIV infection are at a very early stage of development. Given that there is an enormous level of HIV antigen production at all stages of infection, it is likely that therapeutic vaccination against HIV will be unsuccessful.

Further reading

Barre-Sinoussi, F., Chermann, J. C., Rey, F., *et al.* (1983). Isolation of a T-cell lymphotropic retrovirus from a patient at risk for acquired immunodeficiency syndrome (AIDS). *Science*, **220**, 868–71.

Blattner, W. A. (1991). HIV epidemiology: past, present, and future. *FASEB*, **5**, 2340–8.

Bloom, B. (1996). A perspective on AIDS vaccines. *Science*, **272**, 1888–90.

Centers for Disease Control. (1981). Pneumocystis pneumonia. *MMWR*, **30**, 250.

Centers for Disease Control (1992). 1993 revised classification system for HIV infection and expanded surveillance definition for AIDS among adolescents and adults. *MMWR*, **41** (RR-17): 1–19.

Cheng-Mayer, C., Seto, D., Tateno, M., and Levy, J. A. (1988). Biologic features of HIV that correlate with virulence in the host. *Science*, **240**, 80–2.

Dalgleish, A. G., Beverley, P. C., Clapham, P. R., *et al.* (1984). The CD4+ (T4) antigen is an essential component of the receptor for the AIDS retrovirus. *Nature*, **312**, 763–7.

Decker, C. F. and Masur, H. (1993). Current status of prophylaxis for opportunistic infections in HIV-infected patients. *AIDS*, **8**, 11–20.

Fahey, J. L., Taylor, J. M., Detels, R., *et al.* (1990). The prognostic value of cellular and serologic markers in infection with human immunodeficiency virus type 1. *New England Journal of Medicine*, **322**, 166–72.

Fischl, M. A., Richman, D. D., Grieco, M. H., *et al.* (1987). The efficacy of azidothymidine (AZT) in the treatment of patients with AIDS and AIDS-related complex. A double-blind, placebo controlled trial. *New England Journal of Medicine*, **317**, 185–91.

Haseltine, W. A. (1991). Molecular biology of the human immunodeficiency virus type 1. *FASEB*, **5**, 2349–60.

Ho, D. D. (1996). Viral counts count in HIV infection. *Science*, **272**, 1124–5.

McMichael, A. J. and Walker, B. D. (1994) Cytotoxic T lymphocyte epitopes: implications for HIV vaccines. *AIDS*, **8**, S155–513.

Mellors, J. W., Rinaldo Jr, C. R., Gupta, P., White, R. M., Todd, J. A., and Kingsley, L. A. (1996). Prognosis in HIV-1 infection predicted by the quantity of virus in plasma. *Science*, **272**, 1167–70.

Nowak, M. A. and McMichael, A. J. (1995). How HIV defeats the immune system. *Scientific American*, **August**, 42–9.

Pantaleo, G. and Fauci, A. S. (1995). New concepts in the immunopathogenesis of HIV infection. *Annual Reviews of Immunology*, **13**, 487–512.

Riehman, D. D. (1996). HIV therapeutics. *Science*, **272**, 1886–8.

Weiss, R. A. (1996). HIV receptors and the pathogenesis of AIDS. *Science*, **272**, 1885–6.

Zinkernagel, R. M. and Hengartner, H. (1994). T cell mediated immunopathology versus direct cytolysis by virus: implications for HIV and AIDS. *Immunology Today*, **15**, 262–8.

4 Acquired immunodeficiency, postviral states and chronic fatigue syndrome

D. Wakefield

Introduction

Immunodeficiency is a common clinical problem and is most frequently acquired or secondary to an underlying disease. Such immunodeficiencies may be transient or permanent, mild or severe. A large variety of diseases, conditions, and therapies may lead to compromised immunity. The most common and important causes of secondary immunodeficiency are outlined in Table 4.1.

On a global scale the most common cause of immunodeficiency is malnutrition. Nutritional deficiency contributes substantially to childhood morbidity and mortality, especially from infectious diseases. Infection in turn may worsen the nutritional state of the host and cause further immunosuppression, predisposing to more frequent, severe, and complicated infections.

In the developed world the most common causes of secondary immunodeficiency are infections, malignancy, metabolic diseases, and drugs (Table 4.1). The importance of secondary immunodeficiencies lies in the fact that such states predispose to opportunistic infections. In the assessment of an individuals immune status it is important to appreciate the influence of age on immune function.

Ageing and immunity

The immune system undergoes dramatic change from infancy to old age. These extremes of life are often associated with significant depression of the immune systems capacity to respond to antigen. Newborn and especially premature infants have depressed T- and B-cell immunity. Immunoglobulins IgM and IgA levels are relatively low and there may be depressed IgG levels in premature children as a consequence of decreased placental transfer of maternal immunoglobulin. Prematurity is also associated with decreased phagocytosis, chemotaxis, and complement levels.

Thymic involution begins after puberty and with advanced age there is a gradual depression of T-cell function and a concomitant increase in B cells and immunoglobulin levels. There is a decrease in the absolute number of T lymphocytes (CD3), involving both CD4+ and CD8+ T-cell subsets, accompanied by an increase in the number of activated T cells (CD3 HLA DR+). The proportion of helper (CD4) and suppressor T (CD8) cells is not altered with ageing. Studies in mice and humans of the immunoregulatory capacity of monocytes/macrophages have shown that these cells have a reduced capacity to synthesize interleukins with advance in age. A decline in activity of IL-1 may contribute to the decreased T-cell and macrophage proliferative capacity seen with ageing. There is also a decrease in delayed-type hypersensitivity (DTH) skin responses, anergy, and in responses to T-cell dependent antigens. Ageing is also associated with a linear increase in the number of B cells and an increase in the number of natural killer (NK) cells and of T cells able to mediate non-major histocompatibility complex (MHC) restricted cytotoxicity. Normal ageing in humans has recently been shown to be accompanied by a reduced control over production of the multifunctional cytokine IL-6. Experiments in aged mice indicate that significant changes also occur in other T-cell cytokines with age and allergic symptoms tend to improve. The production of IgE declines with age and allergic symptoms tend to improve.

An important consequence of immune changes with ageing is the decreased response to vaccination in the elderly and falling antibody levels, e.g. to tetanus toxoid. This has been shown to be associated with a decreased number of specific antibody secreting B cells and decreased potency of these B cells. Old age is associated with an increased frequency of autoantibodies, paraproteins, and lymphoproliferative disorders.

∎ **Table 4.1** Acquired and secondary immunodeficiencies

Aetiology	Condition	Major immune defect
Metabolic disease	Diabetes mellitus; renal failure; cirrhosis; Cushing's syndrome	Decreased lymphocyte transformation test (LTT)[a] Abnormal bacterial killing and chemotaxis
Malnutrition	Kwashiorkor	Lymphopenia; decreased T cells, delayed-type hypersensitivity and T-cell mitogen response; abnormal bacterial killing; decreased C3 and secretory IgA
Infections	*viral*: HIV, measles, hepatitis B virus, cytomegalovirus, rubella	Decreased T-cell function
	bacterial: tuberculosis, leprosy	Decreased T-cell function
	fungal: coccidiomycosis aspergillus	Decreased T-cell function
Surgery and general anaesthesia	Major surgery, splenectomy	Decreased T-cell function and antibody response
Prematurity	Newborn infants	Lymphopenia; decreased T cells and LTT; abnormal bacterial killing; chemotaxis; decreased IgM, IgA, and complement abnormalities
Infiltrative diseases	Lymphoma; leukaemia	Lymphopenia; decreased T cells and LTT; abnormal bacterial killing and chemotaxis Variable immunoglobulin and complement levels
	Melanoma	Lymphopenia; decreased T cells and LTT Abnormal bacterial killing and chemotaxis Decreased immunoglobulin and complement;
Genetic	Down syndrome	Lymphopenia; decreased T cells and LTT.
	Sickle cell anaemia	Impaired primary and secondary antibody response
Immune (autoimmune) disease	Rheumatoid arthritis; systemic lupus erythematosus; Immunosuppressive therapy	Lymphopenia; decreased T cells and LTT Increased immunoglobulin and complement Corticosteroids Lymphopenia; transient decreased T cells and LTT abnormal bacterial killing; chemotaxis, decreased immunoglobulins
	Cytotoxics	Decreased T- and B-cell number and function Neutropenia
	Cyclosporin	Decreased T- and B-cell function
	Radiation	Decreased T- and B-cell number and function
	Phenytoin	Decreased IgA and cell mediated immunity

[a]LTT is also known as lymphocyte or T-cell proliferation assay.

Genetic, metabolic, and morphological studies reveal impressive evidence of quantitative changes in immune cells with advancing age. At the cell membrane level older humans have been shown to have fewer IL-2 receptors on antigen or mitogen activated T cells than young humans. As IL-2 is essential for activated T and B cells to proliferate the age-related reduction in IL-2 receptors probably contributes to the age-related decline in T-cell proliferation, especially as IL-2 synthesis also diminishes with increasing age. Metabolic changes in immune cell function have also been reported. Decreased levels of nicotinamide adenosine dinucleotide (NAD) and adenosine triphosphate in mitogen-stimulated T cells of old humans suggest impaired ability of antigen or mitogen-stimulated old cells to generate energy. Decreased NAD levels in mitogen-stimulated T cells suggests a decreased ability to repair DNA with increasing age, because NAD is the main substrate for synthesis of polyadenosine diphosphate-ribose, which is involved in DNA synthesis. Further studies indicate that the second messenger activities of cyclic aderosine monophosphate also diminish in older humans. Several functional changes have been detected in nuclei of T cells of older humans, including decreased ability to repair ultraviolet light-induced damage of DNA, increased breaks in DNA strands and decreased transcription of the IL-2 gene.

Immunodeficiency of nutritional origin

Severe protein calorie malnutrition in infants leads to the syndrome of kwashiorkor, in which hypoproteinaemic oedema, skin and hair abnormalities are associated with frequent infections. The complex interactions between nutrition, infection, and immunity are poorly understood and the precise role of each factor is difficult to ascertain. Infections induce profound metabolic alterations resulting in negative nitrogen balance. Protein energy malnutrition, whatever the cause, results in an immune deficiency characterized by impaired DTH, decreased cytokine production, T-cell lymphopenia, and decreased T-cell response to specific antigens and non-specific mitogens. Serum immunoglobulin levels are normal or elevated and antibody responses to most vaccines are normal. Secretory IgA levels, IgA plasma cells in jejunal biopsies, and specific IgA levels are decreased. C3 levels are usually reduced as a consequence of reduced hepatic synthesis and increased consumption, but other complement proteins are normal. Neutrophil chemotaxis and serum opsonic activity are normal but bacterial killing capacity is markedly reduced. Such alterations of immunological parameters can be induced by malnutrition itself but are commonly observed in populations also exposed to a heavy load of infectious agents from birth.

Surgery, anaesthesia, and burns

Surgery, general anaesthesia, and burns lead to an acute depression of immunity. Patients with an existing primary or secondary immunodeficiency are particularly at risk. Splenectomy in particular results in a lifelong risk to the patient of infection by encapsulated bacteria (e.g. *Pneumococcus*) as a result of defective opsonization.

A severe immunodeficiency affecting humoral and cell-mediated immunity is associated with extensive full thickness burns and places the patient at great risk of death from infection. Several factors contribute to this including profound protein loss, increased catabolic rate, increased endogenous corticosteroids, and a break in the integument.

Metabolic diseases

Metabolic diseases such as diabetes mellitus, chronic renal failure, and cirrhosis are among the most common debilitating diseases to affect humans. Morbidity and mortality associated with these diseases is to a large extent due to infections. This is turn can be attributed to the depressed immunity often associated with these metabolic diseases. The causes of the compromised immunity observed in patients with these diseases is multifactorial and not fully understood. Both cellular and humoral immunity are affected (Table 4.1). Diabetics are prone to recurrent bacterial and fungal infections as a result of defective opsonization. Patients with the nephrotic syndrome and cirrhosis are predisposed to bacterial sepsis, particularly pneumococcal and *Escherichia coli* peritonitis, respectively.

Infection and immunity

Infectious diseases not only complicate secondary immunodeficiencies but may also cause them. The acquired immune deficiency syndrome (AIDS) epidemic has given dramatic proof to the ability of viruses to suppress the immune system dramatically, but it is important to realize that a large variety of microbial agents may depress immunity. The effects of common viral, bacterial, and parasitic infections on immunity are summarized in Table 4.1.

One of the most widely studied areas is the effects of herpesviruses and their ability to depress cellular immunity. A recent study suggests that the herpes group virus; (Epstein–Barr virus, EBV; cytomegalovirus, CMV) induced immunosuppression may result from an inhibition of cytokine production after direct interaction of the virus with major histocompatibility components. This suppression appears to be of clinical significance primarily in patients with underlying immune deficiencies.

Patients infected with CMV, for example, can undergo a prolonged depression in peripheral blood lymphocyte blastogenesis and γ-interferon production in response to *in vitro* stimulation with CMV and other viral antigens. In contrast, NK cell and antibody responses appear to be relatively normal. Cellular immunity increases in association with resolution of symptoms and cessation of viral excretion. CD8+ T cells have been linked to CMV-induced immunosuppression of T-cell responses during clinical CMV infection, in that they depress mitogen-induced blastogenesis in mononucleosis patients. These inhibitory effects may be due to decreased production of IL-1 by monocytes and IL-2 by T cells.

The immunosuppressive effects of EBV are evidence in adults with acute mononucleosis and are similar in nature to those of CMV; depression of lymphocyte responses to mitogens and antigens, cutaneous anergy, with a relatively intact antibody response and autoantibody production. CMV-induced immunosuppression is usually less severe and less prolonged than that caused by EBV. In addition many of the herpesviruses have evolved mechanisms for interfering with MHC class I restricted antigen presentation to cytotoxic T lymphocyte (CTL).

Infiltration and neoplastic diseases

A large number of conditions depress immunity as a direct result of infiltration of the bone marrow, lymphoid tissue, and thymus. The most important of these include the leukaemias, lymphomas, plasma cell dyscrasias, and sarcoidosis. This heterogeneous group of diseases often dramatically compromise immunity producing serious clinical consequences. The clinical manifestations of these diseases may be dominated by the effects on immune function. Acute and chronic leukaemias are associated with depression of T-cell responses (decreased DTH and mitogen responses) and variable effects on B-cell function. Chronic lymphocytic leukaemia for example, is associated with hypogammaglobulinaemia and increased bacterial infections. Immunity may also be compromised as a result of treatment with chemotherapy, irradiation, or splenectomy.

Hodgkin's disease is associated with variable suppression of T-cell responses as demonstrated by DTH and phytohaemagglutinin antigen (PHA)-induced proliferation and either normal or increased immunoglobulin levels, often with depressed specific antibody responses. Multiple myeloma is also associated with dramatic changes in T- and B-cell functioning. There is often a functional hypogammaglobulinaemia despite the presence of high levels of serum immunoglobulin, including paraproteins. There is a decreased antibody response and consequent increased infection rate, particularly bacterial pneumonia.

Drug-induced immunodeficiency

With the advent of a large number of potent drugs and therapies has come the realization that the use of these agents is often associated with profound immunosuppression. Iatrogenic disease is now one of the most frequent causes of secondary immunodeficiency. Corticosteroids and cytotoxic drugs in particular are associated with marked immunosuppression (see Table 4.1).

Clinical features of secondary immunodeficiency

Chronic and severe immunodeficiency is associated with an increased incidence of infections, malignancy, allergy, and autoimmunity (Table 4.2).

Infections

Infections are the most common manifestation of immunodeficiency. The type of infection depends on the nature of the associated immune defect. Table 4.1 summarizes the major immune abnormalities observed in patients with secondary immunodeficiencies. Table 4.4 outlines some of the common infective problems seen in this group of patients. In general, patients with defective humoral immunity are predisposed to recurrent extracellular bacterial infections as a result of defective opsonization and complement-mediated killing of these micro-organisms. In contrast, patients with predominant abnormalities in T-cell-mediated immunity suffer from recurrent infections with obligate intracellular bacteria, viral, fungal, and protozoa.

∎ **Table 4.2** Clinical features of Immunodeficiency

Recurrent infections
  Chronic
  Incomplete resolution
  Refractory to treatment
  Unusual micro-organisms
  Reactions to live vaccines
Growth failure/retardation
Chronic diarrhoea
Rashes: eczema, *candida*
Allergies
Autoimmune diseases
Malignancy

∎ **Table 4.3** Common infections in secondary immunodeficiency

Immunodeficiency	Micro-organisms	Features
Immunoglobulins (IgG, IgM)	Pyogenic extracellular bacteria, *strep., staph., Haemophilus influenzae*. Viruses: enterovirus, VZV pneumocystis	Defective opsonization and killing, recurrent infection: lung, CNS, gastrointestinal tract
Secretory IgA	Pyogenic extracellular bacteria: *strep. staph., Haemophilus*, Gram-negative bacteria, fungi, *Giardia*	Mucosal infections of respiratory and gastrointestinal systems. Phenytoin or D-penicillamine therapy cause IgA deficiency
T cells	Intracellular microbes bacteria: *Mycobacteria, Listeria, Legionella, Salmonella, Nocardia.* fungi: *Candida, Histoplasmosis, Cryptospridiosis, Mucor mycosis* DNA viruses: herpes simplex virus, VZV, cytomegalovirus, papova, protozoa: *Toxoplasmosis, Cryptosporidiosis, Pneumocystis*	Decreased T-cell numbers or function leads to defective activation of intracellular killing of pathogens. Recurrent, often severe infections: lung, CNS, gastrointestinal tract, skin
Neutropenia	Gram negative enteric and pyogenic bacteria: *E. coli, Pseudomonas, Klebsiella*, Staph. *Candida, Aspergillus, Mucor mycosis*	Impaired phagocytic capacity. Septicaemia, pneumonia, bacterial endocarditis, anorectal abscesses
Splenectomy	Pyogenic encapsulated bacteria: *Strep. pneumoniae, H. influenzae, N. meningitidis*	Defective opsonization and phagocytosis. Septicaemia

VZV, varicella zoster virus.

∎ **Table 4.4** Special problems in the immunocompromised host

Problem	Microbial pathogen	Site of infection
Febrile and neutropenic	Gram-negative bacteria: *pseudomonas, klebsiella, E. coli*	Blood, lung, GIT, anorectal, urine, heart
Pneumonia	Oral flora, viral, *Pneumocystis*	RLL and basal segments
CNS infection	*Listeria, Pseudomonas, Strep. Pneumonia, Staph. aureus*, viral, cryptococcal	Meningitis, cerebritis, lung abscesses.
Fungal infections	*Candida, Aspergillus, Cryptococcus, Mucor*	GIT, lung, meninges
Disseminated viral infection	Cytomegalovirus, herpes simplex virus, varicella zoster virus	Skin, GIT, CNS, lung

GIT, gastrointestinal tract.   RLL, Right lower lobe

The indications for investigating patients with recurrent infections are outlined in Table 4.5.

Malignancy

Immunocompromised patients are prone to develop certain malignancies, particularly involving cells of the immune system. Such neoplasms have been described in patients undergoing organ transplantation, with autoimmune diseases treated with immunosuppressive agents, and second malignancies occurring in patients given cancer chemotherapy.

∎ **Table 4.5**   Recurrent infections. Indications for investigation

1.   Recurrent major bacterial infection — pneumonia, meningitis, osteomyelitis, septicaemia.

2.   Severe recurrent infections — bronchitis, otitis media, abscesses, diarrhoea.

3.   Opportunistic infections — *Pneumocystis carinii*, fungi.

4.   Clinical features of a classical immunodeficiency syndrome, e.g. thrombocytopenia, ataxia.

5.   Relative of patient with immunodeficiency.

6.   Unexplained leucopenia and/or lymphopenia <1000 cm^3.

There is a threefold increase of various neoplasms in organ transplant recipients compared with age-matched controls. These malignancies occur in a relatively young adult population whose average age at the time of transplantation is 40 years. On average malignancies appear 60 months after transplantation, but certain neoplasms appear at fairly distinct time intervals after transplantation; Kaposi's sarcoma presents an average of 23 months, lymphomas at an average of 37 months and carcinomas of the vulva and perineum at an average of 100 months.

The most common neoplasms occurring in solid organ transplant patients are those involving the skin and lip. Carcinoma of the lip is increased up to 29-fold compared with the normal population. Squamous cell carcinomas are the most frequent skin cancer in transplant recipients and occur on average 30 years younger than in the general population. In an Australian study a fourfold increased incidence in melanomas has been reported. These cutaneous neoplasms are more frequent, more aggressive, and more likely metastasize than squamous cell carcinomas in normal subjects.

The incidence of non-Hodgkin's lymphoma (NHL) in transplantation patients is 28–49-fold greater than in age-matched controls. Three-quarters of these neoplasms are B-cell lymphomas. Virological studies have indicated that the genome of the EBV is commonly isolated from these lesions. Some NHLs have regressed completely after drastic reduction of immunosuppresive therapy or administration of the antiviral agent acyclovir.

There is a 14-fold increase in carcinoma of the cervix, possibly due to human papillomavirus (HPV) compared with control subjects. Although rare, Kaposi's sarcoma is increased in renal transplant patients 400–500-fold.

Similar increases of neoplasms of the same type has also been observed in patients receiving immunosuppressive therapy for autoimmunity, and those receiving chemotherapeutic treatment for an initial malignancy. For example, patients with rheumatoid arthritis, systemic lupus erythematosus (SLE), and Sjögren's syndrome have shown a marked increase in the incidence of NHL. This neoplasm appears to be increased in patients who have received azathioprine, cyclophosphamide, or chlorambucil for at least a 3 month period. The development of bladder cancer following cyclophosphamide therapy is well recognized with a 13–100-fold increase in patients given this drug for non-malignant disease.

Autoimmune and allergic disease

It is not so widely recognized that immunodeficiency may predispose to autoimmunity. This disease association has been extensively studied in patients with human immunodeficiency virus (HIV) infections where a variety of autoimmune diseases including Sjögren's syndrome, idiopathic thrombocytopenic purpura, and haemolytic anaemia have been described. Similarly, allergic reactions occur with an increased frequency in patients with secondary immunodeficiency and this is exemplified by patients with AIDS in whom allergic reactions, particularly to drugs, is a common clinical problem.

Diagnosis of secondary immunodeficiency

In adults, the majority of cases of immunodeficiency are secondary, and the underlying disorder is usually obvious from a careful clinical appraisal of the patient (Fig 4.1). For example, diabetes, renal failure, and cirrhosis are usually long-standing clinical problems before the features of immunodefiency develop. Similarly, surgery, general anaesthesia, burns, and drug therapy are readily recognized entities often associated with the abrupt onset of a severe, acute immunodeficiency syndrome. In contrast, infiltrative diseases, infections, and autoimmune diseases may be less apparent and complications secondary to a defect in the immune system may provide the initial insight into the presence of one of these conditions.

Recognition of typical clinical features of immunodeficiency

The most important step in the assessment of a patient with a secondary immunodeficiency is to think of the possibility. Secondary immunodeficiency is commonly missed, overlooked, or not considered in the assessment of the patient. Infections are by far the most common complications of both primary and secondary immunodeficiency. Such infections are often due to a selective group of micro-organisms (Tables 4.3 and 4.4).

Such infections may be frequent, severe, complicated, resistant to therapy, slow to resolve, and recurrent (Table 4.5). The nature of the infection is principally determined by the underlying immune defect (Table 4.3). As secondary immunodeficiency syndromes often involve abnormalities of both the humoral and cellular arms of the immune system it is important to assess the exact nature of the underlying immune abnormalities.

Assessment of nature and severity of infections

It is imperative in immunocompromised patients to determine precisely the exact nature and extent of associated infections. This requires microbiological confirmation by culture, serology, and direct detection of the organism by histological or molecular biological techniques. It is important to appreciate that multiple infections may occur simultaneously (Fig. 4.1, Tables 4.3 and 4.4).

Assessment of nature and severity of primary disorder

The patient's history and clinical features should direct the appropriate investigations. Table 4.1 outlines the major immunological defects associated with common causes of secondary immunodeficiency. It is important to assess both the functional as well as quantitative aspects of the components of the immune response. Thus T-cell function (e.g. DTH, cytotoxicity, proliferation to antigen and mitogen, cytokine production) and B-cell function (antibody synthesis, proliferation) should also be considered as well the number of T and B cells in the peripheral blood. A guide to the assessment of patients with compromised immunity is outlined in Table 4.6.

Management of secondary immunodeficiency

The management of secondary immunodeficiency is principally directed at treatment of the primary disease, removal of complicating or exacerbating factors and immune restoration. Unfortunately, achievement of these aims is not always possible. An approach to the treatment of the common secondary immunodeficiency syndromes is summarized in Table 4.7. It is possible to treat the cause of an acquired immunodeficiency effectively, under a number of circumstances. Malnutrition for example, is amenable to treatment with adequate restoration of a balanced protein calories intake. Similarly, a variety of nutritional deficiencies may be rectified and lead to immune restoration. Zinc deficiency, for example, has been widely studied. Animal studies have shown that zinc deficiency diminishes monocyte- and T-cell dependent immune functions, and zinc therapy reverses these defects. In elderly humans zinc supplements have been shown to elevate immune responsiveness.

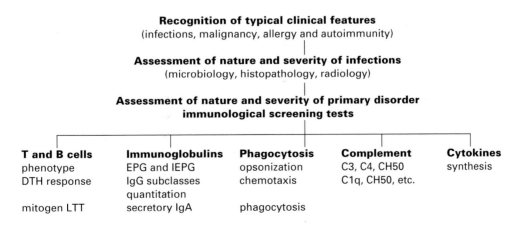

Recognition of typical clinical features
(infections, malignancy, allergy and autoimmunity)

Assessment of nature and severity of infections
(microbiology, histopathology, radiology)

Assessment of nature and severity of primary disorder
immunological screening tests

T and B cells	**Immunoglobulins**	**Phagocytosis**	**Complement**	**Cytokines**
phenotype	EPG and IEPG	opsonization	C3, C4, CH50	synthesis
DTH response	IgG subclasses quantitation	chemotaxis	C1q, CH50, etc.	
mitogen LTT	secretory IgA	phagocytosis		

❙ **Fig. 4.1** Approach to the diagnosis of secondary immunodeficiency.

❚ **Table 4.6**   Assessment of immunity in immunocompromised hosts

Defect	Screening test	Advanced test
Phagocytic	Full blood count and differential, cell morphology	Phagocytosis Chemotaxis Bacterial killing and opsonic activity Nitroblue tetrazolium test
T-cell/macrophage	Lymphocyte count and morphology Delayed-type hypersensitivity skin test X-ray thymus	T-cell subsets Lymphocyte transformation Cytokine assays Lymph node biopsy
Immunoglobulin	Serum immunoglobulins Isohaemaglutinins Antibodies to vaccines	Secretory immunoglobulins Immunoglobulin subclasses B-cell quantitation, immunoglobulin synthesis
Complement	CH50, C3, C4, C1q	CH50, other C components Opsonization

❚ **Table 4.7**   Treatment of acquired and secondary immunodeficiencies

Aetiology	Example	Management
Metabolic disease	Diabetes mellitus, renal failure, cirrhosis, Cushing's syndrome	Maximize medical therapy, correct biochemical abnormalities, treat infections, prophylactic immunization
Malnutrition	Kwashiorkor	Adequate protein calorie, vitamin and mineral replacement: correct abnormalities, treat infections, prophylactic immunization
Infections	Viral: HIV, measles, rubella, CMV	Antiviral therapy, prophylactic immunization, immunotherapy
	Bacterial: tuberculosis, leprosy	Antibiotics, prophylactic immunization
	Fungal: coccidiomycosis	Antifungals, immunotherapy
	Major surgery, splenectomy	Prophylactic immunization (e.g. pneumococcal)
Surgery and general anaesthesia		Symptomatic and supportive (SS) treatment
Prematurity	Newborn infants	SS treatment
Infiltrative diseases	Lymphoma, leukaemia	Chemotherapy: prophylactic immunization (e.g. herpes zoster virus, CMV), bone marrow transplantation, SS treatment
	Myeloma	Chemotherapy, prophylactic immunization, immunoglobulins, SS treatment
Genetic	Down syndrome	Prophylactic immunization Symptomatic and supportive treatment
	Sickle cell anaemia	Prophylactic immunization. SS treatment
Immune (autoimmune) diseases	Rheumatoid arthritis, systemic lupus erythematosus	Stop immunosuppressive drugs. Prophylactic immunization. SS treatment
Immunosuppressive therapy	Corticosteroids, cytotoxics	Stop drug. Prophylactic immunization SS treatment
	Radiation	Stop radiotherapy. Prophylactic immunization. SS treatment

CMV, cytomegalovirus   SS, symptomatic and supportive treatment

Infections commonly exacerbate the immune deficiency that may be secondary to another underlying disease process. Thus it is imperative that aggressive treatment of all infections in immunocompromised hosts be rapidly instituted. Effective therapy is now available for most bacterial and fungal infections, and an increasing array of viral infections. Such infections may require high-dose and long-term therapy (e.g. tuberculosis) to bring about disease remission. Under some circumstances prophylactic long-term antimicrobial therapy may be indicated (e.g. CMV infections, tuberculosis, chronic candidiasis).

Immunosuppression as a result of the use of cytotoxic drugs is best managed by withdrawal of the drug and treatment of any complicating infections or other disease. A similar approach may be required for immunosuppression complicating infiltrative diseases and malignancies.

Immune restoration

Modulation of the immune response is theoretically possible in secondary immunodeficiency states by cell and tissue grafting, and the use of immune enhancing treatments, although this approach is not widely used. There is the possibility that in patients with refractory immunosuppression secondary to disease processes that cannot be modified may be modulated by the use of bone marrow or thymic grafting.

Intravenous immunoglobulin is beneficial in the treatment of infections in patients with multiple myeloma and chronic lymphocytic leukaemia associated with hypogammaglobulinaemia.

The use of thymic factors, antioxidants and an increasing number of cytokines have been examined with some encouraging results in experimental animals and limited human studies. Thymus α-1 substantially restored T-cell function after intravenous injections in mice. Similarly, clinical trials suggest that incorporating cytokines such as gamma-interferon (IFNγ) or IL-12 into vaccines can enhance immune responses. IFNα may enhance phagocytic capacity in immunocompromised subjects. IFNγ therapy has been used in patients with leprosy and leishmania to help reverse the macrophage killing defect.

The use of antioxidants stems from the concept that in many diseases, and in ageing, damage is induced by metabolically derived free radicals. In experimental animals the use of 2-mercaptoethanol has been shown to enhance the antibody forming capacity of old mice and to abrogate the age-related decline in immune response normally seen with ageing.

Immunization

It is important to immunize patients with well characterized immunodeficiencies against potentially life-threatening infections. Caution should be used in the use of live vaccines, especially in patients with severe T-cell immunodeficiency. These include vaccina, BCG (bacille Calmette-Guérin), live polio vaccine (Sabin), measles/mumps, rubella, and yellow fever vaccine. Unlike live vaccines, inactive or recombinant vaccines may safely be given to patients with defective immunity. However, they do not always induce a protective immunity. Increased immunity to infections may also be achieved by passive immunization (e.g. zoster immune globulin). The indications and contraindications to immunization in patients with secondary immunodeficiency are outlined in Table 4.8.

Chronic fatigue syndrome

Definition

Chronic fatigue syndrome (CFS) is a common clinical condition characterized by profound fatigue, sleep disruption, and neuropsychiatric symptoms. Criteria have been developed for research purposes and to aid in the diagnosis of this syndrome (see Table 4.9). The diagnosis of CFS rests upon the recognition of a characteristic symptom complex and also the exclusion of other relevant differential diagnoses.

Pathogenesis

There is increasing evidence that CFS may arise as a result of an abnormal immune response to a variety of common infections. Although the pathophysiology of CFS remains unknown, circumstantial evidence suggests that the condition may result from a disordered immune response to a precipitating infection or antigenic challenge.

CFS is commonly reported to follow an acute viral infection, although in only a minority of cases is the initial infectious agent documented during the acute illness. In these cases a range of common infections have been implicated as apparent precipitants for CFS, including: varicella, EBV, rubella, mumps, enteroviruses, toxoplasmosis, and brucellosis.

Patients with CFS have been reported to have a variety of immunological abnormalities in their peripheral blood. The most consistently reported abnormalities involve depressed T-cell and NK cell activity. Deficiencies in immunoglobulin subclasses have also been noted. Despite these subtle abnormalities in immune system function, patients with CFS do not

∎∎ **Table 4.8**   Immunization in immunodeficient patients

Immunization	Indications	Contraindication
Pneumococcal	Pre-splenectomy and before chemotherapy	
Haemophilus influenzae	Asplenia, immunosuppressive drugs and disease	Allergy to egg protein
Influenza	Immunodeficiency, heart or lung disease. Age >65 years	Allergy to egg protein
BCG	Immunodeficiency with risk of exposure to tuberculosis	T-cell immunodeficiency
ZIG	Immunodeficiency with exposure to varicella zoster virus	History of reactions to human immunoglobulin. IgA deficiency
CMVIG	Immunodeficiency with exposure to cytomegalovirus. Bone marrow and organ transplantation	History of reactions to human immunoglobulin. IgA deficiency
Polio vaccine	Inactive vaccine (Salk) only should be used in patients with T-cell immunodeficiency	T-cell immunodeficiency, pregnancy Avoid in family contacts of immunodeficient patients
Rubella	Inactive vaccines only should be used in patients with T-cell immunodeficiency	T-cell immunodeficiency, pregnancy
Yellow fever	Not indicated in patients with immunodeficiency	T-cell immunodeficiency, pregnancy

∎ **Table 4.9**   Criteria for the diagnosis of chronic fatigue syndrome

(1)   chronic persisting or relapsing fatigue of a generalized nature, exacerbated by minor exercise, causing significant disruption of usual daily activities, present for greater than 6 months, and

(2)   neuropsychiatric dysfunction including impairment of concentration, evidenced by difficulty in completing mental tasks which were easily accomplished prior to the onset of the syndrome, and new onset of short-term memory impairment, and

(3)   no alternative diagnosis reached from the history, physical examination, and appropriate investigation over a 6 month period

appear to have other clinical manifestations of a secondary immunodeficiency such as opportunistic infections, malignancy, or autoimmunity.

Immunological studies in patients with CFS have examined various aspects of the immune response to antigen, including antibody responses, the number and function of NK and T cells, and cytokine production. These studies in patients with CFS have been hampered by at least two major factors: the probable heterogeneity of the patient groups studied, and difficulties in the standardization of immunological tests.

An abnormal immune response to the infections thought to precipitate CFS may allow antigens to evade immune mechanisms (such as antibody-dependent cell-mediated cytotoxicity) crucial for the effective clearance of the agent from the host. The IgG subclass distribution of antibodies generated *in vivo* in response to viral infections (such as EBV, rubella, and varicella zoster virus) is predominantly restricted to the IgG_1, IgG_2 and IgG_3 when compared with normal subjects. Reduced immunoglobulin levels may occur transiently in acute viral infections, including with EBV, and are likely to be due to alteration in the T-cell control of immunoglobulin production and isotype switching by B cells. Cytokines such as $IFN\alpha$, $IFN\gamma$ and IL-4, are known to modulate immunoglobulin synthesis and may play a part in IgG subclass alterations seen in patients with CFS.

Studies of the antibody response to viruses thought to initiate CFS, have focused particularly on the herpes and enterovirus groups. The pattern of development and persistence of IgG antibodies to these viral antigens was previously proposed to be a diagnostic marker for CFS. However, recent studies confirm that neither the presence nor the titre of IgG antibodies to these viruses has any diagnostic usefulness in CFS, although polyclonal activation of antibodies to the herpesviruses (EBV, herpes simplex, CMV, and human herpes virus type-6) has been demonstrated. This antibody production may result from reactivation of latent viral infection, or altered T-cell regulation of immunoglobulin production.

An association exists between atopy and CFS. A history of atopy (inhalant, food, or drug allergy) and skin test reactivity to food and inhalant antigens were found in 50–80% of patients with CFS. This finding contrasts with the prevalence of skin test reactivity of approximately 20–30% in a population of similar age.

NK cells respond rapidly to acute viral infections by proliferation and the lysis of infected cells. This response precedes specific T-cell activation by several days. After this initial NK cell activation, the resolution phase of acute viral infections such as measles are commonly associated with impaired NK cytotoxicity. Estimations of NK cell numbers in the peripheral blood were variable being found to be low, normal, or elevated in these studies. Some studies have found NK cytotoxicity to K562 cells to be impaired. Psychological disturbances such as anxiety and depression have also been shown to impair NK cell function.

Diagnosis

Clinical

The assessment of patients complaining of chronic fatigue requires a thorough history and careful physical examination. In combination with simple laboratory investigations, this will be sufficient to exclude other medical diagnoses. Characteristically, patients with CFS have no abnormalities on physical examination.

Investigations should be used to rule out other relevant diseases which may manifest with fatigue, including endocrine, metabolic, and neurological disorders (flow chart). Although patients with CFS have been shown to have alterations in laboratory assessments of their immune system, such tests are not helpful in verifying the diagnosis for clinical purposes.

The flow chart (Fig. 4.1) outlines an approach to the assessment of patients with chronic fatigue. Several aspects of this approach are noteworthy. The history and physical examination are directed towards finding clues to possible alternative diagnoses. For example, a history of significant weight loss (>10%) should alert the physician to the possibility of an underlying metabolic disorder such as thyrotoxicosis, a chronic infection such as hepatitis B or HIV, or an occult malignancy. The finding of multiple, localized tender points on musculoskeletal examination, along with prominent symptomatic myalgia and arthralgia is consistent with a diagnosis of fibromyalgia. This is a closely related disorder which overlaps greatly, or may be synonymous, with CFS, differing only in the prevalence and severity of musculoskeletal pain.

Careful evaluation of psychological symptoms is important in assessing patients with chronic fatigue. The most difficult differential diagnosis in such patients is to ascertain whether they have a primary psychiatric disorder (such as depression, somatization disorder, or anxiety neurosis) or a primary chronic fatigue state. Helpful clues from the history include the fact that patients with CSF usually do not have a premorbid history of repeated psychological disturbance. In contrast, patients with primary psychiatric disease often have a long history of psychological distress, drug and alcohol abuse, previous psychiatric consultation, and a family history of a similar psychiatric disorder. In addition, the severity of psychological complaints in patients with primary psychiatric disorders is usually greater than those experienced by patients with CFS. A primary depressive illness is suggested particularly by symptoms such as weight loss, feeling of hopelessness, suicidal ideation, and anhedonia (a loss of pleasure in activities of daily life). It is often helpful to obtain a collaborative history from family members to help verify the extent of associated psychological problems.

Laboratory

Investigations are primarily aimed at excluding alternative medical disorders. In patients with CFS, the blood count, film, differential white cell count, and erythrocyte sedimentation rate (ESR) should be normal. Similarly, renal, liver, and thyroid function tests should be normal. Any alterations in these investigations, such as an elevation of ESR, demands further assessment and investigation. For example, a history of painful, blurred vision and the finding of a pale optic disc may suggest multiple sclerosis, and investigation with sensory evoked responses and magnetic resonance imaging scanning should be performed. Similarly, a history of nocturnal snoring, profound daytime somnolence, hypertension, and the finding of a crowded oropharynx, may suggest obstructive sleep apnoea. Referral for sleep studies may be appropriate.

It is likely that the patients diagnosed as having CFS probably do not have a single underlying disease process. Recent research evidence indicates that patients with CFS demonstrate significant heterogeneity in their symptom profile, natural history, and other characteristics, falling into discernible subgroups in which fatigue is the primary complaint.

Measurements of the number of peripheral blood T cells in the various subsets of patients with CFS have yielded conflicting results. In those studies in which absolute numbers (rather than percentages) of T-cell subsets were determined the number of CD4+ (helper/inducer) and CD8+ (suppressor/cytotoxic) T cells was found to be normal in most studies.

Peripheral blood T cells proliferative capacity in response to mitogen also has been shown to be impaired in patients with CFS. As impaired lymphocyte responsiveness to mitogen has been reported to be prevalent in patients with major depression, a matched control group with non-melancholic depression was included in one study. The lymphocyte proliferation in response to PHA was found to be significantly reduced in patients with CFS in comparison with healthy control subjects and subjects with major depression.

The capacity to mount a DTH response *in vivo* to an intradermally injected antigen depends upon prior exposure to the antigen and effective T-cell (and macrophage) function. DTH skin responses have been used to assess the cell-mediated immune function in patients with CFS. The rates of cutaneous anergy in patients with CFS varies from 21 to 54% and in healthy control subjects from 0 to 15%. Hypoergy was demonstrated in 30–50% of patients with CFS, but was found in only 10% of healthy control subjects or subjects with major depression.

It is important to appreciate that acute viral infection is frequently associated with similar alterations in T-cell number and function to those described in patients with CFS. Infections with measles virus, CMV, and EBV have all been shown to produce a transient increase in the prevalence of cutaneous anergy and impaired lymphocyte proliferation in response to mitogen.

The regulation of a cell-mediated immune response to antigen is critically dependent upon the activity of cytokines which function as intercellular messengers. Although essential for effective immunity, cytokines may also directly produce clinical symptoms. For example, profound fatigue and neuropsychiatric symptoms reminiscent of CFS are common adverse effects in patients with chronic hepatitis or malignancy treated with recombinant IFNα. Of the large number of cytokines examined in the serum of patients with CFS, only transforming growth factor-β was found to be consistently elevated.

Tests of immunity in patients with CFS commonly reveal disturbances. The studies reported suggest an association between CFS and altered immune function, with the pattern of findings being similar to that seen in patients during the resolution phase of an acute viral infection. The data are currently limited both by het-

erogeneity within the patient groups studied and by the lack of standardization of immunological assays. Data establishing a causal link between abnormal immunity and CFS have not been found, which may suggest that the alterations occur secondary to an undefined underlying disease process or other co-factor. The prevalence and magnitude of changes in cell-mediated immunity observed in patients with CFS cannot be adequately explained by the co-occurrence of symptomatic depression.

Treatment

There is no cure for CFS. Treatment is symptomatic and supportive, and based on the patients' major clinical problems. Contrary to widely offered opinion, 'rest' is not a cure for CFS. The consequences of the 'rest cure' are uniformly negative muscle wasting, depression, and social isolation.

Although a recently published controlled trial of rehabilitation therapy for patients with CFS (compared with cognitive–behaviour therapy) did not show greater benefit than clinic attendance alone, this study reinforced the feasibility and safety of a gentle exercise regimen. An individually designed, supervised, and graded exercise programme is advisable to maintain some physical conditioning and aerobic fitness in patients with CFS. Psychological support is important and stress management may also be helpful in selected patients (see Table 4.10).

Sleep disturbance is prevalent in patients with CFS, with the complaint of 'non-refreshing sleep' and hypersomnia being almost universal. Regulation of the sleep cycle may provide significant improvement in symptoms. This may be achieved by sedative hypnotics if sleep is very restless or, if insomnia is a feature, tricyclic antidepressants may also be tried. In addition, simple advice to maintain a regular sleep–wake cycle and avoid daytime sleeping is helpful. Similarly, patients with prominent symptoms of fibromyalgia may benefit from a combination of a tricyclic antidepressant and non-steroidal anti-inflammatory drug. A double-blind placebo controlled trial of low-dose tricyclic antidepressant therapy showed amitryptyline 10–30 mg daily to be effective for patients with fibromyalgia. Patients with significant depression intercurrent with CFS may benefit from the use of antidepressants such as fluoxetine or miclobemide. This therapy may substantially improve mood in selected patients, but tends not to alter the severity of the fatigue.

Several studies have examined the use of immunotherapy in the treatment of CFS. An Australian research group showed significant, but transient benefit

▌ **Table 4.10**   Treatment of chronic fatigue syndrome (CFS)

CFS subtype	Possible treatment
1. Post-infective	Symptomatic, high rate of spontaneous remission
2. Concurrent neuropsychological disturbance	Tricyclic antidepressants for sleep disturbance, muscle pain and depression Consider monoamine oxidase inhibitors or non-pharmacological psychological interventions
3. Fibromyalgia	Trial of low-dose tricyclic antidepressant and/or non-steroidal anti-inflammatory drugs
4. Non-specific features	Symptomatic
5. All cases	A structural programme of individually designed graded physical exercise and psychological support may reduce ongoing disability A supportive treatment framework within which both the doctor and patient can facilitate recovery should be sought

from treatment with intravenous immunoglobulin. Transfer factor therapy was found to be ineffective in the treatment of patients with CFS.

Prognosis

There have been few studies of the natural history of CFS. Research indicates that a considerable percentage of patients with CFS spontaneously improve or recover, particularly those with a recent onset postinfective fatigue syndrome. However, patients with associated depression, somatization disorder, or abnormal illness behaviour may suffer a more protracted course over many years. A recent study indicates that the long-term prognosis in patients with CFS may be more closely related to psychological factors than immunological factors.

Further reading

Chandra, R. K. (1981). Immunodeficiency in under and over nutrition. *Nutritional Reviews*, **39**, 22.

Chao, C. C., Janoff, E. N., Hu, S., *et al* (1991). Altered cytokine release in peripheral blood mononuclear cell cultures from patients with the chronic fatigue syndrome. *Cytokine*, **3**, 292–8.

Geokas, M. C., Lakatta, E. G., Makinodan, T., and Timiras, P. S. (1990). The aging process. *Annals of Internal Medicine*, **113**, 455–65.

Griffen, D. E. (1991). Immunologic abnormalities accompanying acute and chronic viral infections. *Review of Infectious Diseases*, **13**, S129–33.

Hickie, I., Hickie, C., Silove, D., Wakefield, D., and Lloyd, A. (1990). Is there significant immune dysfunction in depressive disorders? *Psychological Medicine*, **20**, 755–61.

Klein, L. J. (1985). Incidence of cancers in rheumatoid arthritis and other disorders after immunosuppressive therapy. *American Journal of Medicine*, **78**, 44–9.

Klimas, N. G., Salvato, F. R., Morgan, R., and Fletcher, M. A. (1990). Immunologic abnormalities in chronic fatigue syndrome. *Journal of Clinical Microbiolology*, **28**, 1403–10.

Landay, A. L., Jessop, C., Lennette, E. T., and Levy, J. A. (1991). Chronic fatigue syndrome: clinical condition associated with immune activation. *Lancet*, **338**, 707–12.

Lloyd, A. R., Wakefield, D., Dwyer, J., and Boughton, C. (1989). Immunological abnormalities in the chronic fatigue syndrome. *Medical Journal of Australia*, **151**, 122–4.

Lloyd, A. R., Hickie, I., Boughton, C. R., Spencer, O., and Wakefield, D. (1990a). The prevalence of chronic fatigue syndrome in an Australian population. *Medical Journal of Australia*, **153**, 522–8.

Lloyd, A., Hickie, I., Wakefield, D., Boughton, C., and Dwyer, J. (1990b). A double-blind, placebo-controlled trial of intravenous immunoglobulin therapy in patients with the chronic fatigue syndrome. *American Journal of Medicine*, **89**, 561–8.

Lloyd, A., Hickie, I., Brockman, A., Dwyer, J., and Wakefield, D. (1991). Serum and cerebrospinal fluid cytokine levels in patients with chronic fatigue syndrome and control subjects. *Journal of Infectious Diseases*, **164**, 1023–8.

Lloyd, A., Hickie, I., Hickie, C., and Wakefield, D. (1992). Cell-mediated immunity in patients with chronic fatigue syndrome, healthy control subjects and patients with major depression. *Clinical and Experimental Immunology*, **87**, 76–9.

Penn, I. (1988). Tumours of the immunocompromised patients. *Annual Review of Medicine*, **39**, 63–73.

Reinherz, E., O'Brien, C., Rosenthal, P., and Schlossman, S. (1980). The cellular basis for viral-induced immunodeficiency: Analysis by monoclonal antibodies. *Journal of Immunology*, **125**, 1269–745.

Rinaldo, C. R. (1990). Immune suppression by herpes viruses. *Annual Review of Medicine*, 331–8.

Sissons, J. G. P. and Borysiewicz, L. K. (1985). Viral immunopathology. *British Medical Bulletin*, **41**, 34–40.

Straus, S. E., Tosato, G., Armstrong, G. *et al.* (1985). Persisting illness and fatigue in adults with evidence of Epstein–Barr virus infection. *Annals of Internal Medicine*, **102**, 7–16.

Straus, S. E., Dale, J. K., Wright, R., and Metcalfe, D. D. (1988). Allergy and the chronic fatigue syndrome. *Journal of Allergy and Clinical Immunology*, **81**, 791–5.

Wakefield, D., Lloyd, A., and Brockman, A. (1990). Immunoglobulin subclass abnormalities in patients with chronic fatigue syndrome. *Paediatric Infectious Diseases Journal*, **9**, S50–3.

Section II

Allergic diseases

5 Allergic rhinitis

A. Kupa and J. Bradley

Definition

Allergic rhinitis is a nasal inflammatory state resulting from immunoglobulin E (IgE)-mediated sensitivity to inhalant allergens such as pollens, dust mites, animal danders, and moulds. Less commonly, food allergens may also cause symptoms. Symptoms include sneezing, itching nose and eyes, increased secretions, and nasal obstruction.

Introduction

Incidence
Allergic rhinitis is predominantly a disorder of children and young adults, but can occur at any age. It affects approximately 20% of the population. Factors that influence the development of allergic rhinitis are:

1. *Environmental.* The incidence is affected by month of birth, viral infection, prevalent allergens in the home and work environment, and the level of exposure to seasonal allergens. The risk of developing hayfever is doubled in persons born in spring. Exposure to parental smoking and atmospheric pollution facilitates sensitization to allergens.

2. *Genes and family history.* Allergic rhinitis is more common in males and is inversely related to family size, the first born being at greatest risk. If both parents are atopic, there is a 50% risk of atopy for each offspring.

Pathogenesis

The sensitized atopic individual has IgE antibodies which bind to high affinity receptors on mast cells and basophils. Exposure of the nasal mucosa to allergen results in mast cell degranulation with release of pre-formed mediators such as histamine, kinins, prostaglandin (PGD_2), leukotrienes, and tryptase, demonstrable in nasal washings following allergen challenge. The resultant inflammatory response is characterized histologically, by submucosal vascular dilatation, oedema, increased numbers of goblet, cells, eosinophils, and other inflammatory cells and clinically by pruritus, sneezing, rhinorrhoea, and congestion.

During the pollen season, the number of circulating and nasal intraepithelial mast cells is increased. The latter are mainly of the mucosal phenotype–chymase negative, tryptase positive. Histamine is probably the major mediator of symptoms and specific anti-H_1 antagonists reduce symptoms, but other mediators such as prostaglandins, leukotrienes, and kinins play a part particularly in congestion.

A variety of cytokines elaborated by T cells contribute to the amplification and regulation of the allergic inflammation. The T-cell response in the nasal mucosa is of the Th2 type with an increased production of interleukin (IL)-4, IL-5 and less interferon (IFN) γ, and detectable mRNA for IL-4 and IL-5 production. The number of antigen presenting cells and IL-2 receptor (CD25) positive T cells is increased, reflecting T-cell activation. IL-5 stimulates eosinophil proliferation and activation, IL-4 is necessary for IgE production by B cells and activates endothelium for eosinophil transmigration, and IL-3, a mast cell growth factor, is critical in allowing movement of unprimed eosinophils into tissues.

Late-phase response (LPR)

Approximately 50% of patients manifest a LPR to allergen, characterized especially by obstructive symptoms and eosinophil and basophil infiltration. Activated eosinophils produce a number of substances which are toxic to nasal epithelial cells: eosinophil cationic protein, major basic protein (MBP), and eosinophil peroxidase (EPO). The spectrum of media-

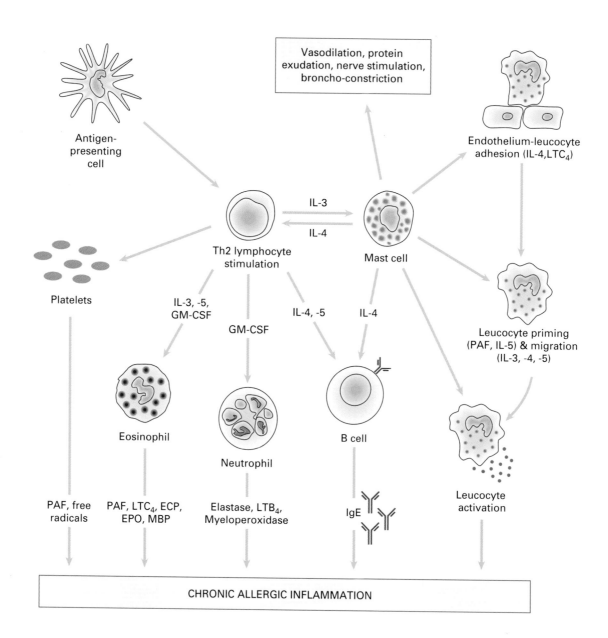

▮ **Fig. 5.1** Cells and cytokines involved in chronic allergic inflammation. PAF, platelet-activating factor; GM-CSF, granulocyte-macrophage colony-stimulating factor. ECP, eosinophil cationic protein; EPO, eosinophil peroxide; MBP, major basic protein.

tors detected during the LPR suggests basophils rather than mast cells are involved because PGD_2 (a mast cell mediator) is absent. During continuous exposure to an allergen, the sensitized patient may become responsive to doses of allergens that are only ~1% of the initial sensitizing dose. The airways which have been 'primed' by allergen exposure are also hyper-reactive to a variety of irritant stimuli, such as smoke, strong smells, temperature and humidity changes, or histamine/methacholine provocative challenge. This phenomenon of *non-specific hyper-reactivity* is analogous to that seen in the lower airways in association with inflammatory changes.

Allergens

Inhalant allergic diseases may be episodic, seasonal or perennial and may produce allergic rhinitis, conjunctivitis, and asthma. Most allergens are 2–60 μm in size — particles 15–25 μm, such as pollen grains, impinge on the conjunctivae as well, but those <15 μm (such as fungal spores) are usually not a cause of conjunctivitis. The allergenic constituents are usually protein and with a molecular weight of 10 000–40 000.

Seasonal allergens are typically grass, weed and tree pollens. The predominant allergens vary with geographical area — ragweed pollen in North America; Timothy and cocks foot grass in the UK and parts of Europe; rye grass in Australia; tree pollens in Scandinavia (birch), Japan (cedar), and Mediterranean climates (olive). Fungal spores may also have a seasonal predominance in temperate zones, e.g. alternaria and cladosporium.

Perennial allergens include house dust mite, cockroach, moulds, and animal allergens. The dust mite thrives in warm humid indoor environments, particularly in mattresses, bedding, carpets, and upholstery. House dust consists of house dust mite organism and faeces, animal dander, insect constituents, vegetable fibre, and other debris. Dog and cat allergens are from saliva, skin dander, and urine.

Occupational allergens include baker's flour, wood dust, isocyanates, and animal allergens.

Ingested (food) allergens such as cow's milk protein are a cause of rhinitis in infants and young children, but are uncommon as a cause of rhinitis in older age groups.

Clinical features

The history is directed at the symptom profile, family history of atopy, associated atopic symptoms such as wheeze or eczema, and a detailed enquiry regarding domestic or work-related allergen exposure, seasonal factors, perceived dietary contributions, and pet exposure. Enquiry about the bedroom environment and bedding type may suggest that dust mite exposure is high.

The major symptoms are sneezing, excess nasal secretion, itching of the nose, eyes, palate and even ears, and nasal obstruction. A symptom diary quantitating the number of sneezes, nose blowings, and duration of symptoms is often helpful. Responses to previous medications should be elicited. With increasing chronicity, the symptom profile may become less irritative and more obstructive with mucus post-nasal drip. Nasal blockage may result in mouth breathing, snoring, sleep apnoea, dryness of the mouth and throat, nasal voice, and loss of smell. In perennial rhinitis, nasal hyper-reactivity is marked. Patients report aggravation of symptoms by non-specific irritants such as cold air, dust, and fumes. In severe allergic rhinitis, patients may feel generally unwell and very tired. There may be a progression of symptoms to asthma at the peak of allergen exposure.

Physical findings

In acute or seasonal allergic rhinitis, there may be reddening of the nose from constant blowing, and irritated conjunctivae or even conjunctival chemosis.

▌ **Table 5.1** Major inhalant allergens

Grasses	*Trees*
Rye	Olive
Timothy grass	Japanese cedar (Japan)
Cocksfoot	Oak (UK and USA), birch, hazel
Ragweed	Silver birch (Scandinavia)
Bermuda grass	
Couch	
Domestic	*Moulds*
House dust mite (*D. pteronysinnus* and farinae)	*Alternaria*
Cat, dog, horse, guinea-pig, hamster protein	*Cladosporium*
Cockroach	

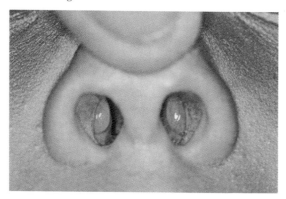

▌**Fig. 5.2** Nasal mucosa in allergic rhinitis with pale shiny swollen mucosa.

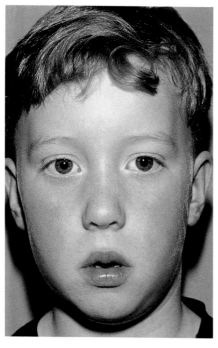

▌**Fig. 5.3** Chronic allergic facies with characteristic open mouth breathing

Examination of the nostrils reveals glistening pale bluish inferior nasal turbinates with clear mucoid secretions. The chronic allergic facies includes: open mouth breathing; dark rings under the eyes due to venous engorgement ('allergic shiners'); dental overbite; transverse nasal crease due to constant rubbing of the nose upwards; the 'allergic salute' (pushing the anterior nares upwards). Nasal passages may be completely obstructed by prominent turbinates. Nasal polyps may occur in association with rhinitis (2%) but

▌**Table 5.2** Classification of rhinitis

Allergic	*Perennial* (non seasonal): e.g. house dust mite, cat, feathers
	Seasonal: grass and tree pollens, moulds
Non-allergic	*Eosinophilic*
	Vasomotor

are more frequent in: males of 30–40 years; those with sinusitis, asthma, and aspirin intolerance; and in children with cystic fibrosis.

Differential diagnosis

Seasonal rhinitis is easily recognized.

The symptom profile of chronic or perennial allergic rhinitis overlaps that of other chronic nasal conditions. Obstruction, rhinorrhea, and nasal hyper-reactivity are features of allergic and non-allergic perennial rhinitis. The latter is defined by negative skin tests and RAST testing (radioallergosorbent test) and is divided into vasomotor and eosinophilic groups. Patients with vasomotor rhinitis have an exaggerated response to physiological or irritative stimuli, e.g. emotional arousal, exercise, changes in ambient humidity, exposure to food smells, or strong perfumes. Occasional patients report nasal congestion after ingestion of wine or amine-rich foods.

Eosinophilic rhinitis resembles allergic rhinitis but there are no identified allergens. There is a strong association between nasal eosinophilia, polyposis, asthma, and aspirin intolerance. Nasal polyps arise in the ethmoidal sinuses in patients with a long history of perennial rhinitis. They present with nasal obstruction, loss of smell, and nasality of voice.

Nasal obstruction may also be due to structural abnormalities, e.g. deviated nasal septum, tumours of the nasophaynx, nose, and sinuses, and vasculitic conditions (Wegener's granulomatosis).

Nasal congestion is seen as a side-effect of α or β adrenoreceptor antagonist drugs, with oral contraceptive use or during pregnancy; and as a rebound phenomenon after topical vasoconstrictor sprays, especially in rhinitis medicamentosa. Cocaine sniffing causes rhinorrhoea and septal perforation.

In children, the differential diagnosis includes adenoidal hypertrophy with persistent obstruction, especially at night; polyposis is associated with cystic fibrosis, infectious rhinitis, and foreign body.

Sinusitis occurs as a complication of perennial rhinitis or polyposis. Symptoms include headache, facial pain, persistent purulent discharge and post-nasal drip, fatigue, and fever. The diagnosis is often missed in children as pain is uncommon and the only symptoms may be night-time cough, fatigue, and irritability. Pneumococci and *Haemophilus influenzae* are common infecting agents.

Investigations

Immediate hypersensitivity prick skin testing to common inhalant allergens is the most appropriate way of defining allergen sensitivities. A standard panel including pollens and mould spores relevant to the area, dust mites, and animal danders should be used. Results should be interpreted in the light of the clinical history as a positive skin test *per se* does not imply clinical disease. Foods are rarely the cause of rhinitis and the result of skin testing correlates less well with the history than that for inhalant allergens. Skin tests can be performed on small children but are contraindicated in severe eczema or dermatographism.

RAST testing correlates well with skin testing and enables determination of levels of specific IgE antibody to allergens. The sensitivity for inhalant allergens is 60–80% and the specificity as high as 90%. Modern tests often contain a mix of allergens and interpretation of positive results may require further screening to individual allergens.

IgE level may be normal in allergic rhinitis, although if asthma or eczema are present it is usual to find an elevated serum IgE. A very low IgE level tends to exclude atopy.

Blood eosinophilia can occur in both allergic and non-allergic rhinitis and its absence does not exclude atopy.

Nasal smear examination may be helpful in distinguishing between infectious and non-infectious rhinitis

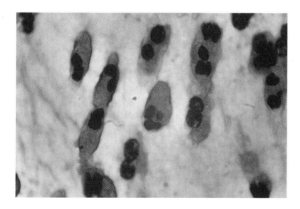

▌ **Fig. 5.4** Nasal exudate smear showing eosinophils.

and in subclassifying perennial rhinitis. This test has variable reproducibility. Samples are obtained by the patient blowing his or her nose on a plastic sheet or by scraping the nasal mucosa with a cotton swab and transferring the smear to a glass slide. The presence of eosinophils suggests that a good response to topical corticosteroids is likely.

Nasal allergen provocation tests are useful in selected clinical situations to confirm suspected sensitivity to an allergen and as a research tool. Results are assessed by symptom scores and/or measurement of nasal airways resistance. Provocative testing can also be used to demonstrate the efficacy of an immunotherapy course. The procedure is time-consuming, potentially dangerous, and not commonly used in clinical practice.

X-rays of sinuses may show sinus membrane thickening, opacification or air fluid levels in sinusitis. Computerized tomography of sinuses with coronal views is a more sensitive investigation and more readily detects ethmoidal sinus change and compromise to osteomeatal units.

Treatment of allergic rhinitis

Allergen avoidance

This is most effective in animal and dust mite allergies. Measures to avoid dust mite exposure include removal of carpets, encasing of mattress and pillows, hot washing of bedding, damp dusting, and perhaps use of newer mitocidal benzoate based or tannate sprays, which denature the dust mite protein. Filtering devices such as electrostatic precipitators and high-efficiency particle arresting filters are helpful in clearing airborne pollens but are of limited usefulness in clearing dust mite allergens.

Drug therapy

Antihistamines

H_1 receptor antagonists have traditionally been used to control itching, sneezing, and rhinorrhoea. Older antihistamines may have sedative and anticholinergic side-effects such as blurred vision and dry mouth and irritability in children and the elderly. The newer highly specific H_1 receptor antagonists terfenadine, astemizole, loratadine, and cetirizine are effective for the irritative symptoms, especially if given prophylactically. They are non-sedative and generally well tolerated.

Terfenadine and astemizole have been reported to cause cardiac arrhythmias (*torsade de pointes*) when used in excessive dosage or in combination with macrolide antibiotics such as erythromycin and ketoconazole.

Levocabastine is a new potent H_1 antihistamine developed for topical use as a nasal spray and eye drops in allergic rhinitis and conjunctivitis. It is effective when applied twice daily and has no adverse effects on mucociliary function.

Nasal decongestants

α-adrenergic agonists (sympathomimetic) drugs offer effective temporary relief of nasal obstruction by vasoconstrictor action on hyperaemic nasal mucosa.

Drugs such as phenylephrine, oxymetazoline, and tramazoline are used as topical agents in sprays or drops with rapid onset of action and duration (3–6 h). Administration of drops is most effective if the patient is in the kneeling or prone position with head down and forwards, so that drops penetrate the osteomeatal complex.

Topical decongestants are contraindicated for long-term use as severe rebound congestion may occur (rhinitis medicamentosa).

Oral decongestants such as pseudoephedrine or phenylpropanolamine are widely available as non-prescription items for treating non-allergic rhinitis. They may cause restlessness, insomnia, tremor, tachycardia, hypertension, and bladder dysfunction. They are contraindicated in patients with hypertension, heart disease, diabetes, hyperthyroidism or those on monoamine-oxidase inhibitor drugs. Proprietary combinations of α-adrenergic agents and antihistamines provide effective control of rhinitis symptoms for many patients especially children.

Sodium cromoglycate

Topical sodium cromoglycate (spray or powder) is of particular value as a prophylactic agent for predictable allergen exposure, e.g. in seasonal or animal-related rhinitis. Its effects are transient, requiring dosages at 3–4 hourly intervals. It has no side-effects apart from causing sneezing in the occasional patient. Patient response to the drug and compliance are variable.

Corticosteroids

Topical corticosteroids, e.g. beclomethasone dipropionate, flunisolide, or budesonide offer highly effective relief of irritative and obstructive symptoms. There is a reduction in the number and activity of inflammatory cells in both early and late-phase responses, and a corresponding decrease in nasal hyper-reactivity. Regular topical corticosteroid used daily or twice a day, pro-vides maximal benefit in a few days and can be continued on a long-term basis without nasal mucosal atrophy, although reassessment of need for medication is appropriate after a few months. The minimal effective daily dose should be used. Long-term topical steroid use is particularly indicated in nasal polyposis.

Systemic absorption of nasal steroids at recommended maintenance dosages is well below that causing adrenal suppression, but the combined absorption of topical steroids for asthma, eczema, and rhinitis in the highly atopic child may reach significance. Side-effects include local burning or irritation, epistaxis, and very rarely nasal septal perforation if the spray is consistently applied to the septum.

Oral corticosteroids may be of great benefit in the severely distressed patient with total nasal obstruction, to achieve rapid symptom relief and permit access for topical medication. Short courses of prednisolone, e.g. 30 mg daily for 3 days tapering to nil over several days, are appropriate. Prolonged oral administration of corticosteroids cannot be justified.

Depot injections of corticosteroids have a prolonged duration of action which may last an entire pollen season, but cause significant adrenal suppression and are used infrequently since the advent of topical steroid sprays.

Ipratropium bromide is an anticholinergic agent which is effective for all types of watery rhinorrhoea. As it has no effect on congestive and irritative symptoms, it is not often used in allergic rhinitis.

Immunotherapy

Conventional immunotherapy is an immunologically specific treatment for allergic rhinitis, of proven efficacy in pollen and dust mite rhinitis. It involves the weekly subcutaneous injection of increasing concentrations of allergen extracts. It is a useful adjunct to drug therapy, often allowing substantial reductions in medical requirements when maintenance therapy is achieved. Immunotherapy should be considered for the patient whose symptoms fail to respond to maximal medical and environmental measures, or whose medication is poorly tolerated. Patients with severe rhinitis may prefer a therapy which modulates their specific immune response and abrogates the need for long-term medication. Patients' symptoms, however, should be sufficient to justify the risks of immunotherapy and the high cost.

Requirements for immunotherapy include: (i) strong provocative or historical evidence of reaction to allergen(s), and (ii) demonstration of specific IgE to the allergen(s) by immediate hypersensitivity skin prick testing or RAST testing.

The likelihood of a response is greatest in patients with a predominant allergen, e.g. grass pollen rhinitis, dust mite, or animal-related rhinitis. Highly atopic patients with multiple inhalant allergies and less well defined symptom profiles are less likely to respond.

Immunotherapy for pollen rhinitis is generally given on a pre-seasonal basis for several years with increasing doses of allergens in sequential courses. Dosage schedules should be flexible and adjusted on an individual basis by an experienced consultant allergist. The maximum tolerated dose is recommended as clinical efficacy is dose related. There are no firm guidelines on duration of treatment. Immunotherapy for perennial aeroallergens such as dust mites may require long-term maintenance.

The most commonly used preparations for rhinitis immunotherapy are pyridine-extracted alum-precipitated extracts which have an excellent safety record. Aqueous allergen extracts may be more effective in some situations such as dust mite sensitivity but are more likely to cause systemic adverse reactions. In recent years allergen extract standardization has improved. Major allergens for many of the most important allergen sources have been identified and molecular weight obtained *(Da)*, e.g. cat — *Fel .dI (32 000)*; mite — *Der. pI (25 371)* and *Der. pII (14 131)*; rye grass — *Lol. pI (27–35 000), pII (11 000), pIII (11 000), pIV (57 000), pV (25–30 000)*. It is likely that future allergen preparations will contain a limited number of major allergens or epitopes produced by recombinant DNA techniques. Modified recombinant allergens may be developed which act directly on T cells without binding antibody and triggering mediator release from mast cells.

Immunotherapy has the potential to induce anaphylaxis, but if firm guidelines are followed, the majority of patients experience only local side-effects such as arm swelling. Immunotherapy should be given in a place where full resuscitative facilities are available. Patients should be observed for 45 min after their injection as virtually all major systemic reactions occur within 30 min.

Immunotherapy is contraindicated in patients with unstable asthma, cardiac disease, hyperthyroidism, beta blocker medication, malignancy, or immunological disorders. Injections should not be given if there is evidence of intercurrent infection or illness or active asthma on spirometric testing. It is unwise to commence immunotherapy in pregnancy as systemic adverse reactions could affect pregnancy outcome.

Surgery

This has a complementary role to pharmacotherapy in allergic rhinitis. Polyps may require surgical removal, although are likely to recur unless long-term topical corticosteroids are instituted. Anatomical obstructions such as deviated nasal septum may require surgical correction. Occasionally, surgical reduction of nasal turbinates is useful in refractory rhinitis. The advent of endoscopic nasal surgery to improve osteomeatal patency has brought considerable relief to many sinusitis sufferers. Vidian neurectomy has been used in some patients with diffuse rhinorrhoea but ipratropium bromide therapy is likely to supercede radical surgery.

Further reading

Bierrnan, C. W., Pierson, W. E., and Donaldson, J. A. (ed.) (1988). International Symposium on Allergy and Associated Disorders in Otolaryngology. *Journal of Allergy and Clinical Immunology*, **81**, 939.

Mygind, N. and Weeke, B. (ed.) (1985). *Allergic and vasomotor rhinitis: clinical aspects.* Munksgaard, Copenhagen.

Naclerio, R. M. (1991). Allergic rhinitis. *New England Journal of Medicine*, **325**, 860–9.

Naclerio, R. M., Baroody, F. M., Kagey-Sobotka, A., Lichtenstein, L. M. (1994). Basophils and eosinophils in allergic rhinitis. *Journal of Allergy and Clinical Immunology*, **94**, 1303–9.

Naspitz, C. K. and Tinkelman, D. G. (ed.) (1990). *Childhood rhinitis and sinusitis, pathophysiology and treatment.* Marcel Dekker Inc., New York.

Pipkorn, U. (1993). Allergic diagnosis and treatment. In *Allergy* (ed. S. T. Holgate and M. K. Church), pp. 18.1–18.10 . Gower Medical Publishing, London.

Solomon, W. R., Mathews, K. P. (1988). Aerobiology and inhalant allergens. In *Allergy: principles and practice*, 4th edn (ed. E. J. Middleton Jr, C. E. Reed, E. F. Ellis, N. F. Adkinson Jr, and J. W. Yunginger), pp. 312–72. Mosby-Year Book Co St Louis, MO.

Vadas, M., Lopez, A., Gamble, J., Khew-Goodall, Y., Smith, W., Bernard, C., *et al.* (1994). Cytokines and allergy. *Journal of Allergy and Clinical Immunology*, **94**, 1289–93.

6 Allergic eye disease

S. Lightman

Definition

The term 'allergic eye disease' is used to describe a number of diseases, predominately affecting the conjunctiva, which occur with increased frequency in people who are atopic. The spectrum encompasses at one end, the non-sight-threatening disorders seasonal allergic conjunctivitis (SAC), perennial allergic conjunctivitis (PAC), and giant papillary conjunctivitis (GPC). Two disorders form the more severe end with potential corneal involvement vernal keratoconjunctivitis (VKC) and atopic keratoconjunctivitis (AKC).

Seasonal allergic conjunctivitis and perennial allergic conjunctivitis

SAC is a part of the symptom complex of hay fever, with pollen being a common allergen and is characterized by mild redness, itching, watering, and discomfort. PAC is a more chronic disorder in which allergy to house dust mite is a significant association. Again, itching and discomfort are a common feature but many of these eyes look only very mildly inflamed. Clinical signs are minimal in both disorders with slight oedema and hyperaemia of the conjunctiva with small papillae.

In both of these disorders, conjunctival biopsy reveals increased numbers of mast cells, neutrophils and eosinophils, in the epithelium and subepithelial stroma. In seasonal disease, the conjunctiva returns to normal after the allergen season so that no increase in cellularity is seen in conjunctival biopsies taken out of season. No increase in collagen is found in contradistinction to the findings in the bronchioli in allergic asthma.

Treatment

Patients are treated by allergen avoidance if possible or with oral antihistamines, together with local mast cell stabilizers. Topical antihistamines are usually of little use. Cromoglycate is effective and is usually given topically in a four times a day dosage. Other more recently introduced drugs include nedocromil and levocabastine both of which have been shown to be effective when given topically, particularly in SAC, and may have advantages in needing less frequent dosage. Topical corticosteroids are not required and have potentially sight-threatening consequences such as induction of cataract and glaucoma. For these reasons they should not be used in these mild disorders which in themselves do not sight-threatening sequelae.

Foreign body associated giant papillary conjunctivitis

This can occur in wearers of all types of contact lenses, in patients with ocular prostheses and in association with exposed sutures, extruding scleral buckles, and cyanoacrylate glue.

Symptoms of discomfort, increased mucus accumulation, itching on lens removal, and reduced lens wearing tolerance occur weeks to months after lens or prosthesis wear has started. The signs are similar to VKC (see below) but there is no corneal involvement and no threat to sight. It differs from VKC in that histamine and eosinophil major basic protein (MBP) levels are not raised in the tears, there is no seasonal variation and it occurs in both sexes and all ages. There may or may not be a history of atopy.

Treatment

This is directed to improvement of lens hygiene, trying different types of lenses such as those with modified edges or made of different materials, reduction in wearing time or using a smaller lens. Offending sutures are removed and cromoglycate has been shown to be effective in the management of GPC. Topical steroid preparations are not indicated for the reasons outlined above except in patients with an ocular prosthesis.

Vernal keratoconjunctivitis

VKC is a seasonal chronic disorder affecting atopic children and young adults in the UK with exacerbations occurring in the Spring, whereas in parts of the Mediterranean, Middle East, Far East, Africa, and South America it is often continuous and may not be associated with atopy. Itching is a predominant feature, with photophobia and discomfort associated with the stringy exudate. Visual loss can occur from associated corneal problems.

Characteristically VKC has large 'cobblestone' papillae on the upper tarsal conjunctiva (Fig. 6.1). When active the conjunctiva is oedematous, infiltrated, and mucus is abundant. Corneal involvement can be mild with punctate epitheliopathy and if the disease is not rapidly brought under control, can progress to corneal macroerosion (Fig. 6.2). This can result in plaque formation when mucus and fibrin are deposited and visual loss can occur.

Histologically, the giant papillae contain an abundance of lymphocytes (Fig. 6.3) (particularly CD4+ T cells), eosinophils with MBP granules seen free in the tissues, mast cells and plasma cells. Thickening of the stroma occurs with extensive deposition of collagen (Fig. 6.4). Some of the T cells express the interleukin-2 receptor and can also be shown to secrete interleukins-3 and -5. Interleukin-5 can activate eosinophils

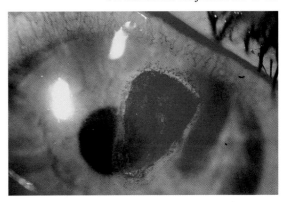

▮ **Fig. 6.2** Corneal macro-erosion stained with rose bengal in active vernal keratoconjunctivitis.

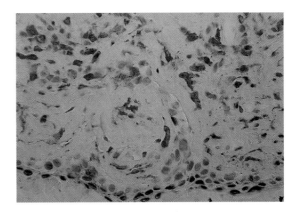

▮ **Fig. 6.3** Giant papillae stained with anti-CD3 monoclonal antibody.

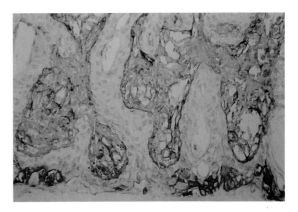

▮ **Fig. 6.4** Giant papillae stained with MoAb for collagen type 5.

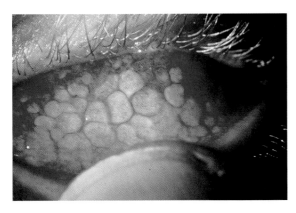

▮ **Fig. 6.1** Large cobblestone papillae on upper tarsal conjunctiva in vernal keratoconjunctivitis.

and MBP is known to be cytotoxic to corneal epithelial cells.

Treatment

A large proportion of patients with VKC need topical corticosteroids when the disease is active but some benefit is also derived from cromoglycate, which does have asteroid sparing benefit. In acute exacerbations intensive topical steroids and cromoglycate are given and the steroids are then tailed off, continuing with cromoglycate once a day for the rest of the year. Topical cyclosporin has also been reported to be helpful. Mucolytic therapy such as acetylcysteine can help and antibiotic prophylaxis is also given topically. Usually intensive topical steroids are required and surgical excision may be necessary if the epithelium does not heal and plaque formation occurrs in the visual axis. In the UK, VKC in children may resolve spontaneously at puberty but can go on to AKC.

AKC is probably the most serious of the 'atopic eye diseases'. It is a life-long, sight-threatening disease characterized by thickened, often keratinized lid margins which are chronically infected by staphylococci. Chronic infiltration of the conjunctiva, often with cicatrization and corneal epithelial defects can result in scarring and neovascularization (Fig. 6.5). Herpes simplex infection is often a problem, and keratoconus, cataract, and retinal detachment can also occur.

Histologically, the conjunctiva is hyperaemic and infiltrated by lymphocytes, plasma cells, and eosinophils. Scarring can also occur particularly in the tarsal conjunctiva. Treatment is aimed at management of the lid margin disease and oral corticosteroids are usually required to control the conjunctival inflammation. Many require additional antiviral treatment while on steroids as herpes simplex infection of the cornea is often a problem and cromoglycate is said to have some steroid sparing effect. Topical cyclosporin has also been found to be helpful in some patients.

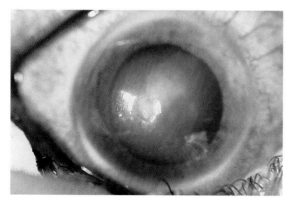

■ **Fig. 6.5** Corneal plaque with stromal scarring in atopic keratoconjunctivitis.

A greater understanding of the pathogenic mechanisms of these diseases should allow more effective therapeutic strategies to be defined for the sight-threatening diseases VKC and AKC. These patients should be managed by an ophthalmologist whereas with the less serious disorders of SAC and PAC can largely be managed by physicians dealing with allergy.

Further reading

Allansmith, M. R. and Ross, R. N. (1988). Giant papillary conjunctivitis. *International Ophthalmology Clinics*, **28**, 309–16.

Allansmith, M. R., Baird, R. S., and Greiner, J. V. (1979). Vernal conjunctivitis and contact lens-associated giant papillary conjunctivitis compared and contrasted. *American Journal of Ophthalmology*, **87**, 544–55.

Baryishak, Y. R., Zavaro, A., Monselise, M., Samra, Z., and Sompolinsky, D. (1982). Vernal keratoconjunctivitis in an Israeli group of patients and its treatment with sodium cromoglycate. *British Journal of Ophthalmology*, **66**, 18–22.

Barishak, Y., Zavaro, A., Samra, Z., and Sompolinsky, D. (1984). An immunological study of papillary conjunctivitis due to contact lenses. *Current Eye Research*, **3**, 1161–8.

Befus, A. D., Bienenstock, J., and Denburg, J. A. (ed.) (1986). *Mast cell differentiation and heterogeneity*. Raven Press, New York.

Buckley, R. J. (1989). Vernal keratoconjunctivitis. *International Ophthalmology Clinics*, **29**, 303–8.

Dart, J. K. G., Buckley, R. J., Monnickendam, M., and Prasad, J. (1986). Perennial allergic conjunctivitis: definition, clinical characteristics and prevalence. A comparison with seasonal conjunctivitis. *Transactions of the Ophthalmological Societies of the United Kingdom*, **105**, 513–20.

Denburg, J. A., Dolovich, J., and Harnish, D. (1989). Basophil, mast cell and eosinophil growth and differentiation factors in human allergic disease. *Clinical and Experimental Allergy*, **19**, 249–54.

El-Asrar, A. M. A., Geboes, K., Misotten, L., Emarah, M. H., Maudgal, P. C., and Desmet, V. (1987). Cytological and immunohistochemical study of the limbal form of vernal keratoconjunctivitis by the replica technique. *British Journal of Ophthalmology*, **71**, 867–72.

El-Asrar, A. M. A., Van den Oord, J. J., Geboes, K., Missotten, L., Emarah, M. H., and Desmet, V. (1989). Immunological study of vernal keratoconjunctivitis. *Graefe's Archives of Clinical and Experimental Ophthalmology*, **227**, 374–9.

Foster, C. S., Rice, B. A., and Dutt, J. E. (1991). Immunopathology of atopic conjunctivitis. *Ophthalmology*, **98**, 1190–6.

Galli, S. J. and Austen, K. F. (ed.) (1989). *Mast cell and basophil differentiation and function in health and disease*. Raven Press, New York.

Gleich, G. J., Frigas, E., Loegering, D. A., Wassom, D. L., and Steinmuller, D. (1979). Cytotoxic properties of the eosinophil major basic protein. *Journal of Immunology*, **123**, 2925–7.

Morgan, S. J., Williams, J., Wails, A. F., Church, M. K., Holgate, S. T., and McGill, J. I. (1991). Mast cell numbers and staining characteristics in the normal and allergic conjunctiva. *Journal of Allergy and Clinical Immunology*, **87**, 111–16.

Sompolinsky, D., Samra, Z., Zavaro, A., and Barishak, R. A. (1982). Contribution to the immunopathology of vernal keratoconjunctivitis. *Documenta Ophthalmologica*, **53**, 61–92.

Tuft, S. J., Kemeny, M. D., Dart, J. K. G., and Buckley, R. J. (1991). Clinical features of atopic keratoconjunctivitis. *Ophthalmology*, **98**, 150–8.

7 Extrinsic allergic asthma

J. H. Alpers, A. J. Frew, P. Bradding, and S. T. Holgate

Definition

There is no single gold standard test for the diagnosis of asthma. In the majority of cases diagnosis is based on history of episodic symptoms of cough, wheeze, shortness of breath, chest tightness, and variable peak flow measurements. Other factors which contribute to the clinical diagnosis are reproducible trigger factors, associated atopic disease (hay fever and eczema), bronchodilator responsiveness on lung function testing, and the degree of histamine/methacholine bronchial hyperreactivity. However, the diagnosis may be difficult in certain situations when the only symptom is cough; when the symptoms are only associated with a single inhalant contact or exercise; a drug-induced cause is invoked, e.g. beta blocker eye drops, gastro-oesophageal reflux with aspiration is the trigger or when upper airways obstruction predominates.

The differential diagnosis of asthma includes benign or malignant tumours of large airways, foreign body inhalation, vocal cord dysfunction, Loeffler's syndrome, Churg–Strauss vasculitis, left ventricular failure, recurrent small pulmonary emboli, drug-induced disease, and recurrent gastro-oesophageal aspiration.

Introduction

Asthma is a common clinical condition which affects individuals at almost any age and is an important cause of respiratory morbidity and mortality. Epidemiological surveys conducted in several different countries have shown the prevalence of asthma to be steadily increasing while death rates attributed to asthma in some countries have increased significantly over the past 30 years. The cause of these temporal trends in asthma prevalence is unclear; in part they represent changes in diagnostic labelling, but where the same definition of asthma has been used, there does appear to have been a true increase in prevalence. Although there is a genetic component to asthma, the rate of increase cannot be explained on a simple genetic basis and most authorities consider that there must be an interaction between a susceptible genotype and one or more changes in the environment. Airborne pollution from motor vehicles, dietary changes associated with affluence, respiratory virus infection in childhood, the increased use of cow's milk bottle feeding in infancy, and indoor pollution have all been blamed. Evidence of a link between domestic concentrations of house dust mite allergens and the likelihood of developing allergic disease in childhood are among the most convincing of these hypotheses.

Much new information on the pathophysiology of asthma has been obtained in the past 15 years particularly through the use of fibreoptic bronchoscopy as a research tool to address the cellular and inflammatory events occurring at the airways mucosa. Application of molecular immunological techniques has also enabled considerable progress to be made in understanding the regulation and expression of immunoglobulin (Ig)E and atopic allergy. These in turn have led to a fundamental reappraisal of the pathophysiological mechanisms of this disease and have provided a firm scientific basis for treatment strategies in this condition.

Genetic factors

Asthma may be loosely divided into atopic and non-atopic forms of the disease. Although there are considerable overlaps, childhood asthma is usually associated with atopic allergy whereas adult-onset asthma often arises in non-atopic individuals. Both allergic and non-allergic asthma appear to have significant inherited components. However, the inheritance of asthma does not obey simple Mendelian laws and family studies suggest that at least two separate components are required before asthma becomes evident. In the case of allergic asthma, these are first the ability to make specific IgE antibodies against relevant airborne allergens and secondly susceptible airways which will go on to develop chronic inflammatory changes when exposed to relevant allergens. Several lines of evidence suggest that the ability to make large amounts of IgE directed against environmental allergens is genetically controlled. IgE responses to simple allergens are often restricted to individuals bearing a particular major histocompatibility complex (MHC) class II haplotype but IgE responses to more complex allergens, e.g. house dust mite and animal danders, are not MHC-restricted. Correspondingly, there are no clear associations of atopic asthma with particular human leucocyte antigen (HLA) types.

Genetic linkage studies have suggested that atopy (defined as one or more skin tests to a common aeroallergen, clinical asthma, rhinitis, or conjunctivitis) may be inherited in association with the gene for the b-chain of the FceRI molecule on the short arm of chromosome 11 but other investigators have been unable to confirm this association. Genetic studies have also found linkage of atopy with polymorphisms in regulatory genes on chromosome 5 where many cytokine genes are clustered. Recent attention has also focused on the role of the intrauterine environment as an important influence on the subsequent development of atopic disease. Whatever the genetics of atopy may turn out to be, it is important to recognize that development of atopy is not sufficient to cause allergic asthma as many individuals have allergic rhinitis or allergic conjunctivitis without clinical asthma or any evidence of increased bronchial hyperresponsiveness (BHR). Nevertheless, atopic allergy is an important cause of asthma and is an important inducer of episodic symptoms in those who are already sensitized to airborne allergens.

When asthma arises in adult life, it may represent reactivation of childhood asthma, in which case atopic allergy is usually demonstrable. Asthma arising *de novo* in adulthood is less frequently associated with atopy. The serum total IgE concentration is usually within the normal range and skin tests to common airborne allergens are negative. Many individuals with late-onset asthma appear to develop the condition for the first time following upper respiratory tract infections. Rhinovirus infection has been linked with the development of asthma on both clinical and epidemiological grounds. Moreover, most individuals with asthma experience acute exacerbations when they develop upper respiratory tract infections. Respiratory viruses are also important in childhood asthma, and a recent epidemiological survey of asthma in school children, using sensitive polymerase chain reaction (PCR)-based isolation techniques, found virus infections in almost 80% of exacerbations. Occupational asthma is an important cause of adult-onset asthma and a wide range of organic and inorganic materials have been implicated.

Bronchial hyperresponsiveness

Asthma is characterized by marked variation in the calibre of the intrapulmonary airways over short periods of time. In addition, asthmatic individuals often report acute episodes of asthma on exposure to non-specific irritants such as cold air, inorganic dusts, cigarette smoke, perfumes, paint, etc. These are not allergic responses but are exaggerated responses of the airways to the non-specific irritant. This phenomenon is termed non-specific BHR and can be formally documented by the response to pharmacological bronchoconstrictors such as methacholine and histamine, or physical stimuli such as exercise or cold air.

In experimental studies, a wide range of non-specific stimuli have been used to induce bronchospasm in asthmatic patients; some agents act directly on the airways smooth muscle, e.g. methacholine, while others act indirectly, either by inducing the release of mast cell mediators, adenosine, hypertonic saline, or through neural reflex mechanisms, sulphur dioxide, bradykinin. Some agents will also induce bronchoconstriction in non-asthmatic individuals, but in general BHR is a characteristic of asthma and in population-based studies, correlates with disease severity. Other pharmacological agents have no direct bronchoconstrictor effect but increase BHR by increasing epithelial permeability or increasing post-receptor sensitivity of smooth muscle. Several mechanisms have been proposed to explain BHR.

Originally, it was thought that the abnormality might lie in the bronchial smooth muscle but the accumulated evidence now indicates that bronchial smooth muscle from asthmatics and normal subjects behaves similarly when studied *in vitro*. Current thinking emphasizes the importance of changes in the geometry of the airways on the response to bronchoconstriction. Thickening of the airways mucosa due to inflammation and oedema has little influence on baseline airways resistance, but when the bronchial smooth muscle contracts, the swollen mucosa continues to occupy the same absolute volume and thus the airways lumen is decreased by a much greater proportion than if the mucosa was not swollen. As resistance is inversely proportional to the fourth power of the radius (Poiseuille's law), a small increase in the thickness of the airways mucosa will have a marked effect on airways resistance in response to a given contraction of

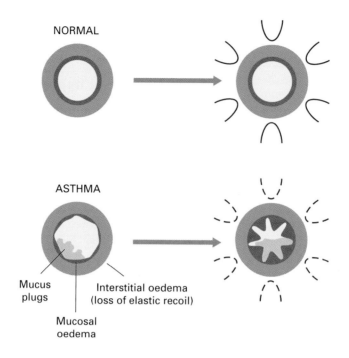

NORMAL

ASTHMA

Mucus plugs

Interstitial oedema
(loss of elastic recoil)

Mucosal oedema

▮**Fig. 7.1** Mechanisms of bronchial hyperresponsiveness. Mucus plugging, epithelial oedema and loss of elastic recoil all contribute to an exaggerated degree of narrowing of the airways to a given dose of bronchoconstrictor. Airways resistance is inversely related to the fourth power of the airways radius.

the bronchial smooth muscle. Intraluminal secretion of mucus and cells will also narrow the lumen and, like mucosal swelling, will have a disproportionate effect on airways resistance when the bronchial smooth muscle contracts. Finally, peribronchial oedema reduces the elastic recoil of the airways and this in turn allows a greater degree of airways narrowing to a given dose of a bronchoconstricting agonist.

Pathology

Until quite recently, virtually all the available information on the histology of asthma was based on post-mortem studies. When individuals die from acute severe asthma, their lungs show widespread obstruction of the small airways with mucus plugs containing fibrin and eosinophils. Death in such cases results primarily from asphyxiation secondary to endobronchial plugging with inspissated secretions rather than bronchoconstriction *per se*. The bronchial epithelium is often damaged and may be shed into the airways. The basement membrane is thickened with subepithelial

fibrosis and there is bronchial inflammation with oedema, vasodilatation and a mixed cellular infiltrate consisting of eosinophils, neutrophils, and T lymphocytes. Ten years ago, it was thought that these changes reflected severe fatal asthma and were not present in milder forms of the disease.

This view has radically changed following a series of studies which have used fibreoptic bronchoscopy to obtain biopsies from asthmatic airways for histological examination. Even in mild asthmatics, bronchial biopsies show inflammatory changes similar to those found in asthma deaths, including leucocyte infiltration, fragility of the bronchial epithelium and subepithelial fibrosis with deposition of collagen beneath the basement membrane

Histological studies of intrinsic, non-allergic asthma and occupational asthma show very similar findings to the biopsy appearances of allergic asthma. In fact, eosinophil and lymphocyte activation are if anything rather more prominent in intrinsic asthma, emphasizing the importance of cellular inflammation as a common feature of all forms of asthma and raising the possibility that intrinsic asthma may represent a

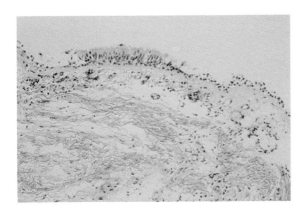

▮ **Fig. 7.2** Histopathology of bronchial biopsy of asthmatic airways, showing patchy loss of epithelium, oedema and a mixed cellular infiltrate.

form of autoimmune disease. These findings have led to the reclassification of asthma as an inflammatory disorder of airways mucosa with BHR and other associated features being viewed as consequences of inflammation rather than primary phenomena.

The inflammatory events in bronchial mucosa

A number of different models have been developed in order to understand the inflammatory process that

exists in asthma. Animal models have generally proved unsatisfactory because they tend to address the process of initial sensitization to allergens rather than the chronic inflammation which is the hallmark of asthma. Interspecies differences in the regulation of IgE production and variation in the ability to produce an eosinophilic response to allergen exposure have led to confusion about the relative importance of different leucocyte types in the generation of airways inflammation. Obtaining good physiological correlates of the inflammatory process has also been difficult, as airways mechanics are fundamentally affected by the anaesthesia which is often required in order to obtain accurate measures of allergen-induced airflow resistance in animals. For maximum relevance and ease of standardization, most investigators have therefore chosen to study these processes in humans and have used allergen-induced bronchoconstriction as a disease surrogate. Evidence obtained from this model has then been validated with a range of observations obtained from reductionist approaches studying individual cell types, chemical mediators, or cytokines. When sensitized asthmatic subjects are exposed to allergen under standardized conditions, they show a range of characteristic patterns of physiological response as assessed by dynamic spirometry.

Bronchoconstriction usually begins to develop within 5–10 min with measurable reductions in forced expiratory volumes (FEVs) and peak expiratory flow

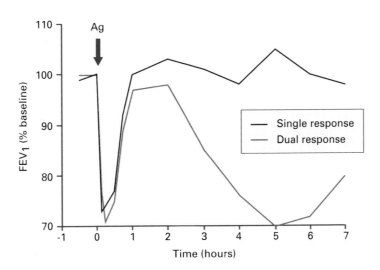

▮ **Fig. 7.3** Patterns of spirometric response to allergen inhalation, showing a single early response and a dual phase response. Ag, antigen.

rates. Generally, this early asthmatic response (EAR) peaks between 15 and 20 min after allergen exposure and then resolves over 1–2 h. Subsequently a proportion of subjects will go on the develop a secondary or 'late-phase' asthmatic response (LAR) with recurrence of their bronchoconstriction between 3 and 9 h after exposure. The LAR usually evolves slowly and can last a few hours or continue for several days. Other reported patterns include a single phase, progressive response in which bronchoconstriction commences within minutes and progresses to a peak at 5–6 h without any intervening period of resolution. Resolution may also be partial while some subjects show isolated late-phase reactions, with bronchoconstriction commencing 2–3 h after exposure, without any detectable immediate bronchospasm as shown by Durham (1990). Subjects who experience LARs often report destabilization of their asthma following challenge and will have increased non-specific bronchial responsiveness for up to 2 weeks after challenge, even though their spirometric values have returned to baseline. Patients who experience an isolated EAR do not usually show alterations in BHR or destabilization of their asthma. Interestingly, the propensity to develop LARs is associated with worse clinical status and patients with seasonal asthma are more likely to develop LARs during or after the natural pollen season than in the winter.

Subjective perception of breathlessness is often greater during the immediate than the late-phase response with a similar fall in forced expiratory flow volume in 1 s (FEV_1). This may be because bronchial obstruction occurs at different sites in the bronchial tree, despite the overall similar degree of change in integrated measures of airflow obstruction such as FEV_1. Studies with helium–oxygen mixtures suggest that the immediate response is associated with turbulent airflow and large airways constriction whereas there is a laminar airflow pattern during the late-phase response, with evidence of widespread small airways narrowing. The increased non-specific bronchial responsiveness that follows allergen challenge starts to develop soon after allergen exposure and can be detected during the resolution phase, within 2–3 h of exposure, in patients who are going to go on to develop LARs. Interestingly, there is no association between baseline bronchial reactivity and the likelihood of developing an LAR rather than an isolated EAR.

Comparative studies have indicated that the magnitude of the EAR depends on two main variables. These are the concentration of allergen-specific IgE and the degree of non-specific bronchial responsiveness. If all other factors are kept constant, it is possible to predict accurately the magnitude of response or alternatively, to predict the dose of allergen which will induce an EAR of fixed magnitude. The factors that determine the magnitude of the LAR are less well defined. There are considerable difficulties in comparing studies from different centres, due to variation in the methodology and end-points used. In most instances, LARs are preceded by EARs, but there is no direct correlation between the magnitude of the EAR and the subsequent LAR. Similarly, there is only a very limited association between serum concentrations of allergen-specific IgE, bronchial responsiveness or cutaneous sensitivity to allergen and the magnitude of the LAR. Nevertheless, within individuals, LARs do appear to be dose-dependent phenomena in terms of the dose of allergen administered. One of the complicating factors in interpreting the literature has been the lack of an agreed definition of the late-phase response. Different centres and investigators have used a variety of different physiological responses and cut-off points. This has led to considerable confusion when trying to assess epidemiological aspects of bronchial responsiveness and the biochemical and cellular correlates of the late-phase response.

Interest in the LAR stems from three important observations: first, the association of LARs with non-specific BHR; secondly, the greater likelihood of developing LARs in patients with more severe forms of asthma; and thirdly the pharmacology of the LAR. In general, drugs which are effective in asthma, such as corticosteroids and the cromones, i.e. sodium cromoglycate and nedocromil sodium, prevent the development of LARs and the associated increase in BHR. In contrast, the immediate asthmatic response is primarily a mediator-driven event, and can be inhibited by pharmacological agents such as antihistamines and prostaglandin synthetase inhibitors, which are less active or inactive against the LAR or clinical asthma

Cellular and biochemical correlates of early and late-phase responses

In patients with allergic asthma, exposure to a relevant allergen causes degranulation of mast cells present in the airways lumen and airways mucosa. This leads to the release of histamine and a range of newly formed mediators which induce bronchoconstriction, oedema, mucus secretion, and vasodilatation. Acute bronchospasm due to allergen exposure closely resembles the bronchospasm induced by inhalation of leukotrienes, prostanoids, or histamine and is considered to result principally from mast cell mediator release without requiring the involvement of other pro-inflammatory leucocytes.

The mechanisms underlying the LAR have received considerable attention since the suggestion by Pepys and colleagues in the mid-1960s that late-phase response to allergen was mediated by immune complex (type III) hypersensitivity. Subsequent studies demonstrated that LARs are IgE-dependent and that allergen-specific IgG antibodies are probably not relevant. In addition to the late effects of mast cell mediators, especially leukotrienes, LARs are associated with the influx of inflammatory cells including neutrophils, eosinophils, lymphocytes, and monocytes, and the consequent development of chronic inflammatory changes in the respiratory epithelium. These inflammatory cells augment the inflammatory response by generating and releasing additional pro-inflammatory mediators, especially mediators which activate endothelial cells and promote microvascular leakage. Most of these processes were studied initially in human skin or in various animal models, although the past few years have seen the extension of these investigations to include bronchoscopic examination of the human respiratory mucosa after inhalation challenge or local endobronchial challenge.

Confirmation of the IgE dependence of the late-phase reaction came principally from human skin studies in which it was demonstrated by Metzger *et al.* (1985) that antibodies directed against human IgE could trigger immediate and late-phase reactions. In further experiments, the LAR was shown to be transferable by serum, and could be attenuated by removing IgE from the serum prior to transfer. The central role of IgE and mast cells was also supported by the demonstration of cutaneous LARs after injection with compound 48/80, a known mast cell secretagogue. Although mast cells release large amounts of histamine, this mediator is not capable of inducing LARs, and in histological studies, induces oedema but little in the way of cellular inflammation

In contrast, the sulphidopeptide leukotrienes LTC_4 and LTD_4 can induce bronchospasm, mucus secretion, and enhanced vascular permeability, while LTB_4 is a very potent chemoattractant for neutrophils, eosinophils, and mononuclear phagocytes

Following allergen inhalation, increased concentrations of both classes of leukotrienes can be detected in bronchial lavage fluid from patients who develop LARs. An integrated measure of sulphidopeptide leukotriene generation can be obtained by measurement of urinary LTE_4, and this increases soon after allergen exposure, although there is no further rise in urinary LTE_4 during the LAR. Platelet-activating factor (PAF) is another potent pro-inflammatory mediator, which is generated by a variety of cell types, although in some cases, e.g. human mast cells, it may be generated but not released. PAF has a range of activities relevant to allergic inflammation; in the skin,

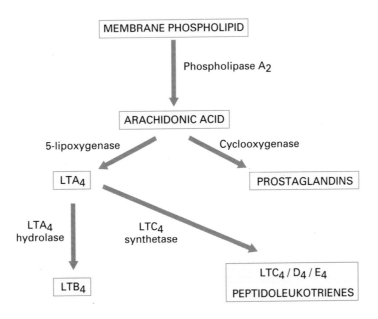

▌**Fig. 7.4** Biosynthesis of leukotrienes (LT) and prostaglandins following mast cell activation.

∎ **Table 7.1** Actions of mast cell mediators

	Leukotrienes	Histamine	Platelet-activating factor	Prostaglandins
Bronchoconstriction	$LTD_4 > C_4 > E_4$	+++	++	PGD_2, PGF_{2a}
Mucosal oedema	LTC_4, D_4	+++	++	PGE_2
Mucus secretion	LTC_4, D_4		++	
Chemotaxis and cellular activation	LTB_4		++++	
Increased NSBR (duration)	LTB_4 transient	No effect	+++	PGD_2 prolonged 30 min only

NSBR = non-specific bronchial responsiveness

PAF induces early and late-phase skin reactions which are associated with neutrophil and eosinophil infiltration. The biological activities of PAF include activation of platelets, neutrophils and eosinophils, contraction of smooth muscle, increased vascular permeability, and increased adhesion of leukocytes for endothelium. Inhalation of PAF induces bronchospasm which is short-lived, but in early reports was linked to subsequent increases in non-specific bronchial responsiveness. However, further investigation have generally been unable to confirm an important part for PAF in asthma.

Mast cells and their mediators seem to be critical for the initiation of the LAR (Table 7.1) but the subsequent events appear to depend on the recruitment and activation of a range of infiltrating leucocytes. In the skin, allergen challenge provokes a rapid accumulation of neutrophils which are followed within 3–4 h by the arrival of eosinophils and CD4+ T cells. In skin biopsies the majority of these eosinophils are activated as demonstrated by expression of the secreted form of eosinophil cationic protein (ECP) on their surface. Upon activation, eosinophils generate LTC_4 and also release their content of basic proteins. Evidence of eosinophil activation can also be found in bronchial lavage fluid, where ECP/albumin ratios are substantially elevated in patients who are experiencing LARs as compared with those who had isolated EARs.

Cellular recruitment and adhesion molecules

Recognition of the inflammatory mechanisms of asthma has led to intense interest in the process of cellular recruitment in asthma. This has also directed attention towards the vascular endothelium as a potential site for novel forms of therapeutic intervention. The proper regulation of the specific and non-specific immune defences requires a set of co-ordinated and precisely regulated mechanisms to control cell–cell interactions. Recruitment and activation of granulocytes and lymphocytes are mediated by a range of surface receptors and their corresponding ligands on endothelium, matrix, and other leucocytes.

There are three main classes of leucocyte–endothelial adhesion molecule, which have been classified according to their structural similarities. These are the selectins, the integrins, and the members of the immunoglobulin supergene family.

Selectins contain an N-terminal lectin-like domain which can bind to carbohydrate elements on the appropriate cellular ligand and are expressed on endothelial cells, platelets, and some leucocytes. P-selectin is mobilized rapidly to the endothelial cell surface within 5 min of exposure to inflammatory stimuli such as histamine, thrombin, or LTC_4 Endothelial P-selectin binds to neutrophils and eosinophils and is thought to be the principal selectin involved in the acute recruitment of granulocytes in the early phases of allergic inflammation. E-selectin (ELAM-1) is an inducible endothelial adhesion molecule, which is synthesized and expressed within 4 h of exposure to inflammatory stimuli such as the cytokines IL-1 and tumour necrosis factor (TNFα). E-selectin binds to the same determinants as P-selectin and its expression is usually transient, disappearing within 24 h of the initial stimulus. L-selectin is a similar molecule expressed on most leucocytes, which serves as a non-specific ligand for granulocytes but in lymphocytes, a differentially glycosylated form is a tissue-specific homing receptor for lymphocytes. Lymphocyte L-selectin binds to a 50 kDa sulphated mucin-like endothelial glycoprotein which is selectively expressed on lymph node high endothelial venules. Under conditions of high shear flow, selectins are the main adhesion molecules able to bind to endothelium. Once bound firmly, members

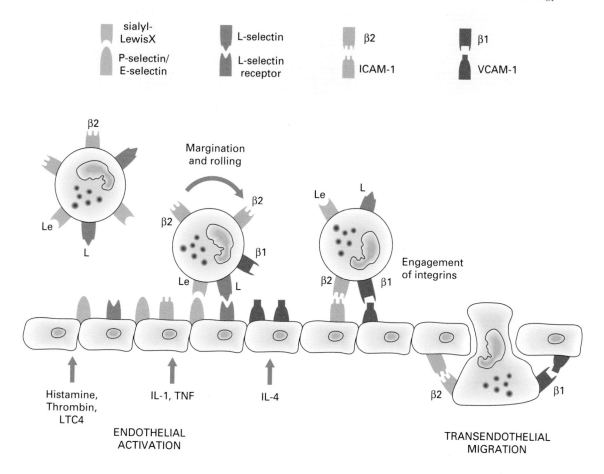

▮ **Fig. 7.5** Overview of leucocyte–endothelial adhesion mechanisms in asthma. E, E-selectin; P, P-selectin; L, L-selectin; LR, L-selectin receptor; Le, sialyl-LewisX; I, ICAM-1; V, VCAM-1; β_1 & β_2, β_1 and β_2 integrins; TNF, tumour necrosis factor.

of the integrin and immunoglobulin supergene family come into play and are required for transendothelial migration.

The β_2-integrins are a family of three heterodimer proteins, with a common β subunit (CD18) and different α subunits (CD11a, CD11b, and CD11c). In humans the genes for the CD11a, CD11b, and CD11c molecules are all located on chromosome 16 while the gene for CD18 is on chromosome 21. The β_2-integrins are only expressed on leucocytes, with CD11a/CD18 (LFA-1) found on all leucocytes; CD11b/CD18 is present on monocytes, granulocytes, and natural killer (NK) lymphocytes while CD11c/CD18 is largely confined to monocytes and granulocytes. Interestingly, the eosinophils and lymphocytes of patients with congenital absence of β_2-integrins are none the less able to migrate into inflammatory sites, indicating that although CD11/18 antibodies can block eosinophil

binding to cultured endothelial cells *in vitro*, β_2-integrins are not essential for eosinophil and lymphocyte migration *in vivo*.

The β_1-integrins are another family of heterodimer proteins with a common β-subunit (CD29) which is paired with one of a range of six different α chains (identified by monoclonal antibodies CD49a–CD49f). The β_1-integrins are widely distributed on most cell types including lymphocytes, neurons, and structural cells (fibroblasts etc.).

Expression of adhesion molecules in allergic disease has been studied in several different contexts relevant to asthma. In atopic asthmatics, local allergen challenge induces infiltration by neutrophils, eosinophils, and T lymphocytes within 6 h.

At the same timepoint, ICAM-1 and E-selectin expression is upregulated on endothelial cells in the bronchial mucosa but there was no change in VCAM-1

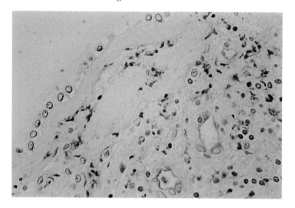

■ Fig. 7.6 Expression of the adhesion molecule ICAM-1 in bronchial mucosa 24 h after local allergen challenge.

expression. In addition, increased ICAM-1 expression is observed on bronchial epithelial cells in the allergen-challenged sites. Another study, using inhalation rather than segmental challenge, found increased endothelial VCAM-1 expression 24 h after allergen exposure but no change in ICAM-1 or E-selectin expression.

Only a limited number of reports have addressed adhesion molecule expression in clinical asthma. Sputum eosinophils of asthmatics express increased numbers of CD11b molecules, and also express ICAM-1 and class II MHC (HLA-DR). This increase in ICAM-1 and β2-integrin expression reflects the activated status of sputum eosinophils as compared with blood eosinophils but whether any of these adhesion molecules is critical to the process of accumulation of eosinophils in the sputum remains to be determined. Indeed, evidence from other *in vitro* studies has suggested that selective eosinophil leucocyte recruitment may be driven by endothelial factors involved in transendothelial migration rather than a selective leucocyte–endothelial adhesion process. Cross-sectional studies of human asthma have shown constitutive expression of ICAM-1, E-selectin and VCAM-1 in allergic asthma, non-allergic asthma, and normal control subjects, with no obvious or statistically significant difference between any of the three groups. Furthermore, 6 weeks treatment with inhaled corticosteroids did not reduce the basal level of expression of these adhesion molecules, even though *in vitro*, corticosteroids can rapidly and significantly reduce ICAM-1 expression on monocytic and bronchial epithelial cell lines. Patients experiencing acute exacerbations of asthma cannot be subjected to bronchoscopy, but increased plasma concentrations of E-selectin and ICAM-1 can be found during the acute and convalescent phase and indicate that endothelial activation is an important feature of clinically relevant forms of acute allergic inflammation.

The therapeutic implications of leucocyte–endothelial adhesion molecules in asthma have been explored in a primate model of asthma. These study findings suggest that ICAM-1 is important in the recruitment of inflammatory cells including eosinophils into the airways, but targeting ICAM-1 alone may not be sufficient to switch off established airways inflammation.

Eosinophils and asthma

The eosinophil is a characteristic feature of asthmatic inflammation and is capable of causing considerable damage to the bronchial epithelium. Tissue eosinophilia is found in asthma of all severities and types, while eosinophils are also seen in the sputum and blood during exacerbations. Most eosinophils present in the airways mucosa are activated, as shown by electron microscopic evidence of partial degranulation and in immunohistological studies by the presence of the secreted form of eosinophil cationic protein on the cell surface. The numbers of activated eosinophils present correlate with indices of disease activity such as methacholine PC20 and are also related to the degree of T-cell activation in the tissue. The eosinophil contains several basic proteins; major basic protein (MBP), eosinophil cationic protein ECP, eosinophil-derived neurotoxin (EDN) and eosinophil peroxidase (EPO) which induce detachment of the bronchial epithelium in experimental models and which can directly induce degranulation of mast cells. Mast cell and eosinophil-derived growth factors [IL-4, transforming growth factor (TGF) β, tumour necrosis factor (TNF) α] can induce the proliferation of myofibroblasts which in turn are probably responsible for the deposition of interstitial collagens beneath the basement membrane. In addition to their effect on epithelial growth and integrity, the eosinophil basic proteins may damage the epithelium by direct effects on the basement membrane which may in turn alter the ability of the epithelium to regulate the water and ion content of the fluid lining the bronchial tree.

Eosinophils are derived from bone-marrow progenitors closely related to the basophil, and eosinophilic myelocytes generally reside in the bone marrow. Eosinophilopoiesis outside the bone marrow occurs only in disease states such as nasal polyposis. Little is known of the mechanisms leading to production of committed eosinophil progenitors from pluripotent stem cells. However, their subsequent proliferation and differentiation is influenced by humoral factors, namely IL-3, IL-5, and granulocyte–macrophage colony-stimulating factor (GM-CSF). These cytokines can induce the production of eosinophils from both human bone marrow cells and cord blood mononuclear cells in culture. Different eosinophilopoietins may support distinct stages of eosinophil growth. Thus, IL-3 and GM-CSF generate myelocytes and metamyelocytes, while IL-5 supports the terminal maturation which follows cessation of proliferation. In addition to their role in eosinophilopoiesis, these cytokines also support the survival of mature eosinophils, and eosinophils chronically exposed to these cytokines in inflamed tissue may have a lifespan of several weeks as compared with an unstimulated lifespan of up to 72 h. Eosinophils possess both high (FcεRI) and low affinity (FcεRII) receptors for IgE which may permit them to participate directly in the response to allergen. IgE-dependent activation of eosinophils from patients with allergic disease leads to selective release of eosinophil peroxidase (EPO) and MBP, but not ECP. Eosinophils from non-atopic subjects are not responsive by this route. IgG and IgA receptors on eosinophils are also stimulate the selective release of granule proteins. Other activating stimuli include complement factors and PAF. PAF is not only one of the most important activators of eosinophils, but is also synthesized and released by stimulated eosinophils. Responses to PAF include chemotaxis *in vitro* and *in vivo*, increased adherence to cultured human umbilical vein endothelial cells, respiratory burst, exocytosis, and increased synthesis of LTC$_4$, which is itself a potent mediator of bronchoconstriction and increased vascular permeability. The respiratory burst results in the generation of potentially toxic oxygen metabolites including superoxide anions, and hydrogen peroxide, which together with EPO, generate the highly tissue damaging hypohalous acids in the immediate environment of the cell. Thus both preformed and newly generated mediators contribute to the tissue damage associated with eosinophil accumulation and activation in allergic disease.

Tissue and blood eosinophilia associated with allergic disease, including asthma, is characterized by the presence of morphologically distinct and functionally activated cells. The appearance of cytoplasmic vacuoles and loss of the dense core of specific granules is associated with secretion of granule contents. The increased capacity of these cells to generate LTC$_4$, superoxide and PAF, their greater adherence to endothelial cells and increased *ex vivo* survival indicates activation has occurred *in vivo*. These cells also have a distinct membrane receptor profile with upregulation of immunoglobulin Fc receptors and increased

expression of the β2-integrin MAC-1, which may contribute to eosinophil recruitment.

Eosinophil functions are upregulated *in vitro* by the eosinophilopoietic cytokines, (see Fig 7.7).

Culture of normal blood eosinophils with IL-3, IL-5, and GM-CSF leads to prolonged survival, enhanced degranulation and adhesion, and augmented LTC$_4$ and superoxide production. It is thus plausible that tissue-derived cytokines, including IL-3, IL-5, and GM-CSF, acting locally and systemically, contribute to tissue eosinophilia via effects on eosinophilopoiesis, eosinophil recruitment and survival. The physical and functional phenotype of eosinophils within the inflammatory environment therefore results from chronic exposure to these cytokines *in vivo*.

Epithelial cells and asthma

The epithelial lining of the conductive airways is the first line of defence against airborne toxins, pathogens, and allergens. In addition to its barrier function, epithelial defences depend on the mechanical clearance of airborne particles (bacteria, allergens, etc.) by the mucociliary escalator. It is frequently disrupted in asthmatics and is the major site of the mast cell and eosinophil-related mucosal inflammatory response. Disruption of the mucociliary escalator also renders the epithelium more vulnerable to airborne infection and insults. In addition to their role as victims, epithelial cells are increasingly being recognized as active participants in these responses and can themselves produce a range of cytokines and other mediators. This, combined with their ability to modulate cell adhesion, emphasizes their potential significance in cellular responses in allergic airways inflammation.

In the regions of the conducting airways where allergens tend to deposit, the epithelium is stratified, comprising basal cells with an overlying columnar cell layer. Epithelial cells require a range of intrinsic adhesion mechanisms to maintain the structural and barrier functions of this layer

These mechanisms can be divided into junctional and non-junctional mechanisms. The tight junction complex found at the apex of the epithelial cells maintains the barrier function of the epithelium between cells. Below the tight junction, the zonula adherens (ZA) junction mediates more dynamic processes particularly during the formation and repair of the epithelium. Desmosomal contacts, formed between cells along lateral and basal aspects of the epithelium, are the major structural link between the epithelial cells. Also at the lateral margin of the cells are gap junctions which facilitate cell–cell communication. Finally, at

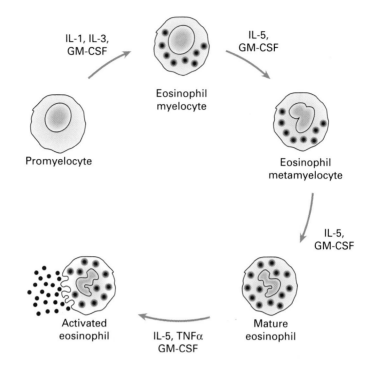

▮ **Fig. 7.7** Cytokine regulation of eosinophil differentiation and activation. GM-CSF, granulocyte–macrophage colony-stimulating factor; TNF, tumour necrosis factor.

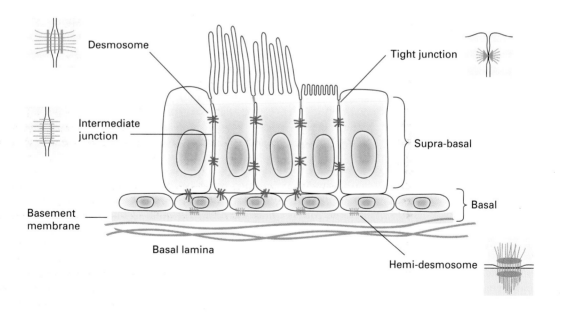

▮ **Fig. 7.8** Schematic diagram of cell–cell adhesion mechanisms in the epithelium (courtesy of Dr P. L. Lackie).

the base of the epithelium are hemidesmosome contacts which link cells in the epithelium to the basement membrane.

In addition to junctional adhesion between cells, there are a wide range of non-junctional adhesion molecules which are found on epithelial cells in the airways. These adhesion molecules characteristically mediate more transient adhesive processes than those of junctional adhesion and include ICAM-1, E-cadherin, CD44, and various integrins. Although these adhesion molecules were originally identified on endothelial cells, they may have different functions in the epithelium.

As the primary site of environmental or pathogen challenge, the epithelium is a target for infiltrating cells mediating the cellular and humoral immune responses. These cells migrate from the vascular system, after extravasation following endothelial cell adhesion. Migration to the epithelium is probably directed primarily by soluble factors including lymphokines and cytokines, some of these, such as IL-8, may be derived from the epithelial cells themselves. Once infiltrating cells are in close proximity to the epithelium, cell–cell adhesion molecules are then involved in proximal signalling. Epithelial cell surface molecules such as ICAM-1, CD44, integrins and HLA-DR may be involved in modulating the response of infiltrating cells. In turn, infiltrating cells modulate cell adhesion molecule expression as shown by the increased epithelial cell levels of ICAM-1 in response to IFNγ and TNFα. Expression of ICAM-1, HLA-DR and CD44 have been reported to be upregulated on epithelial cells in asthma.

Loss of columnar epithelial cells is a characteristic feature of bronchial biopsies from asthmatic subjects and is associated with exacerbation of the disease. Clumps of epithelial cells may be coughed up in sputum and are readily identifiable in bronchial lavage samples from asthmatic subjects. Such epithelial damage probably contributes to non-specific BHR by allowing increased accessibility of the subjacent bronchial smooth muscle. The mechanism causing epithelial loss remains unclear, although eosinophils and their basic proteins have been implicated. Epithelial cells have been shown to produce a variety of pro-inflammatory mediators including the cytokines IL-1b, IL-6, IL-8, and GM-CSF, prostaglandins (PGE$_2$ and PGF$_{2a}$) as well as 15-hydroxyeicosatetraenoic acid (15-HETE), and PAF. In addition, the regulatory peptides endothelin-1 and endothelin-3 are produced by epithelial cells. The precise mechanisms by which these factors may interact to produce symptom exacerbations in asthma remains uncertain.

The epithelial cell is the first barrier encountered by pathogens and provides host cells for many successful viruses, e.g. rhinovirus, respiratory syncytial virus (RSV), and influenza. In the context of inflammatory disease, viral infection of the epithelium is often associated with exacerbation of allergic symptoms. Rhinovirus episodes have been shown to be associated with exacerbation of asthma. The underlying mechanism of this change is unclear, but is likely to involve production of pro-inflammatory mediators such as IL-6, IL-8, and GM-CSF by epithelial cells.

Virus infection and asthma

Viruses have for a long time been thought to play a part in the induction of exacerbations of pre-existing asthma, and possibly also in the precipitation of asthma in previously healthy, susceptible children. Early studies of the part of viral infections in exacerbations of asthma proved inconclusive because of technical difficulties in isolating rhinoviruses and coronaviruses which are the principal viruses involved in acute respiratory infection. In the late 1980s and early 1990s, complete genome sequences were determined for the two human coronaviruses and for several of the over 100 known rhinovirus serotypes. This information permitted the development of accurate and sensitive detection techniques, initially employing cDNA or oligonucleotide hybridization techniques, and more recently, PCR. Using these techniques, recent studies have demonstrated that 85% of exacerbations of asthma in school-age children are associated with respiratory viral infections. In addition, respiratory virus infections are strongly associated with hospital admissions for asthma in both adults and children.

The mechanisms through which upper respiratory viral infections result in exacerbations of asthma remain poorly understood. Recent studies have shown that experimental rhinovirus infection leads to increased numbers of eosinophils and T lymphocytes (CD3+, CD4+) in the bronchial mucosa, in both normal and atopic subjects. However, in the asthmatic subjects, the eosinophil infiltrate persists for at least 6 weeks after infection, whereas in non-asthmatic subjects eosinophil numbers returned to baseline levels by this timepoint. These results suggest that the different pathophysiological response in asthmatics may be explained by a difference in the cytokine profiles of T-helper (Th) lymphocytes activated by viral infections. Normal host immune defence against viral infections induces classical CD8+ cytotoxic T cells (following MHC-class-I-restricted recognition of virus-infected host cells). In addition, NK cytotoxic T lymphocytes are also usually induced.

Cytokines and asthma

Cytokines are soluble proteins released by many inflammatory and structural cells which act in picomolar to nanomolar concentrations to regulate cell function. They are involved in both the regulation of the immune system and in tissue remodelling, with crucial parts in cell growth and differentiation, acute and chronic inflammation, defence against infection, and tissue repair. In general terms they act locally at the site of production but in some instances they may circulate to exert effects at distant sites.

Conventionally, cytokines are classified into a number of families including the interleukins the colony-stimulating factors (CSFs), the interferons, the cytotoxins such as TNFα, and the growth factors. This nomenclature has arisen rather haphazardly depending on the properties of the molecule first described, whereas it is now recognized that most if not all cytokines have multiple effects with a great deal of overlap both within and between the above groups. This apparent redundancy in cytokine networks may ensure there is no failure of many important biological processes. There is an increasing awareness of complex interactions between different cytokines including both synergistic and antagonistic actions. Thus IL-4 synergizes with TNFα in the upregulation of VCAM-1 but inhibits TNFα-induced ICAM-1 upregulation on endothelial cells. Furthermore, one cytokine may induce the production of several others, each with their own individual activities. These observations have therefore led to the concept of cytokine networks and cascades controlling cellular processes rather than individual cytokines.

With the vast and rapidly expanding array of pleiotropic cytokines now identified, and the many cell types likely to be involved in allergic mucosal inflammation, it clear that an extensive number of cytokines may play a part in the pathogenesis of asthma. The presence of atopy is dependent on the presence of mast cell-bound IgE directed against specific aeroallergens, and is intimately related to the development of both cutaneous and mucosal allergic diseases. The isotype switching of B cells from IgG and IgM to IgE synthesis is under the control of IL-4, and is inhibited *in vivo* by administration of neutralizing anti-IL-4 antibody. Many other cytokines also exert actions relevant to the pathogenesis of asthma and are produced *in vitro* by cells known to be present in the bronchial mucosa.

Effects of treatment on cellular infiltration and cytokine expression in asthma

Further evidence supporting the importance of eosinophils and T cells in the pathogenesis of asthma comes from histological studies performed before and after a course of inhaled corticosteroids. This form of treatment is very effective for most forms of asthma, and reduces both non-specific bronchial responsiveness and airways inflammation. When given over a 6 week period, inhaled beclomethasone dipropionate substantially reduced the numbers of eosinophil and activated T cells present in asthmatic airways. Additional evidence comes from a 6 month double-blind placebo-controlled clinical trial of cyclosporin A (a specific inhibitor of T-cell activation) in asthma which showed a clear beneficial effect on spirometric measures in patients with chronic severe asthma.

Conversely, a proportion of patients with severe asthma are 'corticosteroid resistant' in that they show the usual day to day variability of airways calibre and respond to inhaled bronchodilators but are unaffected by 1–2 week courses of oral prednisolone. Corticosteroid-resistant asthma (CRA) is relatively uncommon, but presents difficult problems of management for the clinician. As well as poor or absent effects of oral steroids on physiological parameters of airflow obstruction, these patients show a number of *in vitro* correlates. T lymphocytes from CRA patients show normal proliferative responses to the mitogen phytohaemagglutinin (PHA) but their responses are less sensitive to inhibition by dexamethasone. Similarly, T cells from both steroid sensitive and CRA subjects generate IL-2 and IFNγ when stimulated with PHA and again, cytokine production by cells from CRA show reduced sensitivity to inhibition by dexamethasone. These differences are not due to any difference in glucocorticoid receptor numbers and the CRA T cells can be inhibited by the immunosuppressive agent cyclosporin A.

Corticosteroids are very effective at reducing bronchial mucosal inflammation in many patients with asthma, and it is this effect which is thought to explain their clinical efficacy. However, the mode(s) of action of this class of pharmacological agent in asthma is not yet fully understood. *In vitro*, corticosteroids inhibit the production of many cytokines, although the response of individual cell types may vary. For example, corticosteroids inhibit the production of GM-CSF from human tracheal epithelial cells but not endothelial cells. It therefore seems likely that at least part of the anti-inflammatory action of these drugs in asthma is related to their ability to inhibit cytokine

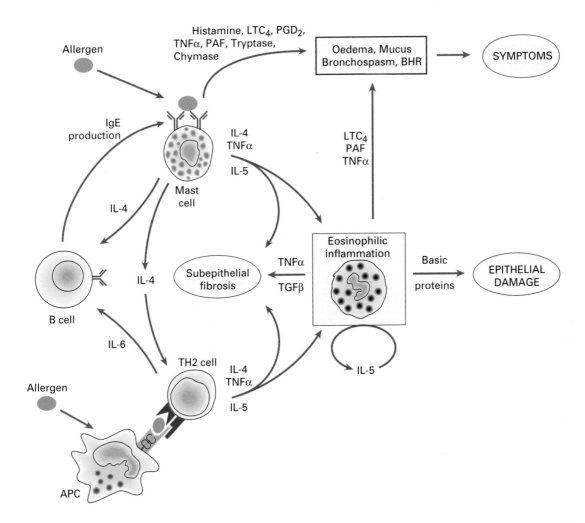

▌ Fig. 7.9 Cytokine networks in asthma. TNF, tumour necrosis factor; PAF, platelet-activating factor; BHR, bronchial hyperresponsiveness; TGF transforming growth factor; APC, antigen-presenting cell.

production. Two weeks treatment with oral prednisolone in symptomatic asthmatic patients leads to a significant reduction in the proportion of cells in bronchoalveolar lavage (BAL) fluid expressing mRNA for IL-4 and IL-5 compared with symptomatic controls treated with placebo. In studies of the late asthmatic response, pretreatment of subjects for 3 days with prednisone 30 mg twice daily inhibits the appearance of cells expressing TGFα, a cytokine which has been implicated in the deposition of collagen beneath the basement membrane. This collagen is type III and type V collagen and is deposited by specialized myofibroblasts whose growth is initiated and regulated by the cytokine TGFβ. Whether this corticosteroid-induced reduction in cytokine expression is due to inhibition of

cytokine synthesis within the bronchial mucosa or simply reflects reduced numbers of cytokine-secreting cells remains to be determined.

When all the available data are considered together, there is much evidence for increased cytokine expression in asthma, particularly for the Th2 cytokines IL-4 and IL-5, which are thought to be particularly important in the pathogenesis of allergic diseases including asthma. As yet there is little information on the effects of administering cytokines directly to the airways, or of specifically inhibiting individual cytokines. It is likely that the expression of many cytokines is suppressed by therapy with corticosteroids both through effects on transcription and translation, and through a reduction in the numbers of cytokine-secreting cells.

∎ **Table 7.2** Possible future targets for therapeutic intervention in asthma

---

Allergen avoidance measures

Novel mediator antagonists (platelet-activating factor leukotriene, D_4 antagonists, etc.)

Mediator synthesis inhibitors (e.g. 5-lipoxygenase inhibitors)

Cytokine receptor antagonists (especially IL-4, IL-5)

Cytokine therapy (e.g. inhaled interferon gamma)

Adhesion molecules

T-cell-directed strategies (novel forms of immunotherapy)

Major histocompatibility complex-directed therapies (competitive peptides)

In the future it may be possible to develop new compounds aimed at inhibiting the local effects of individual cytokines, which may permit dissection of the roles of individual cytokines in asthma, and may provide a novel range of therapeutic agents.

Future implications for the treatment of asthma

Recognition of the inflammatory basis of asthma has already led to a reappraisal of treatment strategies in asthma with increased emphasis on anti-inflammatory treatment, even in very mild forms of the disease. Prospects for new developments in therapeutic intervention have become focused on a small number of likely targets. These include the individual cytokines involved in IgE production (IL-4, IL-13), and in eosinophil differentiation and activation (GM-CSF, IL-5). Strategies directly targeting Th2 cells would also be logical if suitable target molecules can be identified and local forms of therapy made available. Cellular recruitment is another sensible target area and efforts are needed to delineate endothelial adhesion mechanisms which can be blocked without compromising essential elements of the immune system. At the same time, efforts are needed to establish appropriate model systems in which to test these novel approaches to asthma therapy. The comparative biology of IL-5 and IL-13 in the mouse and in humans illustrate the potential differences between human and rodent systems and although primate models have been used to study some aspects of the allergic inflammatory response, these are not practical or justifiable for all laboratories. The principal goal for the next 10 years must be to consolidate existing knowledge and translate research activity into improved health for our patients.

Clinical features

Severity of asthma based on symptoms

Peak flow variability, bronchodilator requirements, symptom grading scores have been devised. Laboratory testing of histamine or methacholine responses can also be used to define severity.

It is important to define within these severity gradings a subgroup of those patients prone to acute severe life-threatening episodes. The patients often exhibit anaphylactic reactions to foods, inhalants, drugs; very labile or brittle airways function as measured by peak flow measurements and histamine inhalation tests; acute severe upper airways obstruction is part of asthma with upper airways closure; and some patients with chronic severe airways inflammation with reversibility. It must also be recognized that even in patients with mild or episodic symptoms may have significant airways pathology as defined by bronchial biopsy.

Episodic asthma may be mild or severe but it is crucial in the history taking to evaluate the importance of potentially life-threatening symptoms such as sudden onset of severe dyspnoea, voice loss, very low peak flow measurements, cyanosis, effort syncope, and upper airways closure.

In episodic asthma, symptoms may be seasonal associated with inhalant allergy to grass and tree pollens in the spring, moulds during the autumn and house dust mite produces perennial symptoms with peaks during the winter. Isolated episodes can also be associated with occupational symptoms, food ingestion, e.g. metabisulphite, gastro-oesophageal reflux, and drugs.

▌ **Table 7.3** Asthma Management Plan

1. Assess severity.
2. Achieve optimal lung function.
3. Maintain optimal lung function by:
    avoiding trigger factors;
    preventer and reliever medication.
4. Written action plan.
5. Educate.
6. Monitor and review.

Treatment and management

The principles of asthma management

These have been formulated by the Thoracic Society of Australia and New Zealand as a six-point Asthma Management Plan, and by the American Thoracic Society and the British Thoracic Society who have also provided detailed statements on asthma assessment and management. Evaluation of these plans, assessing outcomes of the co-management principles between patient and doctor and the definition of 'best practice' guidelines will require continuous review. Long-term studies of outcome measures for persistent asthma in light of recent advances in drug therapy are not yet available. An Asthma Management Plan has been formulated

Objectives in overall asthma management

The aims of treatment of chronic persistent and severe asthma are to improve morbidity (symptoms, quality of life, and work capacity); to avoid mortality; to provide action, crisis/emergency plans and to prevent decrements in long-term lung function (British Thoracic Society 1990).

The application of improved management will reduce hospital admissions, attendances to doctors, and reduce costs to the community.

Particular objectives are:

(1) To improve lung function and reduce the potential for chronic airways pathology and future decrements of ventilatory capacity. Therapy should aim to increase peak flow and reduce its variability, especially the severe nocturnal dips, reduce air trapping, overinflation, increase exercise capacity,

and decrease BHR. All these physiological improvements are achievable in the majority of patients.

(2) Avoid trigger factors such as house dust mite with attention to environmental controls. Other useful measures include reducing temperature variations, indoor heating leaks (open fires, leaking furnaces), cigarette smoke, 'sick building' fumes, indoor moulds (damp areas, indoor plants), and animals (cats, dogs, and birds). Attention to the outdoor macro-environment is more difficult but reduction in grass pollen, cold air, air pollution, and occupational triggers can sometimes be achieved.

Additional measures to improve overall care of asthma are:

1. Treat nasal obstruction and chronic sinusitis.
2. Weight loss if obese.
3. Exercise programmes, e.g. swimming.
4. Psychological support, relaxation training, avoidance of panic, stress management techniques.
5. Education concerning the disease and its treatment.
6. Unproven methods may have an occasional part for certain individuals such as special breathing techniques, hypnosis, acupuncture, meditation, and naturopathic therapies.

Drug therapy in asthma

Anti-inflammatory agents

Inhaled corticosteroids (preventers)

Asthma is an inflammatory disease, therefore anti-inflammatory drugs are primary therapy in all chronic persistent asthma. These drugs have been the major therapeutic advance in the maintenance treatment of asthma in the last two decades. There are a wide variety of formulations of inhaled corticosteroids, with subtle pharmacokinetic differences relating to hepatic metabolism and metabolite activity. However, considering the nature of drug deposition and kinetics within the lung to steroid receptor sites of bronchial mucosal cells it is unlikely these differences are significant in clinical practice. Major preparations in use are beclomethasone dipropionate, budesonide, and fluticasone. Budesonide is rapidly cleared with a half-life of 2.5 h and has some delivery advantage through the use of a Turbuhaler and dry powder delivery system which contains no additives or CFCs. It also is available in a nebulizing suspension. Fluticasone may have a reduced side-effect profile as it has no oral bioavailability.

The use of a spacer and mouth rinsing is essential for all inhaled corticosteroids to reduce the incidence of oral candidiasis and dysphonia. Systemic absorption will occur even with the best precautions and in high-dose inhaled corticosteroid use greater than 1600–2000 μg a day, osteoporosis in adults, skin changes and growth retardation in children can certainly occur though individual tolerance is present.

These drugs are best given twice a day to improve compliance and for maintenance therapy 200–1600 μg twice daily will be required depending on severity of asthma, peak flow response, and BHR. For chronic persistent symptoms 6 months or even permanent therapy is required with regular review to reduce doses if clinically appropriate. Inhaled budesonide may also have a part in moderately acute severe asthma by the nebulized route using a mouth T piece and reservoir bag. Inhaled corticosteroids can lower the risk of fatal and near fatal asthma.

Inhaled corticosteroids will certainly reduce BHR and the effects may be seen within 3–6 months and are maintained, although on cessation of the drug a return to similar BHR can occur. The anti-inflammatory part of inhaled corticosteroids is further confirmed by biopsy evidence of reduction in inflammatory markers such as reduction in T-helper cells, and increase in ciliated epithelial cells, decrease in eosinophils, stabilization of small vessel micro-leakage and oedema, reduction of mediator release, and inhibition of the growth of mast cells. These changes will provide long-term benefit in asthma control.

Oral prednisolone

This is essential therapy for acute severe asthma and maintenance therapy for chronic asthma with persistent airflow obstruction unresponsive to regular inhaled corticosteroids and β_2-agonists. In acute and emergency situations prednisolone can be given in high doses 30–40 mg as single dose for 5 days with slow reduction over the next 10 days depending on clinical response, peak flow measurements, symptoms and β-agonists usage. The clinical response is noted at 2 h, peaking at 8 h and has a maximal pharmacological effect after 16 h. Using single day dosing this regimen allows some adrenal pituitary axis recovery. Emergency pack prednisolone crisis plan management should be routine for all asthmatics with chronic or sudden acute symptoms. For maintenance therapy an alternate day regimen is the ideal and doses of 10–20 mg is generally preferred because of reduced side-effect profile than even small daily doses of 7.5 mg per day. Steroids should be very rarely given in twice daily dosage because of the marked increase in side-effects. The only side-effects reported from high-dose short-term therapy is the occasional fluid retention and

headache and in general short course therapy is very well tolerated.

Sodium cromoglycate

This is an alternative first-line anti-inflammatory drug for children to be used in conjunction with β_2-agonists on a regular maintenance basis for chronic persistent asthma. It can be delivered by dry powder inhalation 20 mg four times a day or metered dose inhaler 8 mg four times a day or can be nebulized for children under 2 years of age. The drug is not metabolized, has a rapid onset of effect which generally lasts 2–6 h. Frequent dosing of four times a day is preferred particularly during seasonal contact with inhalant allergens, e.g. grass pollens when its prophylactic effect is best seen. The above doses can also be increased significantly without side-effects during periods of high-allergen exposure. Additional indicators in adults includes exercise-induced asthma, cold air-induced asthma, post-viral bronchial reactivity, and cough-induced by ACE inhibitor drugs. The more recently formulated inhaler Intal forte (5 mg/puff) can be used with no side-effects. The pharmacological basis for sodium cromoglycate's part in asthma control is still unclear. It was initially thought to be a mast cell stabilizer but the beneficial effects may be related to its part as a vagal inhibitor and an inhibitor of chloride transport. A related preparation nedocromil sodium can provide benefit for maintenance of asthma control (Ruffin *et al.* 1987).

Bronchodilators (relievers)

β_2-agonists

This group of drugs are effective therapy for symptomatic control of acute asthma, used ideally on an as needed basis for acute breakout symptoms when preventative anti-inflammatory therapy is suboptimal. Their action is primarily on β_2-receptors on bronchial cells causing smooth muscle dilatation but there is some clinically significant mild anti-inflammatory effects as well. There is also some evidence they can increase ciliary beat frequency and inhibit mediator release. The number of β_2-receptors is reduced with age and the severity of asthma and can be increased with corticosteroid therapy. The bronchial response will depend on airways calibre, aerosol size, the presence of sputum, and delivery symptoms of the drug. If asthma is severe the duration of effect tends to be shorter. The response is rapid in the first 10 min peaking at 2 h and decaying after 6 h. However, new long-acting preparations, e.g. salmeterol, formoterol, are now available which require only 12 hourly dosing. The side-effect profile of all β_2-agonists is well recognized and includes tremor which tends to decrease with time, tachycardia up to additional 10–20 beats per min and occasional cardiac arrhythias. The CFCs from metered dose inhalers may produce a gag effect and throat dryness and occasional paradoxical bronchoconstriction from metabolites has been described. Present concerns with excessive β_2-agonist use has been the epidemiological evidence from Canada suggesting an increased mortality when these drugs are the sole therapy for asthma, particularly for those with high-dose preparations, e.g. fenoterol.

There may be a class effect which is not yet fully elucidated, although fenoterol has been particularly incriminated. All β_2-agonists can cause hypokalaemia with the development of a rebound increase in bronchial reactivity may occur following cessation of treatment. Permanent dilatation of airways without anti-inflammatory cover in association with inhaled allergen contact may increase the underlying inflammatory response and worse asthma control.

The following guidelines are suggested for β_2-agonist use:

1. Sole therapy is not advised except if asthma is mild or intermittent.
2. The use with anti-inflammatory inhaled steroid should be on an as needed or twice daily basis for additional symptom control.
3. Use in sudden acute breakout symptoms is effective.
4. In general avoid high doses per puff and per day.
5. The use of long-acting drugs such as salmeterol, formoterol, and bambuterol are effective for 'round the clock' symptom control in chronic persistent asthma in addition to inhaled corticosteroids particularly for nocturnal symptoms and may further reduce BHR.
6. Oral preparations such as bambuterol can be given on a once daily basis. The bronchodilator activity of the long-acting preparations in slightly slower in effect.

Adrenaline

This drug has no part in maintenance therapy but in acute severe life-threatening asthma it is still the drug of choice and can be given by self-injectable syringe intramuscularly in those asthma patients prone to anaphylactic type episodes either to inhalants, food additives, or drug reactions; 0.5 ml of 1:1000 solution by intramuscular injection repeated half hourly as required in the emergency setting can be lifesaving therapy.

Methylxanthines

These drugs, particularly theophylline and aminophylline used to be first-line therapies but have now been generally relegated to a secondary role in the management of asthma. They are bronchodilators; can inhibit mediator release, increase mucociliary clearance and can improve contractility of fatigued respiratory muscles. These are, however, many side-effects particularly gastrointestinal, central nervous system irritability, hypotension, tachycardia, and arrhythmias. There is a wide individual variation in tolerance and effect with a relatively narrow therapeutic toxic ratio and a half-life of 5–8 h. Intravenous aminophylline still has a part in acute asthma, although recent studies have questioned its value. There are significant commonly used drug interactions, with theophylline such as erythromycin, ciprofloxacin, cimetidine, phenytoin, and allopurinol and serum levels are affected by smoking and cardiac failure. Maintenance therapy with slow release oral theophylline may still have a limited part, particularly in those patients who have reactions or side-effects to inhaled β_2-agonists.

Ipratropium bromide (Atrovent)

This preparation is an anticholinergic which has effect on vagal airway fibres, reducing vagal tone and irritant receptors. It is synergistic with β_2-agonists in its bronchodilatation effect and can be particularly useful for the irritable cough of asthma and additive to inhaled corticosteroids in those patients with excess mucus secretion. For acute asthma breakout symptoms it is best delivered as a nebulizer solution 500 μg 4 hourly with a β_2-agonist.

The use of large volume spacers for metered dose inhalers (MDI)

These are valuable for those patients with poor inhaler technique and can increase airways deposition from 10 to 20%. Spacers also reduce oropharyngeal deposition as large particles sediment out. They are particularly useful for high-dose inhaled steroids and can reduce oral candidiasis and dysphonia and eight puffs of a MDI in a spacer are equivalent to nebulizer therapy in acute severe asthma generally allowing penetration of smaller particles into the tracheobronchial tree. A further advantage is some evaporation of potentially irritant CFCs reducing the gag effect of MDIs.

Occupational asthma

Definition

Asthma caused by exposure to agents in the working environment with transient persistent or permanent airflow obstruction.

Occupational asthma may be the most common occupational lung disease in many countries. Estimates

∎ **Table 7.4** Causes of occupational asthma: inciting agents

Chemicals
  Isocyanates
  Platinum salts
  Tungsten carbide
  Resins
  Reactive dyes
  Insecticides
  Formaldehyde

Animal origin
  Laboratory animals
  Organ extracts
  Glue workers
  Insects

Plant origin
  Wheat dust
  Castor beans
  Wood dust
  Fungal spores

up to 2–15% of the asthmatic population have occupationally induced disease. Asthma may be induced in a previously healthy individual with permanent increase in bronchial hyperreactivity and persistent airways inflammation. Occupational agents may also aggravate pre-existing asthma, both on an irritant or hypersensitivity basis. More recently, the term 'reactive airways dysfunction syndrome' (RADS) has been used to describe asthma occurring after single exposure to high levels of a toxic substance.

This syndrome is different from most forms of occupational asthma which require periods of exposure and/or sensitization of weeks or months. In the RADS the onset is abrupt, within 24 h of exposure, and persists for some months. This occupational asthma is important for medico-legal considerations because of the wide range of chemicals that workers are now exposed to and the high prevalence of asthma in most communities. Some of the causes of occupational asthma have been defined

The mechanisms of occupational asthma may be immune sensitization, i.e. an acquired hypersensitivity response with specific IgE or IgG antibodies or the process is non-specific and the exposures to the agent is irritant causing inflammation without clear allergic sensitization. Once established occupational asthma may persist despite the individual being removed from the offending substance. Generally, some improvement will occur following complete removal, persistent symptoms are usual. The characteristic features

are those of direct contact exposure with immediate symptom response. However, delayed responses can occur after leaving work in the evening or even on the weekends and the symptoms tend to improve with a break from work and can progress during the week from Monday to Friday. Early, intermediate, and late reactions have been described.

The occupational exposure may be complicated by established lung disease from cigarette smoking or industrial bronchitis. From a medico-legal standpoint it is important to differentiate occupational asthma due to an inciting agent and that of aggravation of pre-existing asthma by non-specific irritants, e.g. sulphur dioxide dusts, or temperature changes.

Risk factors

(1) atopy, increasing the risk of IgE-mediated reactions;

(2) tobacco smoking, opening up epithelial tight junctions and allowing increased ingress of chemicals or other agents into the airways further contributing to the irritant effects and allergic sensitization; and

(3) sulphur dioxide and other agents in the atmosphere may also contribute to ongoing airways inflammation.

Investigations for occupational asthma include regular peak flow monitoring at home, work, weekends, holidays, with an accurate diary of exposures. At work the measurements should be charted frequently, e.g. 2 hourly. Immunological investigations such as RAST, specific IgE and IgG antibodies on skin tests to inhaled proteins may provide evidence of contact but not necessarily of causation. Occupational settings where these may be of value are exposure to animal danders, some chemicals utilizing hapten protein conjugates, e.g. TDI, insects, grain dusts and moulds.

BHR is generally abnormal during direct exposure to the offending agent and may improve considerably with treatment and spontaneously over time many weeks after the original exposure. Inhalational challenge testing is potentially dangerous and is rarely indicated and requires a laboratory pollution chamber with safety guidelines and controls for both staff and patients.

Treatment of occupational asthma

In ideal circumstances the individual should be removed from the offending agent. However, this is not always possible by virtue of significant financial hardship to that worker. Simple preventative measures include wearing appropriate protection, adequate ventilation systems, extractor fans, laminar flow equipment, reduction of non-specific irritants in the work place, e.g. dust sulphur dioxide, cold air. The general management of established asthma is no different from non-occupational causes requiring regular preventative anti-inflammatory inhaled corticosteroid drugs and intermittent use of bronchodilator therapy.

The prognosis in occupational asthma depends on the agent, the degree of exposure in many situations and continuing airways inflammation is the rule rather than the exception. Bronchial biopsies may show chronic inflammatory changes and increased numbers of eosinophils may be present in BAL fluid. BHR often remains persistently abnormal, as described in western red cedar asthma where 60% of individuals had a long duration of exposure before the onset of symptoms.

Asthma — special problems

Asthma in pregnancy

Because of the increasing prevalence of asthma in many communities the association of asthma and pregnancy is therefore common and accounts for 5% of maternal deaths, the third commonest cause behind cardiac disease and cerebral haemorrhage.

The effect of pregnancy on asthma

The physiological changes in pregnancy include a decrease in functional residual capacity and residual volume, total lung capacity and vital capacity are unchanged, minute ventilation increases, arterial P_{CO_2} falls, gas transfer can fall but arterial hypoxaemia is not normally a feature. Acute asthma is unusual during labour or delivery, although the role of prostaglandins in initiating labour has been associated with acute asthma in the later stages of pregnancy with increased intra-abdominal pressure. Gastro-oesophageal reflux can occur and occasionally mimic asthma symptoms particularly with chronic nocturnal cough. Airways hyperresponsiveness generally improves, although in individual cases unpredictable events can occur. In general the more severe asthma prior to pregnancy the more difficult will be symptom control during pregnancy.

The effect of asthma on pregnancy

Prospective studies have shown that asthma is associated with high rates of pre-eclampsia and Caesarean section but major outcomes were no different to non-asthmatic women including birth weights, perinatal deaths, Apgar scores, neonatal respiratory difficulties or congenital malformations. However, undertreated severe asthma can increase fetal and maternal complications.

Specific management of asthma in pregnancy is important as good control will protect the fetus from hypoxia. This is more important than any potential drug side-effects to the mother or fetus. Common drugs used in the management of asthma such as oral and inhaled corticosteroid preventative therapy, cromoglycate, β_2-agonists and even theophyllines are safe throughout pregnancy. High-dose oral steroids has been associated with an increase in stillbirth, although this may still be an acceptable risk in a severe asthmatic. The above drugs cross the placenta and in general the potential for drug side-effects will increase as dosage increases. Antibiotics, penicillin, cephlosporins, and erythromycin appear to be safe but tetracyclines and chlorambutol are contraindicated. Breast feeding needs to be encouraged in asthmatic mothers and has been associated with reduced atopy in offspring if prolonged. Most drugs will appear in breast milk including theophylline, about 70% of the maternal blood concentration. In studies of beclomethasone dipropionate for severe asthma during pregnancy the incidence of congenital malformations, spontaneous abortions, stillbirths, and neonatal deaths were no greater than expected as were the average birth weights.

Asthma and diet

Ten per cent of asthma patients may react adversely to a variety of dietary constituents. In particular these are:

(1) known irritants — to the airways, sulphur dioxide, metabisulphite. (preservatives E220, 221, 222);

(2) food additives — tartrazine and colouring agents (E102);

(3) foods that contain histamine;

(4) nitrites, monosodium glutamate; and

(5) immune-mediated reaction to food proteins, e.g. eggs, milk, fish.

The mechanisms for these reactions which may be life-threatening often are not known considering the complex interaction of absorption and mucosal factors. True food sensitization is relatively rare whereas reactions to additives, preservatives, antioxidants, or flavour enhancers is common. Metabisulphites as preservatives are common in many foods including sparkling and cask wines, beer, preserved fruits, seafoods, prepared 'dips', pickles, and cordials. The mechanism of the often intense bronchoconstriction occurring quite rapidly after ingestion is the release of sulphur dioxide, which is then inhaled from the throat or eructation from the stomach. Other reactions can be delayed and the temporal relationship with food ingestion and the worsening of asthma symptoms can be difficult to ascertain. The mechanism of tartrazine-induced asthma may be mast cell degranulation.

The investigations of food allergies requires a careful history, dietary diary, peak flow monitoring, and a trial of specific elimination diets noting the effect on symptoms, peak flow measurements. Skin testing and RAST testing may be useful for IgE-mediated responses but these are much less common. Food challenge in hospital or laboratory setting may occasionally be necessary requiring double blinding with gradually increasing doses of the food or other agent to be challenged.

Treatment ideally requires identification of the offending agent and elimination in the diet but may be difficult because of the vast array of food mixtures and additives. However, in those patients with documented sensitivity to tartrazines, metabisulphite, and sulphur dioxide a strict elimination diet may be rewarding and occasionally life saving. Ketotifen and oral Intal can also provide some protection.

Near-miss asthma deaths — patients at risk

In the last 5 years there has been reports of increasing mortality in asthma in many countries (Jackson *et al.* 1988). Acute severe life-threatening episodes may occur even in mild asthma but certain subgroups of patients are at risk as detailed below.

1. Anaphylactic episodes:
   (i) ingestants — metabisulphite, monosodium gltamate, tartraz
   (ii) drugs — aspirin and non-steroidal anti-inflammatory drugs;
   (iii) inhalants — sulphur dioxide, smoke, chemicals, and sprays; and
   (iv) injectants — bee stings, penicillin.

2. The brittle patient with hyperactive airways with wide chaotic peak flow patterns coupled with poor understanding of the disease, inadequate medication, and reduced sensing of severity.

3. Abnormal ventilatory control, hypoxia and/or hypercapnoea including sleep-disordered breathing.

4. Those at particular risk for respiratory arrest are obese females with glottic closure, panic reactions,

and chronic unrecognized hypoxaemia in association with exercise.

5. Asthma complicated by collapsible large airways, lobar collapse with excess mucus production, tension pneumothorax, tachyarrhythmias, beta blocker induced asthma, and excessive sedation.

6. Special clinical situations such as reactions to local anaesthetics, scuba diving, and recurrent angioedema of pharynx and tongue.

Further factors that may contribute to asthma mortality have recently been defined by a number of studies and include the following: underdiagnosis, poor perception of the illness by patient and doctor, poor patient education, lack of crisis plan, lack of objective measurements of severity, such as peak flow charting, inappropriate therapy, and under-recognized anaphylactic events to foods or drugs.

Further reading

Bardin, P. G., Johnston, S. L., and Pattemore, P. K. (1992). Viruses as precipitants of asthma symptoms. II. Physiology and mechanisms. *Clinical and Experimental Allergy*, **22**, 809–22.

Beasley, R., Roche, W. R., Roberts, J. A., and Holgate, S. T. (1989). Cellular events in the bronchi in mild asthma and after bronchial provocation. *American Review of Respiratory Diseases*, **139**, 806–27.

Bentley, A. M., Meng, Q., Robinson, D. S., Hamid, Q., Kay, A. B., and Durham, S. R. (1993a). Increases in activated T lymphocytes, eosinophils and cytokine mRNA expression for interleukin-5 and GM-CSF in bronchial biopsies after allergen challenge in atopic asthmatics. *American Journal of Respiration and Cellular and Molecular Biology*, **8**, 35–42.

Bentley, A. M., Robinson, D. S., Menz, G., Storz, C., Durham, S. R., Cromwell, O. *et al.* (1993b). Expression of the endothelial and leukocyte adhesion molecules ICAM-1, E-selectin and VCAM-1 in the bronchial mucosa in steady state and allergen-induced asthma. *Journal of Allergy and Clinical Immunology*, **92**, 857–68.

Bernstein, M., Day, J. H., and Walsh, A. (1982) Double blind food challenge in the diagnosis of food sensitivity in the adult. *Journal of Allergy and Clinical Immunology*, **70**, 205–10.

Bradding, P., Roberts, J. A., Britten, K. M., Montefort, S., Djukanovic, R., Heusser, C. H., *et al.* (1994). Interleukins-4, -5, -6 and TNF-α in normal and asthmatic airways. Evidence for the human mast cell as an important source of these cytokines. *American Journal of Respiration and Cellular and Molecular Biology*, (in press).

British Thoracic Society Research Unit of the Royal College of Physicians, Kings Fund Centre, National Asthma Campaign (1990). Guidelines for the management of asthma in adults. 1 — Chronic persistent asthma. *British Medical Journal*, **302**, 651–4.

Brooks, S. M., Weiss, M. A., and Bernstein, I. L. (1985). Reactive airways dysfunction syndrome (RADS). Persistent asthma syndrome and high level irritant exposures. *Chest*, **88**, 376–84.

Chan-Yeung, M. and Lam, S. (1986). Occupational asthma — state of the art. *American Review of Respiratory Diseases*, **133**, 688–703.

Chan-Yeung, M., McLean, L., and Paggiaro, P. L. (1987). Follow up study of 232 patients with occupational asthma, caused by Western Red Cedar (Thuja Plicatar). *Journal of Allergy and Clinical Immunology*, **79**, 792–6.

Cookson, W. O. C. M., Sharp, P. A., Faux, J. A., and Hopkin, J. M. (1989). Linkage between IgE responses underlying asthma and rhinitis and chromosome 11q. *Lancet*, **i**, 1292–5.

Corrigan, C. J., and Kay, A. B. (1992). T cells and eosinophils in the pathogenesis of asthma. *Immunology Today*, **13**, 501–7.

Djukanovic, R., Roche, W. R., Wilson, J. W., Beasley, C. R. W., Twentyman, O. P., Howarth, P. H. *et al.* (1990). Mucosal inflammation in asthma. State of the art. *American Review of Respiratory Diseases*, **142**, 434–57.

Djukanovic, R., Wilson, J. W. Britten, K, M., *et al.* (1992). Effect of an inhaled corticosteroid on airway inflammation and symptoms in asthma. *American Review of Respiratory Diseases*, **145**, 669–74.

Durham, S. R. (1990). Late asthmatic responses. *Respiratory Medicine*, **84**, 263–8.

Durham, S. R, Graneek, B. J., Hawkins, R., and Newman-Taylor, A. J. (1987). The temporal relationship between increases in airway responsiveness to histamine and late asthmatic responses induced by occupational agents. *Journal of Allergy and Clinical Immunology*, **79**, 398–406.

Ernst, P., Spitzer, W. O., Suissa, S. *et al.* (1992). The risk of fatal and near fatal asthma in relation to inhaled corticosteroid use. *Journal of the American Medical Association*, **268**, 3462–4.

Frew, A. J. and Kay, A. B. (1990). Eosinophils and T-lymphocytes in late-phase allergic reactions. *Journal of Allergy and Clinical Immunology*, **85**, 533–9.

Frigas, E. and Gleich, G. J. (1986). The eosinophil and the pathophysiology of asthma. *Journal of Allergy and Clinical Immunology*, **77**, 527–37.

Goeras, S. N., Liu, M. C., Newman, W., Beall, L. D., Stealey, B. A., and Bochner, B. S. (1992). Altered adhesion molecule expression and endothelial cell activation accompany the recruitment of human granulocytes to the lung after segmental allergen challenge. *American Journal of Respiration and Cellular and Molecular Biology*, **7**, 261–9.

Gundel, R. H., Wegner, C. D., Torcellini, C. A., and Letts, L. G. (1992). The role of intercellular adhesion molecule-1 in chronic airway inflammation. *Clinical and Experimental Allergy*, **22**, 569–75.

Hargreave, F., Dolovich, J., Newhouse, M. (1990). The assessment and treatment of asthma: A conference report. *Journal of Allergy and Clinical Immunology*, **85**, 1098–111.

Jackson, R. T., Sears, M. R., Beaglehole, R., and Rea, H. H. (1988). International trends in asthma mortality 1970–1985. *Chest*, **94**, 914–18.

Meredith, S. K., Taylor, V. M., and McDonald, J. C. (1991). Occupational respiratory diseases in the United Kingdom. *British Journal of Industrial Medicine*, **48**, 292–8.

Metzger, W. J., Hunninghake, G., and Richerson, H. (1985). Late asthmatic responses: inquiry into mechanisms and significance. *Clinical Reviews in Allergy*, **3**, 145–65.

Montefort, S., Holgate, S. T., Howarth, P. H. (1993). Leucocyte–endothelial adhesion molecules and their role in bronchial asthma and allergic rhinitis. *European Respiratory Journal*, **6**, 1044–54.

Ninan, T. K. and Russell, G. (1992). Respiratory symptoms and atopy in Aberdeen schoolchildren: evidence from two surveys 25 years apart. *British Medical Journal*, **304**, 873–5.

Pattemore, P. K., Johnston, S. L., and Bardin, P. G. (1992). Viruses as precipitants of asthma. I. Epidemiology. *Clinical and Experimental Allergy*, **22**, 326–36.

Rea, H. H., Scragg, R., Beaglehole, R., *et al.* (1986). A case control study of deaths from asthma. *Thorax*, **41**, 883–9.

Ruffin, R. E., Alpers, J. H., Pain, M. C., *et al.* (1987). The efficacy of nedocromil (sodium tilade) in asthma. *Australian and New Zealand Journal of Medicine*, **17**, 557–61.

Sandford, A. J., Shirakawa, T., Moffat, M. F., *et al.* (1993). Localisation, of atopy and α-subunit of high affinity IgE receptor (FceRI) on chromosome 11q. *Lancet*, **341**, 332–4.

Schatz, M., Harden, K., Forsythe, *et al.* (1988). The course of asthma during pregnancy, post partum and with successive pregnancies: A prospective analysis. *Journal of Allergy and Clinical Immunology*, **81**, 509–17.

Sears, M. R., Robin Taylor, D., Print, C. B., *et al.* (1990). Regular inhaled beta-agonist treatment in bronchial asthma. *Lancet*, **366**, 1391–6.

Wierenga, E. A., Snoek, M., De Groot, C., Chretien, I., Bos, J. D., Jansen, H. M., *et al.* (1990). Evidence for compartmentalisation of functional subsets of CD4+ T lymphocytes in atopic patients. *Journal of Immunology*, **144**, 4651–6.

Woolcock, A. J., Rubinfeld, A. R., Seale, J. P., *et al.* (1989). Thoracic Society of Australia & New Zealand Asthma Management Plan. *Medical Journal of Australia*, **151**, 650–3.

8 Systemic Anaphylaxis

R. J. Heddle and P. J. Roberts-Thomson

Definition

Systemic anaphylaxis is the most dramatic clinical consequence of immunoglobulin (Ig) E-mediated release of chemical mediators from mast cells and basophils. By definition it involves rapid onset of effects in multiple target organs and is potentially life-threatening. It might be viewed as a negative outcome of the powerful biological amplification systems which animals have evolved to meet survival needs.

A clinically identical syndrome, using the same pathways of biological amplification, can occur through physical or chemical activation of mast cells and basophils without mediation of IgE and such reactions are known as anaphylactoid reactions.

Anaphylaxis and anaphylactoid reactions are, in the acute phase, medical emergencies. They present challenges to the clinician in terms of diagnosis of trigger factors, in patient management, in minimizing recurrences, and in reducing the consequences of any further reactions.

Pathology

Onset of anaphylaxis is usually within minutes and rarely beyond the first hour after exposure to the trigger. Death may occur within minutes of onset of the reaction but with intervention is often delayed and may occur hours or days later. Post-mortem studies of patients who have died from acute anaphylaxis have revealed varying findings including:

1. non-inflammatory oedema of the upper airways, e.g. laryngeal oedema;

2. bronchoconstriction of lower airways with increased mucosal secretions, submucosal oedema, vascular congestion, and eosinophilic infiltration;

3. pulmonary oedema and occasionally pulmonary haemorrhage and atelectasis;

4. intravascular volume depletion, enhanced vascular permeability with leakage of plasma, peripheral vasodilution, and myocardial pallor;

5. extensive congestion of liver, spleen, and bowel wall;

6. dermal swelling and vasodilation;

7. when death has been delayed, ischaemic changes in target organs such as heart, bowel, and kidneys.

Sometimes the respiratory features are more prominent (70%) while in other patients the cardiovascular effects dominate (25%). Occasionally, autopsy findings show no significant pathological changes suggesting that an arrhythmia may have caused the collapse. Delayed mortality and morbidity is thought to occur due to impaired perfusion of vital organs in the acute stages but may possibly reflect a bipolar pattern of the anaphylactic reaction.

Pathogenesis

The pathophysiological manifestations of systemic anaphylaxis are attributed to the physiological and pharmacological effects of the sudden and massive release of a number of preformed and newly synthesized mediators from mast cells and circulating basophils. Other poorly recognized mechanisms and mediators are also probably involved.

Gross mast cell degranulation can occur through two generalized mechanisms: IgE dependent and non-IgE dependent. IgE-dependent degranulation is initiated by allergens cross-linking two specific and adjacent IgE molecules attached to their εRI receptor found in the surface membrane of mast cells (or basophils). This cross-linking leads to mast cell activation and degranulation. This signal transduction process involves a complex series of biochemical steps involving activation of membrane phospholipases with the production if inositol triphosphate and diacylglycerol, activation of phosphokinase C with subsequent phosphorylation of a variety of cytoplasmic proteins, changes in cyclic adenosine monophosphate/guanosine monophoshate ratio and the development of cystosolic Ca^{2+} fluxes. At a later stage nuclear transcription occurs with the synthesis of a variety of cytokines. As a consequence of these transduction signals and subsequent biochemical changes the granules of the mast cell are translocated to the cell surface, the granule membrane fuses with the surface membrane and the

granule content is discharged into the extracellular microenvironment. The granules contain a number of preformed phlogistic substances. The most important of these is the biogenic amine histamine which has potent bioactivities causing vasodilation, increased vascular permeability with plasma leakage and oedema, bronchial constriction, mucosal hypersecretion, hypersecretion of gastric acid, enhanced bowel motility, and increased parasympathetic reflex activity.

Histamine is a potent inducer of P-selectin on endothelial cells. Other preformed substances found within granules include tryptase, chymase, carboxypeptidase A, heparin-proteoglycan, and chemo-

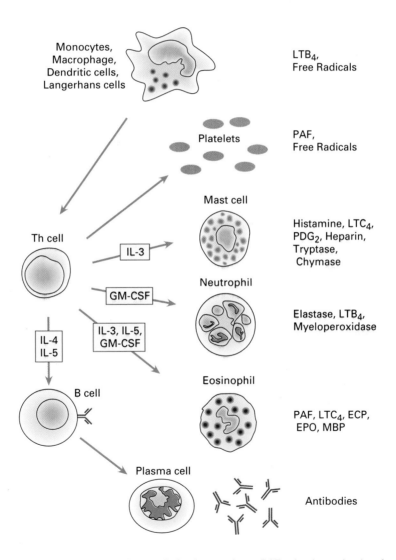

∎ **Fig. 8.1** Cells and mediators involved in anaphylactic reactions. PAF, platelet-activating factor; MBP, major basic protein; GM-CSF, granulocyte–macrophage colony-stimulating factor; EPO, eosinophil peroxidase.

tactic factors. Subsequent to mast cell activation a number of newly formed substances are also released. These include membrane phospholipid-derived mediators (e.g. prostaglandins, leukotrienes, and platelet-activating factors) and following nuclear transcription, a number of specific cytokines: (e.g. interleukin (IL) 3, IL-4, IL-5, IL-10, granulocyte–macrophage colony-stimulating factor, interferon γ, IL-1, IL-6). There is also evidence that tumour necrosis factor α and IL-4 may be preferentially stored in the preformed state is the mast cell and released early in the reaction. The sum total of all these preformed and newly synthesized mediators is to cause profound biological effects on the various shock organs and to lead to the gross clinical manifestations observed in anaphylaxis.

A number of allergens have been identified in initiating IgE-dependent mast cell degranulation. These include a variety of proteins, polysaccharides, haptens, and drugs, and are listed in Table 8.1. The nature of non-IgE-mediated gross mast cell degranulation is less well understood. It appears that a number of chemical mediators or physical triggers can directly activate mast cells without involving the IgE/IgE receptor complex (Table 8.2). These include the complement breakdown or 'anaphylactoid' peptides C3a and C5a, a number of cytokines, drugs including aspirin, non-steroidal anti-inflammatory drugs (NSAIDs), and radiocontrast media and the physical triggers of exercise, cold, heat, and UV exposure.

Anaphylaxis is 'idiopathic' when no specific trigger factors can be identified.

■ Table 8.1   Allergens identifies in IgE-mediated anaphylaxis'

Proteins
Foods, e.g. eggs, cow's milk, nuts, crustaceans, molluscs, legumes,
Venom, e.g. bee, wasp
Vaccines, e.g. measles, influenza, tetanus toxoid
Hormones, e.g. insulin, adrenocorticotrophic hormone, thyroid-stimulating hormone
Antiserum, e.g. horse, anti-venenes, antithymocyte, antilymphocyte globulin
Enzymes, e.g. streptokinase, chymopapain
Latex, e.g. surgical gloves, endotracheal tubes
Allergen extracts, e.g. house dust mite, grass pollens, animal danders

Haptens
Antibiotics, e.g. penicillin, cephalosporins
Muscle relaxants
Vitamins, e.g. thiamine
Cytotoxics, e.g. cisplatin, cyclophosphamide, cytosine arabinoside
Opiates

Polysaccharides
Dextran
Iron dextran
Polygeline

■ Table 8.2   Mast cell activation

IgE dependent
Fc∈R1 cross-linking with allergen

Non-IgE dependent
Fcμ RIII cross-linking with aggregated IgG
Fc∈R1 cross linking by auto-antibody to Fc∈R1 peptides
　substance P
　leucocyte-derived peptides
　collagen degradation products
Cytokines
　chemokines — α-family IL-8
　　　　　　　— β-family MCP-1, MIP-1a, RANTES IL-3
　granulocyte–macrophage colony-stimulating factor
Complement products
　C3a, C5a
Drugs
　opiates, cytotoxics, aspirin, non-steroidal anti-inflammatory drugs, radiocontrast media
Physical factors
　exercise, cold, UV exposure

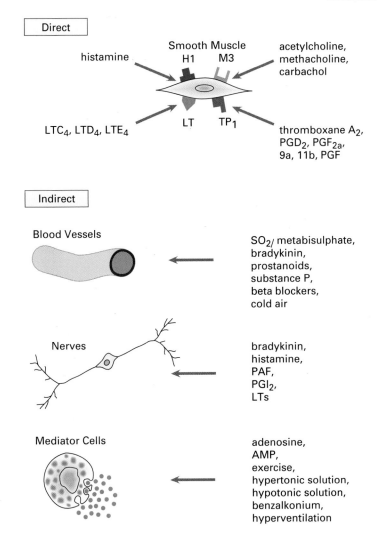

▮ **Fig. 8.2** Anaphylaxis is due to direct effects of agents on smooth muscle, and indirect effects on blood vessels, nerves, and mediator cells. LT, leukotrienes; AMP, adenosine monophosphate; PAF, platelet-activating factor.

Recent studies on chronic urticaria suggest that autoantibodies to the FeεRI receptors are important mast cell activators in some subjects.

Clinical manifestations

Common manifestations are a rash, often urticarial, rhinitis and conjunctivitis, angioedema, particularly of face, upper airways and extremities, asthma, vomiting, diarrhoea and abdominal colic, uterine cramps, and hypotension. Other features may be cyanosis, cardiac arrhythmia, vascular collapse, loss of consciousness, and death. The timing of reactions and the predominant manifestations vary widely but onset is usually within 30 min of exposure.

Biphasic responses, are well recognized and appear to be a frequent occurrence in severe IgE-mediated food reactions. In these an initial onset of symptoms is followed by a relatively symptom-free period, before recurrence of manifestations, often in severe form. Some individuals have a protracted anaphylaxis which may require vasopressor and ventilatory support for days or weeks.

The clinical manifestations are superimposed upon any pre-existing medical problem and this may

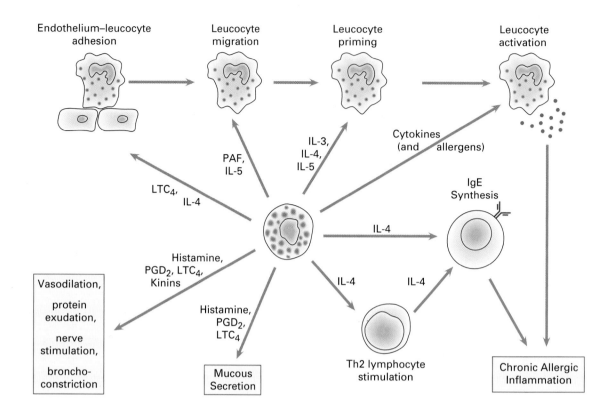

∎ Fig. 8.3   The role of the mast cell in acute and chronic allergic reactions. PAF, platelet-activating factor.

account for the observation, that, although anaphylaxis to insect stings is far more common in children, adolescents, and young adults, deaths occur disproportionately in older subjects. In individuals with vascular risk factors, events such as myocardial infarction and stroke are occasional complications of anaphylaxis.

Insect sting anaphylaxis

This dramatic event probably causes undue fear because of the apparently random nature of the triggering events and the perceived lack of control of the subject and families over the events. The death rate from stinging insect allergy is probably somewhat higher than official estimates, which are usually of the order of 1:5 000 000 subjects per year, because there are cases of sudden death where the contribution of an insect sting has not been recognized. Nevertheless, it is highly probable that stinging insect allergy is a much less frequent cause of death from anaphylaxis than food or drug allergy.

While a substantial minority of an exposed population have allergic antibodies to stinging insect venom (15% in Australian population living in a Mediterranean-type climate), probably only 1% of a population will have experienced a previous immediate generalized reaction to a stinging insect. Only a small proportion of those reactions will have been life-threatening. Unfortunately, 25% of subjects dying as a result of an insect sting have had no prior warning of their hypersensitivity.

The most important stinging insects causing anaphylaxis are members of the order Hymenoptera and include the honey bee, wasps (polistes), yellow jacket (Vespula), and the hornet. There are wide geographic variations in the relative importance of such insects, and there are other stinging insects which appear important in anaphylaxis in specific locations, e.g. *Myrmecia pilosula* (Jack jumper ant) in heavily vegetated, hilly areas of eastern and southern Australia and the fire ant (*Solenopsis invictor*) in south-eastern USA.

Common adverse reactions to stinging insects include large local reactions, often maximal at 24–48 h and immediate generalized reactions, which may be purely cutaneous, or show any or all of the more dangerous features of anaphylaxis. Such reactions usually start within 30 min of a sting and are usually uniphasic. Less common reactions, usually evolving over days or weeks, include serum sickness and delayed hypersensitivity reactions.

The nature of adverse reactions to multiple stings is not well understood, but while subjects encountering extremely large numbers of stings may suffer from toxic reactions, the presence or absence of allergy appears to be an important determinant of outcome after multiple stings.

Only immediate generalized reactions appear to have positive predictive value for anaphylaxis following future stings. Individuals who had respiratory involvement or hypotension after a sting have a substantial chance of recurrence of a similar or worse reaction from a bee sting within the next few years. However, only a low percentage of individuals who have had immediate generalized reactions confined to the skin will develop major cardiovascular or respiratory involvement on subsequent stings. Older sensitized adults, particularly male, and those working in isolated rural settings appear to be at increased risk of death from stinging insect allergies.

For an individual who had an immediate generalized reaction to a honey bee sting the chances of recurrence of a similar or worse reaction vary from about 60% (older studies) to 25% (more recent studies). The longer the interval before the next sting, the less the likelihood of a further reaction but this decline in sensitivity varies greatly between individuals and cannot be predicted precisely by the currently available skin or blood tests.

Anaphylaxis to stinging insects does not appear to correlate closely with atopy. A family history of honey bee sting anaphylaxis is significantly more common in the population attending bee venom immunotherapy clinic than in the general population.

Anaphylaxis resulting from food allergy

Life-threatening IgE-mediated reactions to food proteins probably cause many more deaths than anaphylaxis to stinging insects. Unfortunately, the importance of severe IgE-mediated reactions to foods tends to be overlooked by the inappropriate application of the word 'food allergy' to cover diverse food intolerances. Anaphylactic reactions to foods usually commence within 30 min of ingestion and very frequently the subject has immediate oropharyngeal and abdominal symptoms. Subsequent manifestations are those seen in other forms of anaphylaxis, although biphasic and protracted reactions appear to be unfortunately common in the context of food allergy.

IgE-mediated food allergy occurs in atopic individuals and most commonly presents in early childhood, with severe anaphylactic reactions generally occurring in childhood and early adult years. If less frequent presentation in later life reflects attrition of sensitivity or more effective avoidance strategies is not known. It is established, however, that a number of infants lose clinical hypersensitivity to some food proteins in early life. Clinical and published experience suggests that children and adults manifesting allergy to peanuts, tree nuts (e.g. Brazilnut, hazelnut, or walnut) or seafood (e.g. prawns) can expect persistent hypersensitivity.

Although the list of foods documented as causing IgE-mediated anaphylaxis is large, only a few foods account for the majority of reactions. In early childhood, egg, cows milk, and soya proteins are prominent but beyond infancy peanuts, tree nuts, and seafoods account for many of the most severe reactions. Unfortunately, the amount of food necessary to produce anaphylaxis may be extremely small and traces on utensils or in food production plants have been shown to be able to induce anaphylaxis in a few individuals. This, and a trend towards use of complex preprepared food and cuisine render avoidance difficult.

The vast majority of subjects experiencing anaphylaxis to food proteins will have strong positive skin tests and/or *in vitro* tests for IgE antibody to the food protein.

Some subjects with recurrent or chronic urticaria and/or angioedema and others with asthma have their symptoms reproduced by blind challenges with small biologically active chemicals found in foods, either naturally (e.g. salicylates, biogenic amines, and glutamates) or as additives (e.g. preservatives, colouring agents, antioxidants, glutamates). Occasionally, such reactions are of anaphylactoid proportions. These reactions are not IgE mediated and are not associated with positive skin or *in vitro* tests for IgE antibodies.

Anaphylaxis triggered by physical factors

Anaphylactic episodes can, in some patients, be associated with exposure to cold (e.g. diving into cold sea) or with exercise.

Cold-induced anaphylaxis, a rare condition, is considered to be an extreme form of cold-induced urticaria and presumably reflects the massive mast cell degranulation on sudden exposure to cold.

Exercise-induced anaphylaxis (EIA) is a more common condition that occurs during or shortly after a period of moderate to intense physical activity, e.g. running, cycling, squash, etc. It is not invariably a consequence of exercise and a number of modifying co-factors are recognized:

(1) ambient temperature (more common in warm weather or following hot shower);

(2) higher humidity;

(3) following recent meal (perhaps related to ingestion of specific food allergen, salicylates, azo dyes, preservatives, or recent aspirin or NSAID ingestion);

(4) inhalation of allergen during exercise or in women related to the menstrual cycle.

The severity of the symptoms in EIA varies considerably. In some instances symptoms may be mild and include pruritis, urticaria, and angioedema developing during or after the physical activity, while on another occasion they may be more severe with addition of upper respiratory tract obstruction, bronchospasm, profuse cutaneous flushing, and sweating and vascular collapse.

Idiopathic anaphylaxis

Idiopathic anaphylaxis is a systemic allergic reaction in which an exhaustive clinical history and intensive laboratory testing reveal no known cause for the reaction. The diagnosis is reached by exclusion of other causes of anaphylaxis. Idiopathic anaphylaxis may occur as a single isolated episode or, more commonly, in a recurrent form. In the recurrent form prolonged remission between episodes may occur, and the severity of each reaction varies ranging greatly.

Patients with idiopathic anaphylaxis have elevated levels of plasma tryptase and plasma and urinary histamine during acute episodes, confirming the involvement of activated mast cells in this reaction. Idiopathic anaphylaxis may be as a consequence of the summation of a number of interactive mast cell activating factors (e.g. combination of dietary, neurohumoral, hormonal, physical, and other factors). Observations that anti-FcεRI antibodies play some part in recurrent or chronic uriticaria suggest that they may have a part in idiopathic anaphylaxis. The prevalence of atopy in patients with idiopathic anaphylaxis is raised (50%), and sometimes extensive prick skin testing to food allergens together with a relevant history may reveal an unsuspected food as the cause. The course of idio-

pathic anaphylaxis is highly variable, although the long-term prognosis for treated patients is generally good.

Drug-induced anaphylaxis

Many drugs, acting either as haptens or complete antigens, are prominent causes of IgE mediated anaphylactic reactions (Table 8.1). Many other drugs provoke anaphylactoid reactions (Table 8.2), while others (e.g. opiates) appear in some individuals to produce IgE-mediated anaphylactic and in others anaphylactoid reactions.

Acute management of an anaphylactic reaction

First aid

Stop administration of the causal agent or in cases of insect sting remove the venom sac and sting by scraping with a flat surface (e.g. a knife or coin). The patient should remain supine and be transported to the nearest emergency medical facility.

Definitive therapy

Examination of the patient is needed to assess the severity of the reaction; the vital signs noted and the presence of a generalized rash, upper or lower airways obstruction should be sought for and documented.

If mild bronchospasm appears to be the only important manifestation (it is important to distinguish bronchospasm from stridor), an aerosol or nebulized bronchodilator agent may be given. If signs or symptoms progress despite this treatment or if there is any evidence of upper airways involvement (e.g. dysphagia, dysphonia, sense of choking, or stridor), moderate or severe bronchospasm and/or circulatory involvement, (central cyanosis, hypotension, collapse) supplementary oxygen and parenteral adrenaline should be given immediately. Intramuscular administration probably provides the best combination of maximal efficacy with minimal side-effects in most circumstances, 0.3–0.5 ml of a 1 in 1000 solution should be given (0.01–0.015 ml/kg in children). This dose can be repeated at 5–10 min intervals according to the response.

Intravenous adrenaline should probably be reserved for patients with severe shock or respiratory involvement, or where intravenous access plus cardiac monitoring facilities are in place, as the use of intravenous adrenaline has been associated with cardiac arrhythmias and myocardial death. Only the 1 in 10 000 solution should be used, and this should be infused at a rate of maximum 1 ml/min until a satisfactory response occurs. In severe cases, an adrenaline infusion (5–15 μg/min) may be required for several hours after initial resuscitation. Respiratory administration of adrenaline, by means of a metered dose aerosol or by way of endotracheal tube, may be effective.

Basic supportive therapy including airways maintenance, supplementary oxygen, and intravenously administered fluids, preferably with the use of colloidal solutions such as polygeline or stable plasma-protein solution, must not be forgotten. The importance of intravenously administered colloidal solutions cannot be overemphasized and the initiation of an infusion at the earliest possible phase of a major reaction is recommended. In addition, in extreme cases, cardiopulmonary resuscitation and more advanced life-support techniques also may be required.

Although recent evidence suggests that corticosteroid agents may have a beneficial part in preventing late-phase reactions in anaphylaxis, there is little evidence to support their use in the acute situation. Likewise, H_1-antagonist agents may inhibit the recurrence or shorten the duration of angioedema. However, the administration of corticosteroid or antihistamine agents must never delay or replace the more definitive measures that are outlined above, especially in severe cases.

Patients who have suffered from an anaphylactic reaction require intensive supervision for a least 4 h after onset of the reaction, even when they appear to have recovered fully. This allows for appropriate management of biphasic reactions. Patients with reactions should be referred to an appropriate specialist for further evaluation, as appropriate avoidance measures, Medic-Alert bracelet and Action Plan (e.g. self-administration of adrenaline) may prevent a recurrence.

Management, investigation, prophylaxis, and education

Insect sting anaphylaxis

For those with local or generalized cutaneous reactions only advice about avoidance measures, sting removal (for honey bee stings only), and immediate seeking of medical care should suffice. Oral H_1 antihistamines may shorten the duration of reactions. Unfortunately, there is little evidence that *in vitro* assays for IgE antibody to venoms or skin testing with

∎ **Table 8.3** Medical management of anaphylaxis

Stop administration of causal agent
Adopt supine position with legs elevated
Assess severity
Adrenaline
Establish airways and 100% O_2 (ventilate if necessary)
Intravenous fluids
Assess progress and monitor for at least 4 h

venoms alone can predict a small percentage of these individuals likely to suffer an anaphylactic reaction to a future sting. Sting challenges are demanding of resources, in the case of the honey bee vary greatly in the dose of venom delivered and may themselves affect the hypersensitivity status for the next sting. In some cases where the relatively low risk of a cardiorespiratory reaction to a future sting might be seen as posing a major risk (e.g. older males, those with underlying cardiovascular or respiratory problems or those living in remote areas) and in all cases with a history of cardiorespiratory reactions, provision of adrenaline for self-administration (e.g. Epi-pen auto-injector) should be considered.

Generally, venom immunotherapy should be reserved for individuals who have experienced an immediate generalized reaction to a sting from a clearly identified insect, who have experienced respiratory and/or circulatory manifestations as part of that reaction and who have IgE antibodies to the venom demonstrated by *in vitro* assay or skin testing. There is a low incidence of false negative responses on *in vitro* assays for venom-specific IgE antibodies and a negative assay should always lead to skin testing. Immunotherapy should be performed with due consent, and where there are trained personnel and appropriate equipment for resuscitation immediately available. It is highly effective, reducing greatly the incidence of anaphylactic reactions to future stings. Maintenance immunotherapy until there is evidence of loss of IgE antibodies to the venom by *in vitro* assay or skin testing may be appropriate in individuals who have required major resuscitation. However, there is a growing consensus that for many individuals, 3–5 years of monthly or 6 weekly maintenance immunotherapy leads to substantial protection persisting for many years even if, when the immunotherapy is ceased, there are persisting IgE antibodies to the venom. It appears that there may be a higher relapse rate if immunotherapy is discontinued earlier.

Food-related anaphylaxis

If the subject is atopic, the history suggests an immediate reaction to a food protein known to induce anaphylaxis, and particularly if there have been immediate oro-pharyngeal symptoms, an IgE-mediated anaphylactic reaction to a food protein is probable. If there remains any doubt skin testing or, if that is not available, RAST testing (radioallergosorbent test) to the likely food proteins may be useful. Small positive skin test reactions and weak to moderate *in vitro* reactions to food proteins are often clinically irrelevant.

If the responsible food item can be identified it should be avoided. However, even motivated patients sometimes accidentally eat the responsible food. Patients should be provided with an Action Plan which stresses self-administration of adrenaline (e.g. Epi pen auto-injector), seeking immediate care at the nearest emergency facility and observation for at least 4 h (in order to cover a biphasic reaction). Education regarding the food allergy should extend to the family and friends.

Sometimes the reaction to the food may be anaphylactoid and depend upon a cumulative dose ingested over a period of time and are not predictable in terms of any blood or skin tests. The diagnosis may be far more difficult in these cases. The severity or recurrent nature of episodes may dictate that investigation by a unit experienced in elimination diet and controlled blind substance food challenges is indicated. These patients need the same emergency measures and Action Plans as those with IgE-mediated food anaphylaxis.

At a public health level, legislators and the food industry need to appreciate the significance of trace quantities of allergenic proteins in foods and of appropriate labelling. Legislators should protect non-medically trained persons who in appropriate circumstances administer adrenaline via auto-injectors specifically designed for lay-person use.

Anaphylaxis triggered by physical factors

A carefully taken history is the key investigation. There is a correlation between the rapidity with which urticaria develops in response to exposure to an ice-block wrapped in plastic (to exclude aquagenic urticaria) and the liability of the subject to anaphylaxis on sudden cold exposure. Cholinergic urticaria can usually be identified by the development of a very fine, centripetal, urticarial rash when the subject commences sweating, but also can be confirmed by satellite urticaria developing around the site of an intradermal injection of methacholine. In selected cases there may be a case for exercise testing, but

these investigations are best performed by units with experience in such tests. Food may be a facilitating factor in exercise anaphylaxis, and there is need for skin testing and/or elimination diet in some cases. Interpretation is particularly difficult in this multifactorial situation.

Patients with physical urticaria/physical anaphylaxis should be cautioned about avoidance measures, ceasing the activity at onset of any symptoms. They should have an Action Plan including provisions for intramuscular adrenaline and urgent transfer to emergency medical care. Prophylactic use of an H_1 antagonist may be helpful, but patients should be aware that such agents may partially inhibit rather than prevent a reaction.

Occasionally cold urticaria proceeding to cold anaphylaxis is a manifestation of an underlying disease. Investigations into this possibility have been discussed in the chapter on urticaria.

Drug-induced anaphylactic-anaphylactoid reactions

Immediate hypersensitivity skin testing or *in vitro* assays for specific IgE antibodies are applicable only to IgE-mediated anaphylactic reactions and are then limited in their predictive values by difficulties in reproducing such *in vivo* events as the formation of reactive metabolites and protein binding. Nevertheless, skin testing regimens with useful predictive value have been established for specific drugs, e.g. β-lactam antibiotics, muscle relaxants, chymopapain, and latex (refer to Chapter 11 on Drug reactions).

The prime management of drug-induced anaphylactic and anaphylactoid reactions is avoidance and a warning bracelet is appropriate. Written information describing exactly the nature of the previous drug reaction and any relevant investigation should be readily available.

In unusual circumstances, the risks of anaphylaxis on re-exposure may be balanced by the clinical advantages of the drug and in that situation expert advice regarding the risks/benefits of cautious drug challenge in an intensive care setting with H_1 antagonist and corticosteroid cover or, where available (e.g. penicillin or aspirin), induction of tachyphylaxis should be sought. It is to be stressed that these procedures are to be performed only in high-dependency settings by those with special expertise.

Idiopathic anaphylaxis

All individuals should be given an Action Plan, emergency bracelet, and considered for self-administration of adrenaline.

Further reading

Bochner, B. S. and Lichtenstein, L. M. (1991). Anaphylaxis. *New England Journal of Medicine*, **324**, 1785–90.

Dann, L. (1994). Acute anaphylaxis. *Australian Family Physician*, **23**, 159–61.

Harvey, P., Sperber, S., Kette, F., Heddle, R. J., and Roberts-Thomson, P. J. (1984). Bee-sting mortality in Australia. *Medical Journal of Australia*, **140**, 209–11.

Lucke, W. C. and Thomas, H. (1983). Anaphylaxis: Pathophysiology, clinical presentations and treatment. *Journal Emergency Medicine*, **1**, 83–95.

Roberts-Thomson, P. J., Harvey, P., Sperber, S., Kupa, A., and Heddle, R. J. (1985). Bee sting anaphylaxis in an urban population of South Australia. *Asian Pacific Journal of Allergy and Immunology*, **3**, 161–4.

Roitt, I., Brostoff, J., and Male, D. K. (ed) In (1996). In *Immunology*, 4th edn. Mosby, London, pp. 22.2–22.17.

Shelter, A. L. and Austen, K. F. (1984). Exercise induced anaphylaxis. *Journal of Allergy and Clinical Immunology*, **73**, 699–704.

9 Food allergy

J. Bradley

Introduction

Reaction to food has been recognized since ancient times when reaction to cows' milk was recognized by Hippocrates. However, it has been a confused area of clinical medicine for several decades. One reason for this is that 'food allergy' is frequently misused to describe any kind of idiosyncratic adverse reaction to food instead of being used only in relation to immunologically mediated hypersensitivity reactions. Lack of lactase or alcohol dehydrogenase produce symptoms after ingestion of milk or alcohol but this is not food allergy. Accurate clinical diagnosis has also been a long-standing problem in this field. Recognition that foods could sometimes induce immunological hypersensitivity dates back to the discovery of anaphylaxis at the turn of the twentieth century. Early in this century systematic studies had documented the salient clinical features of food allergy in children.

Definition:

1. *Food allergy* (food hypersensitivity) usually means immunoglobulin (Ig) E-mediated but can include non-IgE-mediated immune responses to food.

2. *Food intolerance* is used to define abnormal response to food due to non-immunological mechanisms: idiosyncratic, metabolic, pharmacological, and toxic.

Food allergy

Ingelfinger in 1948 gave three criteria, which remain the cornerstone of our clinical definition of true food allergy to the present day:

(1) consistent reproduction of symptoms by blind provocation;

(2) functional changes or lesions in the target organs;

(3) demonstration of an immune mechanism in pathogenesis.

In the vast majority of cases, true food allergy is IgE-mediated. Other mechanisms of hypersensitivity have been postulated; for example, formation of immune complexes with activation of the complement cascade, or T-cell-mediated reactions, but evidence for their existence is weak. Gluten sensitivity in patients with coeliac disease is the only well-recognized exception.

Prevalence and natural history of food allergy

The true prevalence of food allergy in the community is difficult to estimate accurately, but is highest in infancy (~4–6%), falling to ~1–2% during early childhood, and less than 1% in adults. These figures reflect the observation that most children cease to suffer from food allergies as they grow towards puberty.

The natural history of food allergy depends on three principal factors: age at onset, type of food(s) involved, and severity of the initial reaction. As a rule, the later the onset of a food allergy the less likely that clinical sensitivity will be lost. While most infants sensitive to cows' milk can tolerate reintroduction by 2 years, children diagnosed as having a food allergy after the age of 3 years are less likely to outgrow the problem. Children are more likely to stop reacting to milk, soy, wheat, and egg allergies as they grow older, whereas reactions to peanut and fish allergies are more often severe and persistent.

Food intolerance

Non-immunological reactions are more common than true food allergies, especially in adults, but are more difficult to diagnose. In most cases, they are attributable to pharmacological idiosyncrasies to a variety of natural dietary chemicals and/or food additives, and probably act via neurogenic rather than immunological pathways. In susceptible individuals, intolerances to xenobiotics of this kind exhibit clinical behaviour which is suggestive of receptor-mediated actions: dose-dependence, withdrawal effects, supersensitivity, and tachyphylaxis, depending on the circumstances of exposure; and cross-sensitivities with pharmacologically related substances. Many foods in the daily diet may be involved, and as reactions are often delayed by several hours, recognition of the connection between symptoms and specific foods can be difficult.

Clinical manifestations of food intolerances are generally more comparable with drug side-effects or idiosyncrasies than to allergies. They can be gastrointestinal, cutaneous, and/or neuropsychiatric, and may include non-specific constitutional symptoms such as headache, malaise, lethargy and myalgia. However, certain reactions, although not immunologically mediated, are clinically indistinguishable from true allergic reactions. The best examples are urticaria and angioedema. Although acute urticaria is a classical manifestation of IgE-mediated allergic reactions, the more common 'hives' of childhood and chronic 'idiopathic' urticaria in adults are non-immunological reactions often triggered by food chemicals. Diagnosis in such cases rests on the use of a carefully controlled elimination diet and systematic oral challenge testing with the substances.

Pathogenesis of food allergy

The normal function of IgE antibodies is to protect the host from parasitic infestation by activating mast cells which are located principally in the skin and mucous membranes. Binding of parasite antigens by IgE leads to release of inflammatory mediators from mast cells, attraction of eosinophils, and killing of the invading organism. Approximately 30% of the population has a genetic tendency to atopy, i.e. produce exaggerated IgE responses to a variety of common environmental antigens. Atopic individuals often have high total serum IgE levels and a family history of allergic disorders (hay fever, asthma, and/or eczema), and about half will experience allergic symptoms at some time during their life. Most individuals with food allergy are atopic but the converse is not necessarily true. Atopic individuals generally do not develop clinical symptoms of food allergy even when food-specific IgE antibodies are present, suggesting an important part for

other, as yet poorly understood factors which contribute to target organ reactivity in symptomatic individuals. Sensitization usually occurs early in life. Intact food protein molecules are known to be capable of crossing the gastrointestinal tract mucosa in sufficient quantities to elicit an immune response, and healthy individuals commonly have low levels of food-specific IgG, IgM, and IgA antibodies. IgE production usually begins in infancy after introduction of formula baby food and solids, and may be enhanced by factors which cause local damage or increase permeability, such as infection or inflammation. Exclusive breast feeding appears to have a protective effect. However, in highly atopic families sensitization can occur *in utero* or in fully breast-fed infants as a result of exposure to antigens in the maternal diet.

Sensitization in a genetically susceptible person begins when antigen is processed by specialized antigen-presenting cells (APC) at the mucosal surfaces. Antigenic peptides bound to human leucocyte antigen (HLA) class II are transported to the APC cell surface where they form a molecular complex which is presented to CD4+ T cells. Due to the nature of the microenvironment CD4+ Th2 cells are activated to produce interleukin (IL) 4, IL-5, and interferon (IFN) γ and interact with antigen-specific B cells to trigger the production of IgE antibodies. Once sensitized, continuing production of specific IgE antibodies leaves the individual at risk of developing an allergic reaction on subsequent re-exposure.

Common food allergens

The foods that cause immunological reactions have common properties: they are heat and acid stable glycoproteins of molecular weight 18–36 kDa. Although atopic individuals can make IgE antibodies to almost any food, only a small number are commonly responsible for causing clinically significant allergies. In 80–90% of children with food allergy egg, peanut, milk, fish, and soya and wheat account for about 90% of reactions confirmed by double-blind placebo-controlled food challenge, and in most cases only one or two foods are involved. In adults, peanut, fish, and shellfish are more prevalent as offending foods. Allergies to egg, milk, and wheat tend to be outgrown.

The prevalence of a specific food allergy also depends on the eating habits of the population. For example, peanut allergy is much more common in the USA and Britain than in Sweden. Similarly, rice allergy is not uncommon in Japan but is rare in Western countries.

Why some foods are more allergenic than others is unknown. The antigenic components of several have been studied in detail and have a number of features in common. They are glycoproteins with molecular weights between 10 and 40 kDa, and are heat and acid stable. In milk, the major allergens are casein and β lactoglobulin, but allergic individuals can also make IgE antibodies to α lactalbumin, bovine serum albumin, and bovine immunoglobulin. Soya, often recommended as a milk substitute, ovalbumin and ovomucoid are also major allergens, as are codfish and shrimp.

Peanut is probably the most potent of the common food allergens. Highly atopic children are at special risk of sensitization and in extreme cases, even the smell of a peanut can provoke urticaria and angioedema around the face and eyes and/or wheezing.

Food 'families' and cross-reactivity

This was first proposed in the 1930s, supported by uncontrolled clinical observations and skin test results, and tables of food 'families' have been reproduced. It is often suggested that peanut-allergic individuals should also avoid other members of the legume family such as peas, beans, lentils, and soya bean. However, clinical cross-reactivity between two or more members of a food 'family' rarely occurs.

Clinical features and diagnosis

Clinically significant food allergy is principally a childhood disorder. It usually occurs against an atopic family background, in children with a history of eczema and/or gastrointestinal symptoms. Most children grow out of the problem before puberty, so that presentation in adult life is uncommon.

The increased susceptibility of children may be due to immaturity of the immunological and gastrointestinal systems. Several studies have suggested that exclusive breast feeding may produce oral tolerance and prevent food allergy and atopic dermatitis. Low concentrations of IgG, IgM, and IgA food specific antibodies are found in normal subjects. Higher levels are found in those with inflammatory bowel disease.

The IgE-mediated responses of food allergy present with clinical features which are dependent on the site of mast cell degranulation and activation. Acute reactions may begin with swelling, burning, or itch around the mouth and throat, followed by vomiting, abdominal cramps, and diarrhoea, and if there is

spread of allergen or a greater release of mediators generalized urticaria, bronchoconstriction, and rarely, fatal anaphylaxis. Severe anaphylaxis most frequently is associated with ingestion of shellfish, fish, peanuts, and nuts.

In asthmatics, acute attacks can occasionally be precipitated by foods, e.g. flour, eggs, and garlic, but in most cases this is due to the non-specific irritant effect of sulphite preservatives rather than to a true food allergy. Chronic eczema or recurrent abdominal symptoms can sometimes be triggered by unrecognized allergy to a frequently ingested food, e.g. milk, eggs, wheat, and chocolate, particularly in children.

Food-induced migraine occurs and may be accompanied by rhinitis, conjunctivitis, urticaria, and/or angioedema.

Diagnosis

A full history, including a family history is needed.

Properly performed skin prick tests or radioallergosorbent tests (RAST) are sensitive and reliable methods for detecting specific IgE antibodies to suspected allergens. A positive result is of no clinical significance in the absence of relevant symptoms. In contrast negative skin tests have a high predictive value in excluding food allergy as a cause of symptoms. In equivocal cases the most definitive test is a double-blind placebo-controlled oral food challenge which must be carried out under careful supervision. Skin testing may not be advisable in some circumstances; e. g. extensive skin disease and prolonged dermatographism. In these RAST may be useful, although it is considered less sensitive than skin tests

Allergies and intolerances

Many foods which are well-recognized allergens can also provoke non-immunological reactions, and this can be a cause of confusion in clinical evaluation. For example, patients with food intolerance can react adversely to toxins in fish and preservatives in shrimp, or lactose in milk. Shrimp is usually implicated as a result of symptoms occurring during or immediately after a meal. These reactions may be due to the combined presence of sulphite preservatives, colourings, and natural salicylates and not to IgE-mediated responses. Fresh shrimp can contain sulphites because it is used as a preservative by fishing boats and markets.

Treatment

The only proven treatment is avoidance of the allergen once the diagnosis of food allergy in made. However, if the offending allergen is present in a number of foods care must be taken to ensure that the patient gets a balanced diet.

For those patients who have had food-induced anaphylaxis examination of food and food labels to detect potential sources of hidden food allergens in necessary. Instruction in the use of self-administered adrenaline is also needed, and syringes of adrenaline and antihistamines should be readily available.

Oral allergy

Oral allergy syndrome describes the occurrence of oropharyngeal symptoms immediately after ingestion of a food, followed by cutaneous, respiratory, and/or gastrointestinal symptoms within an hour. The majority of patients are adults, and 80% have a history of symptomatic food allergy developing in childhood. Early symptoms included a sensation of tingling in the lips or mouth, throat tightness, lip tightness and/or swelling, and oral mucosal blebs, occurring after ingestion of small amounts of offending food, followed by nausea, vomiting, abdominal pain, conjunctivitis, asthma, and/or urticaria if larger quantities were ingested. Positive skin and RAST tests with fish, egg, milk, and nuts correlate well with immediate clinical reactions, while tomato, orange, and other plant allergen tests correlate less well.

Eosinophilic gastroenteritis

This is a rare disorder which can occur at any age, the peak prevalence being in early adult life. It is characterized by mucosal thickening and eosinophilic thickening and eosinophilic infiltration of the stomach and/or bowel wall, causing recurrent or chronic abdominal symptoms, and accompanied in severe cases by malabsorption, ascites, and iron-deficiency anaemia. Most patients are atopic, with high IgE levels and peripheral blood eosinophilia. Definitive diagnosis depends on the finding of a marked eosinophilic infiltrate on gastric or small-bowel biopsy. Dietary restriction can sometimes help to control symptoms. Corticosteroids are the therapy of choice, often leading to dramatic clinical improvement. Oral disodium cromoglycate and ketotifen have been used successfully.

Standard antihistamines have proven to be of little benefit.

Asthma

Foods can sometimes trigger exacerbations of asthma, most commonly due to the irritant effect of sulphite preservatives. In the most sensitive individuals the concentration of sulphur dioxide released in the oropharynx during ingestion of sulphite-preserved foods can be sufficient to trigger acute bronchoconstriction.

Food-induced anaphylaxis

Occurs usually in those who are highly atopic with histories of asthma, eczema, and/or rhinitis. Idiopathic anaphylaxis is an uncommon disorder usually presenting in adult life and characterized by recurrent anaphylactoid episodes of unknown cause. A series of 102 patients were each skin prick-tested with a battery of 790 foods at the Mayo Clinic. Of 32 with positive results, seven were identified in whom the skin test findings correlated with open challenge reactions to one or more previously unsuspected foods. Most of the allergens concerned were unusual ones: aniseed, cashew, celery, flaxseed, hops, mushroom, mustard, shrimp, sunflower seed, and walnut.

Food-dependent exercise-induced anaphylaxis is a recently recognized variant of the same condition. In most cases, symptoms are only triggered if exercise takes place following the ingestion of a specific food. Simple avoidance of the relevant food before exercise is often effective in preventing attacks, but in some cases temperature, humidity, degree of exertion, and alcohol ingestion may be contributory factors requiring attention.

Further reading

O'Hehir, R. E., garman, R. D., Greenstein, J. L. and Lamb, J. R. (1991). The specificity and regulation of T cell responsiveness to allergens. *Annual Reviews of Immunology*, **9**, 67–95.

Loblay, R. H. (1993). Food Allergy in adults-state of the art. *Recent advances in clinical nutrition*, **3**, 153–63.

Min, K-U. and Metcalfe, D. D. (1991). Eosinophilic gastroenterits. *Immunology and Allergy Clinics of North America*, **11**, 799–813.

Pastorello, E. A., Stocchi, L., Pravettoni, V., Bigi, A., Schilke, M. L., Incorvaia, C., and Zanussi, C. (1989). Role of the elimination diet in adults with food allergy. *Journal of Allergy and Clinical Immunology*, **84**, 475–83.

Sampson, H. A. (1991). Immunologic mechanisms in adverse reactions to foods. *Immunology and Allergy Clinics of North America*, **11**, 701–16.

Sampson, H. A. (1988). IgE mediated food intolerance. *Journal of Allergy and Clinical Immunology*, **81**, 495–504.

10 Recurrent urticaria and angioedema

A. Kupa

Definition

The lesions of urticaria are raised, well demarcated, intensely pruritic papules or weals, a few millimetres to many centimetres in size, either erythematous or pale in colour, often with associated erythematous flare. They evolve rapidly and may become confluent to form giant urticaria. Acute urticarial lesions tend to resolve within hours, while the lesions of recurrent urticaria tend to persist for up to 24 h.

Angioedema is swelling of subcutaneous or submucosal tissues, often occurring around the head and neck, palms of hands, soles of feet, or genitalia. The overlying skin appears normal, and the patient usually complains more of discomfort than itch. Angioedema is associated with urticaria in about 45% cases.

Episodes of urticaria/angioedema lasting less than 6 weeks are termed acute, and are most commonly seen in children or young adults, often in relation to allergic reactions or infections. The term chronic urticaria refers to urticaria/angioedema which has been recurring on a frequent basis for more than 6 weeks.

Introduction

Prevalence

Urticaria and angioedema have a cumulative lifetime prevalence of 15–25%.

Pathogenesis

The principal finding in urticaria and angioedema is oedema of the dermis or subcutaneous tissue, respectively. The mast cell plays a pivotal role in the genesis of urticaria and angioedema. Preformed mast cell mediators such as histamine, heparin, and neutral pro-

teases are released with resultant increase in vascular permeability, vasodilation, and itch. The histology of acute urticarial lesions is characterized by dilated capillaries, interstitial oedema, and eosinophilia but very little perivascular cellular infiltrate, reflecting the transient or fleeting nature of the lesions. Biopsy of chronic urticarial lesions reveals more extensive perivascular mononuclear infiltrate. There may be a 10-fold increase in mast cell numbers and a fourfold increase in mononuclear cells which are mainly T cells. It is likely that T-cell and monocyte lymphokine release have potent amplification effects leading to increase in mast cell numbers, and a lowering of the mast cell threshold for degranulation. In addition, a decrease in histamine clearance from the skin of chronic urticaria patients has been demonstrated Fig. 10.1).

Mast cell degranulation can be triggered by many factors — immunoglobulin (Ig) E cross-linking by allergen or anti-IgE antibody; physical factors such as temperature changes, pressure, vibratory stimuli, exercise; drugs such as opiates, aspirin, and non-steroidal anti-inflammatory drugs (NSAIDs); food chemicals including natural salicylates and benzoates; components C3a and C5a of the complement system; hyperosmolarity as seen with radiocontrast media (Fig. 10.1).

IgE-mediated mast cell degranulation is of rapid onset and exquisitely sensitive. In contrast, direct mast cell degranulation by opiates, cyclooxygenase inhibitors or food chemicals is often delayed for some hours and tends to be dose dependent, so that a cumulative intake of such agents may be required before the threshold for mast cell degranulation is exceeded.

Acute urticaria/angioedema

Acute urticaria/angioedema occurs commonly in children and young adults. The precipitating cause is often readily apparent, as in IgE-mediated hypersensitivity

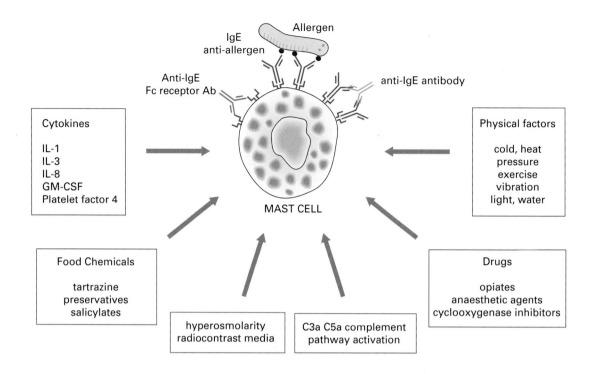

■ **Fig. 10.1** Causes of mast cell activation and production of urticaria. Ab, antibody; GM-CSF, granulocyte–macrophage colony-stimulating factor.

responses to ingested food allergens such as egg, milk, nuts, seafood, or drug allergens such as penicillin.

Contact reactions appear within a few minutes to an hour after exposure to the allergen. Immunological contact urticaria is commoner in atopic subjects. A history of swelling of the lips or tongue follows ingestion of the offending food: nuts, fish, eggs, or fruit. Inhaled allergens such as grass or tree pollens occasionally cause a contact urticaria, generally but not always in association with respiratory symptoms. Contact with other substances such as plants, animals, latex products, foods, and semen can also cause a contact urticaria in sensitized individuals. Injected allergens, drugs, or insect stings may lead to systemic hypersensitivity reactions including urticaria/angioedema.

Viral infections are a common cause of transient urticaria, presumably on the basis of antigen–antibody interaction and complement-mediated mast cell degranulation. Urticaria is a well recognized prodromal symptom of hepatitis B and Epstein–Barr virus infection.

Urticaria due to complement-mediated mast cell degranulation is a feature of serum-sickness syndromes after administration of foreign protein or drugs. Immune complex deposition and complement activation are the underlying mechanisms for urticaria after administration of blood products or immunoglobulin.

Life-threatening angioedema reactions may be a consequence of therapy with the angiotensin-converting enzyme (ACE) inhibitor class of drugs.

Chronic urticaria/angioedema

This is defined as urticaria/angioedema which is present continuously or intermittently for more than 6 weeks. It accounts for more than 70% of all cases of urticaria. Chronic urticaria/angioedema is a disabling condition, and is occasionally potentially life-threatening if the upper airways are involved. In many cases no cause is found despite careful assessment. It is unusual for chronic urticaria to be due to IgE-mediated sensitivity.

▮ **Table 10.1** Causes of urticaria

Acute IgE-mediated
  foods: shellfish, fish, nuts, berries, milk, beans,
    fruits.
  bee and wasp stings
  penicillin
  transfusion of blood or blood products

Physical factors
  pressure,
  cold
  heat
  sunlight
  vibration
  exercise

Immunologically mediated type III immune complex
  in viral disease, e.g. hepatitis
  in autoimmune disease
  after drugs: penicillin, sulphonamides, thiouracil

Non-immunological causes
  Aspirin
  non-steroidal anti-inflammatory drugs naproxen,
  indomethacin, etc.
  radiocontrast media
  local anaesthetics
  food constituents and additives: salicylates,
    tartrazines, benzoates, sulphites

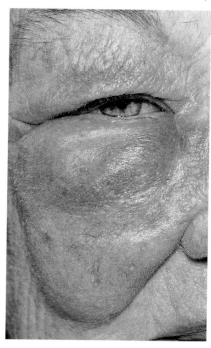

▮ **Fig. 10.2** Angioedema involving the periorbital region following diet rich in salicylates.

Food chemicals (naturally occurring salicylates or food additives such as nitrites, benzoates, metabisulphite, and colourings) play a significant part in many cases of unexplained chronic urticaria. Medications such as aspirin or NSAIDs are also well recognized causes of direct mast cell degranulation. A history of aspirin-induced urticaria in a patient with chronic urticaria provides a strong clue to possible food chemical intolerance.

Chronic urticaria may be the presenting feature of systemic disease. There is an association between autoimmune hyper- and hypothyroid conditions and chronic urticaria. There is increasing evidence that chronic urticaria may have an autoimmune basis in some cases. Autologous serum from chronic urticaria patients causes a weal and flare response when injected intradermally. Recent studies have suggested that the latter response is due to IgG autoantibodies directed against the high affinity IgE receptor on mast cells. The resultant cross-linking of IgE receptors leads to mast cell degranulation. Lymphoproliferative disorders and connective tissue disorders such as systemic lupus erythematosus (SLE), rheumatoid arthritis, and

Sjögren's syndrome, may present with troublesome urticaria and/or angioedema secondary to immune complex deposition and complement-activated mast cell degranulation.

In recurrent angioedema without urticaria, congenital or acquired C1 inhibitor deficiency is a potential cause. Chronic infections (viral, bacterial, fungal, parasitic) may lead to chronic urticaria but this is a less common cause than suggested in older literature.

Vasculitic urticaria (urticarial vasculitis)

Twenty to 30% of patients with chronic urticaria have an underlying vasculitis. The urticarial lesions in such cases:

(1) tend to persist for more than 24 h, typically from 3 to 7 days;

(2) are tender or burning rather than pruritic;

(3) leave a bruised or stained appearance as they fade.

(4) angioedema also tends to be prolonged in such patients

Systemic symptoms such as arthralgias and arthritis (in 75%), abdominal pain, nausea and vomiting, malaise,

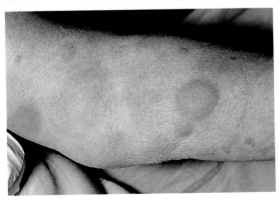

▮ **Fig. 10.3** An urticarial eruption with typical elevated red margin and paler areas.

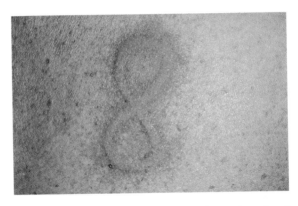

▮ **Fig. 10.4** Dermatographism. The elevated weal and surrounding flare induced by writing the figure 8 firmly on the skin.

or fever may be present. Although renal disease is rare microscopic haematuria and proteinuria may occur, particulary if there is an associated disorder such as SLE. Evidence of this inflammatory state is seen in an elevation of the erythrocyte sedimentation rate (ESR) and C-reactive protein.

Biopsy of the lesions (preferably from fresh and 1 day old lesions) reveals a perivascular inflammatory infiltrate and positive immunofluorescence for immunoglobulins (usually IgM) and complement, consistent with immune-complex-mediated leucocytoclastic vasculitis.

Vasculitic urticaria may be associated with hypocomplementaemia (McDuffey's syndrome), especially in those cases where there is an underlying connective tissue disorder. It is not possible to distinguish clinically between the cutaneous lesions of hypocomplementaemic and normocomplementaemic urticarial vasculitis. Urticarial vasculitis and acquired complement deficiency due to a C3 nephritic factor has also been described. Chronic urticaria associated with a monoclonal IgM paraprotein, fever and bone pain is termed Schnitzler's syndrome.

Physical urticaria

The physical urticarias comprise a heterogeneous group of disorders which accounts for about 20% of all cases. It is not uncommon for patients to have several types of physical urticaria, often in addition to chronic urticaria. Reproducible wealing is produced by the specific physical stimulus.

Dermatographism

In approximately 5% of the population, stroking or scratching the skin results in a weal and flare response.

In a proportion of such patients, the resultant itch is very troublesome, although lesions resolve quickly. Symptomatic dermatographism is often associated with idiopathic chronic urticaria or other physical urticarias. The threshold for response to skin stroking can be determined by using a dermatographometer, an instrument which delivers a standardized stroke pressure. The latter is useful in quantitating clinical responses to therapy in clinical trial situations. In clinical practice, simple scratching of the skin is usually sufficient to confirm the diagnosis of dermatographism (see Fig. 10.4).

Pressure-induced urticaria/angioedema

Pressure-induced urticaria/angioedema may be of immediate or delayed onset. Patients with idiopathic urticaria frequently notice exacerbation of urticaria by sustained pressure of clothing, e.g. belt line. Delayed pressure urticaria/angioedema is a distinct entity occurring 4–6 h after pressure, e.g. prolonged sitting on a hard bench leading to swelling of buttocks, or palm swelling after gripping of hand-held tools. Prolonged angioedema of genitalia after sexual intercourse has also been described. Patients may feel systemically unwell with fever, arthralgias, and leucocytosis. Biopsy of urticarial lesions reveals a perivascular mononuclear infiltrate consistent with a late-phase cutaneous reaction.

The diagnosis is confirmed by the effect of pressure, e.g. a 5–7 kg weight suspended in a bandage, over a shoulder, arm, or thigh,

Cold urticaria syndromes

Patients with this uncommon condition develop urticaria or angioedema on exposure to cold stimuli.

Facial swelling, generalized urticaria, and hypotension or shock may result from total body immersion in cold water. Pharyngeal or tongue swelling may follow ingestion of cold food. Weals generally are of abrupt onset and last 4–6 h, sometimes longer. Rarely, cold urticaria has a delayed onset, as in familial delayed cold urticaria of autosomal dominant inheritance, characterized by the development of pruritic erythematous swellings of the skin 9–18 h after cold exposure. Most cold urticaria syndromes are acquired (acquired cold urticaria or ACU) rather than familial.

The diagnosis is generally confirmed by application of a cold stimulus to the skin, e.g. ice cube, for 5 min, resulting in a weal and flare response (cold stimulation test or CST) corresponding in shape to the ice cube. There is a correlation between the time taken to elicit a weal, and the severity of the ACU. Patients with induction of weal in less than 3 min are more likely to have severe systemic reactions with hypotension. The extent and duration of exposure to cold stimulus also correlate with severity of reactions. About 20% of individuals with ACU have a negative CST but develop urticaria or systemic symptoms after immersion of a forearm in icy water or after cooling of core body temperature in a cold environment.

ACU may be secondary to a variety of disorders, such as: cryoglobulinaemia; infectious diseases such as infectious mononucleosis, varicella, hepatitis, syphilis; cold agglutinin disorders; and leucocytoclastic vasculitis. Passive transfer of cold urticaria activity with purified monoclonal IgG cryoglobulins has been demonstrated. Mast cell degranulation via complement activation or via anti-IgE autoantibodies are likely mechanisms. Clinical features such as Raynaud's phenomenon, purpuric rashes, arthritis, or leg ulcers may point to an underlying systemic disorder such as cryoglobulinaemia.

In primary ACU serum factors have also been demonstrated, either IgE autoantibodies directed against a cold-dependent skin component, or more probably, autoantibodies of IgM or IgG class directed against IgE on mast cells.

Cholinergic urticarias

Cholinergic urticaria presents as multiple small urticarial papules surrounded by intense flare. The extremely pruritic lesions develop on the trunk and limbs after activities leading to increased core body temperature and sweating (such as vigorous exercise), or hot showers. Neurogenic mechanisms result in mast cell degranulation, with subsequent rise in plasma histamine levels. An intradermal injection of methacholine may reproduce the lesions, or the diagnosis may be confirmed by a supervised exercise test.

Exercise-induced urticaria

Generalized urticaria after exercise is also seen in the entity '*exercise-induced anaphylaxis*' (EIA). Systemic mast cell degranulation may also lead to stridor, wheezing, or hypotension. The urticarial lesions tend to enlarge and coalesce and are not related to core body temperature elevation. EIA may be food or aspirin dependent, i.e. the person only experiences exercise-related symptoms after eating certain food (to which specific IgE is often demonstrable) or aspirin/NSAID. The multifactorial nature of mast cell degranulation is illustrated in such cases, where individual activities, such as exercise or eating a particular food, are uneventful, but the two stimuli combined exceed the threshold for mast cell degranulation.

Other physical urticarias

Other physical urticarias include: solar urticaria in which hives develop after exposure to sunlight; heat-induced urticaria; aquagenic urticaria, which is induced by contact with water, e.g. a tepid shower; and vibratory urticaria.

Management of chronic urticaria and angioedema

A detailed history and examination of the patient form the cornerstone of management. A description of the lesions, degree of itch, and time course is helpful in discriminating between chronic urticaria and urticarial vasculitis. In the latter the lesions tend to last longer than 24 h, are generally less pruritic and often fade leaving a bruised or stained appearance which may last days or weeks. The severity of angioedema episodes should also be assessed, as an emergency management strategy may be required. Thyroid disorders, connective tissue disorders, and lymphoproliferative disorders should be specifically excluded.

Physical factors such as heat and pressure aggravate many patients with chronic idiopathic urticaria. Specific questioning regarding the part of cold exposure, exercise, pressure, and sun or water exposure may point to one of the physical urticarias as the predominant problem.

A detailed dietary history should be taken, looking for evidence of high intake of foods rich in natural salicylates (such as citrus, stone or berry fruits, tomatoes, capsicum, tea, peppermint, honey), preservatives such as benzoates, metabisulphite; colourings, or natural amines. Correlation of urticarial outbreaks with dietary factors is difficult when the onset of urticaria occurs hours after food ingestion. Careful enquiry should be

▌ **Table 10.2** Elimination diet A

Low salicylate/Low preservatives/Low artificial colouring diet

The aim of this diet is to keep the intake of salicylates, preservatives, and artificial colours to a minimum.

Salicylates occur naturally in many fruits and vegetables, herbs and spices, and are frequently used in artificial flavourings, perfumes, toothpaste, and medications (aspirin).

Preservatives are added to food to prolong shelf life. For example, benzoates are used in fruit juices; sorbate or sulphur dioxide in dried fruits, fruit salads, and sausage mince; nitrites in processed meats; propionate in yeast products; and antioxidants in oils and margarines.

Colourings such as tartrazine, erythrosine and sunset yellow are commonly used in commercial foods.

Food list and medications

Foods allowed	Foods to avoid
Beverages Decaffeinated coffee, milk, cocoa, milo, malt, mineral water, unpreserved lemonade and tonic water, whisky, gin, vodka.	Tea, fruit juices, commercial soft drinks and cordials, cider, wine, liqueurs, beer.
Bread Any plain unpreserved breads, rolls, muffins or crumpets. Home made pastry.	Breads which contain dried fruits, preservatives or mould inhibitors. Coloured and preserved pastries.
Flour All flours except corn based flowers. Wheaten cornflour e.g. Fielders, Parsons or Kream, uncoloured pasta e.g. spaghetti.	Cornmeal, polenta. Canned baked beans, canned spaghetti. Gravox, Bonox. Maize cornflour, e.g. Wades.
Cereals All cereals except corn. Commercial breakfast cereals which do not contain dried fruit, corn or colouring.	Breakfast cereals which contain dried fruit, corn or colouring, eg. muesli, Sultana Bran, Crunchy Granola, Froot Loops.
Biscuits Plain home made and commercial biscuits (using allowed ingredients).	Home made or commercial biscuits which contain dried fruit, cream filling, spices and colourings.
Cakes Plain home made cakes and sponges (using allowed ingredients).	Home made and commercial cakes which contain dried fruit, artificial cream filling, spices and colouring.
Meat Beef, lamb, veal, pork, mince, poultry (no skin), rabbit.	Meats containing preservatives, colourings, herbs and spices, e.g. bacon, ham, corned beef, sausages, sausage mince, sausage rolls, meat pies, frankfurts, devon salami, processed chicken, meat paste, self basting turkey, seasoned chicken.
Fish Fresh, frozen or canned fish and seafood.	Coloured or preserved fish products, e.g. fish fingers, fish marinades, Prawns.

The information used in this diet chart was researched and compiled by Anne Swain, Dietitian at the Royal Prince Alfred Hospital, Sydney. Further details from Department of Clinical Immunology, RPAH, Sydney.

▎ **Table 10.2** *Continued*

Food list and medications

Foods allowed	Foods to avoid
Eggs	
Eggs	Custard powder, custard mix.
Dairy foods	
Butter, all cream, all plain milks (including UHT, condensed powdered and evaporated. Plain and vanilla. yoghurt. Icecream — home made or commercial vanilla, chocolate, banana and pawpaw flavoured without colouring. Cheese.	Artificial 'cream' in commercial cakes. Flavoured milks. Other flavoured and fruit yoghurt. Coloured or flavoured icecream, iceblocks, and gelato. Cheese which contains preservatives, e.g. individually wrapped cheese slices, cheese spreads, tubs of cottage and ricotta cheeses.
Fats	
Butter, dripping, margarine and oils — safflower and sunflower without antioxidants. Home made salad dressings.	Copha All other oils and margarines. Commercial salad dressings.
Fruit	
Pears, Golden Delicious apples (1 per day only), paw paw bananas. Fruit can be fresh, frozen or canned (in syrup or water). Pick ripe fruit and do not eat skin.	All other fruits. Dried fruits (including pears). Canned fruits in natural juice or nectar (including pears).
Vegetables	
Large white potato (no skin). Beans (French, string). Brussel sprouts, cabbage, celery, chives, choko, parsley, common lettuce (Crisphead), peas, Mung bean sprouts, leeks, swede, shallots, garlic. Dried legumes, e.g. lentils, soybeans, chick peas, split peas.	Pontiac (red) potato, new potato. Broad beans. All other vegetables. Dehydrated vegetables, e.g. Deb mashed potato, Surprise beans.
Soups	
Home made soups from allowed ingredients.	Commercial soups and sauces. Stock cubes, Gravox, Bonox.
Desserts	
Home made desserts from allowed ingredients, e.g. steamed puddings, vanilla junket, egg custard.	Commercial desserts.
Lollies and chocolates	
White milk bottles, white jelly beans, white marshmallows, plain caramels (Columbine), plain toffees (Callard & Bowser), milk chocolate, dark chocolate, and carob.	Liquorice, chewing gum. Commercial, coloured, mint or fruit flavoured lollies and chocolates.
Nuts and chips	
Cashews (raw, dry roasted) unpreserved plain potato crisps and homemade potato chips.	Other nuts. Snack foods and potato crisps. Commercial hot potato chips.
Jams, sugars and sweets	
Golden syrup, maple syrup, pear jam (home made), sugar (white, brown, icing, castor), malt.	Honey. All other jams, conserves and jellies (including lemon butter). Liquid artificial sweeteners.
Condiments	
Parsley, garlic, soy sauce, salt, vanilla essence, citric acid.	Herbs, spices, e.g. pepper, mint, pickles, vinegar, tomato paste, tomato sauce etc, meat pastes, fish pastes, flavouring syrups and essences, Bonox, Marmite, Promite, Vegemite, mustard.

∎ **Table 10.2** *Continued*

Food list and medications	
Foods allowed	**Foods to avoid**

Toiletries and sunscreens
Use: Unscented soaps, shampoos and conditioners where possible and unflavoured toothpaste.
          Hamiltons Sunscreens.
Avoid: Contact with perfumes, scented deodorants and cosmetics, pressure pack sprays, household cleaning
          agents, cigarette smoke and other strong smells.

Medications
Use: Elevit RDI adult vitamin tablets (optional).
          White medications where possible. Colouring can be washed off the surface of tablets by rubbing gently
          under running water.
          Coloured capsules can be opened and the powdered contents taken in a spoonful of Golden Syrup.
Avoid: All coloured medications and vitamins. Read the labels carefully.

made regarding medication, particularly 'over-the-counter' preparations such as analgesics or vitamin supplements which may contain aspirin or colourings.

Investigations

Transient or acute urticarias of uncertain cause often do not require specific investigations. Confirmation of food or drug allergy may require immediate hypersensitivity (IHS) prick skin testing in a controlled setting. A negative prick skin test for a food or drug allergen has excellent negative predictive value for anaphylaxis to that substance.

Relevant tests in chronic urticaria and/or angioedema include:

1. Complete blood picture — looking for anaemia (? systemic disease); lymphopenia (? SLE) or eosinophilia (? allergic reaction or parasitic infection).

2. ESR and C-reactive protein (CRP) — tend to be elevated in vasculitic urticaria.

3. C3, 4 — often depressed in vasculitic urticaria.

4. Thyroid function tests and thyroid autoantibodies.

Other tests which may be relevant in chronic urticaria, as indicated by clinical findings include:

    antinuclear antibody;
    serum electrophoresis;
    cryoglobulins;
    cold agglutinins;
    hepatitis B or EB virus serology
    liver function tests
    faecal microscopy and culture;

    chest X-ray;
    skin biopsy if lesions persist >24 h or if bruising and/or raised CRP/ESR;
    examination of urinary sediment.

Total IgE level, IHS prick skin tests and RASTs do not generally contribute to the diagnosis of chronic urticaria does not reveal a cause.

Treatment and management

In more than 50% of patients, chronic urticaria is idiopathic, i.e. a careful clinical and investigative examination does not reveal a cause. Such patients warrant a 3 week trial of a diet excluding foods rich in salicylates, colourings, and preservatives (Table 10.2). If there is no improvement, a further 2 week trial of a rigid elimination diet comprising several meats, rice, pears, lettuce, potatoes, parsley, water, sugar, and cold pressed safflower oil should be tried. If there is no response to this diet, it is unlikely that dietary factors are significant (Table 10.3). If the urticaria resolves with dietary measures, challenge with capsules containing food chemicals or foods can be undertaken on a daily basis, in an attempt to reproduce symptoms. (Table 10.4). If the patient has never had a life-threatening episode of angioedema, it is safe to challenge on an out-patient basis. In-patient monitoring is essential if there is a history of severe angioedema. Sequential in-patient challenge over 48 h may be helpful in excluding dietary causes of urticaria, but will not necessarily pinpoint the causative agent if a positive reaction occurs, because of the variable time course for such reactions. The more appropriate single daily in-patient challenge is time consuming and expensive.

▌ **Table 10.3**   Strict Elimination diet: to be used if salicylate/preservative/colouring restriction fails.

Foods allowed	Foods to avoid
Meat	
Lamb, veal, and poultry (no skin or fat)	Corned beef, ham, bacon, pork offal, sausages. Chicken skin and fat, fish, seafood, well browned meat and gravy made from browned pan juices or commercial gravy powders.
Eggs	
Eggs	
Fats	
Cold pressed safflower or sunflower oil (no antioxidants)	Other oils and oils which contain antioxidants. Margarine, butter, bream, cheeze, yoghurt, olive oil.
Vegetables	
Common lettuce (crisphead), inside leaves only. Parsley (fresh), sprinckled through food only. Large white potatoes (no skin).	Other lettuce. Commercial potato crisps and chips. Pontiac (red) potatoes. New potatoes. All other vegetables.
Fruits	
Pears — fresh, very ripe and thickly peeled. Pears in sugar syrup not juice or natural juice.	Unripe pears. All other fruit including dried fruit. Golburn Valley and SPC canned pears in juice or nectar.
Cereals	
White rice, rice flour, rice noodles, rice vermicelli. Organically grown brown rice, tapioca, sago. Wheaten cornflower. Arrowroot flour, potato flour. Rice bubbles, rolled rice, rice flakes, unprocessed bran, brown rice cakes.	Other cereals, bread and biscuits. Common brown rice. Maize cornflour.
Sugars	
White sugar, brown sugar, golden syrup, homemade pear jam.	Honey, raw sugar. Artificial sweeteners.
Condiments	
Salt, citric acid, fresh parsley (sprinkle only). Homemade french dressing (cold pressed oil and citric acid to taste)	Herbs and spices (e.g. pepper). Vinegar and lemon juice.

An alternative approach involves the reintroduction of foods in a graduated fashion or specific challenges with foods rich in salicylates, preservatives, or colourings. Dietetic advice is essential for such protocols and particularly for the institution of very rigid elimination diets, for which vitamin and calcium supplementation are recommended.

Dietetic assistance is also invaluable in tailoring a diet according to the results of challenge protocols.

If dietary measures are unsuccessful, treatment with the non-sedative antihistamines (H₁ receptor antagonists) is appropriate. The latter are generally well tolerated and highly effective for most patients with chronic urticaria. *Astemizole, cetirizine, loratadine,* and *terfenadine* have all been shown to reduce histamine-induced weal and flare responses. If one antihistamine has not proven helpful, it is worth trying an alternative, as individual responses vary.

Astemizole has an active metabolite which contributes to the therapeutic effect, which is prolonged for weeks as the drug reaches a plateau or steady state. *Terfenadine* and *loratadine* have shorter elimination half-lives. Hepatic metabolism of terfenadine and astemizole may be affected by other drugs such as erythromycin and ketoconazole, and the resultant higher levels of drugs have, rarely, been reported to cause *torsades de point* cardiac arrhythmia. Patients on astemizole and terfenadine should be advised of possible interactions with antibiotics.

∎ **Table 10.3** *Continued*

Foods allowed	Foods to avoid
Beverages Decaffeinated coffee beans. Decaffeinated instant coffee. Water, soda water, plain mineral water. Homemade pear juice (blend a can of pears and syrup, then add water or mineral water to taste). Homemade lemonade (2 cups sugar dissolved in 2 cups water and add 1 teaspoon citric acid. Dilute with soda water, mineral water or tap water).	All other coffees including cereal coffees (e.g. Ecco). Tea, including herbal teas. Cocoa, milk. Fruit juices, cordial, soft drink, Alcohol. Golburn Valley pear juice. Any chocolate flavoured drinks.
Cooking aids Bicarbonate of soda, cream of tartar, baking powder (before use), gelatine (boil powder in water).	Other cooking aids.
Medications Panadol, Panadeine, Codeine (white tablets only when necessary). Savlon antiseptic cream.	*All medications* not prescribed by your doctor. (e.g. Aspirin, Disprin, Alka Seltzer, Vincents, etc.). *All medications* which contain flavouring or colouring. *Cough lozenges* and syrups. *Oil of Wintergreen* (e.g. Dencorum, Deep Heat, Tiger Balm, Muscle Balm, etc.) Methanol, Eucalyptus, Vicks Vaporub, Tea Tree Oil.
Toiletries Unflavoured toothpaste *or* Sensodyne (red pkt) *or* a mixture of salt and soda *or* ordinary salt, *or* brus-ing well in plain water is effective. Non-allergenic or lightly perfumed cosmetics, toiletries and moisturizers can be used with caution (eg. Sunlight, Neutrogena). Roll on deodorant, preferably unperfumed. Sunscreen.	*Flavoured* toothpaste. *Aerosols and pressure pak products* should be avoided. *Perfumes and strongly perfumed* cosmetics, toiletries and moisturizers are to be avoided.

Cetirizine is a derivative of hydroxyzine, which has a well established role in the management of resistant chronic urticaria cases. Levels of cetirizine may be elevated in renal failure. Cetirizine blocks both early and late phase allergic reactions and has been reported to be of particular value in delayed pressure urticaria which is generally resistant to most H_1 receptor antagonists.

Doxepin, a tricyclic antidepressant and potent H_1 receptor blocker, is often useful in troublesome chronic urticaria.

In resistant urticaria, the addition of an H_2 receptor blocker such as ranitidine, cimetidine, or famotidine may occasionally be of benefit. Other medications such as ketotifen, nifedipine, and danazol have been reported to be of benefit in some cases.

Recent reports of anti-IgE receptor antibodies in severe chronic urticaria suggest that a proportion of such patients have an autoimmune basis for their urticaria. Plasmapheresis has been used efficaciously in such cases. Corticosteroids (prednisolone 1 mg/kg or less) may provide dramatic relief of urticaria but the long-term maintenance or alternate day therapy which is sometimes required carries the risk of steroid side-effects.

Chronic urticaria in euthyroid patients with thyroid autoantibodies may respond to thyroxine therapy.

Urticarial vasculitis

Urticarial vasculitis is generally not very responsive to H_1 receptor antagonists, but it is appropriate to try such medications first. Cetirizine, its parent drug hydroxyzine, or doxepin provide relief in some cases.

Corticosteroid therapy may afford good relief of symptoms, tapering to a low-dose alternate day schedule for prolonged benefit. Medications which have demonstrated efficacy in selected cases include colchicine, dapsone, and hydroxychloroquine. Immunosuppressive agents such as azathioprine or cyclophosphamide may be required in patients who require high doses of prednisolone therapy to control symptoms.

∎ **Table 10.4**   Urticaria/angioedema challenge capsule series

Substance	Quantity	Capsule code
Wheat starch	Control (540 mg)	A
Tartrazine	1 mg	B1
Tartrazine	10 mg	B2
Tartrazine	30 mg	B3
Sodium benzoate	500 mg (2 × 250 mg)	C
Hydroxybenzoic acid	200 mg	D
Brewer's yeast extract	600 mg	E
Aspirin	50 mg	F1
Aspirin	100 mg	F2
Aspirin	300 mg	F3
Sodium metabisulphite	5 mg	G0
Sodium metabisulphite	10 mg	G1
Sodium metabisulphite	50 mg	G2
Sodium metabisulphite	500 mg	G3
Sodium salicylate	600 mg (2 × 300 mg)	H
Sodium nitrite	100 mg	I
Sodium nitrate	100 mg	I+
(BHA) (antioxidant)	50 mg	J
(BHT) (antioxidant)	50 mg	J+
Tyramine	140 mg	K
Phenylethylamine	4 mg	L
MSG	0.5 g (1 × 500 mg)	M1
MSG	1.0 g (2 × 500 mg)	M2
MSG	2.5 g (5 × 500 mg)	M3
MSG	5.0 g (10 × 500 mg)	M4

Guidelines: capsules are taken sequentially, ceasing after an adverse reaction until discussed with the clinician. Subjects with a history of severe urticaria/angioedema or of asthma should be tested under medical supervision.
The unmodified sequence is not suitable for subjects with severe asthma or asthma, which is exacerbated by aspirin, bisulphite, or artificial colouring.

Physical urticarias

Management of the physical urticarias is predicated on avoidance of the precipitating factors where possible. Responses to H_1 receptor antagonists vary considerably.

Dermatographism generally has a modest or good response to the non-sedative antihistamines, with reduction in weals and itch, although flaring is still evident after trauma.

Delayed pressure induced urticaria/angioedema tends to be resistant to antihistamines, although cetirizine, which blocks early and late phase allergic reactions, is effective in some cases. Corticosteroid therapy may be required in high dosage before any benefit is seen.

Cold urticaria: The most effective management strategy is to avoid cold exposure, especially total body immersion in cold water. Patients with ACU should be advised never to swim unaccompanied.

Pharmacological prophylaxis with H_1 receptor antagonist antihistamines is useful in the majority of cases. Cyproheptadine alone, or in combination with H_2 receptor antagonists, has been widely used, in dosages varying from 2 mg daily to 4 mg three times a day, depending on patient tolerance. Low-dose doxepin is another useful agent. The non-sedative antihistamines such as terfenadine or astemizole are preferred options in some patients. Corticosteroid therapy has no place in management.

Induction of cold tolerance by progressive exposure of the body to cold stimuli on a daily basis is of proven benefit, but there is poor patient compliance with regimens requiring a daily cold shower on a long-term basis.

Cholinergic urticaria may be difficult to prevent, although hydroxyzine in high doses has been the drug of choice in the past. It is likely to be superceded by the non-sedative H_1 receptor antagonists, including cetirizine.

Exercise-induced anaphylaxis. Management strategies include: avoidance of food, aspirin, or NSAIDs

∎ **Table 10.5**   Food salicylate content

Negligible	Low	Moderate	High	Very high
Fruit				
Pear (peeled)	PAWPAW	pear (with peel)	PASSIONFRUIT	sultana (dried)
BANANA	golden delicious	loquat	mulberry	*prune
	apple	custard apple	tangelo	raisin (dried)
	pomegranate	red delicious	grapefruit	currant (dried)
		apple	AVOCADO	RASPBERRY
		persimmon	peach	REDCURRANT
		LEMON	MANDARIN	loganberry
		FIG	granny smith apple	BLACKCURRANT
		rhubarb	nectarine	youngberry
		mango	watermelon	date
		tamarillo	lychee	CHERRY
			kiwi fruit	blueberry
			jonathan apple	ORANGE
				boysenberry
				guava
				blackberry
				cranberry
				apricot
				strawberry
				rockmelon
				*GRAPE
				PINEAPPLE
				PLUM
Vegetable				
potato (peeled)	green bean	*broccoli	EGGPLANT	*TOMATO
lettuce	red cabbage	sweet potato	watercress	PRODUCTS
celery	brussel sprout	parsnip	cucumber	gherkin
cabbage	mung bean sprout	*MUSHROOM	BROADBEAN	endive
bamboo shoot	green pea	carrot	alfalfa sprout	champignon
Swede	leek	beetroot		radish
dried beans	shallot	marrow		olive
dried peas	chive	SPINACH		capsicum
red lentils	choko	onion		zucchini
brown lentils		cauliflower		chicory
		turnip		hot pepper
		asparagus		
		sweet corn		
		pumpkin		
Nuts				
poppyseed	CASHEWS	PISTACHIO		ALMOND
		PINENUT		waterchesnut
		MACADAMIA		
		WALNUTS		
		BRAZIL		
		SESAME		
		COCONUT		
		PEANUTS		
		HAZELNUTS		
		PECANS		
		SUNFLOWER		
		SEEDS		

The information used in this diet chart was researched and compiled by Anne Swain, Dietitian at the Royal Prince Alfred Hospital, Sydney. Further details from Department of Clinical Immunology, RPAH, Sydney.

∎ **Table 10.5** *Continued*

Negligible	Low	Moderate	High	Very high
Sweets				
white sugar	golden syrup	molasses		licorice
maple syrup	caramels			peppermints
COCOA				honey
carob				
Herbs and spices				
	vanilla		cinnamon	cayenne
	garlic		cardamon	aniseed
	parsley		black pepper	sage
	saffron		pimiento	mace
	MALT VINEGAR		ginger	curry
	*SOY SAUCE		allspice	paprika
	tandoori		clove	thyme
			nutmeg	dill
			caraway	turmeric
			WHITE VINEGAR	*WORCESTER
			bay leaf	SAUCE
			white pepper	*VEGEMITE
				*MARMITE
				rosemary
				oregano
				garam masala
				mixed herbs
				cumin
				canella
				tarragon
				mustard
				five spice
				mint
				dill
Beverages				
Coffee	Coffee	Coffee		
Andronicus instant	Harris instant	Harris Mocha		
Pablo instant	Bushells instant	International		
Decaffeinated	Bushells Turkish	Roast instant		
	Robert Timms	Moccona instant		
	Instant	Nescafe instant		
	Tea	Tea		Tea
	camomille	decaffeinated		all brands
		fruit		peppermint
		roseship		
	Cereal coffee	Cereal coffee		Cereal coffee
	dandelion	Reform		Natures cuppa
	ecco			
	bambu	Other		
		Rosehip syrup		
Other		fruit juice		
Aktavite		COKE		
Milo				
Ovaltine				
Alcohol		Alcohol		Alcohol
gin		CIDER		*LIQUEUR
whiskey		BEER		*PORT
vodka		*SHERRY		*WINE
		*BRANDY		*RUM

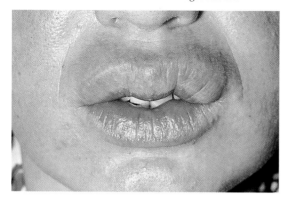

❚ **Fig. 10.5** Hereditary angioedema affecting the upper lip.

prior to exercise; prophylactic use of H_1 receptor antagonists and provision of a preloaded adrenaline syringe for emergency self-injection in life-threatening angioedema or collapse.

Angioedema due to hereditary or acquired deficiency of C1 inhibitor

Hereditary angioedema (HAE) is an uncommon condition presenting as recurrent episodes of angioedema involving skin or mucous membranes of respiratory or gastrointestinal tracts. Urticaria is not a feature of HAE. Involvement of the oropharynx can result in respiratory obstruction, sometimes fatal. Attacks of angioedema may be precipitated by minor trauma such as dental procedures. Patients may present with acute abdominal pain, nausea, or vomiting, secondary to oedematous bowel obstruction. Angioedema is of sudden onset and persists for hours or days.

Genetics

Inheritance is autosomal dominant, with incomplete penetrance.

Pathogenesis

The cause is a qualitative or quantitative defect in C1INH, a glycoprotein which inhibits enzymes of the complement, fibrinolytic, and kinin formation pathways. C1INH is an α_2 protein, which is normally present in the serum in a concentration of 18–22 mg/dl. The protein in encoded by eight exons on chromosome 11.2–q13 and is co-dominantly expressed. It is a serine protease inhibitor of:

(1) activated complement components and is highly competitive for C1r and C1s);

(2) the contact activation pathway of kinin-forming pathway (kallikrein);

(3) intrinsic fibrinolytic pathway (factors XIIa and XIIf).

Conformational changes occur when the C1/INH serpin reactive loop moves from the surface to the internal region upon binding to a serum protease, and an inhibitory activity occurs. C1INH inhibits the proteolytic activity of C4 and C2 in classical complement activation. In the fibrinolytic pathway C1INH inhibits the amplification pathway for factor XII proteolysis, production of plasmin, and formation of bradykinin from kininogen.

HAE type I (85%) is due to a change in the genome sequence that impairs mRNA transcription or translation for a functional protein. HAE type II (15%) has changes that allow transcription and translation of a non-functional product. Deletions, rearrangements, and single base mutation the C1INH gene have been described.

Deficiency of C1INH results in uncontrolled complement activation, because it is the only inhibitor of activated C1r and C1s, and of generation of vasoactive bradykinin. Elevated levels of bradykinin have been implicated in the pathogenesis of the non-pruritic angioedema in this condition. In type I HAE (85% of cases) there is a marked decrease in levels, usually between 5 and 30% of normal, of antigenically and functionally normal C1INH due to decreased synthesis and increased metabolism. It is now possible to diagnose the defect at birth in these families. In type II (15%) HAE, CINH is dysfunctional due to point mutation in the reactive site. Serum C4 is reduced between attacks and becomes even lower or absent in attacks; C2 may be normal between attacks, but falls in attacks of HAE. In an attack there is a fall of factor XII, an increase in kallikrein and in plasmin–α_2-antiplasmin complexes due to activation of complement, fibrinolytic, and kinin pathways. Two products of these pathways have kinin activity: bradykinin which in attacks is produced as a result of increased kallikrein activity, and possibly a degradation product of C2b.

Estimation of C4 level provides a useful screening test for HAE because the C4 level is depressed even when the patient is asymptomatic, therefore it will signal the possibility of HAE in the presence of antigenically normal amounts of CINH in type II families.

Treatment

For prevention and maintenance attenuated androgens (danazol and stanozolol) are used in post puberty

■ **Table 10.6** Complement levels in recurrent angioedema

Cause	C1INH (Antigenic)	C1INH (Functional)	C1	C4	C3
Hereditary					
HAE I	Reduced	Reduced	Normal	Reduced	Normal/reduced
HAE II	Normal	Reduced	Normal	Reduced	Normal/reduced
Acquired					
with paraprotein	Reduced	Reduced	Reduced	Reduced	Normal/reduced
with anti-C1INH antibody	Normal/reduced	Reduced	Reduced	Reduced	Normal/reduced
Idiopathic recurrent	Normal	Normal	Normal	Normal	Normal
Vasculitic	Normal	Normal	Reduced	Reduced	Reduced

cases. Androgens increase transcription, translation, and secretion of C1INH. It is necessary only to raise the C1INH level to 50% normal in order to reduce substantially the severity and frequency of attacks. Usual doses are danazol 400–600 mg/day stanozolol or 4–6 mg/day. The minimal dose to control clinical symptoms, and not the laboratory results, should be used. Serum transaminase levels should be examined periodically to monitor for androgen-induced hepatitis.

Antifibrinolytic drugs are also useful prophylactic agents in some patients.

In acute attacks, passive replacement of C1INH can be life-saving. Infusions of fresh frozen plasma, or, more recently, C1INH concentrates, have been used successfully in emergency treatment of angioedema and prophylactically prior to dental procedures, oral surgery or intubation. Adrenaline is not helpful in emergency management.

Acquired C1INH deficiency (AAE) presents in later life in association with lymphoproliferative disorders of B cell lineage or with autoimmune disorders. Two possible mechanisms for reduced C1INH levels have been described.

1. Activation of C1 by complexes of anti-idiotypic antibodies specific for malignant B-cell monoclonal immunoglobulin, leading to massive consumption of complement components including C1INH.

2. Blocking of C1INH by autoantibodies specific for a variety of epitopes on the C1INH molecule.

AAE type I may respond to attenuated androgens and treatment of the underlying lymphoproliferative disease. C1INH concentrates are useful in acute attacks.

AAE type II responds to lowering of the level of anti-C1INH antibody by measures such as plasmapheresis or cytotoxic therapy.

Further reading

Casale, T. B., Sampson, H. A., Hanifin, J., Kaplan, A. P., Kulczycki, A., Lawrence, I. D., *et al.* (1988). Guide to physical urticarias. *Journal Allergy of and Clinical Immunology*, **83**, 758–763.

Champion, R. H. (1988). Urticaria — then and now. *British Journal of Dermatolology*, **119**, 427–36.

Champion, R. H., Greaves, M. W., Kozba Black, A., and Pye, R. J. (1985). *The urticarias*. Churchill Livingstone, Edinburgh.

Current management of urticaria and angioedema — Round table educational (1991). *Journal of American Academy of Dermatology*, **25**, 146–204.

Greaves, M. W. (1991). The physical urticarias. *Clinical and Experimental Allergy*, **21**. (Suppl.), 284–9.

Greaves, M. W. (1995). Chronic urticaria. *New England Journal of Medicine*, **332**, 1767–71.

Hide, M., Francis, D. M., Grattan, C. E., Hakimi, J., Kochan, J. P., and Greaves, M. W. (1993). Autoantibodies against high affinity IgE receptor as a cause of histamine release in chronic urticaria. *New England Journal of Medicine*, **328**, 1599–604.

Huston, D. P. and Bressler, R. B. (1992). Urticaria and angioedema. *Medical Clinics of North America*, **76**, 805–40.

Mehregan, D. R., Hall, M. J., and Gibson, L. E. (1992). Urticarial vasculitis: A histopathologic and clinical a review of 72 cases. *Journal of the American Academy of Dermatology*, **26**, 441–8.

Wanderer, A. A. (1990). Cold urticaria syndromes: historical background, diagnostic classification, Clinical and laboratory characteristics, pathogenesis, and management. *Journal of Allergy and Clinical Immunology*, **85**, 965–81.

11 Drug allergy and reactions

J. Bradley

Definition

Reaction to the administration of a drug is a significant problem in medical practice. Drug reactions are diverse, have varied clinical presentations, and are frequently associated with acute or chronic diseases.

Although the term 'drug allergy' is commonly used, reactions to drugs rarely involve type I, allergic or immediate hypersensitivity. Most are due to idiosyncracy, intolerance, or immune responses other than type I reactions.

The true type I response :

(1) is seen in those who have been previously exposed to the drug;

(2) is mediated by drug-specific immunoglobulin (Ig)E antibodies;

(3) is due to release of chemical mediators;

(4) occurs within 30 min and subsides within hours.

Introduction

Major types of drug reactions recognized and studied in detail include those to penicillin, local anaesthetics, insulin, and vaccines as well as reactions to aspirin and sulphites.

Drugs of small molecular size possible mechanisms of stimulating an immune response include haptenation, covalent linkage to other proteins, dehaptenation (reversal of attachment by plasma enzymes), and the production of reactive metabolic products through microsomal reactions. Through haptenation, different epitopes on drugs are emphasized. Drugs of this type include: penicillin; sulphonamides, thiazides, hypoglycaemics; cephalosporins; antituberculous drugs; anticonvulsants; muscle relaxants; thiopental and quinidine.

Drugs of large molecular size can act as complete antigens, e.g. insulin; chymopapain, aspariginase; adrenocorticotrophic hormone and other hormones but contaminants in commercial preparations can also cause problems. It is important to determine if a reaction to a drug is immunological, and if it is IgE mediated. With drug allergy all of the above considerations render *in vitro* analysis difficult and, in contrast to atopy, skin testing meets with variable success. It is most useful with sensitivity to proteins such as insulin and chymopapain. RAST testing (radioallergosorbent test) which is available for various small molecules including β-lactam antibiotics, sulphonamides, trimethoprim, and isoniazid as well as other protein determinants, may not distinguish between major and minor epitopes of importance. A lymphocyte proliferation test, although useful for some drugs, has not found general relevance. *In vitro* lymphocyte toxicity assays for hypersensitivity to anticonvulsants involve exposure of donor lymphocytes to microsomal metabolites of the drug, followed by the assessment of lymphocyte toxicity. Other tests of potential use are assays for: mast cell tryptase; C5a and C3a; assessment of classical and alternative pathways of complement activation for immune complex-associated mechanisms; measurement of prostaglandin D_2 for mast cell activation. The clinical presentation and the type of drug may well determine the test of choice.

Incidence

The exact frequency drug reactions is unknown but in the USA is approximately 1–2 million annually. As many as 30% of patients in hospital may have a drug reaction of some type. It has been estimated that approximately 2% of admissions are due to adverse drug reaction and 0.2% are life-threatening.

Drugs

Some drugs are more likely to give rise to problems. A 10 year review in Sweden by Kauppinen and Stubbs (1984) revealed that antimicrobials especially β-lactam antibiotics were responsible for 42–53%, aspirin and non-steroidal anti-inflammatory drugs (NSAIDs) for 14–27% and central nervous system (CNS) depressants for 10–12% of drug reactions. It has been estimated that the risk of a reaction to an antibiotic is increased three times if there has been a previous reaction.

Dose and route of administration

Frequent intermittent administration is more likely to produce an IgE-type response. Once an IgE response has developed a second, or subsequent, exposure to a much smaller amount can produce a massive response with systemic anaphylaxis. Topical (local) administration is more likely to produce sensitization, followed by intramuscular and intravenous with oral administration producing the least.

Genetic factors

The incidence in women of cutaneous drugs reactions is 35% greater than in men. Age may be a factor for some drugs, e.g. adults have a higher incidence than children of allergic reactions to penicillin.

Human leucocyte antigen (HLA) has an influence in hydralazine-induced systemic lupus erythematosus where HLA-DR4 is increased. Gold and penicillin nephropathy have been linked to HLA-B8 and -DR3.

The rate of metabolism in the liver may have an effect. Slow acetylators are more likely to develop reactions to procainamide isoniezid procainamide and quinidine. Reaction to sulphonamide has also been linked to this phenotype.

Beta blockers

An increased incidence of reactions to radiocontrast media and also to penicillin has been linked to concurrent beta blocker administration.

Infection

Infection with Epstein–Barr virus (EBV) increases the risk of a maculopapular skin eruption with Ampicillin from 5% in the the normal population to 70–100%. In the normal population trimethoprim–sulphonamide skin reactions occur in 3%, but this increases to 12% in human immunodeficiency virus (HIV), and to 30–70% in acquired immune deficiency syndrome (AIDS) patients.

Immunopathogenesis

For an immune response to occur it is often necessary for the drug or its metabolite to combine with a plasma or tissue protein to produce a hapten–protein complex.

Most drugs or their metabolites are <1000 KdA. The ability to form strong covalent bonds between drug and protein is important, and high hapten to carrier ratios favour IgE production. The minimum size of a drug determinant is at least three amino acids.

Immune responses to drugs

Type I anaphylactic reaction

Generalized systemic anaphylaxis is the most dramatic and life-threatening reaction. It occurs in those previously exposed to the drug or its parent group of drugs and is mediated by IgE antibodies to drug determinants. Several organs may be involved. The reaction may be mild with itching pruritis, erythema, and urticaria/angioedema, or it may be that of the classic extensive reaction with oral, laryngeal and/or pharyngeal oedema, vasodilatation, hypotension, loss of conciousness and circulatory collapse, gastrointestinal upset, asthma, and sudden death.

Most frequent causes of anaphylactic reactions include β-lactam antibiotics, xenogeneic serum, blood products, and neuromuscular blocking agents.

Anaphylactoid reactions

These are due to non-IgE-mediated mast cell stimulation, and can be just as severe as type I anaphylactic reactions. The clinical features are the same. The pathogenesis is different. Some drugs, e.g. aspirin and NSAIDs, radio contrast media can act directly on mast cells to induce release of their mediators. In other situations the reaction is due to activation of the complement sequence and production of anaphylatoxins C3a and C5a, which then cause the release of mediators from mast cells. Some blood products may do this e.g. the older preparations of immunoglobulin which contained aggregated immunoglobulin.

Type II reactions

An example is penicillin-induced haemolytic anaemia. This occurs after exposure to large amounts of penicillin and an IgG antibody is produced directed against the drug determinant present on the surface of the red cell or the determinant–cell membrane complex. The cell is destroyed by complement activation or phagocytosis

Type III reactions

The formation of immune complexes and complement activation leads to deposition on vascular endothelium or circulating cells. It typically occurs 1–3 weeks after drug therapy commences and may persist for some time after the drug is discontinued. The clinical features of severe reactions are usually fever, malaise, urticaria, and arthralgia. The complement system is activated and levels of serum C4 and C3 are reduced.

Drugs commonly responsible for type III reactions are: xenogeneic sera, sulphonamides, β-lactam antibiotics, streptomycin, thiouracil, hydantoin, and aminosalicylic acid.

Type IV

These type of reactions are now less frequent and are associated topically applied drugs, or occupational exposure to these drugs, e.g. nurse or pharmacists with penicillin-induced dermatitis.

Organ-specific manifestations of drug reactions

Skin

The most frequent manifestation are maculopapular, erythematous, and morbilliform eruptions. These are often associated with reactions to β-lactam antibiotics, sulphonamides, and anticonvulsants. However, erythema multiforme (EM), exfoliative dermatitis, and phototoxic, photosensitive, vesicular bullous eruption may also occur in drug reactions. Pruritis, urticaria/angioedema are frequent in drug reactions but may be due to allergic or non-allergic mechanisms (e.g. aspirin and NSAIDs).

Erythema multiforme has a typical 'target' rash that may occur with erythema, urticaria, or a maculopapular rash. There may also be systemic manifestations as in the *febrile mucocutaneous syndromes*: *Stevens–Johnson syndrome* which consists of EM, fever, signs of toxicity, and involvement of two or more mucous membranes; *Lyells syndrome*, a more severe form where epidermis sloughs and mortality rate may be as high as 35%. Drugs particularly associated with this type of reaction are sulphonamides and trimethoprim–sulphamethoxazole, barbiturates, phenytoin, aspirin, and NSAIDs.

Fixed drug eruptions are rare. Any part of the body may be affected, usually as an eczematoid area, and many drugs have been associated including gold, sulphonamides, β-lactam antibiotics, and barbiturates.

Lung

Pulmonary manifestations of drug reactions are well recognized. The most well recognized was the reaction to nitrofurantoin in which Interstitial infiltrates which could progress to pulmonary fibrosis, associated with eosinophilia occurred. Other drugs responsible are bleomycin, phenytoin, and methotrexate.

Liver

Liver problems have occurred with oestrogens, chlorpromazine, phenytoin, halothane, sulphonamides, and acetoaminophen.

Blood

The binding of a drug, its metabolite, a drug–antibody complex or an altered cell surface membrane determinant may induce a cytopenia. Haemolytic anaemia has been caused by penicillin, quinine, quinidine, and nitrofurantoin. Platelet membrane glycoproteins have been the target in thrombocytopenia induced by quinine, quinidine, and sedormid.

Diagnosis of drug allergy

This is made primarily on the clinical history, although there are a few specific tests of value. It should be remembered that drug allergy accounts for only about 10% of adverse reactions to drugs.

There are typical features that suggest a drug allergy:

(1) the signs and symptoms are those of type I reactions and therefore similar to those caused by other agents (food, insect stings, etc.);

(2) minute doses of the drug may trigger the attack;

(3) there has been previous exposure to the drug or to a cross-reacting drug or possible, unrecognized, subclinical exposure to the drug or related compounds;

(4) the features develop soon after the drug is given and are different to the usual pharmacological actions of the drug.

In the history it is important to establish the temporal relationship between the signs and symptoms and the administration of the drug; a complete documentation of all drugs taken previously and any possible adverse effects.

▌ **Table 11.1**   Intradermal skin test for drug allergy

Penicillin	Cephalosporins	Antituberculous drugs
Quinidine	Anticonvulsants	Penicillamine
Insulin	Local anaesthetics	Muscle relaxants

Laboratory investigations

Intradermal skin tests. These are primarily for detection of specific IgE antibodies to the drug or its by products and are the only immunological test that have a strong predictive value. For most drugs the antigenic determinants are not known. Most drugs have a low molecular weight and they or their metabolites form a macromolecular complex usually with a host protein. Skin tests are of value for some drugs that are proteins, e.g. insulin, foreign antisera, and chymopapain. They are also of value for some drugs used in anaesthesia, and for the major determinant of penicillin (benzyl-penicilloyl: BPO).

Prick testing should be done first. Varying dilutions of the drug from 1/1000 are used. A positive response read at 20 min is a weal of 2 mm or greater than the saline control. If the prick tests are negative then the tests are repeated by 0.05 ml intradermally consecutively at dilution from 1/10 000 to 1/100 at intervals of 20 or more minutes. Although the tests are usually without problems anaphylaxis may occur and therefore the tests should be done by personnel experienced and trained in dealing with anaphylaxis. False negative results may occur due to a reagent that is not appropriate, or after a severe anaphylactic response, i.e. within 2 weeks of the test, which temporarily depletes IgE antibodies and mast cells.

In vitro tests. are generally less specific and less sensitive than skin tests but have the advantage that the adverse effects of skin tests are avoided.

RAST . Drug-specific IgE antibodies may be measured by RAST but the test is less sensitive than skin tests. Tests are commonly available for penicillin, cephalosporins, sulphonamides, trimethoprim muscle relaxants, and anaesthetics.

The *leucocyte histamine release* is not diagnostically reliable.

Serum tryptase assays may be helpful.

Patch tests. This may be helpful in type IV drug reactions to topical medications or preservatives, e.g. neomycon or parabens. The chemical is applied directly to the skin and may induce localized dermatitis after 24–48 h.

Common problems

Penicillin

The best studied drug reaction are those to penicillin because it is responsible for more allergic reactions than any other drug. The real incidence of all immunological reactions to penicillin is unknown. It may be ~ 8%, but it varies, e.g. while 8% of those treated with ampicillin develop a morbilliform or maculopapular skin rash if there is an EBV infection the incidence of skin rash approaches 100%.

In decreasing frequency the manifestations of immune reponses to penicillin are: skin rashes, fever, bronchospasm, vasculitis, exfoliative dermatitis, Stevens–Johnson syndrome, anaphylaxis. These manifestations vary with regards to time of onset. Reactions that take place within the first 3 days are: anaphylaxis, urticaria, angioedema, bronchospasm. In the period afterwards skin rashes, haemolytic anaemia, neutropenia, and Stevens–Johnson syndrome serum sickness may develop.

Anaphylaxis to penicillin is rare occurring in 0.04% of those treated, and is fatal in 0.001%.

Pathogenesis

When benzylpenicillin is metabolized the β-lactam ring of penicillin opens to form a covalent bond with serum proteins thus producing the penicilloyl ('major') determinant, which is recognized by more than 95% of penicillin antibodies. The minor determinants including benzylpenicilloate and penicilloate are produced by other interactions. Because these determinants are generated by interaction it is of no value to skin test with penicillin only. Skin tests have no value for predicting non-IgE-mediated reactions to this drug, e.g. drug fever, serum sickness-like state, haemolytic anaeamia, dermatitis, and maculopapular exanthems.

Anaphylactic reactions are most likely to occur between 20 and 50 years but can occur in the elderly and children. Two-thirds of fatal reactions occur in those who have had penicillin before but without a reaction. They are more frequent with parenteral than oral administration of the drug. With time patients may lose their allergy. Reaction to other antibiotics is 10 times more likely in those with penicillin allergy. BPO compound is the major determinant and accounts for 95% of the metabolites of penicillin. Minor determinants may also give rise to anaphylactic reactions. BPO-polylysine and freshly prepared penicillin (which detects minor determinant reactivity) can be used for skin testing.

The predictive value of skin testing is now recognized. In those who have a positive history but skin tests are negative there are no anaphylactic reactions and ~1% developed pruritis or transient urticaria. An Oral challenge with penicillin is then given under observation. Those who have negative skin tests and negative oral challenge may be given penicillin therapeutically.

If RAST to BPO and benzyl penicillin are used it will detect ~ 80% of reactive patients. However, there are still 20% false negatives. Therefore administration of the drug to those negative to these tests, if necessary, should be done very cautiously.

If penicillin therapy is necessary in patients who give a positive skin test to penicillin oral or parenteral desensitization can be performed.

Amoxycillin and ampicillin

The maculopapular rashes commonly seen in patients with EBV and Cytomegalovirus infections and chronic lymphocytic leukemia are not usually IgE mediated, unless there is an urticarial element to them. They last about a week.

Cephalosporins and other β- lactam antibiotics

These share a common β-lactam strucure with penicillin. However, estimates of cross-reactivity vary from 10 to 50%. Therefore the percentage of penicillin-reactive patients who react to cephalosporin may be the same as to other antibiotics. In choosing an antibiotic for these patients preference is given to drugs known to tolerated, and third-generation cephalosporins are less likely to produce allergic reactions than the first or second generation. Of the newer β-lactams carbapenems cross-react with minor penicillin determinants but monobactams do not.

Other antibiotics

Sulphonamides and other drugs may give rise to reactions. Trimethoprim–sulphamethoxazole induces a skin rash in 3% of HIV-negative and 30% of HIV-positive patients. Sulphonamides used in inflammatory bowel disease give macular skin rash and/or drug fever reactions in 2% cases. Cross-reaction with drugs related to the sulphonamides: diuretics, oral hypoglycaemic drugs, and diaxozide may occur.

Streptokinase

About 17% of those treated develop allergic reactions. A skin test usually detects those at risk.

Chymopapain

This derivative of papaya is used in contact lens solutions, for treatment of disc herniation, as a meat tenderizer, and in beers. Anaphylaxis occurs in about 1%. The non-medical use may induce sensitization and allergic reaction may occur on the first medical use. Skin test and RAST may be helpful.

Radiocontrast media

Reactions are more common when ionic media are used. and anaphylactoid reactions develop in ~2% of those exposed. While reactions tend to be mild, death has been reported. IgE has not been incriminated; reactions may occur on first administration; specific testing does not appear to be of value but pretreatment with antihistamine and steroids appears to reduce the risk.

Local anaesthetics

Most of the reactions to local anaesthetics are toxic or vasovagal. Immune reactions account for the minority (<1%) reactions and these are dermatitis, urticaria, angioedema, and anaphylaxis. Skin testing preparations should not contain adrenaline, and may be followed by incremental increases in subcutaneous doses.

General anaesthesia

Drug allergic reactions occurring during general anaesthesia and producing urticaria, bronchospasm, tachycardia, hypotension, and collapse have an incidence of ~1:10 000 and a fatality rate of 4–6%. They may be due to allergy to: muscle relaxants, e.g. suxamethnium, d-tubocuranine, gallamine; or thiopental and amytal sodium which have the ability to act as complete allergens by virtue of their quaternary ammonium determinants. Some reactions may be due to opiates used at the same time. Skin tests may be performed and are reliable in identifying susceptible patients; they do not produce a positive response in the non-allergic patient.

Insulin

Insulin allergy has decreased since the introduction of recombinant human insulin. Bovine and porcine insulin differ from human insulin by three and one amino acid. This may cause IgG and IgE antibodies to be produced. Some reactions to human recombinant insulin may be due to cross-reactivity with previously produced antibody to animal insulin.

There is an allergic response which usually is local. This may be helped by antihistamines. Systemic reactions occur rarely and may need densitization. Allergy may be confirmed by skin test or RAST

Vaccines

In some vaccines (measles–mumps–rubella, yellow fever) there is a small amount of egg protein. Reactions to this is rare even in those who have egg allergy but skin tests, prick and intradermal, can be done as a precaution.

Anti-inflammatory drugs

Reactions to these drugs operate through non-IgE 'pseudoallergic' mast cell degranulation and present as asthma and urticaria. Aspirin is the classic drug to produce reactions of this type but all the drugs that produce this reaction, (e.g. NSAIDs), are cycloxygenase inhibitors and may push arachidonic acid products from the cyclooxygenase to the lipoxygenase pathway. Those who react should avoid aspirin and NSAIDs. Paracetamol is a safe alternative as an analgesic.

Management

A full clinical history of the reaction and all drugs administered is absolutely necessary. If allergy is suspected alternative drugs are used. This usually means giving drugs that are not immunologically cross-reactive. However, with cross-reacting drugs the reaction is incomplete, e.g. many patients with penicillin allergy will tolerate cephalosporins even though they share a β-lactam structure with penicillin. In these situations the cross-reacting drug is exhibited in increasing doses commencing with a very small dose intially.

Test by skin and or RAST

In general, if these tests are negative give a small test dose only when there are all facilities to deal with an anaphylactic reaction.

If tests are positive do not use the drug unless absolutely necessary to do so. If used densensitization with well recognized protocol is mandatory.

This requires informed consent facilities for treating a general anaphylactic reaction and experienced medical staff. The drug is administered in increments from a very small dose up to a therapeutic dose at 20–30 min intervals.

Further reading

Van Arsdel, P. P. Jr. Classification and risk factors for drug allergy. (1991). *Immunology and Allergy Clinics of North America*, **11**, 475–92.

Blanca, M., Vega, J. M., Garcia, J. *et al.* (1990). Allergy to penicillin with good tolerance to other penicllins: study of the incidence in subjects allergic to beta-lactams. *Clinical and Experimental Allergy*, **20**, 475–81.

Levenson, D. E., Arndt, K. A., Stern, R. S. (1991). Cutaneous manifestations of adverse drug reactions. *Immunology and Allergy Clinics of North America*, **11**, 493–507.

Moscicki, R. A., Sockin, S. M., Corsello, B. F., Ostro, M. G., Bloch, K. J. (1990). Anaphylaxis during induction of general anaesthesia: subsequent evaluation and management. *Journal of Allergy and Clinical Immunology*, **86**, 325–332.

Toogood, J. H. (1988). Risk of anaphylaxis in patients receiving beta blocker drugs. *Journal of Allergy and Clinical Immunology*, **81**, 1–5.

Section III

12 Insulin-dependent diabetes

L. C. Harrison, R. S. Schmidli, N. Petrovsky, and M. C. Honeyman

Introduction

Insulin-dependent diabetes (IDD), or type 1 diabetes, is due to the selective autoimmune-mediated destruction of β cells in the pancreatic islets of Langerhans, with consequent insulin deficiency causing hyperglycaemia. Autoimmunity to β cells is thought to be triggered, in genetically susceptible individuals, by environmental agents such as viruses or possibly chemotoxins. The major genes conferring susceptibility to IDD are in the major histocompatibility complex (MHC) on human chromosome 6, in particular those encoding class II human leucocyte antigen (HLA) proteins at the DR, DQ, and possibly DP loci. In Caucasoids, the highest risk alleles are represented by the haplotype DR 3, 4; DQ 2, 8, where DR4 and DQ8 are in linkage disequilibrium (Table 12.1). There is evidence that class I MHC alleles also confer risk. MHC proteins probably play a direct, determinant part in binding and presenting peptides to autoreactive T cells involved in β cell destruction. The difference in risk between identical twins and HLA-identical siblings (Table 12.2) implies that non-MHC genes also confer risk.

■ Table 12.1 Human leucocyte antigen class II haplotypes and lifetime risks of insulin-dependent diabetes (caucasoids)

Haplotype	Family	General population
DR4-DQ8/DR3-DQ2	1/5	1/25
DR4-DQ8/DR4-DQ8	1/10	1/60
DR4-DQ8/Other	1/10	1/60
DR4-DQ8/DR2-DQ1	1/100	1/500
DR3-DQ2/DR3-DQ2	1/20	1/350
DR3-DQ2/Other	1/40	1/400
Other	1/80	1/5000

■ Table 12.2 Lifetime risks of insulin-dependent diabetes mellitus

Age of diagnosis in proband

Parents	2.2 ± 0.6%
Children	5.6 ± 2.8%
Siblings	6.9 ± 1.3%
Siblings	
HLA non-identical sib	1.2%
HLA haploidentical sib	4.9%
HLA identical sib	15.9%
Identical twin	30–40%

HLA, human leucocyte antigen.

Several lines of evidence (Table 12.3) indicate that environmental factors play a dominant part in the genesis of IDD. For example, the concordance of IDD in identical twins is no more than 40%. Furthermore, no more than 20% of HLA identical siblings and 10% of HLA haploidentical siblings of IDD probands develop IDD, although they share all or half of the high-risk alleles, respectively. In unrelated individuals with high-risk class II HLA alleles the lifetime risk of IDD is no more than 5%. The incidence of IDD shows a 40-fold gradient from a high in Scandinavia and Finland (where it approaches 40 per 100,000 per annum) to a low in Japan, despite equivalent standards of living. Environmental factors including handling, diet, lighting, living conditions, and viral infections influence the natural history of disease in the animal models of spontaneous IDD, the non-obese diabetic (NOD) mouse and the diabetes-prone Bio-Breeding (BB) rat. In humans, early cessation of breast feeding and introduction of cows' milk to infants has been implicated in the aetiology of IDD, although the epidemiological evidence for this, and equally for specific

∎ **Table 12.3**   Role of environmental factors in the genesis of insulin-dependent diabetes

Most genetically-susceptible persons do not develop diabetes. They include:
~ 60% of monozygotic twins with a diabetic twin
~ 90% of persons with a haploidentical diabetic sibling
~ 95% of persons with high risk major histocompatibility complex alleles

Geography is an important determinant of incidence
Difference between countries (Finland/Japan = 36/1)
Incidence of migrants approaches that of adopted country (i.e. Japanese in Hawaii, French in Canada, Jews in Montreal)
Rapid changes in regional incidence (2.5-fold in Finland in 30 years).

Some diabetogenic agents have been identified

Viruses
Rubella (congenital) in humans and rabbits
Coxsackie B4 in several humans and in mice
Encephalomyocarditis in mice
Venezuelan encephalitis in mice, hamsters, and monkeys
Reovirus 1 and 3 in mice

Chemotoxins
'Vacor' (rodenticide) (*N*-3-pyridylmethyl-*N*-*P*-nitrophenyl urea) in humans
Streptozotocin (2-deoxymethyl-nitrosurea-glucopyranose) in animals
Alloxan (mesoxalylurea) in animals

immunity to cows' milk proteins in IDD, is far from convincing.

Pathogenesis

The classic textbook description of the clinical onset of IDD is of polyuria, polydipsia, and weight loss over days to weeks. However, the underlying islet lesion that leads to IDD progresses for months to years, except possibly in very young children, before culminating in the loss of most β cells and subsequent clinical features (Fig. 12.1). It is difficult to follow the course of β-cell destruction in humans due to the inaccessibility of the pancreas, although an 'end-stage' picture has been revealed from the analysis of rare post mortem and pancreas isograft specimens, as well as from pancreas needle biopsy specimens obtained from recently diagnosed Japanese patients. The histological appearance resembles that in the rodent models, namely a mixed mononuclear cell infiltrate of the islets, termed insulitis, in which CD8+ T cells predominate in the end-stage. However, the rodent models also reveal that insulitis evolves from a stage of islet cell hyperexpression of class I MHC molecules associated with activated macrophages, to peri-islet infiltra-

tion predominantly by CD4+ T cells, followed by intra-islet infiltration with increasing numbers of CD8+ T cells concomitant with β-cell destruction (Fig. 12.2). This is the picture of a delayed-type hypersensitivity (DTH) lesion. Besides lymphocytic insulitis, evidence for the autoimmune basis of IDD is summarized in Table 12.4.

Studies of mouse and human T-cell clones, and of several mouse models of parasitic and autoimmune diseases, have defined two major functional subsets of CD4 T cells, Th1 and Th2, on the basis of the cytokines they elaborate. Th1 cells produce interleukin (IL) 2, interferon (IFN) γ, and tumour necrosis factor (TNF) β, and mediate cellular immunity or DTH, e.g. to intracellular micro-organisms and to tumours; Th2 cells produce IL-4,-5,-6,-10 and -13 required for B-cell differentiation and antibody production and mediate humoral immunity to soluble antigens and toxins, and allergic responses. The categorization of immune responses into either Th1 or Th2 is a convenient oversimplification. In the case of IDD, both cellular and humoral responses to islet antigens are present. Nevertheless, the 'quality' of insulitis and its propensity to progress to β-cell destruction could depend on the balance of Th1 and Th2 cells within the lesion. This concept, as a framework for understanding immunopathology, is depicted in Fig. 12.3.

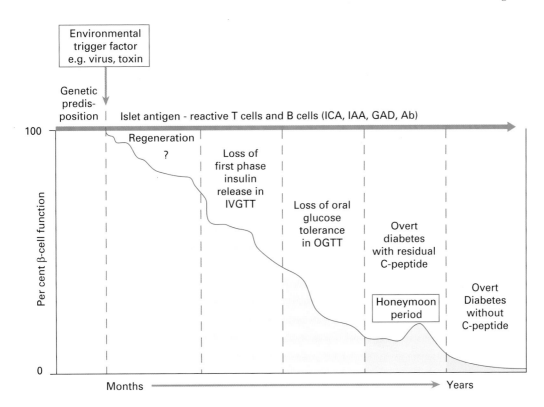

▌Fig. 12.1 In the majority of cases, clinical presentation of insulin-dependent diabetes is preceded by a pre-clinical phase of autoimmune-mediated β-cell destruction recognized by the presence of circulating antibodies, e.g. islet cell antibodies (ICA), insulin autoantibodies (IAA), antibodies to glutamic acid decarboxylase (GAD) and antibodies to tyrosine phosphatase, IA-2. T-cell reactivity to insulin, GAD and IA-2 have also been documented in the pre-clinical phase. IVGTT, intravenous glucose tolerance test; OGTT, oral glucose tolerance test.

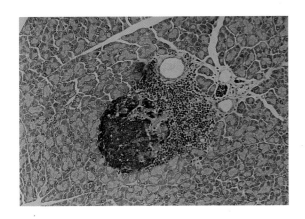

The primary antigenic stimulus to β-cell autoimmunity remains unknown. Several islet antigens are recognized as targets of the immune response in IDD (Table 12.5). Only the target antigen(s) of islet cell

▌Fig. 12.2 The islet is surrounded and infiltrated from its vascular pole by macrophages, CD4+ T cells, some B cells, and CD8+ T cells, which invade and selectively destroy the insulin-producing β cells. In this photomicrograph, the β cells are stained brown by reaction with anti-insulin antibody–horseradish peroxidase and chromogen and the tissue section counterstained to highlight the nuclei (blue) of the infiltrating cells.

antibodies (ICA) that are detected by indirect immunofluorescence on frozen sections of human pancreas (Fig. 12.4), insulin, glutamic acid decarboxylase (GAD), and the more recently described tyrosine phosphatase IA-2 meet criteria that justify their designation as islet antigens. These criteria include immune responses to antigen which are disease-specific, precede the onset of clinical disease and correlate with other indices of disease pathology. ICA may be accounted for predominantly by antibodies to GAD

■ **Table 12.4**   Evidence for the autoimmune basis of insulin-dependent diabetes

1. Mononuclear cell infiltration of islets (insulitis) in recent-onset diabetes, recurrent diabetes after pancreas isograft between human leucocyte antigen identical twins and rodent models (non-obese diabetic mouse and BioBreeding rat).

2. Adoptive transfer of diabetes with T cells in rodent models.

3. Prevention of diabetes in rodent models by anti-T-cell monoclonal antibodies (to CD4, CD8, class II major histocompatibility complex) and drugs (cyclosporin).

4. Increase in remission rate in recent-onset patients given immunosuppressive drugs (azathioprine ± glucocorticoid, cyclosporin).

5. Islet antigen-reactive T cells and antibodies which antedate clinical disease.

6. Suppression of disease development in mice by induction of immunological tolerance to islet antigens.

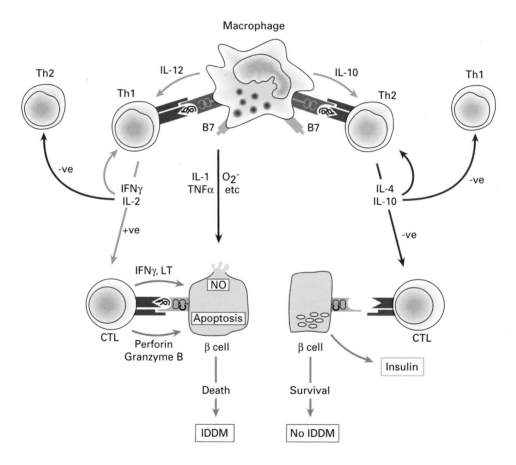

■ **Fig. 12.3**   β-cell destruction can be conceptualized as the outcome of an interplay between Th1 and Th2 subsets of islet antigen-specific T cells in the insulitis lesion. Th, T-helper CD4+ lymphocyte; CTL, cytotoxic T lymphocyte; NO, nitric oxide; O_2^-, oxygen-free radical; IDDM, insulin-dependent diabetes mellitus; LT, leukotriene.

and IA-2. Insulin (or its precursor, proinsulin) is the only antigen that is β-cell specific, but localization of an antigen to the β cell is not necessarily a prerequisite for the selectivity of β-cell destruction. For example, β cells could be differentially sensitive to inflammatory mediators such as free radicals or nitric oxide; on the

▌ **Table 12.5** Islet cell antigens in IDD

Antigen	Localization	Autoantibody assay	Autoantibody prevalence
ICA (islet cell antibody) antigen (= GAD + IA-2 + ?)	All islet cells	Indirect immunofluorescence on frozen sections of human pancreas	70–80% of subjects with recent-onset IDD.
Insulin	β cells	Immunoprecipitation of ^{125}I-insulin	40–50% of subjects with late pre-clinical and recent-onset IDD, predominantly younger children.
Glutamic acid decarboxylase (GAD)	β cells? all islet cells (also in neurons, testis, ovary, and other sites)	Immunoprecipitation of recombinant or native protein, or of enzymatic activity; ELISA using recombinant protein	70–80% of ICA positive first-degree relatives and recent-onset IDD subjects
'37 kDa/40 kDa' tryptic fragments, derived from the tyrosine phosphatases IA-2α and β	β cells? all islet cells	Immunoprecipitation of 35S-methionine-labelled islet proteins and trypsin treatment Immunoprecipitation of recombinant IA-2	70–80% of pre-clinical and recent-onset IDD subjects, especially children with more rapid progression to clinical disease

Other candidate antigens, proposed on the basis of incomplete evidence, include carboxypeptidase H (52 kDa neuroendocrine secretory cell granule protein), glucose transporter type 2 (55 kDa), heat shock protein (65 kDa), peripherin (58 kDa), ICA69, bovine serum albumin.
IDD, insulin-dependent diabetes.

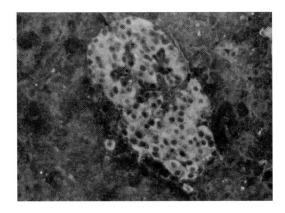

▌ **Fig. 12.4** Fluorescein-stained islet in a frozen section of human pancreas. The section was reacted with serum from a patient with recent-onset insulin-dependent diabetes (IDD), washed and then reacted with fluorescein isothiocyanate-labelled antihuman globulin. Islet cell antibodies react with all islet cells. They are detected in 70–80% of persons with recent-onset IDD, 3–5% of first-degree relatives of persons with IDD and <1% of the general population.

other hand, selective destruction by cytotoxic T cells would only require that a peptide be presented uniquely by β-cell class I MHC proteins. The peptide could either be derived from an infecting virus or be endogenous, but not necessarily β-cell specific, and be either presented aberrantly under conditions of β-cell dysfunction or cross-react (molecular mimicry) with a microbial peptide which has elicited an immune response elsewhere in the body.

Markers of preclinical insulin-dependent diabetes

First-degree relatives of persons with IDD, who are 'at-risk' and in a preclinical phase of the disease, can be identified by the presence of circulating antibodies or T cells to islet antigens (Fig. 12.1; Table 12.4). In the pre-clinical phase, β-cell failure can be detected by the loss of first phase insulin release in the intravenous glucose tolerance test (IVGTT), although this test has poor reproducibility. Screening of relatives and, more recently the general population, for immune and metabolic markers, is now being undertaken on a research basis in many centres internationally. Preclinical diagnosis is important for education and counselling, and to avoid morbidity and hospitalization associated with acute presentation, gain insight into the natural history, help identify environmental causes, and identify those persons who will be the best candidates for intervention therapy to prevent clinical disease.

Antibodies

ICA are detected in 70–80% of subjects with recent-onset IDD, and antedate the onset of symptoms. However, because there is a low prevalence of ICA in normal subjects (~1%), the positive predictive value is not sufficiently high for ICA to be of clinical use in the general population. Predictive studies are therefore based on first-degree relatives, in whom the risk of IDD is considerably higher. As up to 30% of first-degree relatives who develop IDD do not have ICA, there has been interest in increasing the predictive value of ICA by improving the assay and by incorporating additional risk factors. The predictive value of ICA is influenced by ICA titre and by age, with high titre ICA and young age denoting a higher risk of IDD. Despite standardization of method and unit of measurement internationally, the ICA assay remains semiquantitative. However, because of its relatively high sensitivity and specificity it remains the initial test used in almost all screening and intervention studies.

Low-titre insulin autoantibodies (IAA) are detected in up to 50% of subjects overall at diagnosis, their prevalence and level being inversely related to age. In a Scandanavian study, 43% of children and 4% of adults had IAA at diagnosis, despite similar ICA levels. In the absence of ICA, IAA is not predictive for IDD; nevertheless, the combination of antibodies in first-degree relatives denotes a higher risk than ICA alone.

In attempting to identify IDD antigens, in the 1980s, Steinnun Baekkeskov observed that a rat islet protein of 64 kDa was immunoprecipitated by sera from 80% of children with recent-onset IDD. Efforts to identify the 64 kDa antigen by direct sequencing and cDNA library screening were unsuccessful and it was not until 1990 that the antigen was identified as GAD. This was a result of the association noted between IDD and stiff-man syndrome, a rare neurological disorder in which GAD had been shown to be an antigen. GAD is the major inhibitory neurotransmitter in the central nervous system, and is presumed to function in the islets as a paracrine factor. It has two isoforms of 65 and 67 kDa (GAD65 and GAD67), encoded by separate genes. GAD65 is the predominant form in human islets, whereas mouse islets contain predominantly GAD67 and rat islets both GAD65 and GAD67.

GAD antibodies (GADAb) occur in up to 80% of subjects with recent-onset IDD and antedate the onset of clinical disease. Using recombinant GAD65 and GAD67, several groups have shown that GAD autoantibodies in humans preferentially react with GAD65. A strong correlation exists between ICA and GADAb positivity and preabsorption of IDD sera with native GAD or recombinant GAD65 reduces ICA staining of islets or even abolishes it in a small subset of ICA-positive subjects. The latter correlates with a 'restricted' pattern of ICA staining of β cells only, with high-titre ICA and GADAb, and with a relatively slow progression to IDD. One study was not able to demonstrate that GADAb added to the predictive value of ICA; nevertheless, first-degree relatives with antibodies to multiple islet antigens appear to be at higher risk.

The most recent addition to the stable of islet autoantigens is a novel protein tyrosine phosphatase. It was initially termed ICA512 after being isolated from an islet cDNA library by immunoscreening with IDD sera, and subsequently cloned from a human insulinoma subtraction library and termed IA-2. Recombinant IA-2 is recognized by some 70% of recent-onset IDD sera and blocking experiments have shown that IA-2 antibody may comprise a portion of ICA in subjects who are positive for ICA but negative for GADAb. Initial studies indicate that IA-2 antibody may be more predictive of progressive preclinical disease than GADAb. Antibodies to 37 and 40 kDa tryptic fragments of islet proteins precipitated by IDD sera had previously been shown to be markers for the development of IDD in identical twins and patients with polyendocrine autoimmunity. The 40 kDa fragment is now thought to be a component of IA-2, and the 37 kDa fragment probably derives from a closely related tyrosine phosphatase.

T Cells

Evidence for T-cell immunity in IDD (Table 12.4) includes the demonstration of T-cell reactivity to islet antigens *in vitro*. Altered reactivity to a porcine pancreatic extract was first demonstrated in IDD subjects over 20 years ago by the leucocyte migration inhibition test; intracutaneous injection of this extract in IDD subjects also induced a classic DTH reaction. Subsequently, peripheral blood mononuclear cells (PBMC) from IDD subjects at diagnosis were shown to be cytotoxic against rat islets. Cytotoxicity was reduced by co-incubation of PBMC from IDD and healthy subjects, suggesting that healthy subjects have regulatory or protective cells. A range of islet preparations was then used in conjunction with T-cell proliferation assays to identify islet-specific T cells in the blood of IDD subjects. PBMC responses to whole human islets and fetal pig islets (FPI) or islet homogenates were shown to be increased in recent-onset IDD subjects and their 'at-risk' first-degree relatives. PBMC responses to insulin were weak and detected in less than half of the ICA positive relatives. A possible explanation for the apparent low frequency of insulin-reactive T cells is that the dominant T-cell epitope is in proinsulin rather than insulin. This is supported by evidence that PBMC in a majority of ICA-positive relatives proliferate in response to a peptide that spans the B chain of insulin and the connecting (C) peptide of proinsulin.

PBMC from IDD subjects or 'at-risk' first-degree relatives have also been shown to exhibit increased proliferative responses to either full length GAD65 or a glutathionine-S-transferase fusion protein containing the central portion of GAD67. Interestingly, an inverse relationship noted between the levels of GAD-reactive T cells and GADAb in 'at-risk' relatives raises the possibility that deviation of immunity to GAD towards either a cellular (Th1) or a humoral (Th2) response may be critical in determining the natural history of preclinical IDD. This concept is also supported by the finding that specific immunoglobulin (Ig) G subclasses to GAD are significantly correlated with non-progression to diabetes in at-risk relatives (IgG2 ± IgG4; Th2), or with recent-onset diabetes (IgG1 ± IgG3; Th1).

T-cell assays with PBMC are unphysiological, have poor reproducibility and do not characterize the responding T-cell population. To be applied to the preclinical diagnosis of IDD, T-cell assays must be robust and convenient, reproducible, sensitive and specific. T-cell cytokine production is a convenient and reliable means to detect T-cell activation that allows characterization of the responder cells, e.g. into Th1 or Th2 subsets. Cytokine-based assays can also be performed under more physiological conditions with whole blood, obviating the need to purify PBMC. Such assays may enable one to determine the predictive value of islet antigen-reactive T cells, map T-cell epitopes, and quickly assess new candidate islet autoantigens.

Prospects for prevention and cure

Based on rapidly emerging knowledge of immunological mechanisms, there is a strong expectation that IDD can be prevented and cured. This view is supported by studies in the rodent models of IDD, particularly the NOD mouse, in which a variety of intervention treatments reduce the incidence of IDD and islet transplantation restores insulin production and even prevents vascular complications.

In the absence of known environmental trigger agents in the vast majority of cases and the means to modify genetic susceptibility, primary intervention is not feasible. Currently, attention is focused on modifying the ongoing preclinical disease process by either immunotherapy and/or treatment to enhance β-cell resistance to immuno-inflammatory mediators. Both semispecific immunomodulatory agents, e.g. cyclosporin A, monoclonal antibodies to immune cell surface markers or to particular cytokines, and specific agents, e.g. islet antigens given transmucosally or by other routes to induce immunological tolerance, decrease the incidence of IDD in NOD mice. Controlled trials have demonstrated that conventional immunosuppressive agents, either non-specific (azathioprine) or semispecific (cyclosporin A), increase the frequency and duration of remissions in humans with recent-onset IDD. These potentially toxic agents are, however, not justified in asymptomatic, at-risk individuals, many of whom are children. In relation to β-cell resistance, nicotinamide, which replenishes intracellular levels of nicotinamide adenine dinucleotide, has been shown to delay the onset of diabetes in the NOD mouse. *In vitro*, nicotinamide inhibits cytokine-mediated damage to β cells, at least in part, by increasing resistance to the inflammatory mediator nitric oxide. Controlled trials of

▪ **Table 12.6** Antigen-based therapeutic strategies for autoimmune disease

Strategy	Target	Modality
T-cell receptor antagonism	Effector T cells	Autoantigen peptide analogues
Deletion or anergy	Effector T cells	Excess, soluble autoantigen
		Soluble autoantigen peptide–major histocompatibility complex complexes
		Autoantigen plus blockade of 'second signal' mole cules
Immune suppression or deviation	Regulatory T cells	Autoantigen given transmucosally
		Autoantigen plus cytokine

nicotinamide in high-risk, ICA-positive first-degree relatives are currently in progress in Europe.

The ethical imperatives for preclinical intervention are a high degree of prediction for the development of clinical disease and the availability of treatment which at least is safe, if not effective. Intervention will initially be limited to the subgroup of first-degree relatives whose levels and/or combination of immune markers place them in the highest risk category, e.g. a more than 50% chance of developing diabetes within 5 years. Screening to detect unrelated, at-risk individuals within the general population is also underway, but the predictive power of immune marker tests decreases markedly in the general population where the prevalence of IDD is at least a log-fold less than in families with an affected first-degree relative.

The requirement for safety underlines the need for specific, targeted immunotherapy to prevent or treat autoimmune diseases like IDD. The specific elements in an immune response are the peptide–MHC molecule complex and the T-cell receptor (TCR) molecule. The generalization of either MHC-based strategies, e.g. blockade by synthetic antagonists or antibodies, or TCR-based strategies, e.g. T-cell or TCR peptide vaccination, is limited by the population heterogeneity of MHC and TCR proteins. In contrast, autoantigen-based therapy (Table 12.6) should be widely applicable. In addition, studies in animal models of autoimmune disease reveal a 'bystander' effect on T-cell responses to several antigens following induction of immunological tolerance to a single antigen.

Replacement of β-cell function for the cure of IDD will entail either transplantation of pancreas or islets, replacement of the insulin gene and its regulatory apparatus or stimulation of β-cell regeneration. Cure is also likely to require concomitant immunotherapy to control graft rejection as well as recurrent or ongoing islet autoimmunity. At present, intact pancreas transplantation is the only successful form of β-cell replacement. The 1 year survival of segmental pancreas grafts exceeds 80%, but the need for continuing non-specific immunosuppression limits this procedure to patients requiring a kidney transplant. For the majority, most hope is pinned on transplantation of xenogeneic islet tissue which is readily available, e.g. from fetal pigs, combined with safer forms of specific immunotherapy, but whether this will be a practical reality remains to be seen.

In conclusion, secondary prevention of IDD is probably a realizable goal within the next decade or two. Safe, specific therapy for islet immunity will also be a prerequisite for curative modalities in established IDD. Preclinical diagnosis and intervention therapy in

IDD may serve as a model for the prevention of other autoimmune diseases such as rheumatoid arthritis and multiple sclerosis.

Further reading

Bach, J-F. (1994). Insulin-dependent diabetes mellitus as an autoimmune disease. *Endocrine Reviews*, **15**, 516–42.

Baekkeskov, S., Anastoot, H. J. and Christgau, S. (1990). Identification of the 64K autoantigen in insulin-dependent diabetes as the GABA-synthesizing enzyme glutamic acid decarboxylase. *Nature*, **347**, 151–6.

Bingley, P. J., Bonifacio, E., and Gale, E. A. M. (1993). Can we really predict IDDM? *Diabetes*, **42**, 213–220.

Bingley, P. J., Christie, M. R., Bonifacio, E., Bonfanti, R., Shattock, M., Fonte, M-T., *et al.* (1994). Combined analysis of autoantibodies improves prediction of IDDM in islet cell antibody-positive relates. *Diabetes*, **43**, 1304–10.

Gerstein, H. C. (1994) Cow's milk exposure and type 1 diabetes mellitus. *Diabetes Care*, **17**, 13–19.

Harrison, L. C. (1992). Islet cell autoantigens in insulin-dependent diabetes: Pandora's box revisited. *Immunology Today*, **13**, 348–52.

Harrison, L. C. (1995). Antigen-specific therapy for autoimmune disease: prospects for the prevention of insulin dependent diabetes. *Molecular Medicine*, **1**, 722–7.

Harrison, L. C., Honeyman, M. C., DeAizpurua, H. J., Schmidli, R. S., Tait, B. D., Cram, D. S., and Colman, P. G. (1993). Inverse relationship between humoral and cellular immunity to glutamic acid decarboxylase in humans at-risk for insulin-dependent diabetes. *Lancet*, **341**, 1365–9.

Honeyman, M. C. and Harrison, L. C. (1993). The immunologic insult in type 1 diabetes. *Springer Seminars in Immunopathology*, **14**, 253–74.

Kikutani, H. and Makino, A. S. (1992). The murine autoimmune diabetes model: NOD and related strains. *Advances in Immunology*, **51**, 285–322.

Mandrup-Poulsen, T., Reimers, J. I., Andersen, H. U., Pociot, F., Karlsen, A. E., Bjerre, U., and Nerup, J. (1993). Nicotinamide treatment in the prevention of insulin-dependent diabetes mellitus. *Diabetes/Metabolism Reviews*, **9**, 295–309.

Payton, M. A., Hawkes, C. J., and Christie, M. R. (1995). Relationship of the 37,000- and 40,000-M_r tryptic fragments of islet antigens in insulin-dependent diabetes to the protein tyrosine phosphatase-like molecule IA-2 (ICA5 12). *Journal of Clinical Investigation*, **93**, 1506–11.

Petrovsky, P. and Harrison, L. C. (1995). Cytokine-based human whole blood assay for the detection of antigen-reactive T cells. *Journal of Immunology Methods*, **186**, 37–46.

Rudy, G., Stone, N., Harrison, L. C., Colman, P. G., McNair, P., Brusic, V., *et al.* (1995). Similar peptides from two β-cell autoantigens, proinsulin and glutamic acid decarboxylase, stimulate T cells of individuals at risk for insulin-dependent diabetes. *Molecular Medicine*, **1**, 625–633.

Schmidli, R. S., Colman, P. G., and Harrison, L. C. (1994). Do glutantic acid decarboxylase antibodies (GADAb) improve the prediction of IDDM in first-degree relatives at-risk for IDDM? *Journal of Autoimmunity*, **7**, 873–9.

Tait, B. D. and Harrison, L. C. (1991). Overview: the major histocompatibility complex and insulin-dependent diabetes mellitus. *Baillière's Clinical Endocrinology and Metabolism*, **5**, 211–28.

13 Thyroid and other endocrine glands

J. Bradley

Thyroid

Introduction

Autoimmune thyroid disease was established by Rose and Witebsky, and Roitt and Doniach when lymphocyte infiltration and thyroid dysfunction was produced in experimental animals and thyroid antibodies were detected in patients with Hashimoto's thyroiditis. The detection in some cases of hyperthyroidism of a long-acting thyroid stimulator (LATS), which was subsequently shown to be an immunoglobulin was further confirmation of the presence of thyroid autoimmunity.

Animal models

Classical experimental autoimmune thyroiditis (EAT) has played a major part in the understanding not only of human thyroid dysfunction but also in autoimmunity in general. Now the development of EAT produced by immunization with thyroid peroxidase (TPO), the production of monoclonal antibodies to thyroid-stimulating hormone (TSH) with stimulatory or blocking functions, and a new spontaneous form of thyroid autoimmunity in the non-obese diabetic mouse (NOD) have added more to understanding of human thyroid disease. Animal work has also added to understanding about tolerance and immune manipulation. In some mice pre-injection of soluble thyroglobulin protects against the development of EAT, and transforming growth factor (TGF) β mediates *in vivo* oral tolerance to antigen in thyroid disease by inhibiting T-cell proliferation to autologous thyroid cells.

Human disease

The autoimmune process probably begins with the activation of CD4+ T cells specific for thyroid antigens. These have been identified and isolated from patients with Graves' disease. Once activated these CD4+ T cells in turn activate CD4+ and CD8+ T cells, and also B cells which secrete thyroid autoantibodies.

Many factors are important in autoimmune thyroid disease: genes, age, sex, race, and hormonal status. In addition, environmental factors are also important: dietary intake of iodine has an influence. In human populations epidemiological link between iodination and thyroid autoimmune disease. The highest prevalence of chronic autoimmune thyroiditis occurs in areas of the highest iodine intake, e.g. USA and Japan, and the percentage of hyperthyroidism due to Graves' disease is ~85% and the recurrence rate after thyroid surgery is greater than in areas of low iodine intake. Children given iodine prophylaxis after the Chernobyl nuclear disaster developed antibodies to thyroid membrane and thyroglobulin.

Following therapy with IFNα thyroid autoantibodies (20%), hypothyroidism (5%), and less frequently Graves' disease may develop. IL-2 and GM-CSF may cause the same effects.

Thyroid antigens

Several thyroid autoantigens have now been identified: thyroglobulin (TG), thyroid peroxidase (thyroid microsomal antigen — TMA), surface and other cytoplasmic antigens and (TSH) receptor (TSH-R). Cloning of genes for the three main thyroid antigens, thyroglobulin, thyroid peroxidase, and TSH-R, has allowed definition of the T- and B-cell epitopes.

Thyroglobulin (TG-660 kDa) is a prohormone, and from it thyroxine and triiodothyronine can be cleaved by TPO-catalysed iodination and coupling of tyrosines. The dominant epitope lies in central (non-hormone region) clones of TG reactive T cells recognize nonamer peptide at position 2553. A major recent development is demonstration that iodinated determinants are responsible for pathogenicity in EAT model.

Thyroid peroxidase (TPO-105 kDa) is identical to thyroid microsomal antigen. EAT can be induced by injecting porcine TPO in complete Freund's adjuvant or by the transfer of T cells from an immunized animal.

In human disease T-cell reactivity is to three regions of TPO: at amino acids 415–432, 439–457, 463–481. These regions stimulated the peripheral blood lymphocytes of 23–37% patients with Graves' disease or autoimmune thyroiditis.

TSH-R is synthesized as a 90 kDa precursor. Patients with hyperthyroidism have stimulatory autoantibodies to TSH-R which activate adenylcyclase, elevate mRNA for TG and TPO and c-*myc* and c-*fos* oncogene products.

In primary hypothyroidism the antibodies block the receptor and are non-stimulatory. Stimulatory and blocking autoantibodies bind to different parts of the molecule. The autoantibody site has been identified as the large extracellular N-terminal region of the TSH-R. This is not present in other receptors and from transfection studies it looks as though this is the primary antigenic site.

In addition, another autoantigen recently recognized is the 64 kDa antigen on cell membrane which is present on thyroid and extraocular muscle.

Thyroid autoantibodies

The TMA (TPO) antibody is present in high titre in primary myxoedema and Hashimoto's disease, and in moderate titre in thyrotoxicosis. Low levels are found in ~ 8% of the normal population Autoimmunity to thyroid antigens may be expressed as destructive inflammation of the gland, and/or antireceptor autoimmunity. Autoantibody to TSH-R is a primary (pathogenic) antibody and it may stimulate or block growth or metabolism.

Autoimmune hyperthyroidism (Graves' disease)

Definition

Autoimmune hyperthyroidism is the commonest form of thyrotoxicosis. It affects about 0.5% of the population with a female to male predominance of 7:1, and can occur at any age but is most common in the 30–40 year age group. The aetiology is unknown but the immune mechanisms have a definite role in the pathogenesis of the disease. An antibody to TSH-R is detected with improved assays in ~90% cases on presentation. The level of TSH-R antibody correlates with disease activity and falls with therapy.

About 0.2% of pregnant women have Graves' disease and occasionally it also occurs in the newborn infant as *neonatal thyrotoxicosis* due to transplacental transfer of immunoglobulin (Ig) G autoantibody. In the affected infant as the pathogenic maternal antibody is catabolized the hyperthyroidism remits within 2–3 months of birth. Maternal thyroid dysfunction in the year following pregnancy may be due to post-partum thyroiditis and should be treated with caution.

Genetic factors

In about half of the patients there is a family history of thyroid disease. Human leucocyte antigen (HLA) DR3 in Caucasians confers a fourfold risk for autoimmune thyroid disease. There is concordance of 50% in monozygotic but <5% in dizygotic twins.

Pathology

The thyroid shows uniform hyperplasia of the cells, little colloid and lymphocytic infiltration. The lymphocytes are CD4+ and CD8+ T cells but, unlike Hashimoto's disease, there is little or no germinal follicle formation in the lymphoid infiltrates. The autoantibodies have various activities. Most have been defined by their action on the thyroid. Thyroid-stimulating antibodies increase cyclic aderosine monophosphate in the cells, increase production of thyroid hormones and cause hyperthyroidism. Other forms of autoantibody to TSH, thyroid growth stimulating antibody, stimulate thyroid growth by increasing thyroid cell division and DNA synthesis but do not increase activity. Other TSH antibodies block, but not stimulate, the TSH-R site and thereby cause hypothyroidism.

Clinical features

The major symptoms are those of thyroid overactivity, ophthalmopathy, and a diffusely enlarged thyroid. In the young sympathetic overactivity is evident but in elderly may not be as obvious, but cardiac symptoms, e.g. dysrhythmias, are pronounced. About half develop exophthalmos and this may precede, coincide with, or follow the hyperthyroid phase. Exophthalmos is due to infiltration of muscles with lymphocytes, myositis, and proliferation of retro-orbital tissue. The skin may be thickened in certain areas, for example, in the pretibial area, *pretibial myxoedema*, hands and feet, by increased production of glycosaminoglycans and mucopolysaccharides. The degree of thyroid overactivity is not related to goitre size, and conversely thyroid growth stimulating antibody correlates with goitre size not thyroid activity (T3 and T4).

Ophthalmopathy can vary from gross clinically evident to that detectable only by computerized tomography. In 5% of cases it is a progressive problem and may threaten sight.

Diagnosis and treatment

Beta blockers may be used to control the sympathetic overactivity. Thyroid overactivity may be blocked by antithyroid drugs, e.g. methimazole or propylthiouracil. It may also be successfully treated by radioactive iodine or surgery. There is no need to use immunosuppression.

For severe cases of exophthalmos high-dose steroids, cyclophosphamide, and cyclosporin A have been used.

Autoimmune thyroid (Hashimoto's) disease

This is more common in women, often in the third to fourth decade, but can occur at any age from childhood onwards. Now it is the commonest cause of goitre in developed countries. While, initially, 75% are euthyroid, 20% hypo- and 5% hyperthyroid about half eventually become hypothyroid. In the USA and UK 40% women and 20% men have some evidence of local thyroiditis at autopsy.

Pathology

The cause is unkown. Animal experiments have demonstrated that the disease can be induced by injection of thyroid in complete Freund's adjuvant and that it can be transferred by T lymphocytes. The thyroid shows lymphoid infitration similar to that seen in Graves' disease but lymphoid follicles are also present. De Quervain's thyroiditis often follows a viral illness and thyroid antibodies are usually transient and of low titre.

Clinical feature

Diagnosis rests on the presence of goitre and/or hypothyroidism or less commonly hyperthyroidism and the serological presence of thyroid autoantibodies. The differential diagnosis is from simple goitre and subacute (De Quervain's) thyroiditis, a condition which often follows a viral illness and in which there is the transient presence of thyroid autoantibodies.

Only 9% of patients are <45 years, but the disease can occur in adolescents and older children. While patients with multinodular goitre and thyroid cancer may have thyroid antibodies in low titre, in autoimmune thyroid higher titres are found: e.g. >1:6400 for antimicrosomal; >200 IU/ml for antithyroid peroxidase. More than 95% patients have antibodies. Despite the presence of thyroid antibodies fine needle aspiration biopsy should be performed on rapidly enlarging goitres or suspicious nodules.

In those with subclinical hypothyroidism there may be progression into overt hypothyroidism, but at a slow rate: ~ 5% per year in women; but faster in men.

Therapy

The level of thyroid hormones (T3 and T4) and TSH are monitored to detect the onset of hypothyroidism. Thyroid replacement is commenced to prevent clinical hypothyroidism Overt hypothyroidism is treated with thyroxine in a dose which normalises the serum thyrotropin concentration.

Post-partum thyroiditis

Some pregnant women (5–10%) may develop variable thyroid function during pregnancy, and for the period afterwards. This is due to an underlying thyroiditis. Autoantibody to TPO (TMA) is present. The condition is subclinical and there may be periods of hyper- or hypothyroidism, or a mixture of both.

Primary hypothroidism

This is the most common cause of hypothyroidism in the elderly population. Thyroid autoantibodies are found in >80%, and antibodies are detected which block both thyroid cell metabolism and growth

There is an antibody and cellular response. Biopsy of the gland shows lymphocyte infiltration fibrosis and atrophy. Intense CD4 and CD8 lymphocytic infiltration is present together with macrophages and plasma cells also, and germinal follicles. Antibody and complement can be demonstrated on the thyroid cells, and the autoantibody blocks cell growth and/or metabolism. Antibodies are detected in >80%, and those to TPO (thyroid microsomal) appear to correlate with Hashimoto's disease activity.

Adrenal

Adrenal insufficiency

The majority (80%) of cases adrenal insufficiency are due to autoimmune disease, and the rest due to tuberculous granuloma or carcinoma. The incidence of autoimmune adrenal cortical insufficiency (Addison's disease) is about 6/100 000, the autoimmune process involving the cortex but not the medulla. It has a peak incidence at 40–50 years with female to male ratio of >2:1.

Pathology

Adrenal glands are small and fibrotic with all the hallmarks of an autoimmune process: lymphoid infiltration, germinal follicles, and occasional plasma cells. Antibodies are detected in about 80% early cases and are directed against cytoplasmic cortical antigens, and also to adrenocorticotrophic hormone receptors. One of the autoimmune targets is a key enzyme used in the steroid biosynthesis of 17α-hydrolase.

A rare form of Cushing's disease — *micronodular adrenocortical hyperplasia* — is similar to Graves' disease in that it is due to an antibody which stimulates cortisol production.

Patients should be tested for other autoantibodies as 40% have another endocrinopathy: of the thyroid in 20%, diabetes in 15%, of the ovary in 8%, and hypoparathyroidism in 4%.

Pituitary

Rarely, autoimmune disease of the pituitary occurs. The first reports were of a lymphocytic hypophysitis associated with thyroiditis. They may present with symptoms of hypopituitarism requiring hormone replacement.

Pituitary antibodies have been most frequently found in the empty sella syndrome and also in association with thyroiditis, Graves' disease, and pituitary disorders. They are detected by their reaction against pituitary tissue, or against cell lines secreting pituitary hormones

Parathyroid

Some cases of hypoparathyroidism, usually in childhood, are due to autoimmunity. Most often it is associated with Addison's disease, ovarian failure, or pernicious anaemia. Autoantibodies to cytoplasmic parathyroid tissue may be detected in idiopathic hypoparathyroidism but their frequency, <30–70%, in this condition is not clearly established. Auto-antibodies are also found to renal tubular parathyroid hormone receptor found in 95% of those with renal failure. This leads to hypocalcaemia and secondary hyperparathyroidism.

Further reading

Dalton, T. A. and Bennett, J. C. (1992). Autoimmune disease and the major histocompatibility complex: therapeutic implications. *American Journal of Medicine*, **92**, 183–8.

Dayan, C. M., Daniels, G. H. (1996). Chronic autoimmune thyroiditis. *New England Journal of Medicine*, **335**, 99–107.

Konno, N., Makita, H., Yuri, K., Iizuka, N., Kawasaki, K. (1994). Association between dietary iodine intake and prevalence of subclinical hypothyroidism in the coastal regions of Japan. *Journal of Clinical Endocrinology and Metabolism*, **78**, 393–7.

Livoli, V. A. (1994). The pathology of autoimmune thyroid disease: a review. *Thyroid*, **4**, 333–9.

Roitt, I. M., Doniach, D., Campbell, P. N. and Hudson, R. V. (1956). Auto-antibodies in Hashimoto's disease (lymphadenoid goitre). *Lancet*, **2**, 820–1.

Tomer, Y. and Davies, T. F. (1993). Infection, thyroid disease and autoimmunity. *Endocrinology Reviews*, **14**, 107–20.

Watanabe, U., Hashimoto, E., Hisamitsu, T., Obata, H., Hayashi, N. (1994). The risk factors for development of thyroid disease during interferon-alpha therapy for chronic hepatitis C. *American Journal of Gastroenterology*, **89**, 399–403.

Vanderpump, M. P. J., Tunbridge W. M. G., French J. M., *et al.* (1995). The incidence of thyroid disorders in the community: a twenty-year followup of the Whickham Survey. *Clinical Endocrinology (Oxford)*, **43**, 55–68.

14 Stomach: Gastritis and pernicious anaemia

I. R. van Driel, P. A. Gleeson and B. H. Toh

Gastritis

Gastritis is one of the commonest pathologies of the human gastrointestinal tract with a prevalence of approximately 70% in some populations. A common classification of gastritis is based upon the region of the stomach affected (Fig. 14.1). Type A is predominantly corpus, type B is mostly antral and type AB is pangastric. Type B gastritis is usually associated with infection of the antrum with *Helicobacter pylori* and is rarely associated with autoimmunity. On the other hand type A gastritis is rarely accompanied by bacterial infection but is commonly accompanied by auto-antibodies directed towards the gastric parietal cell which suggests an underlying autoimmune cause.

Pernicious anaemia

Pernicious anaemia (PA) is the result of severe, chronic atrophic gastritis type A which develops in only a small proportion (10–15%) of subjects with type A gastritis. PA is a megaloblastic anaemia due to vitamin B_{12} malabsorption. Nevertheless, at an estimated incidence of 0.1% in Western adult populations it represents the most common cause of vitamin B_{12} deficiency. The prevalence in different racial groups varies and is highest among white Europeans of northern origin and rare among southern Europeans, Asians, Africans, and Latin Americans.

Clinically, it presents as complaints of pallor and fatigue (~90%), breathlessness (~70%), feelings of lethargy and depression, and some may have paraesthesiae (~30%) and signs of neurological involvement (~5%).

The condition is characterized by gastric mucosal atrophy, loss of parietal and chief cells, intestinal metaplasia, and submucosal lymphocytic infiltration. Megaloblastic anaemia results from deficiency of intrinsic factor essential for dietary vitamin B_{12} absorption from the terminal ileum. There may be accompanying dysmyelination of spinal cord postero-lateral columns (subacute combined degeneration) and peripheral neuropathy if vitamin B_{12} deficiency is prolonged. Gastric neoplasia, attributed to trophic action of secondary hypergastrinaemia, may be a long-term complication.

Laboratory diagnosis rests on demonstration of:

(1) megaloblastic anaemia with low serum vitamin B_{12} levels;

(2) low level of serum pepsinogen I;

(3) chronic but variable atrophic gastritis on gastric biopsy;

(4) total achlorhydria;

(5) autoantibodies to parietal cells in >90% which develop early and persist, and/or to intrinsic factor; and

(6) low Schilling's test which measures absorption of vitamin B_{12}.

It appears that the only life-threatening effect of severe autoimmune gastritis is the lack of vitamin B_{12}. Hence, the therapy of choice is replacement of this vitamin. While corticosteroid treatment has been shown to be of some benefit in reversing the underlying lesion the possible side-effects render this treatment inadvisable.

Genetics

Genetic predisposition is suggested by clustering of PA with other endocrine autoimmune diseases. Gastric autoimmunity rates (but not necessarily clinically apparent PA) are 20–30% in patients with thyroid autoimmunity, insulin-dependent diabetes mellitus, Addison's disease, vitiligo, and primary gonadal failure. In addition, there is a high incidence (13%) of gastric autoimmunity in first-generation PA relatives versus only 1% in controls. Limited studies of PA in monozygotic twins also suggests a role for genetic factors. However, the genetic basis for all these observations remains unknown. A number of studies have investigated the linkage with human leucocyte antigen (HLA) and gastric autoimmunity. An increased frequency of a number of HLA alleles have been reported in some studies but the association is weak and not substantiated in other studies.

Autoantibodies

One of the defining features of autoimmune gastritis and PA is the presence of antibodies to the membranes of parietal cell and to intrinsic factor which is produced by parietal cells (Fig. 14.1). Intrinsic factor autoantibodies are present in approximately 70% of subjects with PA and may either bind to intrinsic factor at B_{12} binding sites (blocking antibodies) or to sites remote from this location (binding antibodies). These antibodies may contribute to intrinsic factor deficiency. Intrinsic factor antibodies rarely occur in gastritic individuals in the absence of PA.

Most studies suggest that parietal cell autoantibodies are found in 90% of patients and 2–5% of the general population suggesting that this is a highly sensitive marker of type A gastritis. However, it should be noted that coincidence between gastritis and autoantibodies and hence sensitivity may vary considerably between different populations.

The molecules recognized by the anti-parietal cell antibodies appear to be predominantly the subunits of the gastric parietal cell proton pump (H/K ATPase) (Fig. 14.2). The proton pump consists of the 114 kDa catalytic α and the 60–90 kDa glycoprotein β subunit. The proton pump, located on secretory membranes of

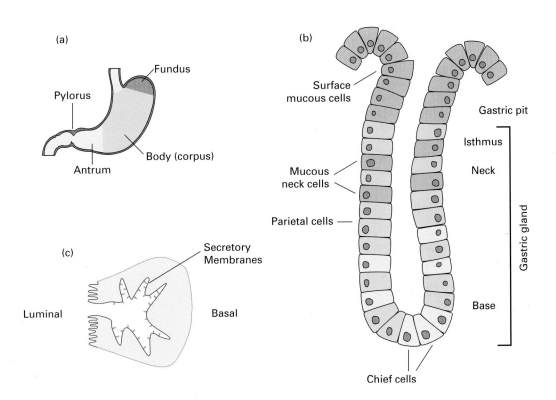

∎ **Fig. 14.1** (A) The stomach; (B) gastric gland; and (C) parietal cell. The shaded areas on the fundus and body of the stomach are the parietal cell containing parts. The parietal cells are a polarized cell type with distinct luminal (apical) and basal membrane surfaces. The secretory membranes which contain the gastric H+, K+ ATPase are continuous with the apical membrane. ACh, acetylcholine; R, receptor.

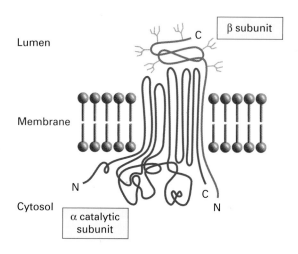

Lumen

Membrane

Cytosol

β subunit

α catalytic subunit

N

C

N

C

■ Fig. 14.2 Schematic representation of the H^+, K^+ ATPase. The α catalytic subunit has 10 transmembrane domains. The β subunit contains six potential *N*-glycosylation on the large extracellular domain.

parietal cells, is responsible for acidification of gastric juice. It was originally proposed that the 94 kDa protein reacting with parietal cell antibodies by immunoblotting was the H/K ATPase α subunit. In addition, patient sera was found to deplete H/K ATPase activity from parietal cell membranes. Reactivity with α subunit was confirmed using purified and recombinant proteins. Reactivity with a lower molecular weight 60–90 kDa protein was also observed. At the time of this observation the existence of the β subunit was unknown. Biochemical and molecular characterization of this protein led to the discovery that it was in fact a previously unknown H/K ATPase β subunit.

Recently, the differences between the antibody binding patterns obtained by different groups was explained. Binding of autoantibodies to the subunits of the gastric H/K ATPase in immunoblotting assays is dependent upon conditions of electrophoresis, which explains differences in the antibody binding patterns of different investigators. Using optimal conditions for the detection of both anti-α and anti-β specificities, antibodies to both subunits were invariably found in anti-parietal cell sera.

The proton pump is sequestered from the circulatory system in cytoplasmic secretory membranes or the luminal face of the parietal cells (Fig. 14.1). Hence, it seems that anti-proton pump antibodies are unlikely to contribute to the destruction of parietal cells. Work in animal models supports this proposition and also implicates T lymphocytes in pathogenesis (see below). Furthermore, individuals with B-cell immunodeficiencies still develop PA.

Cellular involvement

Examination of gastric mucosa of PA patients illustrates a significant increase in CD4 and CD8 T lymphocytes as well as a sixfold increase in non-T lymphocytes that were probably B lymphocytes. Analysis of the mucosal infiltrates in murine experimental autoimmune gastritis (see below) have resulted in similar data. In this system CD4+ T cells increase approximately four-to-fivefold with the onset of gastritis while the number of CD8 cells remains relatively low. A very large increase in the number of B cells occurs relatively late in the disease process. A recent phenotypic analysis of T cells in peripheral blood of PA patients did not detect any significant differences relative to age-matched controls.

Animal models of autoimmune gastritis

Gastric autoimmunity can be induced in mice by either neonatal thymectomy, a combination of thymectomy and treatment with cytotoxic drugs and immunization with purified gastric proton pump. All these models share common features with human gastritis in that there is the production of autoantibodies to the gastric proton pump, destruction of parietal and chief cells and a proliferation of undifferentiated mucosal cells. To date a large amount of work has been performed with the neonatal thymectomy model. These investigations have demonstrated that CD4+ T lymphocytes and not autoantibodies are capable of causing the gastric lesion. These data contradict earlier findings that demonstrated induction of atrophic gastritis in rats upon treatment with immunoglobulin G from PA patients.

Autoreactive T cells appear to be present in mice that do not have autoimmune gastritis but they are kept in abeyance by mechanisms that are not clearly understood. Treatment of mice with cyclophosphamide to reduce the number of lymphocytes and other haematopoietic cells only induces autoimmune gastritis if mice are also thymectomized near the time of drug treatment. This observation implicated the thymus in the prevention of autoimmune disease. Hence, the thymic atrophy which normally occurs with increasing age may be a contributing factor in autoimmunity.

Mouse models have also been important in defining the specificity of T cells that initiate autoimmune gastritis. Transgenic mice have been used to demonstrate that T cells directed to the gastric H/K ATPase β subunit are required for initiation of gastritis. In addition, a T-cell line reactive with a peptide sequence derived from the H/K ATPase a subunit has been isolated. This cell line caused gastritis when transferred to athymic mice after activation.

The clear definition of the autoimmune targets in this disease and the availability of a readily malleable animal model make autoimmune gastritis an ideal model system to investigate the events that initiate autoimmunity and the pathogenic actions of the autoimmune lymphocytes.

Further reading

Alderuccio, F., Toh, B. H., Tan, S. S., Gleeson, P. A., and van Driel, I. R. (1993). An autoimmune disease with multiple molecular targets abrogated by the transgenic expression of a single autoantigen in the thymus. *Journal of Experimental Medicine*, **178**, 419–26.

Callaghan, J. M., Khan, M. A., Alderuccio, F., van Driel, I. R., Gleeson, P. A., and Toh, B. H. (1993). α and β subunits of the gastric H^+/K^+-ATPase are concordantly targeted by parietal cell autoantibodies associated with autoimmune gastritis. *Autoimmunity*, **16**, 289–95.

Carmel, R. (1992). Reassessment of the relative prevalences of antibodies to gastric parietal cell and to intrinsic factor in patients with pernicious anaemia — influence of patient age and race. *Clinical and Experimental and Immunology*, **89**, 74–7.

Gleeson, P. A., Toh, B. H., and van Driel, I. R. (1996). Organ specific autoimmunity induced by lymphopenia. *Immunological reviews*, **149**, 97–125.

Roitt, I. M., Doniach, D., and Shapland, C. (1965). Autoimmunity in pernicious anaemia and atrophic gastritis. *Annals of the New York Academy Science*, **124**, 644–656.

Strickland, R. G. and Mackay I. R. (1973). A reappraisal of the nature and significance of chronic autoimmune gastritis. *American Journal of Digestion*, **18**, 426–40.

Toh, B. H., Gleeson, P. A., Simpson, R. J., Moritz, R. L., Callaghan, J., Goldkorn, I., (1990). The 60–90 kDa parietal cell autoantigen associated with autoimmune gastritis is a β subunit of the gastric H^+/K^+-ATPase (proton pump). *Proceedings of the National Academy of Sciences, USA*, **87**, 6418–22.

Toh, B. H., Gleeson, P. A. and van Driel, I. R. (1997). Pernicious anemia and gastric atrophy. In *The immune diseases*, 2nd edn (ed. N. R. Rose and I. R. Mackay). Academic Press, New York. (In press.)

15 Gastrointestinal disorders

I. C. Roberts-Thomson and A. G. Cummins

Immunology of the gastrointestinal tract

The gastrointestinal tract differs from many other organs in the body in that it is continuously exposed to a vast array of foreign antigens such as food proteins, intestinal micro-organisms, and other environmental antigens. Many of these antigens are degraded within the intestinal lumen by a variety of digestive enzymes in intestinal secretions. Those which escape digestion have only limited access to the portal circulation because of the evolution of several defence mechanisms which constitute an effective barrier to antigen absorption. Some of these mechanisms are immunological such as the secretion of immunoglobulin (Ig) A and IgM into the gut lumen and enhanced secretion of mucus which is mediated by immune complexes. Despite these defences, however, a small amount of dietary protein can be detected in the peripheral circulation after meals, probably because of endocytosis and transport across epithelial cells.

The total mass of lymphoid tissue in the gut exceeds that of any other organ including the spleen. This gut-associated lymphoid tissue differs from the systemic immune system in a variety of areas including antigen uptake and processing, immunoglobulin production, subpopulations of T cells, selective homing properties, and cell-mediated immune responses. In addition to limited antigen absorption through epithelial cells, luminal antigen has access to lymphoid tissue through specialized microfold (M) cells which overlie Peyer's patches. The latter process may be more relevant to particulate bacterial antigens which are at highest concentration in the ileum and colon than to food antigens which are at highest concentration in the proximal small bowel.

The normal lamina propria contains a large population of plasma cells, mostly of the IgA isotype. On release from plasma cells, IgA is usually in the form of a dimer joined by J chain. This polymeric IgA is then selectively transported by the immunoglobulin transporter on the basolateral membrane of enterocytes and is secreted into the bowel lumen with a soluble portion of the immunoglobulin transporter called the secretory piece. In this form, IgA is relatively resistant to proteolytic digestion. Polymeric IgM may also be found in the bowel lumen but is of lesser importance because of lower rates of secretion and higher rates of degradation.

Lymphocytes in the intestine are found in lymphocyte-filled villi and Peyer's patches and are dispersed within the lamina propria and between surface epithelial cells (intraepithelial lymphocytes). The lamina propria contains CD4+ and CD8+ T cells in a ratio of about 2:1, with the majority having the $\alpha\beta$ T cell receptor (TCR). Intraepithelial lymphocytes are a heterogeneous population but 95% are CD7+ (pre-T cell), CD8+, and HML–1+. Varying proportions have the $\alpha\beta$ TCR or $\gamma\delta$ TCR and there is a small population of lymphocytes which are CD7+ and CD4–, and CD8–. There is increasing evidence that the gut epithelium may promote extrathymic T-cell differentiation of both $\gamma\delta$ and $\alpha\beta$ TCR+ cells.

Lamina propria T cells produce predominantly interferon (IFN) γ, IL-2, IL-5, and IL-6 with the IFNγ producing T cells being at highest concentration in the proximal small bowel. Intraepithelial lymphocytes produce transforming growth factor (TGF) β which may be important as an immunosuppressive cytokine. Enterocytes also produce cytokines such as TGFβ and IL-6. There is considerable cytokine 'cross-talk' between the epithelium, lymphocytes, other cells such as fibroblasts and mast cells and even enteric nerves.

Another area of interest involves the role of epithelial cells in the regulation of immune responses to dietary and other antigens. Epithelial cells express class II molecules of the major histocompatibility complex and may present soluble antigen to primed T cells, perhaps causing preferential activation of suppressor T-cell populations.

A central theme in intestinal immunity is that of oral tolerance, a process of downregulation of mucosal immune responses, which is established during weaning and persists throughout life. One attractive hypothesis is that disorders such as coeliac disease and chronic inflammatory bowel disease represent a breakdown of oral tolerance in genetically susceptible individuals. If this hypothesis is correct, reasons for the failure of oral tolerance are unknown but might include the amount of luminal antigen, the chemical nature of the antigen, the site and degree of antigen absorption and the nature of humoral and cell-mediated immune responses.

Coeliac disease

Introduction

Coeliac disease is a chronic inflammatory disorder of small bowel which results in malabsorption of nutrients. The characteristic histologica appearance is that of villous atrophy, crypt hyperplasia, and lymphocytic infiltration of the epithelium and lamina propria. A unique feature of the disease, its induction by dietary gluten, was first suggested by Dicke in the late 1940s when Dutch children, deprived of wheat products, showed improvement in symptoms during the Second World War. The disease has a number of autoimmune-like features including a dense lymphocytic infiltrate in the affected bowel, a strong association with human leucocyte antigens (HLA), responsiveness to corticosteroid drugs and an association with an autoantibody, which has high specificity for the disease.

Epidemiology

The prevalence of disease varies in different parts of the world with a peak of 1:300 on the west coast of Ireland to 1:2000 in the UK, 1:6500 in Sweden and perhaps very low prevalence rates in Asia and Africa. It is likely, however, that the true prevalence is somewhat higher as milder forms of the disease may remain undiagnosed.

The age at diagnosis varies from the first few months of life to the eighth decade; about half of patients are diagnosed as children and the rest as adults. In adults, the ratio of women to men is 2:1 but the female predominance is less obvious in children where ratios approach 1:1 in most studies. It is not known whether or not those patients diagnosed as adults had asymptomatic or undetected coeliac disease as children, or if the intestinal lesion developed in adult life. Occasionally, the diagnosis of coeliac disease is made after the development of anaemia

during pregnancy or because of symptomatic steatorrhoea after gastric surgery (gastrectomy or vagotomy and pyloroplasty).

Genetic factors

In twin studies, the frequency of concordant coeliac disease in identical twins has been estimated at 75%. In family studies, the prevalence of coeliac disease in first-degree relatives of coeliac patients is still debated but may be of the order of 5–10%. Higher prevalence rates have been reported when asymptomatic relatives have been investigated with multiple small bowel biopsies.

There is a strong association with HLA-DQ2. This gene product, a glycoprotein, is encoded by HLA genes within the HLA-D region (subregion DQ) called DQB1*0201 and DQA1*0501. These DQ alleles are functionally expressed, both when encoded in the *cis* position on HLA-DR17 or in the *trans* position on heterozygous DR11/DR7 or DR12/DR7 haplotypes.

About 95% of patients with coeliac disease express HLA-DQ2, even patients from markedly different geographic areas. Furthermore, siblings of affected patients who express HLA-DQ2 have a frequency of coeliac disease of about 30%. On the other hand, symptomatic coeliac disease develops in only a small minority (1% or less) of the general population who express HLA-DQ2. Of the 5% of coeliac patients who fail to express HLA-DQ2, most have the HLA haplotype DR4, DQ8.

Dietary and environmental factors

Many investigators have attempted to isolate the dietary antigens responsible for coeliac disease. Although wheat products appear to be the most toxic, lesser degrees of histological damage can be induced by rye, barley, and oats. The toxic fractions reside in the endosperm (flour), particularly those components which are soluble in 70% ethanol and are collectively termed prolamins. This includes gliadins from wheat, secalins from rye, hordeins from barley and avenins from oats.

By gel electrophoresis, gliadins can be categorized into four major fractions: α, β, γ, and ω with molecular weights ranging from 32 to 58 kDa. These fractions contain several closely related polypeptides with a high content of glutamine and proline. Although the amino acid sequence of several gliadins is now known, the sequences which are toxic still remain unclear, although α-gliadins may be more toxic than other fractions. This issue may be difficult to resolve as several gliadin fractions may activate the disease and sensitivity to fractions may vary in different patients.

Furthermore, some gliadin fractions are impure and there is debate about the assessment of toxicity both *in vivo* and *in vitro*.

Perhaps the most likely scenario is that of a series of prolamins which express certain disease-precipitating epitopic domains of similar or identical structure. Important amino acid sequences may include proline–serine–glutamine–glutamine and serine–proline–glutamine–glutamine.

Other environmental factors may also influence the development of coeliac disease. For example, early exposure to wheat cereals may precipitate the disease in some individuals while prolonged breast feeding has been reported to decrease the severity of disease. Indeed, promotion of breast feeding on the west coast of Ireland (a genetically susceptible population) apparently decreased the prevalence of disease in children from 1:300 to 1:2000.

Another possible factor is a gastrointestinal infection with human adenovirus serotype 12. Kagnoff and colleagues have reported a sequence homology between α-gliadin and the E1b protein of the virus which might trigger immune responses to prolamins. Some support for this hypothesis has been derived from serological and immunological tests (leucocyte migration inhibition assays) but results have been difficult to corroborate in other centres and the issue has not been resolved.

Pathology

The diagnosis of coeliac disease is established by small bowel biopsy. Characteristic features include villous atrophy, crypt hyperplasia, effacement of surface epithelial cells, and a marked increase in lymphoid cells in the lamina propria and in the epithelium (Fig. 15.1). These changes are most marked in the duodenum and jejunum and decrease in severity in the distal small bowel. This variation presumably reflects the luminal concentration of gluten.

In adults, the above histological features are diagnostic of coeliac disease in most settings, although similar changes are occasionally observed in patients with tropical sprue, graft-versus-host disease, and diffuse intestinal lymphoma. In children, other causes need to be considered including viral gastroenteritis, giardiasis, and soy and milk protein allergy. This extended differential diagnosis has led some authors to promote more stringent diagnostic requirements in children including improvement in morphology with a gluten-free diet and a histological relapse after the reintroduction of gluten. Other authors have relied on clinical improvement after gluten withdrawal and the presence in serum of antigliadin or anti-endomysial antibodies.

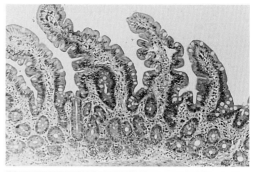
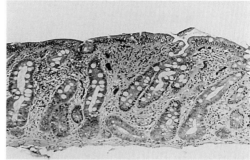

▌Fig. 15.1 Normal jejunal biopsy (above) and biopsy from a patient with coeliac disease (below); the latter showing absent villi, hyperplasia of crypts, changes in surface epithelial cells and increased numbers of inflammatory cells in the lamina propria (haematoxylin and eosin × 80).

Immunohistochemical studies have shown increased numbers of T cells in the lamina propria, largely CD4+ helper cells. There is also an increase in B cells and plasma cells producing IgG, IgM, and IgA with a disproportionate increase in cells producing IgG in relation to those producing IgA. Other cells also increase in number including eosinophils and mast cells. In the epithelium, intraepithelial lymphocytes increase in density and there is an increased proportion of cells positive for the $\gamma\delta$ (TCR) rather than the $\alpha\beta$ TCR. This disproportionate increase in $\gamma\delta$ TCR+ cells persists even in treated coeliacs in whom small bowel morphology returns to near-normal.

Patients with coeliac disease have a risk of malignant neoplasms which is about twice that of the general population. The most striking association is with lymphomas, particularly of the small intestine (enteropathy-associated T-cell lymphoma), but there is also an increased risk for squamous cell cancers of the oesophagus and pharynx. Ulcerative or stricturing jejunitis complicating coeliac disease is likely to be a lymphoma, although the diagnosis may take years to establish with certainty. Enteropathy-associated T-cell lymphomas have the unusual phenotype, CD7+

HML–1+, consistent with a neoplasm of intraepithelial lymphocytes.

'Latent' or 'potential' coeliac disease is a new concept which, in a strict sense, can only be diagnosed retrospectively. It refers to the potential to develop coeliac disease when the initial biopsy is normal but a subsequent biopsy shows typical features of coeliac disease. This has been best described in case reports in twins. Various surrogate markers of 'potential' coeliac disease have been suggested including elevated titres of IgM antigliadin antibody in intestinal fluid and increased numbers of intraepithelial lymphocytes in intestinal biopsies.

Immunopathogenesis

Current hypotheses for the pathogenesis of coeliac disease emphasize the importance of HLA-DQ2 for presentation of antigen to primed T cells and the development of small bowel inflammation as a manifestation of a vigorous cell-mediated immune reaction. Despite substantial progress over the past decade, however, the precise sequence of events remains unclear and there is no persuasive explanation for the development of disease in only a small minority of patients expressing HLA-DQ2.

One model for the association between HLA-DQ2 and coeliac disease predicts that DQ2 facilitates the binding of gliadin peptides to antigen-presenting cells which, in turn, activates a pathogenic population of T cells (Fig. 15.2). Products released by activated T cells then play a major part in the production of small bowel inflammation. Support for this hypothesis comes from recent studies where T-cell clones from coeliac patients have recognized a synthetic α-gliadin when presented with DQ2. The development of coeliac disease in only a minority of patients with HLA-DQ2 might then be explained by other factors such as the duration of breast feeding, the time of introduction of dietary gluten, exposure to gastrointestinal viruses, and variation in the repertoire of immune responses in the mucosa. Although the nature of antigen-presenting cells is still unclear, these seem more likely to be lamina propria cells than epithelial cells as the latter may not express DQ2.

Several observations support the hypothesis that the pattern of mucosal injury in coeliac disease is the result of a cell-mediated immune reaction. These include clinical and morphological improvement with corticosteroids and immunosuppressive drugs and the induction of similar histological lesions in graft-versus-host disease and intestinal allograft rejection (Table 15.1). Furthermore, the lamina propria of coeliac patients contains T cells which appear to respond only to gliadin presented by DQ2. Increased

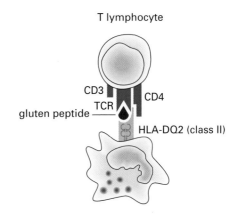

T lymphocyte

CD3 · TCR · CD4 · gluten peptide · HLA-DQ2 (class II)

Macrophage / dendritic cell
(antigen-presenting cell)

∎ **Fig. 15.2** An attractive hypothesis for the aetiology of coeliac disease is that HLA-DQ2 facilitates the binding of gliadin peptides to antigen presenting cells which subsequently activate a pathogenic population of T cells. TCR, T-cell receptor.

∎ **Table 15.1** Markers of delayed-type hypersensitivity reactions in the intestine

Villous hypertrophy followed by atrophy
Crypt hyperplasia
Increased numbers of intraepithelial lymphocytes
Degranulation of mucosal mast cells
Increased epithelial expression of human leucocyte antigen class II (DR) antigens
Activated T cells and macrophages (DR+, IL-2R+)
Increased production of γ interferon by T lymphocytes

numbers of these mucosal lymphocytes and amacrophages are activated as assessed by the expression of interleukin (IL) 2 and these activated cells may be responsible for the elevated concentrations of soluble interleukin 2 receptor (IL-2R) in peripheral blood (Fig. 15.3). The role of antibody in the pathogenesis of disease still remains unclear, although IgM antigliadin antibodies might play a part.

The cytokines which mediate particular components of mucosal injury have not yet been clarified. One possibility is that T cells activate macrophages which release a variety of enteropathogenic cytokines and enzymes that collapse the cellular and acellular (proteoglycan) support for the villus. Other cytokines

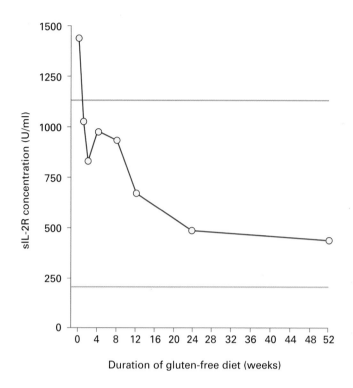

■ Fig. 15.3 Plasma concentrations of soluble IL-2 receptor (sIL-2R) in the peripheral blood of patients with coeliac disease before and after the introduction of a gluten-free diet. The circles are the median values for groups of 10–20 patients. Reference range, 230–1100 U/ml.

such as IFNγ, tumour necrosis factor (TNF), and IL-6 may increase intestinal permeability by interfering with the structure and function of tight junctions between epithelial cells.

Clinical features and diagnosis

Coeliac disease can present in a variety of different ways depending on the age of the patient, and the duration and extent of disease. Symptoms in children tend to be more uniform and include impaired growth, diarrhoea, irritability, bulky stools, anorexia, weakness, and abdominal distension. Some evidence exists for spontaneous improvement in symptoms during the teenage years, perhaps because of enhanced absorption in the ileum. In adults, the most common symptoms are diarrhoea, weight loss, and anaemia. However, a wide variety of other features may occur including peripheral oedema, easy bruising, bone pain, mouth ulcers, amenorrhoea, and psychiatric disturbances.

Disorders associated with coeliac disease include type I diabetes mellitus (30-fold increase), selective IgA deficiency (10-fold increase), and Addison's disease. About 5% of coeliacs have symptomatic dermatitis herpetiformis but most, if not all, patients with dermatitis herpetiformis have gluten sensitivity, often with only mild or patchy changes in jejunal morphology. Hyposplenism occurs in about 40% of patients and is more common in adults, perhaps because prolonged stimulation of mucosal immunity results in suppression of immune responses in the spleen.

Laboratory features

Preliminary investigations prior to small bowel biopsy may reveal anaemia, usually due to a deficiency of iron and/or folic acid. The lymphocyte count is often low and the blood film may show features of splenic atrophy. The serum albumin may also be low while an elevated concentration of alkaline phosphatase suggests osteomalacia. Faecal excretion of fat is usually elevated (>5 g/24 h), and tests of small bowel absorption and permeability are often abnormal including the D-xylose test, lactulose–rhamnose test, and the chromium[51] EDTA absorption test. The sensitivity and specificity of antigliadin antibodies and various autoantibodies will be discussed below.

Dietary antibodies and autoantibodies

Coeliac disease is almost always accompanied by elevated serum concentrations of IgG and IgA antibodies to gliadin and to other food proteins such as β-lactoglobulin, casein, and ovalbumin. In addition, IgM and IgA antibodies are secreted into intestinal fluid. In general, there is a poor correlation between concentrations of serum and intestinal antigliadin antibody. While serum IgA is mostly monomeric in normal individuals, patients with coeliac disease have higher concentrations of polymeric IgA, presumably because of higher rates of mucosal secretion.

Elevated serum concentrations of various food protein antibodies seem likely to be a response to the increase in intestinal permeability associated with mucosal inflammation. One mechanism which may minimize this response involves the formation of IgA and IgM complexes in extracellular fluid which are actively transported into epithelial cells. Subsequently, antigen and antibody are dissociated, antigen is degraded and antibody is secreted back into the intestinal lumen.

Some data are now available on the sensitivity and specificity of IgG and IgA antigliadin antibodies in coeliac disease. IgG antigliadin antibody measurements are more sensitive (95%) but not specific whereas IgA antigliadin antibody measurements are more specific but less sensitive. In one epidemiological study in children aged 11–15, 2% had elevated concentrations of IgG antigliadin antibody but only 0.3% had elevated concentrations of IgA antigliadin antibody. The majority of the latter group were confirmed as having coeliac disease by small bowel biopsy. In other studies, elevated titres of antigliadin antibody have been documented in Crohn's disease, human immunodeficiency virus (HIV) enteropathy, and intestinal bacterial overgrowth. Although these studies are of interest, there is a need to develop reference standards and to establish age-specific antigliadin antibody cut-offs to accommodate the fall in antigliadin antibody titres with age.

The role of antigliadin antibody in the pathogenesis of coeliac disease still remains unclear. IgA antigliadin antibody seems unlikely to have a part in intestinal inflammation as IgA does not bind complement and coeliac disease can occur in the presence of IgA deficiency. This may not apply to IgM where complement activation may occur, particularly with the hexameric polymer.

The autoantibody of coeliac disease is directed against an extracellular matrix protein which has not been purified as yet but is not collagen. The presence of antibody in serum is assayed by immunofluorescence using various tissue substrates. The antibody was first described as antireticulin (referring to the reticular network around muscle bundles) and was detected coincidentally when testing for antismooth muscle antibody. An alternative technique using monkey oesophagus or human umbilical cord detects anti-endomysial antibody. Both antireticulin and anti-endomysial antibodies are directed against the same tissue antigen in the intestine. Purification of the antigen should permit the development of an ELISA assay (enzyme-linked immunosorbent assay) in the near future.

Anti-endomysial antibodies appear to be highly sensitive and specific for coeliac disease (90–100%). However, results of tests are less reliable in young children (<1 year) and anti-endomysial antibody (an IgA class antibody) is absent in selective IgA deficiency. Titres of both anti-endomysial antibody and antigliadin antibody tend to parallel the severity of mucosal changes and, because of this, antibody may also be absent in treated coeliacs whose mucosal architecture has returned towards normal.

Treatment

The treatment of coeliac disease consists of a gluten-free diet for life. This results in resolution of symptoms and reduces the longer-term risk for development of cancer. The role of a gluten-free diet in patients with gluten sensitivity but without symptoms remains unclear, although epidemiological studies suggest that they are also at higher risk for a variety of cancers.

In symptomatic coeliac disease, treatment with a gluten-free diet often results in near-normal jejunal morphology in children after 3–6 months but this is less common in adults, perhaps because of greater difficulty with compliance with the diet. Corticosteroid and immunosuppressive drugs also result in clinical and morphological improvement but their use is restricted to patients with severe symptoms and/or a poor initial response to a gluten-free diet. The requirement for drug therapy, however, should raise the possibility of development of an enteropathy-associated T-cell lymphoma.

Inflammatory bowel disease

Introduction

The term 'inflammatory bowel disease' or 'chronic inflammatory bowel disease' is normally used to encompass the idiopathic inflammatory disorders of ulcerative colitis and Crohn's disease. These diseases are relatively common in Western countries but rare in much of the developing world. At present, the aetiology of these disorders remains unclear and there is continuing debate as to whether ulcerative colitis and Crohn's disease are separate diseases or different manifestations of similar pathogenic mechanisms.

Support for the possibility that these disorders result from altered mucosal immunity largely rests with responsiveness to corticosteroids and other immunosuppressive drugs. Autoantibodies do exist but are neither sensitive nor specific for the disorders. Furthermore, associations with other autoimmune diseases and with particular HLA antigens are relatively weak. The purpose of this section is to provide an overview of the two disorders with emphasis on immunological features and immunopathogenesis.

Epidemiology

Neither ulcerative colitis nor Crohn's disease is a new disorder; both were described in the nineteenth century, although Crohn's disease carries the name of Dr B. B. Crohn who introduced the term 'regional ileitis' in 1932. Although data on annual incidence rates can be criticized, incidence rates for ulcerative colitis appeared to increase between 1930 and 1970 to a peak of 10–15 per 100 000 population per year in many Western countries. Crohn's disease appeared to be rare prior to 1950 but increased in a similar way through to 1980 reaching a peak of 3–6 per 100 000 population per year. Over the past decade, these rates have either stabilized or decreased.

The highest incidence rates have been reported in white populations in Europe including Scandinavia. In Europe and the USA, ulcerative colitis may be more common in Jews than in other racial groups. For Crohn's disease within the USA, prevalence rates per 100 000 population for Hispanics (4.1) and Asians (5.6) were much lower than for whites (43.6) and blacks (29.8). Countries with a low incidence of inflammatory bowel disease include Japan and eastern Europe and much of Asia, Africa, and South America.

In high-risk populations, the incidence of inflammatory bowel disease peaks between the ages of 20 and 40 years. However, more recent epidemiological studies have emphasized a bimodal distribution with a second peak in those over the age of 60 years. Women are more frequently affected than men with a female to male ratio of about 1.5:1. In patients developing disease after the age of 60, males predominate for ulcerative colitis whereas females predominate for Crohn's disease.

Although many studies have explored environmental factors which may predispose to inflammatory bowel disease, the only consistent associations relate to non-smoking and ulcerative colitis, and smoking and Crohn's disease. Weak associations have been found between Crohn's disease, use of oral contraceptives, and a high dietary intake of sugar. Gastrointestinal or other infections do not appear to precipitate the onset of disease but may play a part in exacerbations of intestinal inflammation. Reliable data in relation to breast feeding are difficult to obtain but early weaning has been associated with both ulcerative colitis and Crohn's disease in some studies.

Genetic factors

Persuasive evidence exists for a genetic component to susceptibility for inflammatory bowel disease. For example, the proportion of patients with a positive family history for inflammatory bowel disease is usually in the range of 10–20% and the risk for development of disease in siblings is increased by about 30-fold. Crohn's disease appears to be more familial than ulcerative colitis, although it is common for affected families to have some individuals with ulcerative colitis and others with Crohn's disease.

In twin studies, the concordance rate (both twins affected) for monozygotic and dizygotic twins has been estimated at 67 and 8%, respectively, for Crohn's disease and 20 and 0%, respectively, for ulcerative colitis. Interestingly, there are no reports of monozygotic twins where one has ulcerative colitis and the other has Crohn's disease. Children may be at relatively high risk for development of disease when both parents are affected but spouses of affected patients have a similar risk to that of the general population. Higher than expected frequencies of inflammatory bowel disease have been reported in the genetic disorders of Turner syndrome and Hermansky–Pudlak syndrome.

No significant associations have been found between inflammatory bowel disease and polymorphic genetic markers including red blood cell antigens, red cell enzymes, and serum proteins. In regard to HLA typing, results have been inconsistent but some studies show an increase in HLA-DR2, HLA-B5, and the haplotype HLA-B5/DR2. This issue has not been clarified by HLA typing of affected families, although it is still possible that HLA antigens predispose to particular subsets of patients with inflammatory bowel disease. When ulcerative colitis is associated with ankylosing spondylitis and sclerosing cholangitis, significant associations exist between spondylitis and HLA-B27 and between sclerosing cholangitis and HLA-B8, -DR3 and -DRw52a. One study has reported an association between Crohn's disease and inherited polymorphism in the third component (C3) of the complement system.

Pathology

In ulcerative colitis, inflammation is largely confined to the mucosa and extends proximally from the anal margin to involve a variable length of colonic mucosa. Terms such as proctitis, proctosigmoiditis, left-sided colitis, and total colitis describe involvement of the rectum, rectosigmoid region, descending colon and the entire colon, respectively. Although the extent of disease remains relatively stable in the majority of patients, a minority show proximal extension of inflammation with the passage of time.

In active colitis, microscopic features include a dense inflammatory infiltrate in the lamina propria, epithelial cell necrosis, a reduction in the goblet cell population, crypt abscesses, and mucosal haemorrhages (Fig. 15.4). Some of these features resolve with colitis in remission but residual changes include a decrease in crypt density, short crypts, thickening of the muscularis mucosa, and focal collections of chronic inflammatory cells. The presence of persistent dysplasia is associated with an increased risk for the

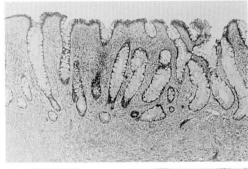

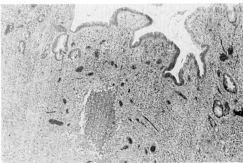

▎**Fig. 15.4** Rectal biopsy from a patient with ulcerative colitis in remission (above) showing normal colonic crypts and only a mild increase in inflammatory cells in the lamina propria. The rectal biopsy below shows severe ulcerative colitis with destruction of crypts, goblet cell depletion, a mucosal abscess, and a marked increase in inflammatory cells in the lamina propria (haematoxylin and eosin × 40).

development of colon cancer. In long-standing disease, the colon is short and loses its normal haustral pattern because of changes in intestinal muscle, perhaps aggravated by mucosal fibrosis.

In contrast to ulcerative colitis, inflammation in Crohn's disease involves all layers of the bowel wall and may be associated with granulomas and deep fissuring ulceration. Inflammation is often discontinuous with abnormal areas separated by normal mucosa. The small bowel alone is affected in about 30% of cases while 25% have colitis alone and the remainder (45%) have ileocolitis. Rarely, patients have involvement of the proximal small bowel, stomach, oesophagus, and oral mucosa. Transmural inflammation usually leads to the development of adhesions and may result in inflammatory masses, abscesses, and fistulae to adherent bowel, skin, or other organs.

The microscopic appearance is variable and involves transmural inflammation, lymphoid aggregates, granulomas, mucosal ulceration, submucosal fibrosis, and hypertrophy of nerves in the submucosa and myenteric plexus. In segments of bowel removed at surgery, granulomas can be found in the mucosa or muscle layers in about 70% of specimens while 25% have granulomas in regional lymph nodes. These granulomas have a variety of morphological appearances ranging from 'microgranulomas' to large, well-formed granulomas which contain giant cells and large numbers of epithelioid cells.

In both ulcerative colitis and Crohn's disease, the inflammatory cell infiltrate in the lamina propria largely consists of neutrophils, macrophages, lymphocytes, and immunoglobulin-producing B-cell blasts and plasma cells. The increase in immunoglobulin-producing cells is usually greater than the increase in T cells and particularly involves cells producing IgG. Increases in IgM cells tend to be more prominent in Crohn's disease than in ulcerative colitis. Changes in IgG and IgA subclasses have also been found including IgG1 cell expansion in ulcerative colitis and IgA1 cell expansion in both disorders, the latter reflecting a systemic type of immune response. There is also evidence for decreased expression of J chain by mucosal B cells and for decreased expression of the secretory piece by surface epithelial cells.

In regard to the expansion of T cells, monoclonal antibodies to CD4 and CD8 have not revealed significant alterations in the proportion of the two subsets, either in the lamina propria or in the epithelium. However, increased numbers of CD4+ T cells express the activation marker IL-2R, particularly in Crohn's disease. The TCR expression of intraepithelial lymphocytes in both Crohn's disease and ulcerative colitis appears to be similar to that in normal colonic epithelium.

Immunopathogenesis

The immunological theory for the pathogenesis of inflammatory bowel disease is only one of a number of hypotheses which have been generated to account for the development of intestinal inflammation. Other hypotheses promote an infective aetiology (particularly for Crohn's disease), submucosal vasculitis with mucosal ischaemia (Crohn's disease) and metabolic hypotheses such as a deficiency in the ability of gut epithelial cells to metabolize luminal nutrients (ulcerative colitis) and the generation of elevated concentrations of bacterial peptides, which stimulate mucosal leucocytes (ulcerative colitis). Additional factors may involve changes in mucous glycoproteins secreted by epithelial cells and susceptibility factors associated with decreased exposure to gastrointestinal pathogens in much of the developed world.

In the immunological hypothesis, intestinal inflammation is viewed as a defect in generating and sustaining mucosal oral tolerance (Fig. 15.5). In contrast to coeliac disease, it is proposed that the antigenic stimuli involve luminal bacteria or their products which are in highest concentration in the distal gastrointestinal tract. In Crohn's disease, the earliest lesion may involve epithelial expression of HLA-DR antigens overlying Peyer's patches and lymphoepithelial follicles followed by aphthous ulceration. This is associated with activation of mucosal lymphocytes as determined by expression of IL-2R and elevated serum concentrations of soluble IL-2R. In ulcerative colitis, the cells responsible for elevated levels of soluble IL-2R appear to be macrophages rather than T cells.

The development of mucosal inflammation may be due to the local production of pro-inflammatory cytokines (IL-1, IL-6, IL-8, TNFα), other mediators [platelet-activating factor, leukotriene (LT) D_4, prostaglandin (PG) E_2] and the phlogistic action of IgG complement-fixing antibodies. There may also be downregulation of the immunosuppressive cytokines, IL-4, IL-10, IL-13, and TGFβ. These events aggravate the inflammatory cell infiltrate which now includes

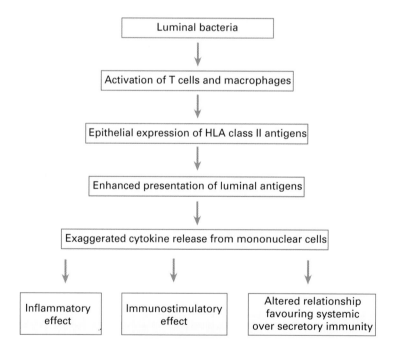

∎ **Fig. 15.5** An immunological hypothesis for the development of inflammatory bowel disease based on the failure of oral tolerance with the development of pathogenic immune responses to luminal bacteria or their products.

lymphocytes, macrophages, mast cells, eosinophils, and neutrophils. Other injurious events then follow which involve proteolytic enzymes, myelo- and eosinophil peroxidases, oxygen radicals, and nitric oxide. In most studies, faecal levels of inflammatory mediators such as leukotrienes and prostaglandins have been higher in ulcerative colitis than in Crohn's disease. Almost all drugs which are effective in inflammatory bowel disease have been shown to modulate immune activity including sulphasalazine (decreases IL-1, IL-8, and TNFα).

As noted above, some differences in humoral immune responses have been demonstrated between ulcerative colitis and Crohn's disease. At a cellular level, immunological events mediated by T lymphocytes appear to be more important in Crohn's disease, while activated macrophages and neutrophils may have a greater part in ulcerative colitis. At a clinical level, complete remission of Crohn's disease has been reported in a patient who became infected by HIV. In animal experiments, an ulcerative colitis-like disease develops in 'knockout mice' which lack particular cytokine genes. While this is understandable for immunosuppressive cytokines such as IL-10 and TGFβ which may mediate oral tolerance, it also occurs in mice lacking IL-2, perhaps supporting the hypothesis that this disease is not mediated by T cells.

Thus far, no hypothesis clearly accounts for the intestinal and extra-intestinal manifestations of inflammatory bowel disease. Furthermore, the initial events leading to intestinal inflammation remain unclear. However, persuasive evidence supports the view for involvement of the immune system in a self-perpetuating cycle which can be influenced by the use of immunosuppressive drugs. Recent reports of clinical responses to anticytokine antibodies raise the possibility of newer forms of immunotherapy which are more specific and effective, perhaps without the side-effects of agents currently in use.

Clinical features

The typical symptoms of ulcerative colitis are those of diarrhoea, rectal bleeding, and abdominal pain. The severity of diarrhoea is largely determined by the extent and severity of inflammation. Some patients with proctitis will have rectal bleeding as the major symptom, while others with limited disease may have diarrhoea plus blood, mucus, and pus as well as the passage of small formed stools. At presentation, 25% of patients will have proctitis or proctosigmoiditis, 50% will have left-sided disease, and 25% will have total colitis.

At sigmoidoscopy, the rectal mucosa has a red 'granular' appearance with prominent contact bleeding. Blood and mucus are usually obvious in the lumen. Superficial ulcers may be present in patients with severe disease while others with long-standing inflammation may have pseudopolyps or rectal narrowing. The extent of disease is normally determined by colonoscopy or barium enema X-ray.

Rare colonic complications include massive haemorrhage, the development of a toxic megacolon (sometimes associated with perforation) and the longer-term risk for development of colon cancer. Although the precise risk of colon cancer is still debated, this risk increases after 10 years of disease and is highest in patients with total colitis. Extra-intestinal manifestations, often associated with active disease, include various forms of arthritis (20%), skin lesions (5%), eye lesions (5%), biliary and hepatic disorders (5%), thromboembolism, and renal calculi.

In Crohn's disease, symptoms vary depending on the site and severity of inflammation. Common symptoms include diarrhoea, abdominal pain, fever, and weight loss. Rectal bleeding is much less common than in ulcerative colitis. Patients with ileal disease may have features of a partial small bowel obstruction or fistula formation or may present with an abdominal mass or abdominal abscess. Features of anorectal Crohn's disease include skin tags, fissures, fistulae, and abscesses.

Diagnosis

The diagnosis of Crohn's disease rests on the demonstration of inflammation in the small or large bowel, sometimes after exclusion of various infectious causes of colitis. Although colonoscopy and the double-contrast barium enema X-ray provide complementary information, colonoscopy permits serial biopsies and is more likely to be diagnostic in mild disease. Colonoscopic features include aphthous ulcers, linear ulcers, skip lesions, contact bleeding, 'cobblestoning', and strictures. Extra-intestinal manifestations are similar to those of ulcerative colitis apart from a lower frequency of hepatic and biliary manifestations such as sclerosing cholangitis.

In both ulcerative colitis and Crohn's disease, anaemia is usually due to blood loss but may be caused by chronic inflammation or by deficiencies of folic acid or vitamin B_{12}. The majority of patients also show elevation of erythrocyte sedimentation rate (ESR) and C-reactive protein. Protein loss from the gastrointestinal tract largely accounts for a depressed serum albumin and may be documented by elevated faecal concentrations of inflammatory proteins such as α_1-

antitrypsin. Colonic inflammation can also be demonstrated by nuclear medicine scans using labelled white blood cells. For research studies in Crohn's disease, attempts to quantitate disease activity have not been entirely satisfactory but range from a simple index of symptoms as proposed by Harvey and Bradshaw to a more complex formula such as the Crohn's disease activity index of the National Cooperative Crohn's Disease Study.

Antibodies and autoantibodies

Both ulcerative colitis and Crohn's disease have been associated with a bewildering array of changes in humoral and cell-mediated immune responses. Several of these changes such as antibodies to food proteins seem likely to be epiphenomenona which reflect enhanced absorption of dietary components as a result of mucosal inflammation. Antibodies to milk proteins have been of interest in light of reports of improvement in ulcerative colitis with a milk-free diet, but no consistent differences in prevalence or titre have been demonstrated in relation to control groups.

Most studies have found that patients with inflammatory bowel disease have a higher prevalence and/or titre of antibodies to a variety of commensal gut bacteria including *Escherichia coli*. Furthermore, cellular hypersensitivity to *E. coli* has been demonstrated in peripheral blood lymphocytes using a leucocyte migration inhibition assay, particularly in patients with ulcerative colitis. The presence of circulating antibodies to a variety of pathogenic micro-organisms including *Campylobacter*, *Yersinia*, and atypical mycobacteria have generally failed to show a convincing association with inflammatory bowel disease. Negative results have also been obtained in Crohn's disease when mycobacterial remnants have been sought by DNA hybridization.

In regard to autoantibodies, both diseases have been associated with raised IgG antibody titres to colon epithelial antigens. This phenomenon is more common in ulcerative colitis where anticolon antibodies cross-react with a bacterial component common to most Enterobacteriaceae. Indeed, anticolon antibodies can be induced in animals by immunization with *E. coli* in adjuvant but such animals do not develop colitis. Another autoantibody is directed against mucopolysaccharide found in goblet cells in both the large and small intestine. Additional autoantibodies are directed against lymphocyte membrane antigens (antilymphocyte antibodies) and against enzymes contained within the cytoplasmic granules of neutrophils (ANCA). Elevated titres of ANCA are more common in ulcerative colitis than in Crohn's disease and may be detected in up to 80% of patients during exacerbations

of inflammation. Autoantibodies associated with established autoimmune disorders appear to have a similar frequency in inflammatory bowel disease to that in the general population. Indeed, coexisting autoimmune disease is rare in Crohn's disease (2%) but somewhat more common in ulcerative colitis (6.6%), particularly thyroid disease, coeliac disease, and autoimmune haemolytic anaemia.

Treatment

The medical treatment of ulcerative colitis and Crohn's disease largely involves corticosteroids, sulphasalazine, and various aminosalicylates. When inflammation involves the distal colon, corticosteroids can be given by suppository, foam, or enema. Sulphasalazine has a particular part in the maintenance of remission of colitis but may be less effective when Crohn's disease involves the small bowel. The demonstration that the active constituent of sulphasalazine was 5-aminosalicylic acid has led to the development of a number of new aminosalicylates including mesalazine and olsalazine. These drugs have not been shown to be superior to sulphasalazine but are free of side-effects associated with the sulphapyridine component of sulphasalazine. Immunosuppressive drugs used in the treatment of patients with difficult or advanced disease include azathioprine, cyclosporin A, and methotrexate. Elemental diets have a part in the management of patients with Crohn's disease but may be ineffective in ulcerative colitis. Surgical treatment becomes necessary in about 80% of patients with Crohn's disease but is much less common in ulcerative colitis.

Further reading

Coeliac disease

Catassi, C., Ratsch, I-M., Fibiani, E., Rossini, M., Bordicchia, F., Candela, F., *et al.* (1994). Coeliac disease in the year 2000: exploring the iceberg. *Lancet*, **343**, 200–3.

Ferguson, A., Arranz, E., and O'Mahony, S. (1993). Clinical and pathological spectrum of coeliac disease — active, silent, latent, potential. *Gut*, **34**, 150–1.

Ferreira, M., Davies, S. L., Butler, M., Scott, D., Clark, M., and Kumar, P. (1992). Endomysial antibody: is it the best screening test for coeliac disease? *Gut*, **33**, 1633–7.

Gjertsen, H. A., Lundin, K. E. A., Sollid, L. M., Eriksen J. A., and Thorsby, E. (1994). T cells recognise a peptide derived from α-gliadin presented by the coeliac disease-associated HLA-DQ ($\alpha1*0501, \beta1*0201$) heterodimer. *Human Immunology*, **39**, 243–52.

Halstensen, T. S., and Brandtzaeg, P. (1993). Activated T lymphocytes in the celiac lesion: non-proliferative activation (CD 25) of CD4+ α/β cells in the lamina propria but proliferation (Ki-67) of α/β and γ/δ cells in the epithelium. *European Journal of Immunology*, **23**, 505–10.

Howdle, P. D. and Blair, G. E. (1992). Molecular biology and coeliac disease. *Gut*, **33**, 573–5.

Kagnoff, M. F. (1993). Immunology of the intestinal tract. *Gastroenterology*, **105**, 1275–80.

Kagnoff, M. F. (1992). Celiac disease. A gastrointestinal disease with environmental, genetic and immunologic components. *Gastroenterology Clinics of North America*, **21**, 405–25.

Marsh, M. N. (1992). Gluten, major histocompatibility complex, and the small intestine. A molecular and immunobiologic approach to the spectrum of gluten sensitivity ('celiac sprue'). *Gastroenterology*, **102**, 330–54.

O'Farrelly, C. and Gallagher, R. B. (1992). Intestinal gluten sensitivity: snapshots of an unusual autoimmune-like disease. *Immunology Today*, **13**, 474–6.

Van Berge-Henegouwen, G. P. and Mulder, C. J. J. (1993). Pioneer in the gluten free diet: Willem–Karel Dicke 1905–1962, over 50 years of gluten free diet. *Gut*, **34**, 1473–5.

Inflammatory bowel disease

Brandtzaeg, P., Halstensen, T. S., Kett, K., Krajci, P., Kvale, D., Rognum, T. O., *et al.* (1989). Immunobiology and immunopathology of human gut mucosa: humoral immunity and intraepithelial lymphocytes. *Gastroenterology*, **97**, 1562–84.

Brandtzaeg, P., Halstensen, T. S., and Kett, K. (1992). Immunopathology of inflammatory bowel disease. In *Inflammatory bowel disease* (ed. R. P. MacDermott and W. F. Stenson), pp. 95–136. Elsevier Science Publishing Co., New York.

Duchmann, R., Kaiser, I., Hermann, E., Mayet, W., Ewe, K., Mayer Zum Büschenfelde, K.-H. (1995). Tolerance exists towards resident intestinal flora but is broken in active inflammatory bowel (IBD). *Clinical and Experimental Immunology*, **102**, 448–55.

Fiocchi, C. (1992). Cytokines. In *Inflammatory bowel disease*, (ed. R. P. MacDermott and W. F. Stenson), pp. 137–62. Elsevier, New York.

Isaacs, K. L., Sartor, R. B., and Haskill, S. (1992). Cytokine messenter RNA profiles in inflammatory bowel disease mucosa detected by polymerase chain reaction amplification. *Gastroenterology*, **103**, 1587–95.

James, S. P. (1988). Cellular immune mechanisms in the pathogenesis of Crohn's disease. *In Vivo*, **2**, 1–8.

Jewell, D. P. and Snook, J. A. (1990). Immunology of ulcerative colitis and Crohn's disease. In *Inflammatory bowel diseases*, (ed. R. N. Allan, M. R. B. Keighley, J. Alexander- Williams, and C. Hawkins), pp. 127–46. Churchill Livingstone, Edinburgh.

MacDermott, R. P. and Stenson, W. A. (1988). Alterations of the immune system in ulcerative colitis and Crohn's disease. *Advances in Immunology*, **42**, 285–322.

Matsuura, T., West, G. A., Youngman, K. R., Klein, J. S., and Fiocchi, C. (1993). Immune activation genes in inflammatory bowel disease. *Gastroenterology*, **104**, 448–58.

Meucci, G., Vecchi, M., Torgano, G., Arrigoni, M., Prada, A., Rocca, F., *et al.* (1992). Familial aggregation of inflammatory bowel disease in Northern Italy: a multicentre study. *Gastroenterology*, **103**, 514–19.

Toyoda, H., Wang, S-J., Yang, H-Y., Redford, A., Magalong, D., Tyan, D., *et al.* (1993). Distinct associations of HLA class II genes with inflammatory bowel disease. *Gastroenterology*, **104**, 741–8.

16 Liver

R. Ghalib and M. Peters

Introduction

Autoimmune diseases of the liver are uncommon. However, there are a number of distinct autoimmune diseases that predominantly affect the liver, and non-autoimmune diseases of the liver may have immunological manifestations. The symptoms of many chronic liver diseases may be identical and a detailed history and physical examination are critical to making an accurate diagnosis. Thus, it is essential to understand the subtle distinguishing features between the various aetiologies of chronic liver diseases and the use of serological and immunological testing. This chapter will describe the specific autoimmune diseases and then the immunological manifestations of more common liver diseases.

Autoimmune chronic active hepatitis

Introduction

Idiopathic autoimmune chronic active hepatitis (AICAH) is a rare clinical syndrome with an unknown aetiology, characterized by a number of immunological phenomena. There are three types of AICAH characterized by the presence of certain autoantibodies.

1. *Type I* has a bimodal age distribution: ages 10–30 and ages 50–70 years.
2. *Type II* occurs in younger children, although it can be seen in women over 40 years.
3. *Type III* is seen in older women. Approximately 75% of all patients are females. The younger peak appears to be decreasing and the older increasing.

Pathology

Histological findings on liver biopsy include a variable degree of portal fibrosis with increased lymphocytes and plasma cell infiltration, piecemeal necrosis, and chronic aggressive hepatitis. Lobular injury is patchy and therefore sampling error may occur.

Immunological response

Patients with AICAH are characterized by markedly elevated levels of serum immunoglobulin (Ig) G (90%). The autoantibodies present differ between the types of AICAH (Table 16.1) and include antinuclear antibody (ANA), antibody to soluble liver antigen (SLA), antiliver–kidney microsomal (LKM) antibody and smooth muscle antibody (SMA).

1. *Type I or classical AICAH* is characterized by the presence of smooth muscle or antinuclear antibodies, hypergammaglobulinaemia (IgG), associated autoimmune disorders, and an increased incidence of human leucocyte antigen (HLA) A1-B8-DR3.
2. *Type II (anti-LKM1)* is characterized by the presence of antibodies to liver/kidney microsomes, an antibody which is directed against cytochrome P450 IID6.
3. *Type III* is characterized by the presence of antibodies to soluble liver antigen, which are probably directed against cytokeratin.

Other immune abnormalities include alterations in the number and ratio of CD4+ and CD8+ T cells. In contrast to patients with primary biliary cirrhosis and hepatitis B, patients with AICAH do not have abnormal complement activation. Increased antibodies to certain viruses such as measles and rubella and bacteria such as *Escherichia coli* and *Salmonella* has been noted especially in type I, suggesting molecular mimicry as a pathogenic factor. Patients with hypergammaglobulinaemia may have falsely positive antibody test to hepatitis C (HCV). This can be excluded by confirmatory testing such as recombinant immunoblot assay (RIBA) II or HCV RNA. While the two diseases are not generally linked, in some regions of the world (Italy), patients with AICAH frequently have associated HCV.

Clinical features

Patients may present with malaise, anorexia, fever, jaundice, hepatomegaly, and even ascites. Other autoimmune diseases may be associated with this entity including inflammatory bowel disease, rheumatoid arthritis, or thyroid disease. Younger patients may appear to have acute hepatitis, but 50% already have cirrhosis at presentation.

Treatment and prognosis

There are excellent long-term studies proving the value of prednisone and azathioprine in treatment of AICAH. Spontaneous resolution rarely occurs. The combination of prednisone and azathioprine leads to remission in 70% of patients at 2 years. However, relapse is common and most patients should be maintained on low-dose immunosuppression (azathioprine alone or in combination with low-dose prednisone). Prednisone alone is effective, especially if used in high doses but the side-effects are more frequent. Other immunosuppressives have been used (cyclosporin and FK506) with some success but there are limited data available as yet.

Poor prognostic indicators include aspartate aminotransferase (AST) more than five to 10 times normal; the histological features of bridging fibrosis, cirrhosis, or multilobular necrosis; and clinical features of ascites, encephalopathy, varices, or associated ulcerative colitis. However, with appropriate therapy many patients may have a near-normal lifespan. Liver transplantation is an option in severely symptomatic patients, those who fail to respond to immunosuppression, or have life-threatening complications not amenable to other therapy. Hepatocellular carcinoma is rare.

Primary biliary cirrhosis

Introduction

Primary biliary cirrhosis (PBC) is a progressive cholestatic disease of unknown aetiology. More than 95% of the patients are females. The peak age for presentation (40–60 years) is decreasing, as many asymptomatic patients with elevated serum alkaline phosphatase are being found with the increased use of automated blood testing.

Pathology

There is a progressive destruction of bile ducts by lymphocytes and macrophages, and formation of granuloma. The lymphocytes are mainly CD4+ T cells in the centre of the portal tracts, and CD8+ T cells near the damaged bile ducts and in areas of piecemeal necrosis. B cells are less frequent but IgM producing cells are found in the inflammatory infiltrate around bile ducts.

Histopathological findings on liver biopsy have been classified into four stages:

(1) 'florid bile duct lesion' of interlobular bile ducts with lymphocytic and plasma cell infiltrate;

(2) biliary fibrosis with atypical duct proliferation;

(3) biliary fibrosis with decrease in ducts; and

(4) biliary cirrhosis with loss of small to medium size bile ducts.

Major histocompatibility complex (MHC) class II is not expressed on normal bile duct epithelium. However, in PBC damaged ducts and adjoining apparently normal ducts express MHC class I and II. The cause of bile duct damage is not clear but the increased expression of MHC may serve as means of antigen presentation, and provide a target for the immune response.

Immunological response

Serum IgM is particularly elevated relative to the other immunoglobulins and is a characteristic feature for PBC which may differentiate it from other chronic liver disorders. *The antimitochondrial antibody (AMA) is found in more than 95% of the patients, and its absence virtually excludes the diagnosis.* The titre of this antibody does not correlate with disease severity. AMA lacks diagnostic specificity as it is also found in non-hepatic disease such as syphilis, myocarditis, drug-induced disorders, and other autoimmune disorders. Several mitochondrial antigens have been identified as targets. Antibodies against the E2 component and protein X, which is a polypeptide that is tightly bound to E2, are specific for PBC. The E2 component of the mammalian pyruvate dehydrogenase complex (PDH), is one of three related multienzyme complexes located in the inner mitochondrial membrane. The other two are 2-oxyglutarate dehydrogenase complex and branched chain 2-oxo acid dehydrogenase complex.

Other autoantibodies such as ANA and rheumatoid factor may be positive in PBC. An elevation of the erythrocyte sedimentation rate (ESR) is noted in most patients. Complement activation occurs in PBC. Other immune abnormalities in PBC include diminished T-cell responsiveness. Whether these abnormalities are

Table 16.1 Comparison of autoimmune liver diseases with other liver diseases

CAH	AICAH Type I	AICAH Type II	AICAH Type III	PBC	Viral hepatitis	Alcoholic liver disease
Other autoimmune diseases	+(10%)	+(17%)	<10%	+(28%)	60%	none
Serum Ig elevated	IgG	IgG	IgG	IgM	IgG	IgA
ANA	+(33%)	+(2%)	0	±	30% low titre	<5%
SMA	+(100%)	0	30	±	+ low titre	low titre
AMA	+(8%)	0	22	>90%	–	–
Anti-LKM	0	+(100%)	0	–	+	–
SLA	0	0	+(100%)	–	–	–
Antigen	actin	P450dbl (IID6)	cytokeratin 8/18	PDH	HCV	–
HCV RNA positive	–[a]	–	–	–	100	50%

[a] In some countries (e.g. Italy) older patients with classical AICAH have a high incidence of HCV positively. Otherwise patients are HCV negative. PDH, pyruvate dehydrogenase complex, SLA, soluble liver antigen.

responsible for the bile duct damage or secondary phenomena, is not clear.

Circulating immune complexes have been detected and complement activation is suggested by increased catabolism and synthesis of C1q and C3

Clinical features

The disease may be asymptomatic for several years. The most common symptoms at presentation are fatigue and pruritus. The development of jaundice is usually a late feature and is a bad prognostic sign as the median 10 year survival is about 50%. Because serum cholesterol is usually elevated in these patients, they may have xanthelasma, especially periorbital. Other autoimmune disorders that may be associated with PBC are keratoconjunctivitis sicca (Sjögren's syndrome), seronegative arthritis, scleroderma, and autoimmune thyroiditis. The CREST syndrome is seen in some patients: *c*alcinosis, *R*aynaud's phenomenon, o*e*sophageal dysmotility, *s*clerodactyly, and *t*elangiectasia.

Treatment and prognosis

Multiple therapies have been tried for PBC in the past without significant success, and no treatment has been shown conclusively to stop the progression of the disease. However, ursodeoxycholic acid therapy has recently been shown to improve the clinical (fatigue and pruritus) and chemical parameters in PBC after 6 months of therapy. The earlier stages of PBC appear to respond best. Histological improvement has not definitively been shown. Other immunosuppressive drugs (e.g. methotrexate) may be of use and are being studied at this time. As PBC is a disease that progresses slowly and variably over decades, it has been difficult to assess long-term outcome and clinicians have wisely avoided drugs with serious side-effects. Ursodeoxycholic acid has very few side-effects, none of which are life-threatening and is thus an ideal drug for long-term use.

Primary sclerosing cholangitis

Introduction

Primary sclerosing cholangitis (PSC) is a progressive disease of unknown aetiology, characterized by inflammation and fibrosis of both intra- and extra-hepatic bile ducts. The disease is more common in males under 50 years of age. It is associated with ulcerative colitis (UC) in 75% of the cases.

Pathology

Prominent periductal fibrosis, focal necrosis of ductal epithelium, and increased lymphocytic infiltration surrounding or infiltrating the ducts may be noted on liver biopsy. However, liver biopsy is frequently non-diagnostic. The cholangiographic appearance in PSC is characteristic and reveals multiple strictures resulting in a 'beaded' appearance to the intra- and extrahepatic bile ducts. Eventually, significant narrowing and obliteration of ductal lumina develop with progression to biliary cirrhosis.

Immunological aspects

Hypergammaglobulinaemia is noted in patients with PSC but is less pronounced than that seen in PBC. Autoantibodies are uncommon: antimitochondrial, antinuclear, and antismooth muscle antibodies are positive in less than 10% of patients. Anti neutrophil nuclear antibody has been detected in patients with PSC and inflammatory bowel disease and has been studied as a diagnostic marker for PSC. Recently, models of PSC have been developed in mice with increased CD8+ lymphocytes in the liver. This model may help elucidate the immunological associations and mechanisms of PSC. HLA-B8-DR3 is present in approximately 60% of patients with PSC. Other factors implicated in the pathogenesis of PSC include: portal bacteria, increased absorption of toxins in patients with UC, viral infection, and vascular injury.

Clinical features

The symptoms are similar to other cholestatic disease including pruritus, jaundice, and fatigue. As with PBC, it is a variably progressive disease. Unlike PBC, patients may have recurrent episodes of cholangitis from biliary obstruction and present with fever and abdominal pain. There is a 14% risk of cholangiocarcinoma in patients with PSC.

Treatment and prognosis

The survival of patients with PSC once they are symptomatic is variable. Seventy-five per cent of patients progress to cirrhosis within 5 years after diagnosis. A number of therapeutic modalities have been tried in PSC without significant success in retarding the progression of the disease. These modalities include: bile duct surgery, biliary drainage, colectomy in patients with UC, and immunosuppressive agents. Orthotopic liver transplantation is an option for patients with PSC who have recurrent cholangitis or end-stage liver disease.

Viral hepatitides

Introduction

Acute and chronic hepatitides are diagnosed by the presence of specific antibodies to viral proteins. The prodrome of acute hepatitis may include immune complex deposition with arthritis and glomerulonephritis (GN). The majority (>85%) of all viral hepatitides are inapparent, anicteric infections. A small percentage of cases present as fulminant hepatic failure (<1%) and the degree of chronicity differs between viruses.

After viral infection of the host, there can be various cellular responses with an equilibrium between the host and the virus. The amount of cellular injury thus depends upon the viral load, the rate of viral multiplication, and the host's response to the virus. If a virus is cytopathic, it will destroy the cell in which it resides, leading to cell death. This scenario is rarely seen with hepatotrophic viruses but can be seen in fulminant hepatic failure. In these latter cases, when the host recovers or is transplanted, there is a low chance of viral reinfection because the virus has been eliminated. Hepatitis B virus (HBV) does not appear to be cytopathic; viral particles are noted in the serum during the prodrome of hepatitis at the same time as there are normal liver enzymes, immunocompromised individuals (transplant and chemotherapy patients and neonates) have normal enzymes with virus present in serum and liver. HCV also has a carrier state and cellular damage occurs with significant inflammatory infiltrate. There is some evidence for cytopathic effect; when interferon (IFN) decreases the viral load, enzymes often normalize. However, the pathology and presence of cryoglobulins, autoantibodies, and lymphocyte responses suggest an immunological response to the virus. For hepatocytes extensive cytopathic damage causes fulminant hepatic failure. The virus may pass to other cells or itself be destroyed. It is unclear why some individuals clear the virus from their liver with minimal damage and a strong antibody response while others are unable to produce neutralizing antibody and continue to harbour virus within their hepatocytes. Fulminant hepatic failure may result from powerful immune responses with lysis of all virally infected hepatocytes. If individuals survive fulminant hepatitis B, they do not usually develop chronic disease.

Hepatitis A

Introduction

The hepatitis A virus (HAV) is a small RNA virus in the picornavirus family, classified as enterovirus no. 72. Only one serological type has been identified despite the existence of multiple strains. Transmission occurs via the faecal–oral route. After experimental infection of apes with HAV the antigen appears in the faeces 3–5 weeks later. The incidence of HAV is decreasing worldwide, possibly due to an improvement in living conditions. Control is mainly dependent on good standards of personal hygeine and sewage control. The infection is common in childhood in underdeveloped countries, with the majority of indi-

∎ **Table 16.2**   The hepatitis viruses

Name	Virus family	Particles, shape	Virion size (nm)	Nucleic acid	Nucleotide
Hepatitis A virus	Picornavirus	Naked, spherical, icosahedral	–27	Linear, single-stranded RNA Does not integrate	7480
Hepatitis B virus	Hepadnavirus ('para-retrovirus')	Spherical	42	Circular, partially double-stranded, small portion triple-stranded DNA, RNA	3200
Hepatitis C virus	Flavivirus, pestivirus	Spherical	55	Positive strand RNA immediate Does not integrate	9500
Hepatitis D virus	Plant viroid, virusoids or plant satellite RNA (?)	Spherical, covered with hepatitis B surface antigen	36 (some 40)	Single-stranded circular RNA	~1700
Hepatitis E virus	Calicivirus	Spherical, non-enveloped	32–34	Single-stranded, polyadenylated RNA	~7500

viduals immune by middle age. Infection is usually inapparent, self-limiting, and anicteric, with an overall mortality of 0.01%. It is generally milder in children, with individuals over 40 years of age at greater risk of severe disease.

Pathology

The morphological features on liver biopsy are similar to those of other forms of acute viral hepatitis including ballooning degeneration of hepatocytes, focal inflammation, and Kupffer cell hyperplasia. These changes are noted to be more prominent in the periportal areas in HAV hepatitis compared with hepatitis B.

Immunological response

Radioimmunoassay (RIA) methods and enzyme-linked immunoassay (EIA) are used to measure serum IgG, IgM, and IgA, all of which are elevated in acute HAV (Fig. 16.1). IgM to HAV (IgM anti-HAV) is detected at the onset of symptoms and persists for several months. It is used to diagnose current or recent infection, i.e. <6 months. IgG anti-HAV is also detected at the onset of symptoms, but persists for life. Its presence indicates current or previous infection and provides immunity against reinfection. Both IgG and IgM are secreted in saliva. HAV antigen detection in the stool occurs early in infection and persists for 2 weeks. HAV RNA can be detected in the stools, liver, and serum of patients by the use of hybridization or polymerase chain reaction (PCR) methods. Antibodies against the non-structural domain of the viral polypeptide can be detected in the sera of infected patients early after the increase in alanine aminotransferase (ALT) and remain elevated for 1 year in humans. However, they remain as research tools at the present. Their clinical role in immunity to HAV remains unclear. The pathogenesis of the hepatocellular damage in acute hepatitis A infection remains controversial. It is evident that the virus replicates inside the hepatocytes prior to the symptomatic period and this is followed by the development of immunoglobulins and the acute illness. These observations suggest that the virus is cytopathic and the immune response is secondary to the liver damage. However, hepatocyte necrosis is mainly periportal with predominance of lymphocytes suggesting an immune-mediated hepatolysis. Antibodies to liver cell membrane antibodies (e.g. liver-specific lipoprotein: LSP) are reported in acute HAV infection. However, they are not specific for hepatitis A.

Clinical features

The incubation period is variable ranging 10–50 days and may be followed by clinical findings of acute viral hepatitis, i.e. fever, malaise, nausea, vomiting, dark urine, and abdominal pain. As noted above, many

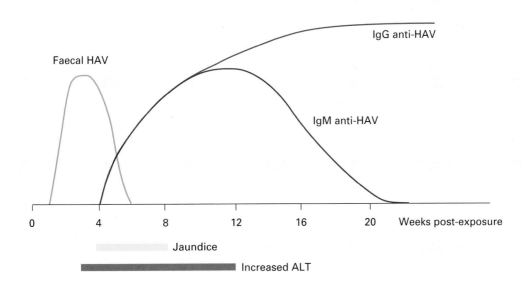

▌**Fig. 16.1** Immunological response with time in hepatitis A. Clinical features include jaundice and elevations in serum aminotransferases (ALT). Laboratory response indicates presence of faecal hepatitis A virus (HAV), serum antibody to HAV, both IgM and IgG.

▮ **Table 16.3**   Modes of transmission of the hepatitis viruses

Name	Method of transmission	Form of hepatitis
Hepatitis A virus (HAV)	Faecal–oral, enteric, water-borne	Acute
Hepatitis B virus (HBV)	Blood-borne, venereal, mother to child transfusion, needle injection, parenteral	Acute, chronic, carrier, primary cancer of the liver
Hepatitis C virus	Blood-borne, parenteral	As HBV
Hepatitis D virus	Same as HBV	Chronic, carrier-associated after HBV infection
Hepatitis E virus	Same as HAV	Acute, high mortality in pregnant women

patients will have a 'flu'-like illness with some diarrhoea and their hepatitis will go unrecognized. Diarrhoea is a prominent feature in hepatitis A when compared with the other forms of hepatitis. Serum transaminases peak prior to onset of jaundice. Most patients make a full recovery usually within 3–4 weeks. Rarely longer symptomatic periods up to 6 months have been reported, but chronic disease never occurs.

Treatment and prophylaxis

There is no specific treatment for hepatitis A. Passive immunization of exposed individuals with pooled human immune serum immunoglobulins provides a high degree of protection (up to 90%) against acute HAV. In some cases, the prophylaxis is followed by a mild clinical infection. Preexposure prophylaxis or immunization is recommended for travellers to areas where hepatitis A is epidemic. For post-exposure prophylaxis, the sooner the prophylaxis is used after exposure the more likely for it to be protective. Active immunization for HAV with a formalin-inactivated vaccine is now available. This induces antibodies in 95% after one dose, and 99% after two doses.

Hepatitis E virus

The hepatitis E virus (HEV) is a single-stranded polyadenylated RNA virus whose genome is 7.5 kb. The virus has a diameter of 32–34 nm. It is similar to HAV in most respects: transmission is faecal–oral; occurs most frequently in epidemic outbreaks in developing countries, particularly in Asia and North Africa; and it never causes chronic disease. The most notable distinguishing features of this virus are:

(1) that although the mortality rate is low in the general population (0.5–3%) it has a high mortality in pregnant women (up to 30%), especially in the third trimester; and

(2) its low secondary attack rate in household contacts.

The prevalence of anti-HEV antibodies varies greatly in different countries: Europe, 2–3%; Spain, 6.8%; Thailand, 70%.

Hepatitis B

Introduction

Approximately 5% of the world's population is infected with HBV which can cause a necro-inflammatory disease of variable duration and severity. Immune responses are responsible for both the clearance of HBV and the disease pathogenesis. Chronic infection with HBV and hepatocellular inflammation may lead to cirrhosis and hepatocellular carcinoma (HCC). A large proportion of the population of Asia and Africa suffer and die from the complications of HBV infection.

HBV is a 42 nm double-stranded DNA virus in the Hepadnaviridae family. It consists an inner core and an outer envelope. The core particle (HBcAg) contains the circular double stranded DNA and DNA polymerase. The outer envelope consists of 22 nm spheres and tubules, known as the hepatitis B surface antigen (HBsAg, initially called the Australia antigen). HBsAg is produced in excess in the hepatocyte, explaining the abundance of 22 nm particles in the serum compared to Dane particles (whole virus). HBeAg is a 'surrogate' marker of viral replication; when present in the serum it reflects viral replication in the liver. HBeAg is an alternatively spliced product of the core gene, 5′ to the start site of core protein replication. When active viral replication is occurring, HBeAg will be made with a signal peptide that allows export through the endoplasmic reticulum and HBcAg is produced which is incorporated into virions. A mutation in the core gene between the two start sites (3′ to HBeAg and 5′ to HBcAg) results in active viral replication but no serum HBeAg. These mutations are clinically relevant because patients may have active viral replication with hepatocellular damage but be seronegative for HBeAg. These patients may also respond to therapy.

HBV is one of the most widespread worldwide infections and has a high prevalence in developing countries. It may be found in all body fluids including serum, saliva, semen, breast milk, but not stool. Transmission is parenteral by blood products, surgical procedures, or contaminated needles, and by sexual contact.

Pathology

Elimination of HBV is due to cytolysis of infected hepatocytes by cytotoxic T cells and removal of infective virus and antibody neutralizes extracellular virus and viral particles thus preventing the spread of infection. The histopathological findings on liver biopsy in acute hepatitis due to HBV are similar to those of acute hepatitis A. In chronic hepatitis B infection, the findings are more variable ranging from normal liver to focal areas of hepatocyte necrosis to disruption of the limiting plate between the portal tracts and parenchyma. Diagnosis relies upon finding HBsAg in the cytoplasm (ground glass cells) and HBcAg in the nucleus. HCC may develop decades after initial infection. HBV has been shown to be incorporated in the host genome. Tumorigenesis may result from induction of oncogenes, an effect on tumour repressors or via the integration into the host genome.

Immunological response

The humoral immune response in hepatitis B is well characterized (Fig. 16.2). The diagnosis of acute hepatitis B is made by detecting IgM anti-HBc which is present in acute infection for 6 months but may recur in lower titres during chronic hepatitis B. The presence of HBeAg indicates viral replication as noted above and most patients with HBeAg in their serum have active hepatocellular damage. HBeAg and anti-HBeAg form immune complexes and thus what is noted in the serum depends upon whether there is antigen or antibody excess. However, the presence of anti-HBe usually indicates loss of viral replication and normalization of aminotransferases. The presence of anti-HBs usually indicates loss of viral replication recovery and immunity against reinfection. In a small percentage of patients with chronic liver disease, non-neutralizing anti-HBs may be present. Serum HBV DNA measured by hybridization is a more direct measure of infection in acute or chronic hepatitis B with active liver disease. HBV DNA by PCR technique is very sensitive and may remain positive for many years after normalization of liver enzymes and loss of other markers of viral replication.

Antiviral cytotoxic T lymphocytes (CTL) are thought to eradicate infection by identifying and killing virally infected cells by recognizing viral pep-

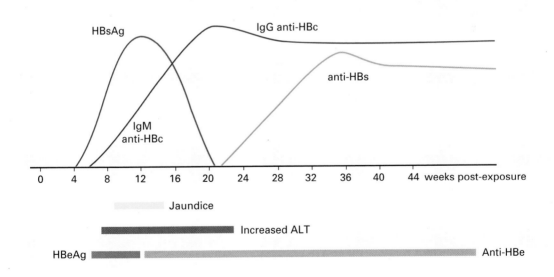

▮ **Fig. 16.2** Immunological response with time in hepatitis B. Clinical features include jaundice and elevations in serum aminotransferases (ALT). Laboratory response indicates presence of hepatitis B surface and e antigen (HBsAg, HBeAg), serum antibodies to HBcAg (anti-HBc) both IgM and IgG, and antibodies to HBsAg (anti-HBs) and HBeAg (anti-HBe).

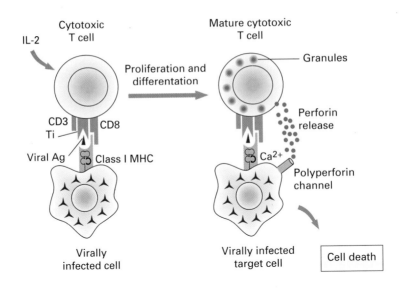

❚ **Fig. 16.3** The role of cytotoxic T cells in removing virally infected T cells. MHC, major histocompatibility complex; Ag, antigen.

tides synthesized in the infected cells and presented by HLA class I molecules. Patients who successfully control HBV during an acute viral hepatitis develop strong, polyclonal, multispecific HLA class I and class II restricted T-cell responses to many antigens of HBV. The virus is eliminated by several pathways:

(1) killing of HBV-infected cells by CD8+ CTL;

(2) elimination of virus from within the cell without killing the cell by the action of cytokines which inhibit gene expression and viral replication by destabilizing viral RNA;

(3) recruitment of non-specific cells, e.g. macrophages which amplify the cytopathic process.

In chronic disease low serum levels of IFNα and-β occur together with reduced MHC class II expression. The response of HBV-specific CD8 T cells to envelope, polymerase, and nucleocapsid antigens is weak and restricted or negative compared with that from patients with acute HBV hepatitis who clear the infection. This and the positive effect with IFNα suggests that the failure to eradicate virally infected cells is a major factor in the genesis of the chronic state, and emphasizes the importance of T-cell immunity and cytotoxicity in control of the disease process. Other factors may be anti-idiotypic antibodies, reduced antibody production and suppressed or altered T-cell responses, e.g. Th2 instead of Th1 cell responses. Recent studies have demonstrated the importance of altered viral peptides which bind the T cell receptor

but do not activate the cell, leading to continued HBV infection.

Clinical features

Acute hepatitis B infection may result in subclinical hepatitis, acute hepatitis with complete recovery, subacute hepatic necrosis, or fulminant hepatitis. During the prodromal phase arthralgias, fever, and vasculitis may occur. In the majority of cases the liver recovers completely.

Chronicity depends upon age of acquisition of HBV infection: neonates who acquire HBV from their mother perinatally have >95% chance of developing chronic infection; children between 40 and 80%, but less than 10% of adults cases progress to chronic infection. Chronic infection present a continuum from a carrier state with normal liver histology to chronic hepatitis and cirrhosis. Patients may fluctuate back and forth from normal histology to mild or severe chronic hepatitis. The risk of HCC is 100 times greater in chronic HBV infection.

Extrahepatic manifestations of hepatitis B are seen in 10–20% of patients. These include a serum sickness-like syndrome, polyarteritis nodosa, membranoproliferative GN, and essential mixed cryoglobulinaemia. All except mixed cryoglobulinaemia are more common in HBV than HCV infection, and will be discussed here.

Serum sickness-like syndrome presents as fever, rash, and polyarthritis. It is a type 3 hypersensitivity reaction (Arthus) secondary to immune complex formation and complement activation. HBsAg has been detected in synovial membrane and fluid. It is seen in the prodrome of acute infection and symptoms subside rapidly after the onset of jaundice.

Polyarteritis nodosa is a multisystem necrotizing vasculitis affecting small and medium-sized arteries especially of the kidney, musculoskeletal system, liver, and gastrointestinal tract. Thirty per cent of patients with polyarteritis nodosa have associated HBV infection. Immune complexes involving HBsAg have been found in serum and involved tissue.

Membranous GN can be associated with HBV infection especially in children who are HBeAg positive. Immune complexes of HBsAg, HBeAg, and HBcAg and their respective antibodies are found in glomerular and capillary basement membranes. Treatment of these immunological manifestations has included classical immunosuppressives (prednisone, azathioprine, and cyclophosphamide) as well as IFN therapy. Corticosteroids increase HBV replication and is usually avoided in these patients. IFN therapy has led to remission in some patients, the prognosis being better in children than adults.

Prevention and therapy

Active immunization with the hepatitis B vaccine is proven to be safe and effective. Vaccination is now recommended, not only high-risk groups such as health care workers and dialysis patients, but for all individuals. Passive prophylaxis with hepatitis B immune globulin (HBIG) is indicated if viral inoculation has occurred via parenteral, eye, or wound exposure.

There is no effective therapy for acute hepatitis B.

1. *Corticosteroids.* These should be avoided as they increase viral replication and serum transaminases may rebound markedly after withdrawal of therapy. Fulminant failure and death has resulted from use of steroids in patients with HBV infection. In some patients with mild serum aminotransferases and active viral replication, steroids have been used prior to IFN therapy to 'prime' the response. This should only be done by the specialist with great care.

2. *Alpha interferon (IFNα)* In chronic hepatitis B this leads to loss of viral replication in 50–60% of patients. Long-term follow up of these patients reveals increasing normalization of serum aminotransferases, loss of viral markers, and even acquisition of antibody to HBs. Why patients clear virus months or years after IFN therapy is unknown. One hypothesis is that there is a continuing balance between viral replication and host response to the virus. If the host response predominates then T-cell-mediated lysis of virally infected hepatocytes will occur, with clearance of virus from the host. If viral replication predominates then chronicity continues. Those most likely to respond to IFN therapy are females with short duration of disease, low levels of HBV DNA, and high aminotransferases. In countries such as Japan where liver transplantation is not readily available intractable forms of hepatitis have been treated medically with combinations of IFNα with cyclosporin A.

3. *Liver transplantation* for hepatitis B has been associated with relatively poor results because of the high incidence of hepatitis B recurrence post-transplantation. Long-term HBIG therapy has drastically reduced recurrence of HBV post-transplantation.

Hepatitis D

The hepatitis delta virus (HDV) is a small negative-stranded defective (incomplete) RNA virus, which is 36 nm in diameter. HDV only occurs in patients who are infected with hepatitis B because it requires HBsAg for its protein coat. It causes severe acute liver disease and rapid progression to liver cirrhosis. Both EIA and RIA tests for anti-HDV are available. IgM anti-HDV tests are available in Europe. The standard for establishing the diagnosis of chronic δ hepatitis is the detection of HDV antigen in the nuclei of hepatocytes using immunofluorescence and immunoperoxidase techniques.

Hepatitis C

Introduction

HCV was identified in 1988 solely by molecular techniques using sera from non-A, non-B post-transfusion hepatitis to screen a cDNA library prepared from plasma of chimpanzees infected with non-A, non-B hepatitis. It is a single-strand-positive sense RNA virus of 9.4 kb which is responsible for most cases of non-A, non-B hepatitis. The genome has been fully sequenced and contains a single open reading frame which is flanked by untranslated regions at the 5′ and 3′ ends. The open reading frame encodes a large protein which is cleaved into three putative structural proteins: capsid (C), envelope 1 (E1), and envelope 2 (E2). There appear to be six non-structural proteins: NS 2, NS 3, NS 4a, NS 4b, NS 5a, and NS 5b. Like other members of the Flaviviridae, the non-structural proteins are likely to be involved in viral replication.

There is variability in the genomic sequence among different HCV isolates. An international panel has proposed a nomenclature in which the genotypes are designated 1–6 with subtypes a, b, c, etc. There is marked variation in the genotype distribution in different countries:

(1) Scotland (type 1=50%; 2=14%; 3=39%);

(2) Hong Kong (type 1=59%, 2=3% 6=32%);

(3) Egypt (types 1, 2, 3 =0%, 4=90%);

(4) Australia (type 1=50%, 2=13%, 3=33%).

Hepatitis C can be transmitted parenterally with the highest incidence in intravenous drug users, transfused individuals, health care workers, and tattoos. While there is no clear evidence regarding other modes of transmission, it has been found in families and sexual partners, suggesting a low incidence of transmission via intimate contact. Vertical transmission can occur but is uncommon. Occupational exposure has been reported and in a survey 1.75% of New York dentists were HCV positive compared with 9.3% oral surgeons and 0.14% controls. Transmission between patients who had minor surgery has also been reported. Of those with HCV 40% have no known risk factors.

Of patients with acute hepatitis C 50–90% will develop chronic liver disease. In follow-up studies of non-A, non-B transfusion hepatitis about 20% developed cirrhosis within a 10–20 year period.

There is evidence linking chronic HCV infection with the development of HCC. In HCC in Japan, Africa, and Italy 60–80% are HCV antibody positive. In prospective studies of HCV-associated cirrhosis in Japan HCC developed in 10% within 3 years, 20% by 5 years, ~50% by 10 years. However, the contribution of other factors such as smoking, HBV, aflatoxin, and alcohol is not clear.

Clinical features

The acute phase of HCV infection is usually asymptomatic and anicteric, but the transaminase level may fluctuate. HCV RNA can be detected in the serum by PCR within 1–2 weeks of inoculation. About 12 weeks after infection antibodies can be detected. In some the infection may be eliminated, antibody disappears, and there is no long-term problem. However, the majority (90%) fail to clear the virus and develop chronic infection. These may have normal or mildly elevated transaminases and by 6 months the changes of chronic hepatitis may be present.

Essential mixed cryglobulinaemia (EMC) is a vasculitic syndrome presenting as purpura, arthralgias, neuralgia, and GN. The diagnosis is made by finding serum cryoglobulins which may consist of polyclonal IgG, monoclonal IgM, and complement in cutaneous and renal lesions. Ninety per cent of patients with mixed cryoglobulinaemia have HCV and anti-HCV,

but <5% have HBV, in their cryoglobulins. It was only recently that the link between hepatitis C and cryoglobulinaemia was detected. Treatment of the hepatitis C with IFN clears the cryoglobulins and improves non-renal symptomatology.

Membranoproliferative GN is also seen in HCV-positive patients in association with cryoglobulins and is less responsive to IFN therapy.

Porphyria cutanea tarda (PCT) frequently is associated with hepatitis C. The association of alcohol with hepatitis C is common (50%) as is alcohol with PCT. In addition, PCT is associated with iron overload and phlebotomy is the treatment of choice. Iron overload can be noted in hepatitis C, independent of PCT, and studies of the value of phlebotomy in the treatment of hepatitis C are underway.

Immunological response

Anti-HCV is not useful in early diagnosis of acute hepatitis C as only 40% of patients are seropositive and it may not become positive until a year after initial infection. Anti-HCV persists in patients who develop chronic hepatitis. The HCV antibody test is an ELISA (enzyme-linked immunosorbent assay) RIBA can be used as a confirmatory test and results are expressed as 1–4+ positive antibodies to four different HCV antigens, including core, envelope, and non-structural proteins. Active research on antibodies useful in indicating acute disease is underway. HCV RNA may be detected by PCR in the serum and liver of patients with acute and chronic hepatitis C. It is very sensitive but also expensive and labour intensive. However, it is presently the best means for semiquantitative levels of viral genome.

Prevention and therapy

No vaccine is available for hepatitis C. IFNα therapy for hepatitis C results in decreased ALT and HCV RNA in 60% of patients with chronic liver disease. The standard dose for HCV at present is 3 million units three times per week for 12 months. However, most patients (60–90%) relapse after discontinuing treatment. The long-term response therefore is about 20–25%. Those most likely to respond to treatment have low levels of virus, high aminotransferases, and early histological disease (no cirrhosis). Studies of various long-term treatments and other antivirals are being actively pursued. Patients with established cirrhosis have a poor response to IFN. Liver transplantation for end-stage liver disease secondary to hepatitis C is associated with better results than hepatitis B. Despite documented serological and histological recurrence of HCV post-transplantation, graft failure secondary to HCV is uncommon.

Alcoholic-induced liver disease

Introduction

Alcohol liver disease is common. In the UK half the cases of cirrhosis are due to alcohol abuse. Alcohol does not appear to be a direct hepatotoxin. Only a minority of chronic alcoholics develop cirrhosis and there is no direct correlation between amount of alcohol ingested and severity of disease. Elegant studies of differences in isoenzymes reveal that there are genetic as well as environmental factors important in the incidence of alcoholic liver disease. There are also host response differences with some individuals developing fatty liver while others develop alcoholic hepatitis or cirrhosis. It should rarely be a problem to distinguish alcoholic liver disease from other liver diseases. Progression to hepatitis and cirrhosis may occur even after cessation of alcohol abuse.

Hypergammaglobulinaemia is noted in alcoholic liver disease. A moderate elevation of IgA is considered characteristic. IgA deposits have been noted in the liver, skin, and kidneys of these patients. A variety of antibodies has been detected in alcohol liver disease. These include antibodies against ethanol-modified hepatocytes, antibodies against liver cell membrane and against liver-specific protein. None of these antibodies are specific for alcoholic liver disease nor do they correlate with severity of the disease.

Drug-induced liver disease

Drug-induced liver disease mimics all varieties of liver disease. In every case of liver disease, both acute and chronic, a drug history should be carefully sought and evaluated. The symptoms and signs of drug-induced liver injury are variable depending on the degree of liver injury and the type of the drug. Some drugs or their metabolites may be direct hepatotoxins (e.g. acetaminophen); drugs may interact with a structural component or enzyme in the hepatocytes, and hypersensitivity reactions may occur.

Clinically and histologically, the hepatic injury may be classified as hepatocellular or cholestatic:

(1) *hepatocellular* damage which can mimic AICAH has been reported with oxyphenisatin, monoamine-oxidase inhibitors, α-methyldopa, nitrofurantoin, isoniazid, aminosalicylic acid and sulphonamides;

(2) *cholestatic* drug reactions may occur in association with phenothiazines, oral hypoglycaemic agents, and antithyroid drugs such as thiouracil.

Summary

Autoimmune diseases of the liver are not common but can be diagnosed after careful evaluation. Many liver diseases have multisystem manifestations and immunological features as described above. Therapy for viral hepatitis (IFN) can elicit autoimmune phenomena. Finally, other liver diseases can mimic autoimmune diseases of the liver by histology or biochemistry.

Further reading

Cuthbert, J. A. (1994) Hepatitis C: progress and problems. *Clinical Microbiology Reviews*, **7**, 505–32.

Esteban, J. I., Genesca, J., Alter, H. J. (?). Hepatitis C: Molecular biology, pathogenesis, epidemiology, clinical features, and prevention. *Progress in Liver Diseases*, 253–82.

Gershwin, M. E. and Mackay, I. R. (1991). Primary biliary cirrhosis: Paradigm or paradox for autoimmunity. *Gastroenterology*, **100**, 822–33.

Homberg, J., Abuaf, N., Bernard, O., Islam, S., Alvarez, F., Khalil, S. H., et al. (1987). Chronic active hepatitis associated with antiliver/kidney microsome antibody type 1: A second type of 'autoimmune hepatitis'. *Hepatology*, **7**, 1333–9.

Hoofnagle, J. H. and Di Bisceglie, A. M. (1991). Serologic diagnosis of acute and chronic viral hepatitis. *Seminars in Liver Disease*, **11**, 73–83.

Johnson, P. J. and McFarlane, I. G. (1993). Meeting report: International autoimmune hepatitis group. *Hepatology*, **18**, 998–1004.

Johnson, R. J., Gretch, D. R., Yamabe, H., Hart, J., Bacchi C. E., Hartwell, P., et al. (1993). Membranoproliferative glomerulonephritis associated with hepatitis C virus infection. *New England Journal of Medicine*, **328**, 465–70.

Lindor, K. D., Weisner, R. H., MacCarty, R. L., and LaRusso, N. F. (1990). Advances in primary sclerosing cholangitis. *American Journal of Medicine*, **89**, 73–80.

Maddrey, W. C. (1993). How many types of autoimmune hepatitis are there?. *Gastroenterology*, **105**, 1571–5.

Manns, M. (1991a). Cytoplasmic autoantigens in autoimmune hepatitis: molecular analysis and clinical relevance. *Seminars in Liver Disease*, **11**, 205–14.

Manns, M. P. (1991b). Cytoplasmic autoantigens in autoimmune hepatitis: Molecular analysis and clinical relevance. *Seminars in Liver Disease*, **11**, 205–14.

Milich, D. R. (1991). Immune response to hepatitis B virus proteins: relevance of the murine model. *Seminars in Liver Disease*, **11**, 93–112.

Miller, R. H. (1991). Comparative molecular biology of the hepatitis viruses. *Seminars in Liver Disease*, **11**, 113–20.

Misiani, R., Bellavita, P., Fenili, D., Borelli, G., Marchesi, D., Massazza, M., et al. (1992). Hepatitis C virus infection in patients with essential mixed cryoglobulinemia. *Annals of Internal Medicine*, **117**, 573–77.

Ross, B. C., Anderson, D. A., and Gust, I. D. (1991). Hepatitis A virus and hepatitis A infection. *Advances in Virus Research*, **39**, 209–53.

Rothschild, M. A., Berk, P. D., and Lieber, C. S. (1993). Alcoholic liver disease. *Seminars in Liver Disease*, **13**, 109–216.

Snook, J. A., Chapman, R. W., Fleming, K., and Jewwell, D. P. (1989). Anti-neutrophil nuclear antibody in ulcerative colitis, Crohn's disease, and primary sclerosing cholangitis. *Clinical and Experimental Immunology*, **76**, 30–3.

Surh, C. D., Coppel, R., and Gershwin, M. E. (1990). Structural requirement for autoreactivity on human pyruvate dehydrogenase-E2, the major autoantigens of primary biliary cirrhosis. Implication for a confirmational autoepitope. *Journal of Immunology*, **144**, 3367–74.

Zakim and Boyer (eds) (1990). *Hepatology*, 2nd edn. W. B. Saunders, Philadelphia.

Zimmerman, H. J. (1978). *Hepatotoxicity*. Appleton Century-Crofts, New York.

Zinkernagel. R. M. (1993). Immunity to viruses. In *Fundamental Immunology*, 3rd edn, (ed. W. E. Paul), pp. 1211–50. Raven Press, New York.

17 Lung

J. Bradley

Granulomatous disease

There are a number of granulomatous diseases affecting the lungs which differ in aetiology, cause, pathology, presentation, and response to therapy (see Table 17.1).

Table 17.1 Causes of pulmonary granulomatous disease

Infective	Tuberculosis
Non-infective	Hypersensitivity: extrinsic allergic alveolitis
	Vasculitis: Wegener's granulomatosis
	Polyarteritis nodosa
	Churg–Strauss syndrome
	Rheumatoid arthritis
	Foreign body: e.g. talc
Sarcoidosis	

Tuberculosis

In the developed world this is an uncommon but a re-emerging problem, particularly since the advent of human immunodefiency virus (HIV)/acquired immune deficiency syndrome (AIDS). The World Health Organization state that ~20% of the world's population is infected with the tubercle bacillus; three million people die each year from the disease at present and it accounts for about four deaths per 100 000. If there is a poor T-cell response to infection due to malnutrition and poverty, immunosuppression, HIV infection, exposure to active cases then the disease may occur in a generalized or miliary form. If, however, the T-cell response is vigorous the mycobacteria are localized, often in the lung, in a granulomatous process and there

is a good response to therapy, (see Chapter 38 on tuberculosis).

Hypersensitivity pneumonitis (extrinsic allergic alveolitis)

Hypersensitivity pneumonitis (HP) presents as a clinical syndrome of cough and dyspnoea in some individuals who are exposed to organic dusts, chemicals, or drugs and is an immunological, inflammatory granulomatous response involving alveoli, bronchioles, and interstitium. The inciting antigens reach alveoli by inhalation, e.g. organic dusts, but may also do so by bloodstream, e.g. drugs. It is an uncommon disease with a frequency of 1–10% that of asthma.

The incidence of HP is ~7–15% of those exposed to the antigens. The most frequent causes of HP are thermophilic actinomycetes from soil and mouldy hay, but not everyone who reacts develops disease. Of dairy farmers 8% have precipitating antibodies to these inhaled antigens but only 4% have evidence of the disease, 'farmers lung'. In areas of high rainfall and humidity 10% of farmers may be affected. There are many causes of HP including thermophilic organisms, animal and bird proteins, chemicals, e.g. isocyanates, and drugs, e.g. procarbazine, gold, amiodarone hydrochlorothiazide) and they are listed in Table 17.2.

Immunopathogenesis

In the acute phase there is mononuclear cell infiltration which may proceed to non-caseating granuloma formation and an increase in CD8+ T cells. Lymphocytes with CD8+ T cells predominantly and natural killer (NK) cells, macrophages, giant cells, and neutrophils are present in the alveoli. Later if there is repeated

■ **Table 17.2** Hypersensitivity pneumonitis

Antigen	Source	Disease
Animal protein		
Avian serum or faeces	Pigeon, budgerigar, parrot	Pigeon-breeder's lung
		Bird fancier's lung
Animal protein	Rat or other animal urinary protein,	Rodent handler's pneumonitis (lung)
	Chicken proteins	Feather plucker's disease
	Fish meal	Fish meal worker's lung.
	Serum or pituitary protein	Snuff taker's lung
Dusts		
Wheat flour	Wheat weevil	Miller's lung
Coffee bean dust	Coffee beans	Coffee-worker's lung
Cedar, blackwood	Wood dust; *Alternaria*	Wood-worker's lung
mahogany, etc.		
Moulds		
Penicillium casei	Mouldy cheese	Cheese worker's lung
Penicillium frequentans	Mouldy cork dust	Suberosis
Aspergillus fumigatus/clavatus	Mouldy barley	Malt worker's lung; farmer's lung.
Faeni rectivingula	Compost, mouldy hay	Farmer's lung
(Micropolyspora faeni)		
Thermoactinomycetes candidus	Humidifiers	Humidifier lung; sauna taker's lung.
Thermoactinomycetes saccharii	Water in air conditioner	Ventilation lung
Saccharomonospora viridis		
Trichosporon cutaneum	Japanese summer air	'Summer-type' hypersensitivity pneumonitis
Cephalosporium	Sewage	Sewage worker's disease.
Chemicals		
Bordeaux mixture	Vineyards	Vineyard sprayers disease
Di-isocyanates	Plastics	
Pyrethrum	Insecticide spray	

exposure to the antigen obliterative brochiolitis and progressive interstitial pulmonary fibrosis occur.

HP was thought to be caused by immune complexes because of the demonstration of precipitating antibodies, and this was suggested by symptoms that began 4–6 h after exposure to the antigen. But asymptomatic individuals exposed to same antigen may have antibodies but no disease and the pathogenesis is not clear. Lung biopsies in early disease reveal deposition of IgG, IgA, IgM, and C3 in the lesions but the presence of T cells in the lung and bronchoalveolar fluid of humans and transfer of the disease by T cells in animal models suggest that cytokines interleukin (IL) 1, IL-6, tumour necrosis factor (TNF) α, granulocyte–macrophage colony-stimulating factor, arachidonic metabolites, and immune complexes are all involved in the pathogenesis of the disease.

Clinical features

The acute form of the disease presents as cough and breathlessness with signs of systemic illness: fever, rigors, fatigue, headache, and myalgia which occurs 3–8 h after exposure to the antigen. The symptoms can subside in hours or days, but recur on further exposure. In the commoner subacute and chronic forms the main symptoms are a typical non-productive cough and gradually progressive dyspnoea. In the chronic disease weight loss and fatigue may be the presenting features, and at this stage diffuse interstitial pulmonary fibrosis may already be present. Eventually hypoxia and pulmonary hypertension develop. Examination usually reveals moist sounds over basal or entire lung fields especially after recent exposure to the antigen. Diagnosis is made by the history, clinical findings, typical pulmonary function studies, and laboratory findings.

The blood neutrophil count and serum immunoglobulin levels are raised. Precipitating antibody to the antigen aids the diagnosis in that it indicates previous exposure to the antigen, but more have antibodies than have disease. They may occur in 5–25% of those exposed, e.g. pigeon breeders, but in whom no evidence of disease is found. However, the higher the titre the more likely is disease to be present.

Pulmonary function tests usually reveal a restrictive defect with reduced lung volumes but in mild cases the only defect may be D_{LCO} (diffusing capacity for carbon monoxide). Radiological appearances may be normal, diffuse alveolar infiltrates and in the later stages pulmonary fibrosis. However, in the acute stages there may be a diffuse alveolar and interstitial infiltrate. Computerized tomography (CT) may be a more sensitive investigation.

Treatment

Avoidance of the causative antigen is most important. In farmer's lung 30% of those who have been exposed for more than 5 years develop pulmonary fibrosis and permanent respiratory impairment. To avoid exposure, use of masks, improved ventilation and/or air-conditioning systems may be needed. Corticosteroid may reduce the inflammatory phases seen in acute attacks, but long-term administration is avoided.

Pulmonary fibrosis (fibrosing alveolitis)

Fibrosing alveolitis affects individuals in whom the disease process is triggered by known causes (extrinsic allergic; alveolitis; occupational dust diseases; drugs; ingested of inhaled agents) or by unknown causes (idiopathic or cryptogenic pulmonary fibrosis).

Idiopathic pulmonary fibrosis

Idiopathic pulmonary fibrosis (IPF), also known as *diffuse interstitial pulmonary fibrosis* or *cryptogenic fibrosing alveolitis*, results from the inability to control healing processes within the lung. It can occur at any decade but usually affects patients in the 35–55 year group who present with increasing dyspnoea, finger clubbing, and fine moist sounds (crepitations) over the lower lung fields. No underlying cause for fibrosis is found. The incidence is about three to five per 100 000.

Pathogenesis

The cause is not known but there appears to be an immunological response to unknown antigens. The lung is infiltrated with neutrophils, activated macrophages, and often lymphocytes, involving CD4+ >CD8+ T cells. Major histocompatibility complex (MHC) class II is expressed on alveolar epithelial cells. There are reactive oxygen, enzymes, cytokines (e.g. IL-1; IL-8; TNFα), chemoattractants, and growth factors. Bronchoalveolar lavage (BAL) fluid contain up to 40% neutrophils and eosinophils, increased lymphocytes (up to 15%), and immune complexes which are both free and in macrophages.

Clinical features

IPF often presents with persistent non-productive cough and progressive exertional dypnoea without a wheeze. Finger clubbing is present in some. The course of the disease varies but the process is chronic with 50% of patients dying within 5 years of cor pulmonale, respiratory failure infection, or cancer. It is important to rule out other causes of interstitial pulmonary disease: connective tissue diseases; occupational and environmental diseases, e.g. farmer's or bird fanciers lung, humidifier disease; and drugs.

BAL reveals neutrophils and/or lymphocytes. Those with an increase in lymphocytes appear to be more responsive to corticosteroids and have a better prognosis. Those with neutrophil and/or eosinophils have more fibrosis and are less responsive to corticosteroids. Pulmonary function tests show generally reduced values, and in particular D_{LCO} is reduced.

Lung biopsy provides a definitive diagnosis, excludes neoplastic disease and provides an assessment of the progression of the disease.

Therapy

Because of the bad prognosis with progression to severe pulmonary disease and death immunosuppressive therapy with high-dose prednisolone or combinations of prednisolone/cyclophosphamide is used with objective response in ~20%. For those <60 years with rapidly progressive disease and poor response to this therapy single lung transplantation is considered.

Sarcoidosis

This is a relatively common multisystem non-caseating granulomatous disease of unknown aetiology, which is usually chronic but may be acute. There is involvement of many organs but a high frequency of pulmonary, parenchymal, or thoracic lymph node involvement. Any other organ may be involved but especially lymph nodes, liver, skin, spleen, and central nervous system. The histological picture is that of an epithelioid non-caseating granuloma with some disturbance of the tissue architecture. Spontaneous remission occurs in 50–70%, but the disease may remit and relapse

Introduction

Incidence

Sarcoidosis occurs worldwide but the incidence varies. It is 10–40 per 100 000 in North America and Europe but is more frequent in Scandinavia, and in Irish living in London. It is rare in New Zealand Maoris, in Southeast Asia, in Eskimos, and in Japan (2.5 per 100 000).

Epidemiology

There are genetic and environmental factors. Sarcoidosis is seen more frequently in monzygotic twins than in dizygotic twins, and geographical clustering has been observed.

Pathology

The typical lesion is a granuloma which is no different to those found in other diseases. It consists of epithelioid cells derived from cells of the monocyte–macrophage series, occasional multinucleate giant cells with CD4+ T cells interspersed among the cells. This is surrounded by a zone of predominantly CD4+ T cell with occasional CD8+ T cells. BAL has contributed to our understanding of the disease process by revealing that the CD4+ T cells that form the predominant T-cell in the infiltrates are active and proliferating at two to three times the usual rate. The T cells are of the CD4+, CD45RO+ phenotype, i.e. 'primed' or 'memory' T cells, and they have increased expression of MHC class II and CD2 on their surface. They are activated for they are producing IL-2 and interferon (IFN) γ and have increased expression of IL-2 receptor (IL-2R). There is also evidence that the alveolar macrophages are activated and involved in increased antigen presentation; their surface MHC class II expression is increased as is their production of IL-1 and TNF. In keeping with this antigen-presenting cell (APC) and T-cell activity there is also B-cell overactivity with a polyclonal increase in serum immunoglobulins and presence of circulating complexes

Immunopathogenesis

The granuloma is typical of an 'immune' granuloma and is similar to that seen with chronic beryllium exposure. This suggests the presence of a persisting antigen, but none has been identified. An expansion of the T cells, especially CD4+ cells occurs in the blood and the organs involved, e.g. the lungs.

In about 30% of patients there is an increase in T cells bearing the T-cell receptor (TCR) $\gamma\delta$. and in some of these up to 50% of the T cells are of the $\gamma\delta$ type. In addition, there appears to be TCR restriction for there is predominant use of the Vγ9 and Vδ2 variable region which is also seen in bacterial infections, especially with mycobacteria.

There is evidence that IL-2 and other cytokines are released, and increased expression of IL-2R can be demonstrated in BAL and lung. Other signs of activation are alveolar cells and presence of adhesion molecules, plus B-cell activation. This compartmental effect is usually seen in the lungs, but peripheral blood shows the reverse, i.e. reduced T cells especially CD4 cells, raised immunoglobulin levels, plus an increased incidence of rheumatoid factor, antinuclear antibody, and immune complexes. Delayed hypersensitivity skin tests to tuberculin and recall antigens are reduced or negative. About 60% fail to respond to 100 unit of tuberculin (PPD).

Clinical features

The disease varies. It can be mild and asymptomatic, or severe multisytem with systemic manifestations; chronic or occasionally acute; self-limiting or chronic. The common sites of involvement are lungs, lymph nodes, eyes and skin. In mild cases the diseases may be present asymptomatically as bilateral enlargement of the hilar lymph nodes. In half of these there is no evidence of the disease within 2 years, but the other half continue as a chronic mild illness. However, chronic persistent inflammation may lead to dysfunction, recurring injury, and fibrosis. The mortality rate is ~1–4%.

Criteria for diagnosis of active sarcoidosis:

1. Clinical manifestations: fever, arthritis, erythema nodosum, uveitis, pneumonitis, and cardiac sarcoidosis.

2. Radiological evidence of passage from stage 1 (lymphadenopathy) to stages 2–4. The degree of involvement is assessed by the staging system in

▌ **Table 17.3** Clinical features of sarcoidosis

Acute	Chronic/insidious
Fever	'Dry cough' and/or breathlessness
Hilar lymphadenopathy	Lymphadenopathy
Iritis	Anterior uveitis
Joint pain	Hepatic involvement
Erythema nodosum	Plaques/erythema nodosum
Malaise	Hypercalaemia/hypercalciuria

which stage 1 is bilateral hilar lymphadenopathy; stage 2 is bilateral hilar lymphadenopathy plus parenchymal infiltrates; stage 3 is parenchymal infiltration without bilateral hilar lymphadenopathy. Spontaneous complete remission of disease occurs in 50–80% of cases of stage 1 sarcoid; 30–50% stage 2; and 10–30% stage 3. Disease progression occurs in fewer than 15% of stage 1 whereas in stage 3 the disease is persistent or progresses.

3. Pulmonary function tests (PFTs) are important to determine the extent of the disease, and to follow its course longitudinally. Reduction in vital capacity, total lung capacity, or diffusing capacity for carbon monoxide occur in 40–70% of cases; obstructive defects are present in 20–40% of cases. Serial PFTs are essential to document the extent and course of the pulmonary parenchymal process, but none reliably differentiate inflammation (alveolitis) from fibrosis.

4. BAL and fibre-optic bronchoscopy with BAL has provided insights into the pathogenesis of the lung lesion in sarcoidosis. In active pulmonary sarcoidosis there are increases in the number and per cent of activated CD4+ T cells, reduced suppressor (CD8+) cells and increased CD4+/CD8+ ratio, immunoglobulins, and IgG-secreting cells. The alveolar T cells spontaneously release a variety of lymphokines and express IL-2 R.

5. Serum angiotensin-converting enzyme (ACE). Elevated serum concentrations of ACE occur in 30–80% of patients with sarcoidosis and may correlate with disease activity. The level appears to be less sensitive as an indicator of alveolitis than BAL but may provide a better estimate of the total body granuloma burden.

Treatment

The impact of therapy in altering the course of sarcoidosis remains highly controversial. In mild asymptomatic cases observation only is necessary as spontaneous remissions occur in nearly two-thirds of patients. However, approximately 20–30% of patients develop severe or progressive disease. The presence of any ocular, central nervous system, or myocardial involvement requires immediate therapy as does persistent or progressive pulmonary disease, as assessed radiologically or by PFTs, renal disease, hepatic dysfunction, or skin lesions. Corticosteroids are the main form of therapy and are effective in inhibiting or reversing the disease process by exerting profound inhibitory effects on T cells and APCs. In active disease the main form of therapy is prednisolone usually ~1 mg/kg per day but subsequently this may be reduced to 0.1–0.3 mg/kg per day. The prognosis for those with acute disease is good after treatment with 90% better after 3 months, but chest X-rays may take another 3 months to improve. The chronic, insidious form may progress to generalized disease. Although sarcoidosis responds well to therapy 5% of patients die of the disease. If there is a poor or no response to steroids, methotrexate, azathioprine, or cyclophosphamide may be of value.

NSAIDS are of value in controlling musc loskeletal and cutaneous symptoms in subacute sarcoidosis. Chloroquine may also be useful. In view of the possibility of ocular toxicity all patients should have a full ophthalmic examination before commencing chloroquine and at 3–6 monthly intervals while on the drug.

Further reading

Baughmann, R. P. and Lower, E. E. (1990). The effect of corticosteroid of methotrexate therapy on lung lymphocytes and macrophages in sarcoidosis. *American Review of Respiratory Diseases*, **142**, 1268–00.

Cooper, J. A. D. (1990). Drug induced pulmonary disease. *Clinics in Chest medicine*, **11**, 1–194.

Dreisin, R. B. C. (1993). New perspectives in Wegeners granulomatosis. *Thorax*, **48**, 97–9.

DuBois, R. M., Holroyd, K. J., Saltinin, C., and Crystal, R. G. (1991). Granulomatous processes. In *The lung: scientific foundations*, (ed. R. G. Crystal and J. B. West), pp. 1925–38. Raven Press, New York.

Lynch, J. P. III and Strieter, R. M. (1991). Sarcoidosis. In: *Immunologically mediated pulmonary disorders*, (ed. J. P. Lynch III and R. A. DeRemee), pp. 189–00, J. B. Lippincott, Philadelphia, PA.

Lynch, J. P. III and Hunninghake, G. W. (19??). Sarcoidosis. *Current Therapy in Allergy, Immunology and Rheumatology*, **4**, 243–251.

Meredith, S. D. K., Taylor, V. M., and McDonald, J. C. (1991). Occupational respiratory disease in the United Kingdom 1989: a report to the British Thoracic Society and the Society of Occupational Medicine by the SWORD project group. *British Journal of Industrial Medicine*, **48**, 292–8.

Panos, R. J. and Jing, T. E. Jr (1991). Idiopathic pulmonary fibrosis. In *Immunologically mediated pulmonary diseases*, (ed. J. P. Lynch III and R. A. DeRemee), p. 1. J. B. Lippincott, Philadelphia, PA.

Thomas, P. D. and Hunninghake, G. W. (1987). Current concepts of pathogenesis of sarcoidosis. *American Review of Respiratory Diseases*, **135**, 747–60.

18 Skin

R. StC. Barnetson and A. Gramp

Many skin diseases have an immunological basis, and it will not be possible to cover all which come into this category. In this section the following will be discussed:

1. Autoimmune disease.
2. Immune complex-mediated diseases.
3. Delayed hypersensitivity diseases.
4. Connective tissue diseases of the skin.
5. Skin cancers in which immunological responses play an important part.

Autoimmune diseases

Chronic idiopathic urticaria

Urticaria (Fig. 18.1(a)) is a common condition which results from mast cell degranulation in the skin. When it affects the face and the groin, there is commonly swelling in the subcutaneous tissues, and it is known as angioedema or giant urticaria (Fig. 18.1(b)). The main characteristic of urticaria and angioedema is their transience. They normally last for 1–3 h and then

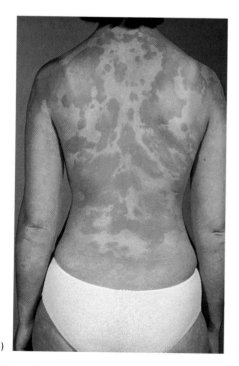

(a)

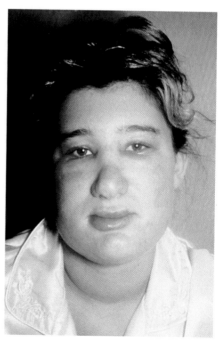

(b)

Fig. 18.1(a) Urticaria. Extensive urticaria on the trunk which may last for 1–2 h. (b) Angioedema, with marked but transient swelling of the lower face.

resolve. There is no other skin condition which will give this history.

There are a number of causes of urticaria. These all involve mast cell degranulation due either to immunological mechanisms via immunoglobulin (Ig) E, or complement activation, or non-immunological mechanisms, which are poorly understood, e.g. physical urticarias and urticaria due to aspirin. IgE-mediated urticaria due to ingestants such as egg and fish, or to insect venoms, is well understood and is discussed further in chapter X on urticaria and urticarial vasculitis (Vasculitis, Chapter X) due to complement activation.

However, the most common type of urticaria to present to a dermatology clinic is chronic idiopathic urticaria, where the cause is unclear. Clinically, it is characterized by urticaria which occurs daily, month after month, and it may initially develop after a virus infection. The urticaria may be localized or widespread. Drugs such as aspirin will exacerbate it, as may food constituents, e.g. salicylates, additives, or colourings such as tartrazine. It usually runs a course of 1–2 years, and then resolves spontaneously. However, in a number of patients, it may continue for many years, occasionally remitting and developing again. In some there may be a seasonal incidence. Some may respond to H_1 antihistamines; others are very recalcitrant to treatment. Recent research suggests that it is due to an autoimmune mechanism, as anti-IgE receptor antibodies have been identified in this condition. These are IgG antibodies against the high-affinity IgE receptor which cross-link the receptors directly. This results in mast cell degranulation with release of histamine and other vasoactive mediators. Chemoattractant substances (e.g. platelet-activating factor (PAF), cytokines) may also be released which induce expression of adhesion molecules (e.g. ICAM-1) which may be responsible for the CD4+ T-cell infiltrate in urticarial lesions.

The treatment of chronic idiopathic urticaria is summarized in Table 18.2.

Pemphigus

This is an uncommon, but important group of blistering diseases, which may result in the death of the patient from septicaemia or fluid and electrolyte imbalance. It tends to affect middle-aged people. The main forms are:

1. pemphigus vulgaris
2. pemphigus foliaceus
3. fogo selvagem (in Brazil)
4. paraneoplastic pemphigus

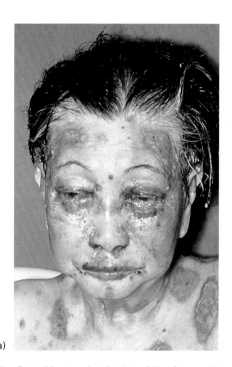
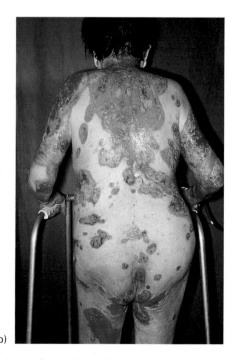

(a)   (b)

▮ **Fig. 18.2** Pemphigus vulgaris: (a) of the face, with erosions of the skin and mucous membranes (eyes and mouth); (b) of the trunk with extensive erosions.

Each is characterized by the formation of IgG autoantibodies to keratinocyte cell surface antigens in the epidermis. This leads to increased conversion of plasminogen to plasmin, which is responsible for the loss of cell adhesion. It is possible that complement may play a part in this as well (as is the case in pemphigoid). Passive transfer of pemphigus antibodies has been induced in neonatal mice, and infants born to mothers with pemphigus may have transient blistering at birth. These diseases are therefore examples of type II hypersensitivity reactions.

Pemphigus vulgaris

This is the most severe form of pemphigus with widespread, flaccid blisters. Drug treatment controls the condition only with difficulty and a number of patients die from fluid and electrolyte imbalance or septicaemia. In pemphigus vulgaris, the blister is formed in the lower epidermis suprabasally. IgG and C3 can be

demonstrated in the epidermis staining the keratinocyte cell surface on direct immunofluorescence of the skin, and IgG autoantibodies in the serum by indirect immunofluorescence. The titre of the autoantibody in the serum is usually proportional to the disease extent. The three polypeptides of MW 210 kDa, 130 kDa (desmoglein-3, the target antigen), 85 kDa in the epidermis to which the autoantibodies bind appear to be different from those in the other three main types of pemphigus.

Clinical features

Pemphigus vulgaris presents in approximately 90% cases with oral erosions, and other mucous membranes may be involved. Later, numerous large blisters (bullae) appear in the skin which may be very widespread. The disease is progressive, unlike bullous pemphigoid which usually resolves spontaneously within 3 years.

Treatment is often unsatisfactory, as the disease is difficult to control. The drugs used are corticosteroids in high dosage (e.g. prednisolone 300 mg daily) or somewhat lower doses, azathioprine, cyclophosphamide, cyclosporin, and gold; in some cases plasmapheresis is helpful.

Pemphigus foliaceus

This is more common than pemphigus vulgaris and may affect any age group. In pemphigus foliaceus the blisters are more superficial, being found in the region of the granular layer of the epidermis. The IgG autoantibodies bind to polypeptides of MW 260 kDa; 160 kDa (desmoglein-1, target antigen) and 85 kDa on the keratinocyte membrane. It is more common than pemphigus vulgaris and may affect any age group. It is usually controlled more easily,

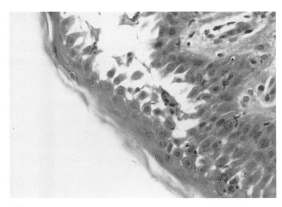

(a)

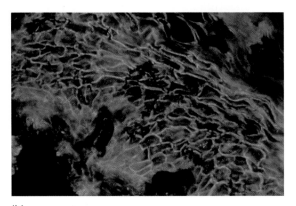

(b)

∎ **Fig. 18.3** (a) Pemphigus vulgaris. Intraepidermal suprabasal blister (haematoxylin and eosin). (b) Pemphigus vulgaris. IgG staining of keratinocytes.

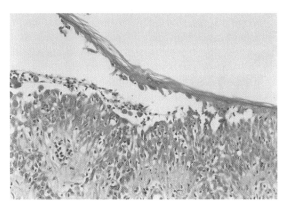

∎ **Fig. 18.4** Pemphigus foliaceus. Intraepidermal sub-cornea/blister (haematoxylin and eosin).

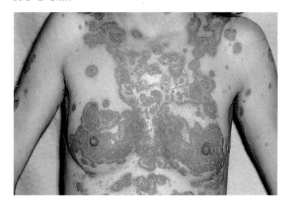

▌ Fig. 18.5 Pemphigus foliaceus on the trunk of a female aged 20 years. There are no intact blisters.

although it runs a chronic course without permanent remission.

Clinical features

Pemphigus foliaceus presents with plaques of erythema resembling psoriasis in the skin which may be present for several years before the correct diagnosis is made. Blisters are few, because being superficial they rupture easily. Eventually the patient may become erythrodermic. Oral lesions are less common (<10%) than in pemphigus vulgaris.

A pemphigus foliaceus-like disease may be caused by a number of drugs including penicillamine, captopril, and rifampicin. The mechanism of this is unclear.

The treatment of pemphigus foliaceus consists of oral corticosteroids in relatively low doses, and azathioprine, which usually control the rash easily.

Fogo selvagem

This is an interesting form of pemphigus, which is common in Brazil. It is also called endemic pemphigus foliaceus. Substantial epidemiological evidence suggests that it is precipitated by an environmental factor, as the vast majority of patients live close to rivers. It is postulated that the disease may be associated with blackfly (*Simulium pruinosum*) bites, but this is far from proven. As in other forms of pemphigus, the disease presents with blistering of the skin, although the mucous membranes are spared. It often progresses to erythroderma with a marked evening pyrexia. About 20% resolve spontaneously.

Paraneoplastic pemphigus

This is a newly described entity, which is usually associated with lymphoma and thymoma. Immunofluorescence findings are different in that as well as intercellular staining for IgG being positive, there is usually granular or linear IgG staining along the basement membrane zone resembling the staining seen in bullous pemphigoid. The antibody binds to urinary bladder epithelium on indirect immunofluorescence of the serum, which is not the case in other forms of pemphigus. The IgG antibodies are produced to a complex of four polypeptides of MW 250 kDa, 230 kDa, 210 kDa and 190 kDa. The disease therefore seems to be different from either pemphigus vulgaris or foliaceus.

Clinical features

As in pemphigus vulgaris, the disease usually starts with oral erosions and mucous membrane involvement (conjunctivae, vaginae, lips) is usually prominent. Later, bulla formation in the skin may be extensive. The course of the disease fluctuates with the activity of the neoplasia. For instance, if the thymoma is removed, or if the lymphoma is treated successfully with chemotherapy, the pemphigus may go into remission. Otherwise, treatment is with oral corticosteroids and the other drug regimens used in pemphigus.

Pemphigoid

Pemphigoid is a similar disease to pemphigus though the blisters are subepidermal, and thus deeper and more likely to remain intact. There are four types of

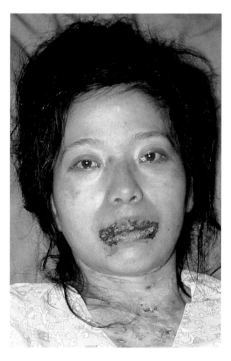

▌ Fig. 18.6 Paraneoplastic pemphigus, usually starts in the mouth, but also involves the skin of the trunk and limbs.

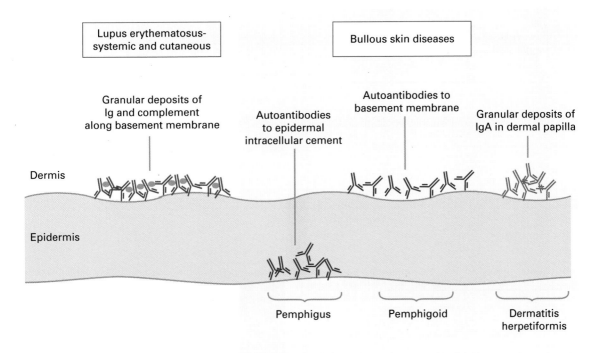

▮ **Fig. 18.7** Characteristic location of immunoglobulin in pemphigus, pemphigoid, lupus, and dermatitis herpetiformis.

pemphigoid; arising from the location of the various pemphigoid antigens (Fig. 18.8):

1. Bullous pemphigoid.
2. Cicatricial pemphigoid.
3. Pemphigoid gestations (herpes gestations).
4. Dermolytic pemphigoid (epidermolysis bullosa acquisita).

Bullous pemphigoid

A disease of the elderly who develop autoantibodies to antigens in the basement membrane zone of the epi-

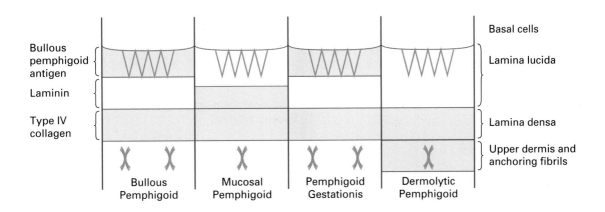

▮**Fig. 18.8** Locations of antigens in four forms of pemphigoid.

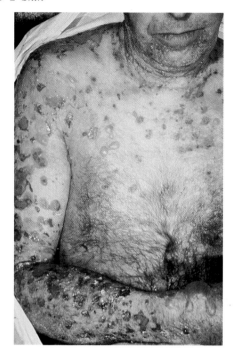

❙ **Fig. 18.9** Bullous pemphigoid, showing extensive erosions on the trunk and right arm, with some intact blisters.

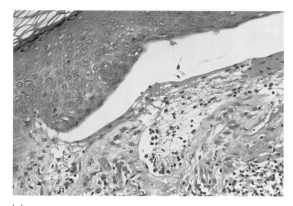

(a)

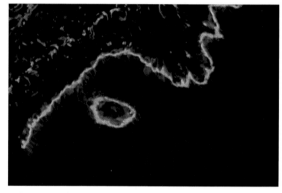

(b)

❙ **Fig. 18.10** (a) Bullous pemphigoid. Subepidermal blister (haematoxylin and eosin). (b) Bullous pemphigoid IgG: staining of basement membrane zone of epidermis.

dermis. Most interestingly for an autoimmune disease, the disease is self-limiting usually resolving within 3 years, although circulating autoantibodies may continue to be present for years after this clinical resolution.

Immunofluorescence studies demonstrate IgG and C3 (sometimes also IgA and IgM) at the basement membrane zone, and it is likely that the blisters are formed due to complement activation. Most patients also have circulating IgG autoantibodies; unlike pemphigus, there is no correlation of the antibody titre with the disease extent.

The bullous pemphigoid antigens are polypeptides located in the hemidesmosomes of the basement keratinocytes of the epidermis, and are thought to be transmembrane molecules with MW 230 and 180 kDa. Pemphigoid blisters have been induced in both guinea-pigs and neonatal mice on passive transfer of auto-antibodies. If salt-split skin studies are performed, fluorescence is seen at the roof of the blister.

Clinically, bullous pemphigoid in the elderly (age group 60–80 characteristically) presents with intact blisters and urticaria-like plaques. They may develop in localized areas such as the shins initially, and then become widespread. Mucous membrane blisters and erosions occur in only 10% of cases. A peripheral blood eosinophilia is common, as are increased concentrations of IgE in the serum (e.g. 4000 ku/l); the cause of the latter is unknown.

The disease responds to low-dose steroids (e.g. prednisolone 40 mg daily initially, decreasing to a maintenance dose of 5–10 mg daily). Azathioprine is a useful steroid sparing agent. The drugs need to be continued for 2–3 years.

Cicatricial pemphigoid (benign mucosal pemphigoid)

This is much less common than bullous pemphigoid. As its name suggests it affects mucosal surfaces such as the mouth, nose, larynx, oesophagus, conjunctiva, glans penis, vagina, and arms. Usually, the eroded areas lead to marked scarring.

Histopathological studies show a subepidermal blister containing lymphocytes containing a few eosinophils, and the evidence suggests that the antigens are within the lower part of the lamina lucida which are polypeptides of MW 230 and 180 kDa as in bullous pemphigoid.

Clinically, the condition presents with erosions or blisters in the mouth, and other mucosae. In the eye, there is initially conjunctivitis followed by the development of adhesions and scarring, and eventual blindness if unchecked. In all the mucosal lesions there is a tendency to formation of adhesions and development of scarring. In some patients, bullae develop in the skin, and the appearance is similar to that of bullous pemphigoid.

Oral corticosteroids are not particularly effective in controlling the condition. Topical or intralesional steroids may be helpful, as may be azathioprine, cyclophosphamide, and dapsone.

Pemphigoid gestationis

This is an interesting form of pemphigoid which occurs in pregnancy, and in females with hydatidiform mole and choriocarcinoma. The patients develop subepidermal blisters, and IgG and C3 may be demonstrated in the basement membrane zone, although IgG is found on direct immunofluorescence in only 25% of cases. However, IgG deposition can be confirmed by immunoelectronmicroscopy, and IgG1 is the predominant subclass compared with IgG4 in bullous pemphigoid. The antigen of MW 180 kDa may or may not be the same as the 180 kDa antigen in bullous pemphigoid, but does seem to be a component of the basal keratinocytes.

When it occurs during pregnancy (about 1:60 000 pregnancies), it usually develops in the second trimester and continues till parturition. There may be a post-partum flare. In subsequent pregnancies it may occur earlier; it is not present between pregnancies apart from immediately post-partum. Erythematous

plaques and bullae develop and the appearance is suggestive of bullous pemphigoid.

If the condition is mild, topical steroids may suffice. Otherwise oral steroids are indicated, and a dose of prednisolone 30 mg daily initially will usually control the blistering, reducing to a maintenance dose until parturition.

Dermolytic pemphigoid (epidermolysis bullosa acquisita)

This is a type of pemphigoid which may be associated with inflammatory bowel disease, and some other malignancies such as thymoma and lymphoma. As in other types of pemphigoid, the patients develop subepidermal blisters, and the antigens have been localized to the anchoring fibrils (target antigen-type IV collagen) in the lamina densa having a MW of 290 and 145 kDa. Immunofluorescence shows IgG and C3 staining at the basement membrane zone, with fluorescence at the floor of blisters induced by sodium chloride (salt-split skin).

Clinically the disease may resemble bullous pemphigoid but there is a tendency to develop erythematous plaques and blisters on the extensor surfaces of the limbs which heal with scarring and milia.

Treatment with corticosteroids, azathioprine, dapsone, and cyclosporin, all have rather variable results. In some patients, the disease is difficult to control with any measures.

Immune complex diseases

Normally immune complexes are removed from the circulation by the reticuloendothelial system. However, in certain circumstances, they may be deposited along the vessel walls, resulting in vasculitis and complement activation. In certain circumstances, immune complexes may be formed extravascularly; examples include erythema nodosum leprosum in lepromatous leprosy, and possibly dermatitis herpetiformis. These are all manifestations of type III hypsersensitivity reactions, and may be divided into *vasculitic* and *non-vasculitic* groups.

Vasculitic immune complex disease

There are several examples of immune complex deposition disease in the skin, which is not surprising when one considers the variables, these include:

1. The site of the vessel. Usually vasculitis affects the lower legs, and this is presumably an effect of gravity.

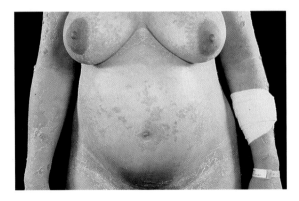

❙ **Fig. 18.11** Pemphigoid gestationis (herpes gestationis), a form of bullous pemphigoid in pregnancy, affecting the trunk.

2. The nature of the vessel (arteriole, venule, capillary) and its size.

3. The size and solubility of the immune complexes.

4. The antibody class within the immune complex.

5. Whether or not the complexes are deposited from a distant site, or formed locally (Arthus reaction).

6. The chronicity of immune complex formation.

The tissue damage which results from immune complex formation and deposition is usually caused by complement activation. When complement is fixed, anaphylotoxins are released as split products of C3 and C5. Chemical mediators are released that include histamines, leukotrienes, prostaglandins, and chemotactic factors for neutrophils which phagocytose the immune complexes and release proteolytic enzymes. Platelets within the vessels aggregate causing thrombosis and ischaemia. The degree of damage depends on:

(1) concentration of immune complexes;

(2) ability of complexes to activate complement;

(3) availability of neutrophils;

(4) availability of effector enzyme systems, e.g. kallikrein, Hageman factor.

Factors involved in the formation and removal of complexes and in the repair of blood vessel damage will influence the course of the clinical disease; immune complexes may continue in the circulation either because of their persistent formation or because of impaired clearance by the reticuloendothelial system.

There are a number of examples of immune complex disease which result in skin manifestations.

Leucocytoclastic vasculitis (allergic vasculitis)

This is the most common form of vasculitis which is characterized by a polymorphonuclear infiltrate and fibrinoid change involving the small dermal vessels. It results from immune complex deposition in the vessels as a result of bacterial infections, viral infections, drugs, connective tissue, and malignant diseases.

The disease may be acute, chronic, or recurrent. Purpura develop, usually on the legs, but also on the arms. There is often accompanying fever and arthralgia. The purpura may develop into haemorrhagic blisters, and ulcers if severe. Urinalysis may reveal microscopic haematuria, due to renal involvement.

Histological examination of the purpura will reveal leucocytoclastic vasculitis, with the presence of nuclear dust. Immunofluorescence studies may show IgG or IgM immune complexes deposited in the

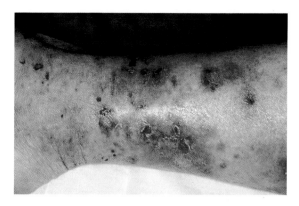

▌ **Fig. 18.12** Allergic (leucocytoclastic) vasculitis, with purpura affecting the lower legs.

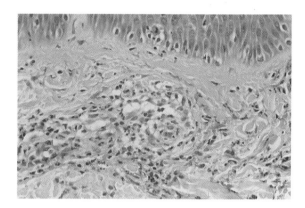

▌ **Fig. 18.13** Leucocytoclastic vasculitis (haematoxylin and eosin).

vessels. Low levels of C3 and C4 are found in the serum.

The condition runs a variable course, but most will resolve spontaneously with 3 months. If there is renal involvement, treatment is mandatory with corticosteroids, colchicine, or dapsone.

Henoch–Schönlein purpura (Fig. 18.14) is a particular form of vasculitis which is associated with the development and deposition of IgA complexes. It is common in children. The causation is unclear, but it probably results from a viral or bacterial infection; some patients have a marked polymorphonuclear leucocytosis. It usually starts with headache, fever, and malaise, which lead on to purpura, arthralgia, and abdominal pains. The purpura affect the external aspects of the limbs, particularly the legs, and may occur in successive waves. The abdominal symptoms include colic, vomiting, diarrhoea, and haematemesis. Renal involvement is common with haematuria and proteinuria.

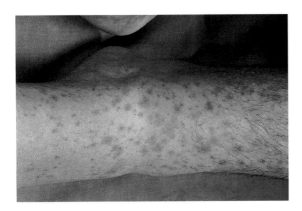

▌ Fig. 18.14 Henoch–Schönlein purpura, affecting the (L) ankle.

Histological examination of the skin reveals a leucocytoclastic vasculitis with IgA deposited in the vessels, and there may be raised IgA concentrations in the serum.

The course is variable, but usually the disease remits in 3–6 weeks but sometimes takes longer. Where there is renal involvement, cytotoxic drug treatment may be indicated.

Erythema nodosum

This condition differs markedly from leucocytoclastic vasculitis, and is due to immune complex deposition in and around vessels of the deep dermis and subcutaneous fat. For some reason it localizes to the shins. It results from a number of conditions: sarcoidosis; yersinosis; deep mycoses; tuberculosis; streptococcal infection; drugs (halides and sulphonamides); enteropathies (Crohn's disease, ulcerative colitis); and malignant disease (e.g. Hodgkin's disease).

It is commonly accompanied by malaise, fatigue, and arthralgia. The erythema nodosum itself presents with tender, red plaques in the skin, which may cause the patient difficulty in walking. After the first week, bruising occurs within the area(s) and this resolves within 6 weeks. The condition may then recur, and these recurrences may continue for several years.

A biopsy will show a lymphocytic vasculitis in the deep dermis and subcutaneous fat. Investigations for causative conditions must be carried out.

Treatment is with bed rest, corticosteroids, or indomethacin.

Polyarteritis nodosa

This is a form of immune complex-mediated disease which affects arteries in a widespread, necrotizing, inflammatory process (see Chapter 30 on Vasculitis). It is a multisystem disorder, which may present with the skin changes with the presence of cutaneous or subcutaneous nodules occurring in groups along the course of superficial arteries, particularly on the legs. Embolization of thrombi may occur leading to infarcts and splinter haemorrhages on the fingers and toes. Other systems involved include the cardiovascular system (hypertension), the kidneys (cortical infarction and glomerulosclerosis), the bowel (gangrene of the intestine), and bones and joints. The diagnosis can be confirmed by skin biopsy which shows arteritis, and ischaemia of the skin. Treatment is with corticosteroids and cytotoxic drugs.

Non-vasculitic immune complex disease

Dermatitis herpetiformis (DH)

This disease is characterized by the development of small, itchy blisters (vesicles) usually in adulthood, on

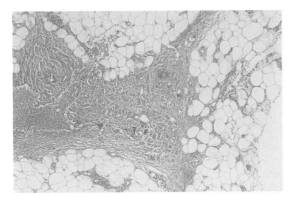

▌ Fig. 18.15 Erythema nodosum showing vasculitis in the panniculus (haematoxylin and eosin).

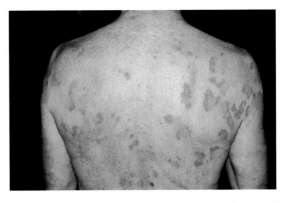

▌ Fig. 18.16 Dermatitis herpetiformis: causing small itchy blisters on the trunk.

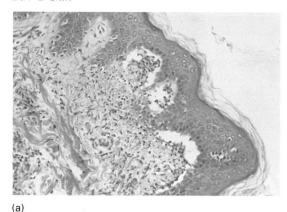

(a)

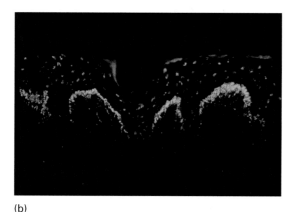

(b)

▮ **Fig. 18.17** Dermatitis herpetiformis. (a) Subepidermal blister (haematoxylin and eosin). (b) Granular IgA staining at the dermo-epidermal junction.

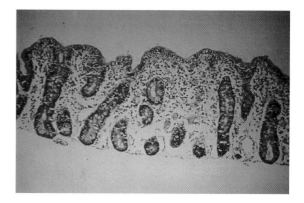

▮ **Fig. 18.18** Dermatitis herpetiformis: villous atrophy of the jejunum.

the elbows, knees, shoulders, and buttocks. The condition is so itchy that usually these blisters have been destroyed by scratching, leaving small erosions. These blisters can be ameliorated by treatment with dapsone or sulphapyridine which seem to have a direct effect on the skin. Microscopy of these blisters demonstrates that they are subepidermal, and direct immunofluorescence microscopy shows granular IgA in dermal papillae at the dermo-epidermal junction.

A majority (about 80%) of DH patients have partial or subtotal villous atrophy of the proximal small intestine, resembling the changes in coeliac disease (Fig. 18.18). Despite this, only about 10% of patients with DH have frank malabsorption. This may result from the possibility that the disease is confined to a small area in the jejunum, compared with much larger areas affected in coeliac disease. More than 90% of DH patients are human leucocyte antigen (HLA) DRW3 as is the case in coeliac disease. It thus seems likely that DH is a variant of coeliac disease, and this is sup-

ported by the fact that in a majority of patients both the jejunal changes and the blisters, after a period of 2 years, clear on a gluten-free diet.

The evidence for DH being an immune complex-mediated disease is as follows:

1. IgA can be demonstrated at the dermo-epidermal junction binding to the dermal microfibrillar bundles. This IgA appears to be derived from the jejunal mucosa because J chain and secretory components have been demonstrated related to the IgA in the skin.

2. IgA complexes can be demonstrated in the serum of some DH patients, and the level of these complexes tends to increase after ingestion of gluten.

The diagnosis of DH is made by skin and jejunal biopsy. These patients have gliadin antibodies in their serum, and also IgA endomysial (smooth muscle) antibodies, and the levels of these antibodies parallel the response to a gluten-free diet.

Treatment is initially with dapsone or sulphapyridine, which are thought to block release of neutrophil chemotactic factors, together with a gluten-free diet. During a period of 2 years, the drug dosage required to ameliorate the blistering will lessen, until the drug can be stopped. There is now evidence that treatment with a gluten-free diet on DH will prevent the development of small intestinal lymphoma.

Delayed hypersensitivity

There are three types of delayed hypersensitivity of type IV hypersensivity reaction: contact, tuberculin, and granulomatous. Both contact and tuberculin hypersensitivity occur at about 48 h.

Contact dermatitis

Contact sensitivity (allergic contact dermatitis) is characterized by an eczematous reaction in the skin at the point of contact. The allergens in this case are usually haptens and may be elements such as nickel and chrome (Fig. 18.19a). The ability to sensitize varies from hapten to hapten; some, e.g. dinitrochlorobenzene (DNCB), will sensitize nearly all individuals. Epicutaneously applied DNCB binds to epidermal proteins through the NH_2 groups of lysine.

Contact sensitivity is primarily an epidermal reaction, dependent on presentation of the hapten via antigen-presenting cells, the Langerhans cells. These are bone marrow derived cells which express CD1 and major histocompatibility complex (MHC) class II molecules on their surface. They endocytose the hapten–protein complex and migrate to the lymph nodes where they present the antigen to CD4+ T lymphocytes (Fig. 18.20). Sensitization takes 10–14 days during which time memory CD4+ T cells are produced.

When the hapten is in contact with the skin post-sensitization, an allergic reaction develops at about 48 h. Keratinocytes in the epidermis play a key part in this reaction, and release a number of cytokines such as tumour necrosis factor (TNF) α and granulocyte–macrophage colony-stimulating factor (GM-CSF). The earliest histological change in the allergic reaction is seen at about 6 h, with the appearance of mononuclear cells around blood vessels and adnexae, with subsequent epidermal infiltration (Fig. 18.21). By 48 h, there is an infiltration of macrophages and between 48 and 72 h most infiltrated cells are CD4+ T cells with a few CD8+ cells. The reaction wanes after 72 h; downregulation depends on migration inhibitory lymphokines, transforming growth factor (TGF) β from dermal mast cells, activated keratinocytes and lymphocytes, interleukin (IL) 1 synthesized by lymphocytes and IL-10 production. The diagnosis is confirmed by applying the hapten to the skin (patch test) and observing the inflammation caused at 48 h. (Fig. 18.19(b)). Treatment is with topical steroids and avoidance of the allergen.

Atopic dermatitis (AD)

AD is a common skin condition, which affects about 10% of the population. In its milder form it affects the flexures, but may be very widespread. It usually presents in early childhood.

The relationship between delayed hypersensitivity and AD is unclear. There are skin changes similar to those of allergic contact dermatitis with infiltration of the dermis with lymphocytes and macrophages, and microvesiculation in the epidermis. There is therefore an eczematous reaction, but contact sensitivity (delayed hypersensitivity) would seem to be a secondary rather than a primary event. This is also true for IgE-mediated hypersensitivity. The part of IgE in AD remains to be elucidated. Patients with AD often have very high IgE concentrations in their serum (up to 100 000 IU/l), but 20% will have normal levels of IgE with negative tests for inhalant and food allergens. The vast amount of IgE produced by AD patients is to inhalants, with the highest levels to house dust mite (*Dermatophagoides pteronyssinus*). These patients often have delayed hypersensitivity tests to the house dust mite in the form of positive patch tests and positive lymphocyte stimulation tests to the mite. A number of patients also have IgE-mediated allergy to foods (e.g. egg, milk, nuts, fish, shellfish), with the development of angioedema and urticaria. Some of

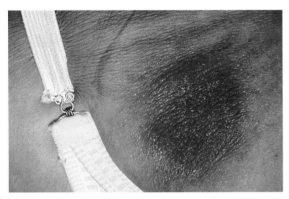

(a)

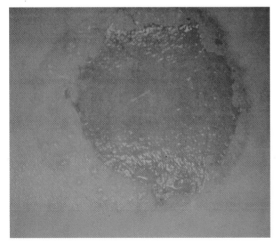

(b)

▌ **Fig. 18.19** Allergic contact dermatitis: (a) caused by nickel in the bra clip, (b) results in a positive patch test to nickel at 48 h.

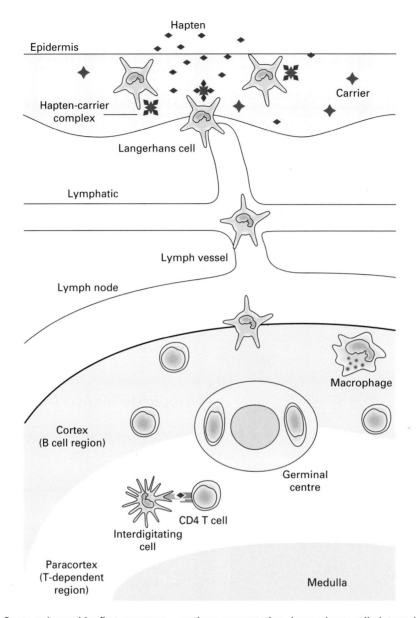

∎ **Fig. 18.20** Contact dermatitis: first exposure —antigen presentation. Langerhans cells internalise the hapten-carrier complex, migrate to regional lymphnode and present antigen to helper T cells.

these patients also have delayed hypersensitivity tests (e.g. positive patch tests to milk).

The treatment of AD is summarized as follows:

(1) avoidance of precipitating factors;

(2) topical steroids;

(3) antibacterials;

(4) emollients;

(5) night sedation;

(6) immunosuppressives for severe disease.

Connective tissue diseases

It is proposed to discuss only those conditions which primarily involve the skin.

1. Lupus erythematosus: discoid and subacute lupus.

2. Scleroderma: localized and generalized.

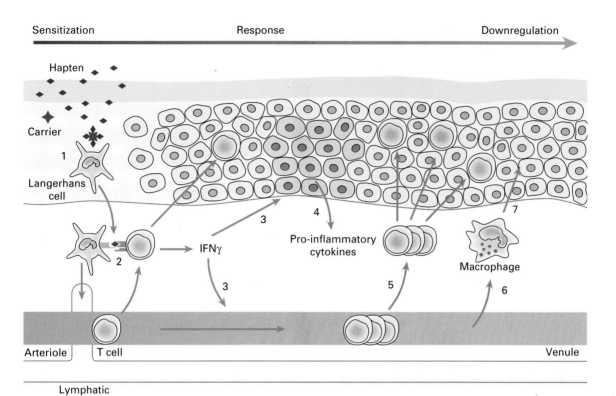

▌Fig. 18.21. Elicitation phase of contact dermatitis. Langerhans cells internalize the antigen and:
(1)   migrate through the dermis and lymphatics to the regional node where they present the antigen to T-helper cells;
(2)   activated CD4+ T cells release IFNγ;
(3)   inducing expression of ICAM-1 on keratinocytes and endothelial cells;
(4)   activated keratinocytes release cytokines, e.g. IL-1, -6, granulocyte–macrophage colony-stimulating factor;
(5)   non-specific CD4+ T cells are attracted to the area;
(6&7) macrophages are attracted to the skin and downregulation occurs associated with prostaglandin E release.

Lupus erythematosus

Discoid lupus erythematosus

This is a benign form of lupus which usually affects the face, and other sun-exposed areas. There may be a history of Raynaud's phenomenon or chilblains. In some, there may also be a history of arthralgia. The rash of discoid lupus usually affects the face, but may occur on the neck, arms, and legs, and in the scalp. There are circumscribed plaques, which are usually bilateral but not symmetrical. Where it affects the scalp, there is scarring alopecia. Within the plaques there is obvious follicular plugging. In some, scarring is prominent and in dark skinned races there may be depigmentation. In lupus profundus, there is a lupus panniculitis.

On histological examination of the skin, there are a number of characteristic features including liquefaction degeneration of the basal layer of the epidermis, hyalinization and fibrinoid change in the subepidermal region, and peri-appendageal infiltrate. IgG or IgM and C3, usually in a granular pattern may be demonstrated at the dermo-epidermal junction. Laboratory investigations may reveal anaemia, leucopenia, or thrombocytopenia. Antinuclear antibodies are found in 35% patients, and antibodies to single-stranded DNA in about 15% cases.

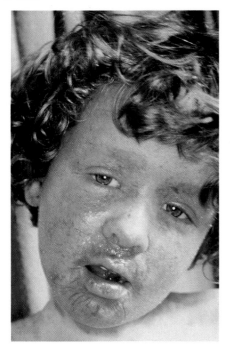

The treatment of discoid lupus depends mainly on adequate sunscreening, potent topical steroids, and antimalarials, e.g. chloroquine, hydroxychloroquine. Usually discoid lupus runs a chronic but benign course with only 6% developing systemic lupus erthematosus (SLE).

Subacute cutaneous lupus erythematosus

This is a 'halfway house' between discoid lupus and SLE. It comprises about 10% patients with lupus. It is characterized by the development of erythematous plaques, some of which have an annular configuration on the upper trunk, and outer aspects of the arms. These resolve leaving areas of depigmentation. There may also be oral ulceration, nail fold dilatation, and reticulate livedo. Some have fever, malaise, and arthralgias.

The histology of these lesions is similar to those in discoid lupus erythematosus. Antinuclear antibodies are found in over 50% patients, with anti-Ro and anti-La antibodies. The prognosis and treatment is similar to that in discoid lupus erythematosus.

∎ **Fig. 18.22** Atopic dermatitis with involvement of the face.

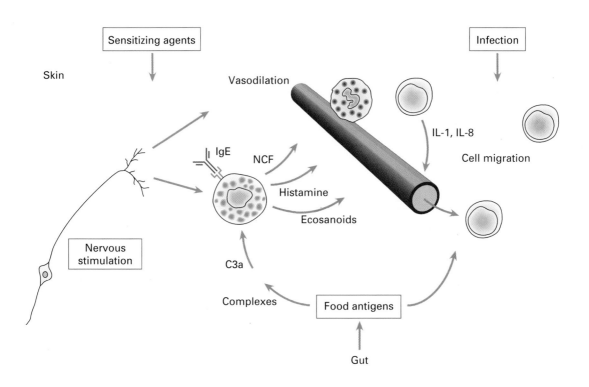

∎ **Fig. 18.23** Factors influencing atopic dermatitis.

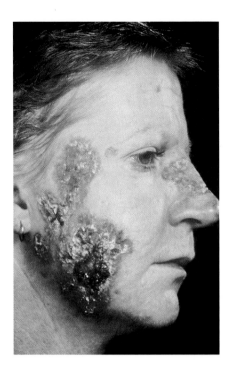

▌ Fig. 18.24 Discoid lupus erythematosus affecting the face.

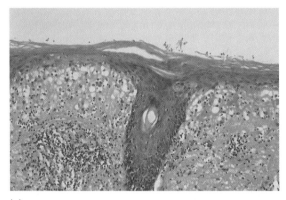

(a)

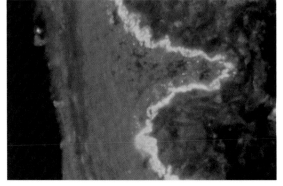

(b)

Scleroderma

This constitutes a spectrum of disease which is discussed elsewhere. As in lupus, it may be a multisystem disease, but in two variants the disease is confined to the skin.

Morphoea and linear scleroderma

This is characterized by localized sclerosis in the skin, i.e. a plaque or linear configuration. It presents as a bluish area in the skin, which undergoes sclerosis becoming an ivory colour. It may be found on the face and scalp, on the trunk, or on the limbs (usually linear on the limbs).

On histological examination there is fibrosis, and IgM and C3 may be found at the dermo-epidermal junction. There are no serological abnormalities. It often resolves spontaneously.

Generalized morphoea

The skin sclerosis usually starts on the trunk and it coalesces to become generalized, joint pains and a history of Raynaud's phenomenon are present in some The disease is very similar to that seen in chronic graft-versus-host disease.

Immunofluorescence of the skin may show IgM and C3 at the basement membrane and in the dermal blood vessels. There may be antinuclear antibodies present in the serum. The disease runs a chronic, progressive course. Steroids are useful in some cases.

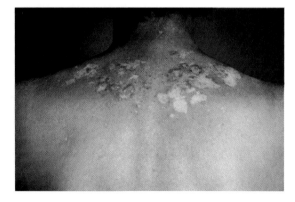

▌ Fig. 18.26 Subacute cutaneous lupus erythematosus affecting the neck and shoulders.

▌ Fig. 18.25 Lupus erythematosus. (a) Peri-appendageal infiltrate, and degeneration of basal layer (haematoxylin and eosin). (b) Granular staining at dermo-epidermal junction with C3.

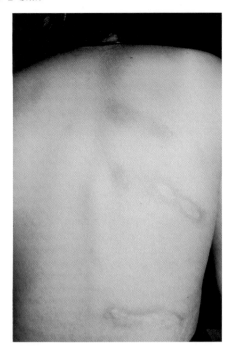

Fig. 18.27 Morphoea, with linear areas of induration on the trunk.

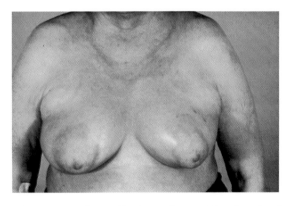

Fig. 18.28 Generalized morphoea, with sclerosis of the skin.

Skin cancer

There are three common types of epidermal skin cancers: malignant melanoma, basal cell carcinoma (BCC), and squamous cell carcinoma. All three epidermal skin tumours, may undergo spontaneous regression and may disappear completely. There is evidence to suggest that this regression is immunologically mediated.

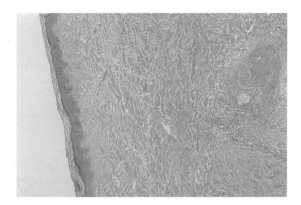

Fig. 18.29 Generalized morphoea (scleroderma) (haematoxylin and eosin).

Malignant melanoma

This skin tumour derived from melanocytes may metastasize early and has a bad prognosis: but in 4% of cases the primary tumour regresses completely leaving residual metastases.

It is likely that more tumours regress completely where there have been no metastases. The incidence of this phenomenon is unknown. However, on histological examination, roughly 25% of tumours show evidence of early or late regression.

Early regression is characterized by infiltration of the tumour by T lymphocytes, which appear to be breaking up the tumour nests. In intermediate and late regression, there is neovascularization and fibrosis with little evidence of active tumour. Studies of regressing tumours have demonstrated that the lymphocytes involved in this regression are activated CD4+ T lymphocytes, and the regression is probably mediated by cytokines. Treatment of metastatic melanoma is at present unsatisfactory, but vaccines

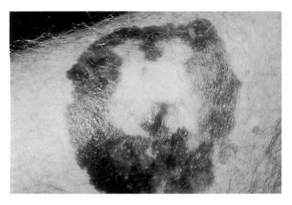

Fig. 18.30 Regressing malignant melanoma showing central depigmentation and regression.

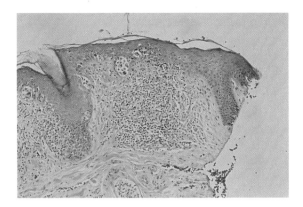

▌ **Fig. 18.31** Regressing superficial spreading melanoma (haematoxylin and eosin).

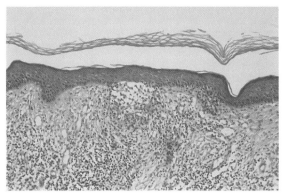

▌ **Fig. 18.33** Regressing basal cell carcinoma (haematoxylin and eosin).

containing cytokines and tumour infiltrating lymphocytes are currently undergoing trials.

Basal cell carcinoma

It is believed that spontaneous regression also occurs in BCC. This is supported by the fact that in trials of interferon α in the treatment of BCC, 20% of tumours in the placebo arm of the trial underwent spontaneous regression. BCC very rarely metastasize, and there has been no description of patients with metastases where the primary has regressed completely as occurs in malignant melanoma. The incidence of spontaneous regression in BCC is unknown, but on histological examination more than 50% of tumours show some evidence of regression. Clinically, regression is most commonly seen in superficial BCCs, where there may be marked central scarring.

The histological features of regression in BCC are similar to those in malignant melanoma: the tumour is

infiltrated by CD4+ T lymphocytes, which appear to be causing fragmentation of the tumour and disruption of the pallisading. There is marked apoptosis, and later there is neovascularization and fibrosis. Regression can be induced artifically by intralesional injections of interferon α.

Squamous cell carcinoma

There are two variants of squamous cell carcinoma which undergo spontaneous regression as part of their natural history, keratoacanthoma and familial self-healing epithelioma (the gene for which is on chromosome 9, as is the case in familial melanoma and naevoid BCC syndrome).

Keratoacanthoma

This is a form of squamous cell carcinoma which grows for about 6 weeks and then undergoes spontaneous regression. However, in immunosuppressed patients, the

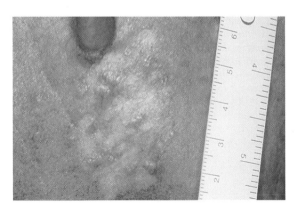

▌ **Fig. 18.32** Regression in a superficial basal cell carcinoma adjacent to the pinna of the (R) ear.

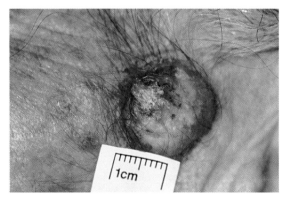

▌ **Fig. 18.34** Keratoacanthoma, which undergoes spontaneous regression as part of its natural history.

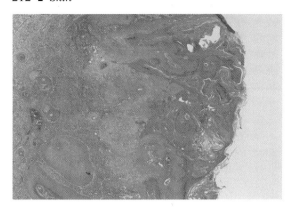

▮ .**Fig. 18.35** Keratoacanthoma, showing central keratin plug (haematoxylin and eosin).

tumour may continue to grow, reaching large proportions, and may metastasize. This is a similar situation to mice which when injected with regressor skin tumour cells, develop a progressor tumour due to the immunosuppressive effects of ultraviolet light.

The histology of clinical keratoacanthoma is very variable. Normally, the picture is of a well differentiated squamous cell carcinoma, with a distinctive configuration, but some have a very poorly differentiated histology. Surprisingly, even those with poorly differentiated histology may be effectively treated by curettage alone without recurrence. A recent study has shown that keratoacanthomas contain significantly more CD4-activated T cells (CD4+) cells infiltrating the tumour, compared with the squamous cell carcinomas, suggesting that these cells play an important part in the regression of the tumour.

Familial self-healing epithelioma

This is an interesting, but rare, condition which is due to an aberrant gene on chromosome 9. These patients have a tendency to develop squamous cell carcinomas on exposed sites in early adulthood. This tendency continues through adult life. The histology of the tumours is typical of squamous cell carcinoma, and does not have the distinctive configuration of keratoacanthoma. As its name suggests, most tumours regress spontaneously; however, a small number may proceed to invasive carcinomas with metastases.

Further reading

Anhalt, G. J., Kim, S. C., Stanley, J. R., Korman, N. J., Jabs, D. A., Kory, M., *et al.* (1990). Paraneoplastic pemphigus. An autoimmune mucocutaneous disease associated with neoplasia. *New England Journal of Medicine*, **323**, 1729–35.

Black, M. M. (1994). New observations on pemphigoid 'herpes' gestationis. *Dermatology*, **189**, 50–1.

Diaz, L. A., Sampaio, S. A., Rivitti, E. A., Martins, C. R., Cunha, P. R., Lombardi, C., *et al.* (1989). Endemic pemphigus foliaceus (fogo selvagem). I. Clinical features and immunopathology. *Journal of American Academy of Dermatology*, **20**, 657–69.

Goodless, D. R., Dhawan, S. S., Alexis, J., and Wiszniak, J. (1990). Cutaneous periarteritis nodosa. *International Journal of Dermatology*, **29**, 611–15.

Hide, M., Francis, D. M., Grattan, C. E. H., Hakimi, J., Kochan, J. P., and Greaves, M. W. (1993). Autoantibodies against the high-affinity IgG receptor as a cause of histamine release in chronic urticaria. *New England Journal of Medicine*, **328**, 1599–604.

Hunt, M. J., Halliday, G. M., Weedon, D., Cooke, B. E., and Barnetson, R. StC. (1994). Regression in basal cell carcinoma: an immunohistochemical analysis. *British Journal of Dermatology*, **130**, 1–8.

Jorizzo, J. L. (1993). Classification of vasculitis. *Journal of Investigative Dermatology*, **100**, 106–10S.

Norris, D. A. (1993). Pathomechanisms of photosensitive lupus erythematosus. *Journal of Investigative Dermatology*, **100**, 58–68S.

Ohadera, Y., Shimuzu, H., Hashimoto, T., Ishiko, A., Ebihara, T., Tanaka, M., and Nishikawa, T. (1994). Difference in binding sites of autoantibodies against 230 and 180 kD bullous pemphigoid antigens on salt split skin. *Journal of Investigative Dermatology*, **102**, 686–90.

Patel, A., Halliday, G. M., Cooke, B. E., and Barnetson, R. StC. (1994). Evidence that regression in keratoacanthoma is immunologically mediated: a comparison with squamous cell carcinoma. *British Journal of Dermatology*, **131**, 789–98.

Tefany, F. J., Barnetson, R. StC., Halliday, G. M., McCarthy, S. W., and McCarthy, W. H. (1991). Immunocytochemical analysis of the cellular infiltrate in primary regressing and non-regressing malignant melanoma. *Journal of Investigative Dermatology*, **97**, 197–202.

Tanaka, T., Furukawa, F., and Imamura, S. (1994). Epitope mapping for epidermolysis bullosa acquisita autoantibody by molecularly cloned cDNA for type VII collagen. *Journal of Investigative Dermatology*, **102**, 706–709.

19 Eye

D. Wakefield and P. McCluskey

Immunological features of the eye

The eye has several unique immunological features that result from its distinctive anatomical, physiological, and biochemical characteristics. The lens and cornea, for example, are avascular and thus ocular antigens reach the vascular system in low concentration by slow diffusion. Antibodies and lymphocytes are thus restricted in their ability to gain access readily to ocular antigens. The anterior chamber of the eye, cornea, and lens are regarded as 'immunologically privileged' sites. Recent studies indicate that immune privilege in the eye is not absolute in that immune responses, such as delayed rejection of allogeneic grafts implanted in the anterior chamber of the eye, are slowly rejected. Lens proteins may act as autoantigens and result in phacogenic uveitis should these antigens reach the systemic circulation and generate an immune response. Similarly, the retina enjoys a considerable measure of freedom from immune surveillance as a result of the blood–retinal barrier. Retinal antigens, such as retinal S antigen and antigens derived from the photoreceptor layer, may act as potent autoantigens in the induction of uveitis. In contrast, the conjunctiva, uvea, and sclera are very vascular structures, easily accessible to cells and molecules of the immune system. They are therefore the principal sites of ocular immunological diseases. The most common and clinically important ocular immune diseases are outlined in Table 19.1.

Contact dermatitis

Introduction
Several types of eczema or dermatitis affect the eyelids, periocular skin, and conjunctiva.

▌ **Table 19.1**   Ocular immune diseases

Anatomical sites	Immunological diseases
Eyelids	Contact and atopic dermatitis
	Keratoconjunctivitis
	Myasthenia gravis
Extraocular muscles	Myasthenia gravis
	Graves' ophthalmopathy
Conjunctiva	Allergic conjunctivitis
	Keratoconjunctivitis
	Bullous diseases
	Sjögren's syndrome
	Sarcoidosis
Cornea	Herpetic keratitis
	Corneal graft rejection
	Bullous diseases
	Amyloidosis
Sclera and episclera	Scleritis
	Episcleritis
Lens	Lens-induced uveitis
Uvea	Uveitis
	Choroiditis
Retina	Retinitis
	Retinal vasculitis
Optic nerve	Optic neuritis
	Multiple sclerosis
	Giant cell arteritis

Contact dermatitis usually occurs under two circumstances. The periocular skin may be inflamed as a result of the application of a direct irritant. The common causes of this include: cosmetics, mascara, eye liner, detergents, and soaps. The second type is a delayed-type hypersensitivity reaction, often as a result of contact with metals, such as nickel and chromium, resins, topical antibiotics, and antihistamines.

Clinical features

Contact dermatitis presents with a marked redness and burning of the skin following exposure to an allergen. There is pruritus often associated with increased lacrimation and photophobia. The disease may be chronic or persistent in nature. The skin may be papular, vesicular, or bullous. The lesions usually become crusted and in the chronic phase develops psoriaform-like scaling plaques. Histologically, there is a spongiform dermatitis.

Immunopathogenesis

The delayed-type hypersensitivity response is mediated by Langerhans cells in the skin which take up antigen(s) and present these to local T cells, resulting in a cell-mediated immune response to the offending antigen(s).

Diagnosis

The diagnosis of contact dermatitis is clinical and is based on the appearance of the skin and history of allergen exposure. Biopsy is rarely necessary.

Therapy

Treatment involves avoiding the offending agent or allergen. Topical corticosteroids may be required in refractory or chronic cases, together with the application of moisturizers.

Atopic dermatitis

Introduction

Atopic dermatitis is a recurrent inflammatory condition of the skin that commonly occurs in genetically predisposed individuals. It is often associated with a personal or family history of eczema, hay fever, or asthma. Atopic children may develop a severe chronic keratoconjunctivitis termed vernal keratoconjunctivitis which burns out following adolescence. Adults may develop a clinically identical severe keratoconjunctivitis termed atopic keratoconjunctivitis.

Immunopathogenesis

The pathogenesis of this disease is believed to involve a type 1 hypersensitivity reaction. Immunopathology of the ocular lesions reveals that there is a marked T-cell infiltrate in addition to the mast cells and polymorphs which are typical of an acute allergic response. There is also prominent subepithelial conjunctival fibrosis.

A variety of systemic immunological abnormalities have been described in patients with atopic dermatitis. Such individuals frequently have elevated serum immunoglobulin (Ig) E levels, T-cell lymphopenia with decreased delayed-type hypersensitivity reactions and lymphocyte transformation.

Clinical features

Atopic keratoconjunctivitis is the most severe form of ocular allergy. The signs are similar to those of seasonal and perennial allergic conjunctivitis except that they are much more florid and severe, chronic, and resistant to simple measures. Severe atopic keratoconjunctivitis is associated with corneal ulceration (shield ulceration) and can lead to corneal scarring and even perforation.

Ocular infections, especially herpes simplex keratitis and staphylococcal blepharitis, occur with increased frequency in atopic individuals. Herpes simplex ocular infection in patients with severe atopy is an extremely difficult management problem.

Patients with atopic dermatitis involving the eyelids and periocular skin should be assessed by an ophthalmologist to determine the extent of ocular involvement and to ensure that there is no corneal involvement. A drug-induced eczematous dermatitis may also involve periocular tissue. This is seen for example in penicillin hypersensitivity reactions. Similarly, photosensitivity reactions may involve the eye. Several autoimmune diseases particularly, systemic lupus erythematosus and polymyositis, may be associated with a periocular inflammatory response and these may occur early in the course of these diseases and provide the first clue to the diagnosis of the underlying disorder.

Therapy

The cutaneous disease should be managed in the same fashion as that for the generalized form of skin disease. This consist of topical application of corticosteroids, the use of moisturizers, antihistamines, and antibiotics for secondary infections. Patients should be encouraged to avoid aggravating and exacerbating factors.

Severe ocular involvement is sight threatening and is an indication for systemic corticosteroid therapy. Systemic steroids may also be necessary at the time of ocular surgery to prevent a severe flare of keratoconjunctivitis. Topical cyclosporin A therapy will be particularly useful for atopic keratoconjunctivitis when an active form of the drug becomes available.

Allergic conjunctivitis

Introduction

Allergic conjunctivitis is a common, recurrent inflammatory disease that occurs frequently in both normal and atopic individuals. There is a seasonal and a perennial form.

Clinical features

Patients often have associated eczema, hay fever, and asthma. Acute allergic conjunctivitis is most common in young children and adolescents and there is a seasonal variation in frequency of the disease, being more common in spring and summer. The usual complaints are pruritus, photophobia, and increased lacrimation.

There is no seasonal variation in the perennial form of allergic conjunctivitis which may also occur in patients with a history of allergies. Symptoms include pruritus, dryness, photophobia, and mild blurring of vision. Slit-lamp examination reveals chemosis, conjunctival injection, and papillae, especially in the upper eyelid (Fig. 19.1). The cornea and anterior chamber are normal in patients with allergic conjunctivitis.

Clinical assessment should involve a careful history to ascertain possible allergens that may precipitate or aggravate the disease. Immediate hypersensitivity skin test (skin prick tests) may help in identifying specific allergens as may a radioallergosorbent (RAST) test.

Immunopathogenesis

The pathogenesis of this disease is believed to be related to a type 1 hypersensitivity reaction in response to aeroallergens. Common allergens include: pollens, grasses, animal dander, house dust and house dust mite, and moulds.

Therapy

The management of allergic conjunctivitis involves allergen avoidance and symptomatic treatment. Hyposensitization may be effective in selected cases. Symptomatic treatment may be achieved with topical application of corticosteroids and antihistamines. These should only be used for short periods of time to avoid side-effects. A short course of oral corticosteroids may provide dramatic symptomatic relief in refractory cases.

Cicatricial pemphigoid

Introduction

Ocular cicatricial pemphigoid (OCP) is a chronic scarring disease of the conjunctiva. Although the eye may be extensively affected by a variety of bullous skin diseases, including Steven–Johnson syndrome and pemphigus, chronic cicatricial pemphigoid is the most common bullous disease to affect the ocular surface.

Clinical features

The disease occurs most frequently in older patients. Cicatricial pemphigoid follows a chronic, insidious course with formation of subepidermal blisters that rupture damaging the conjunctival surface and extensive fibrosis of the conjunctiva with formation of adhesions (symblepharon) between the bulbar and palpebral conjunctiva and resultant loss of the conjunctival fornices (Fig. 19.2). OCP is a blinding disease with a poor prognosis as patients lose vision from corneal scarring and opacity as a result of severe ocular dryness and damage from eyelid and eyelash abnormalities.

The diagnosis is made clinically by the recognition of the typical conjunctival scarring, eyelid deformity,

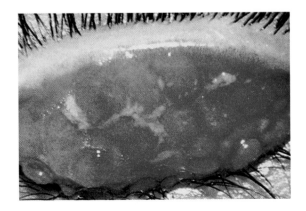

∎ **Fig. 19.1** Allergic conjunctivitis.

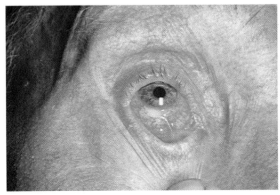

∎ **Fig. 19.2** Ocular cicatricial pemphigoid.

dryness, and hyperkeratosis of the conjunctiva. Biopsy of conjunctival lesions reveals deposition of IgG, IgA, and complement on the basement membrane in the majority of patients. A disease clinically similar to cicatricial pemphigoid may complicate the long-term use of eye drops and is due most commonly to either the preservatives in the medications or glaucoma medications such as pilocarpine and adrenaline.

Immunopathogenesis

Bullous pemphigoid is an antibody-mediated disease. Immunofluoresence studies have demonstrated deposition of immunoglobulin and complement components, together with fibrin, on the basement membrane of the skin and conjunctiva.

Therapy

OCP is a difficult management problem. Systemic immunosuppressive therapy has been shown dramatically to slow the rate of progression of the disease and to decrease visual loss. High-dose systemic corticosteroids halt the progression of the disease but are often associated with significant side-effects in older patients. A variety of immunosuppressive drugs have been used in combination with corticosteroids in this disease. These include azathioprine, methotrexate, cyclophosphamide, and cyclosporin.

The therapeutic approach to patients in the active phase of this disease is twofold. The first phase involves the use of immunosuppressive drugs to halt the progression of blistering and scarring. Secondly, and just as important, are local measures to prevent additional scarring. These include the removal of abnormally directed eyelashes, adequate tear film maintenance, and surgery to correct lid deformities. Ocular surgery is quite hazardous in these patients due to the severe disturbance of the ocular surface and tear film and should be approached carefully.

Corneal transplantation

Introduction

Corneal transplantation remains the most common and successful form of organ transplantation in humans. In optimum circumstances, the success rate is greater than 95%. The remarkable success of this procedure is due to many factors, including: the avascular nature of the cornea, the relative immunological privilege of the anterior chamber of the eye, and the ability to apply potent immunosuppressive therapy locally. The commonest indications for corneal transplantation include: corneal dystrophies such as keratoconus, corneal scars

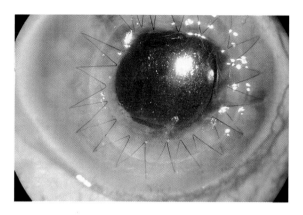

■ **Fig. 19.3** Corneal transplant rejection.

from infection and trauma, and corneal decompensation as a result of previous intraocular surgery.

Clinical features

There are two types of corneal grafts. Partial thickness (lamellar) grafts do not include the donor endothelium, are used for non-visual repair of the cornea and sclera and are not affected by severe graft rejection reactions. Full thickness (penetrating) corneal grafts include the donors endothelium, are the usual form of corneal transplantation and may fail as a result of graft rejection. All patients require topical corticosteroids after corneal graft surgery to prevent rejection. This may be lifelong in patients at high risk of graft rejection, such as those with vascularized corneas or those who have had multiple transplants. Graft rejection may occur at any time following grafting but is commonest in the first year after surgery. Graft rejection directed at the corneal endothelium is the most common and serious reaction as the endothelium is not reconstituted by the cornea and damage will ultimately lead to graft failure (Fig. 19.3). It has a characteristic slit-lamp appearance. There may be an identifiable local (e.g. suture removal) or systemic (e.g. immunization) trigger which precipitates the rejection episode.

Immunopathogenesis

Graft rejection occurs in response to human leucocyte antigen (HLA) and corneal antigens present in the graft tissue that are recognized as foreign by the host. This is particularly likely to occur in patients who have a history of previous graft rejection or who have extensively vascularized corneas. The process of corneal healing and scarring allows access to the cornea of cells of the immune system to the grafted tissue which participate in the immune response and lead to a graft rejection. The process of graft rejections involves humeral and cellular immune responses and has been previously outlined.

Management

As in other organ transplants, increased immunosuppressive therapy may ameliorate graft rejection. In the cornea, intensive topical and periocular corticosteroid therapy will often control graft rejection. Severe or advanced graft rejection may respond to oral or intravenous corticosteroid treatment. High-risk patients benefit from prophylactic therapy using cyclosporin A for 1 year following transplantation.

Sjögren's syndrome

Introduction

Sjögren's syndrome (SS) is a common systemic autoimmune disorder characterized by lymphocyte-mediated destruction of exocrine glands leading to diminished or absent glandular secretion. It may present as a primary disease process or in association with other systemic autoimmune diseases (Table 19.2 and 19.3).

Clinical features

Primary SS has been defined as the presence of keratoconjunctivitis sicca and xerostomia in the absence of another well-defined autoimmune or rheumatic disease. Patients with primary SS frequently have systemic autoimmune manifestations (e.g. autoantibodies and vasculitis), but their symptoms do not satisfy criteria for a diagnosis of an autoimmune disease such as rheumatoid arthritis or systemic lupus erythematosus Secondary SS syndrome can be associated with a variety of autoimmune diseases as outlined in Table 19.3. The exact prevalence of SS is unknown, although it is probably the second most common autoimmune disease after rheumatoid arthritis, which occurs in about 1% of the population. About one-third of patients with rheumatoid arthritis have secondary SS. Several studies have shown that 90% of patients with primary SS are females. Primary SS is commonest in the fifth and sixth decades of life but can occur at any age. The age and sex distribution of secondary SS follows that of the accompanying autoimmune disease. The differential diagnosis of SS is outlined in Table 19.4.

Ocular manifestations

Ocular symptoms occur secondary to atrophy of the secretory epithelium of the major and minor lacrimal glands. While all patients with keratoconjunctivitis sicca are by definition lacking in tear secretion, only 60% complain of dry eyes. About 80% of patients complain of ocular grittiness, burning, or a foreign body sensation. Approximately 50% of patients will complain of red eyes and a third complain of itch. Other complaints include: ocular soreness (57%),

---

▌ **Table 19.2** Diagnostic and distinguishing characteristics of primary and secondary Sjögren's syndrome

Primary
Keratoconjunctivitis sicca with minor salivary gland biopsy showing lymphocytic infiltration.
Extraglandular features may be present, including: pneumonitis, nephritis, neuropathies, etc.
Patients with sicca syndrome alone have a greater frequency of enlarged parotid glands, Raynaud's phenomenon, purpura, lymphadenopathy, myositis, and renal involvement.
HLA-B8 and DR3-positive.
Antinuclear antibodies specific to SS-A and/or SS-B

Secondary
Keratoconjunctivitis sicca with minor salivary gland biopsy showing lymphocytic infiltration, indistinguishable from primary Sjögren's syndrome.
The presence of established rheumatoid arthritis or other connective tissue disease.
Serological and immunogenetic findings consistent with the underlying or associated rheumatic disorder (e.g. HLA-DR4 in rheumatoid arthritis and HLA-DR3 in systemic lupus erythematosus)

Exclusions
Sarcoidosis, lymphoma, pemphigoid, amyloidosis, haemochromatosis
Acquired immune deficiency syndrome (AIDS)
Graft-versus-host disease

HLA, human leucocyte antigen.

▮ **Table 19.3** Autoimmune diseases associated with secondary Sjögren's syndrome

Rheumatoid arthritis
Systemic lupus erythematosus
Progressive systemic sclerosis
Primary biliary cirrhosis
Chronic active hepatitis
Polymyositis
Addison's disease
Autoimmune thyroiditis
Mixed connective tissue disease
Mixed cryglobulinaemia
Hypergammaglobulinaemic purpura

▮ **Table 19.4** Sjögren's syndrome differential diagnosis

Ageing (sicca complex)
Sarcoidosis
Amyloidosis
Autoimmune disease, AIDS (HIV) rheumatoid arthritis, graft-versus-host disease, systemic lupus erythematosus, mixed connective tissue disease, scleroderma

Infection
    Acute bacterial/viral (Epstein–Barr virus, cytomegalovirus, mumps, HIV)
    Chronic (tuberculosis, syphilis, actinomycosis, histoplasmosis)

Neoplasms
    Lacrimal tumours (cysts, epithelial, lymphoreticular)
    Primary salivary tumor
    Malignant lymphoma
    Waldenström's disease

Drugs
    Anticholinergic drugs, tricyclic antidepressants, Diuretics, decongestants

Miscellaneous
    Hyperlipidaemias, bulemia
    Malnutrition, diabetes

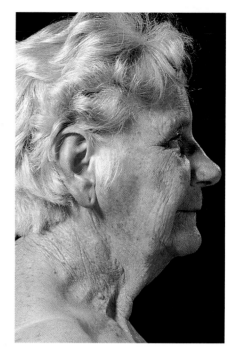

▮ **Fig. 19.4** Sjögren's syndrome: parotid gland enlargement.

diminished visual acuity (32%), and photophobia (53% of patients). Patients often complain of a tenacious, adherent ocular mucus which collects at the inner canthus. Affected patients have difficulty tolerating contact lenses, air-conditioned environments, and characteristically have greater problems in warm, dry climates. Chronic severe dryness produces recurrent corneal ulceration and scarring which may produce significant visual loss. Parotid gland enlargement is common (Fig. 19.4), while lacrimal gland enlargement is uncommon, but well recognized, as is the development of uveitis.

Tear production may be assessed using the Schirmer's test. Schirmer's test can be performed with or without the prior instillation of a local anaesthetic. A Schirmer's test strip is placed in the inferior fornix of each eye. The distance of wetting in each strip is calculated for each eye after 5 min. A distance of less than 5 mm of wetting is considered abnormal. Rose Bengal staining may be used to assess the effects of dryness on both corneal and conjunctival epithelium. A 1% solution of Rose Bengal is instilled into the lower fornix after applying local anaesthesia. Staining of the bulbar conjunctiva or cornea is considered abnormal. Usually multiple erosions over the cornea and conjunctiva are seen and the degree and extent of Rose Bengal staining may be quantified.

A number of abnormalities have been reported in the tears of patients with SS, although these are of no help in the diagnosis. There is an increase in tear osmolality and a reduction in lysozyme, lactoferrin, and IgA concentrations in tear fluid. The levels of

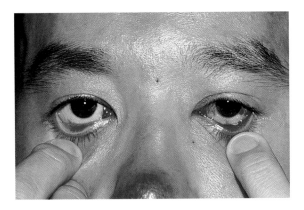

❙ Fig. 19.5 Sjögren's syndrome and keratoconjunctivitis sicca in a patient with HIV infection.

❙ Table 19.5 Products useful in the treatment of xerophthalmia

	Manufacturer	Preservative
Artificial tears		
Liquifilm	Allergan	Chlorobutanol
Liquifilm forte	Allergan	Thimersol
Tears Plus	Allergan	Chlorobutanol
Tears Naturale	Alcon	Benzalkonium
Plasma	Autologous	None
Fibronectin	Autologous	None
Ocular ointments		
Duratears	Alcon	Methylparaben
Lacrilube	Allergan	Chlorobutanol
Lacriserts	Merck	None

ceruloplasmin and IgG remain unchanged or are increased in the tear fluid of such patients.

Human immunodeficiency virus (HIV) infection and SS

SS (predominantly sicca symptoms) has been described in patients with HIV infection (Fig. 19.5) and such an aetiological factor should be considered in appropriate clinical circumstances. This clinical syndrome is usually seen in advanced HIV infection. A lymphocytic salivary infiltrate of predominantly CD8+ positive T lymphocytes may be a manifestation of HIV infection. The numbers of circulating CD8+ lymphocytes and the prevalence of HLA-DR5 are greatly increased in HIV-positive patients with sicca syndrome.

Treatment

The treatment of SS is symptomatic in the majority of patients. Drugs with anticholinergic effects including tricyclic antidepressants, antispasmodics, and antiparkinsonian therapy as well as diuretics, antihistamines, and decongestant preparations should be used cautiously in patients with SS as all of these medication may exacerbate sicca symptoms. Contact lens wear may precipitate symptoms in patients with early SS and is best avoided.

Effective treatment of xerophthalmia is important but difficult, and requires commitment from both patient and physician. The mainstays of treatment are artificial tear-drops and ocular lubricant ointments (Table 19.5). Patients may develop contact irritant or allergic reactions to the preservatives used in these preparations and in these patients single use non-preserved drops are extremely valuable. Some patients respond favourably to topical administration of autologous serum diluted with saline. Recent clinical trials

of topical fibronectin preparations have indicated marked improvement in some patients. Punctal occlusion treatment is a valuable, often underutilized, treatment modality. Tarsorraphy may be required to protect the cornea in severe disease. Secondary infection is common and may be associated with a chronic blepharitis which needs specific treatment with lid hygiene and topical antibiotics.

Corticosteroids and immunosuppressive medications should be reserved for potentially serious systemic complications of SS, such as: myositis, vasculitis, pulmonary, renal, or central nervous system disease, and are rarely required for ocular disease.

Episcleritis

Introduction

Episcleritis refers to inflammation of the episclera, the highly vascular connective tissue which lies superficial to the sclera. Episcleritis is an acute inflammatory disease, abrupt in onset, recurrent in nature, and frequently bilateral. It is a benign disease commonly associated with an allergic diathesis, rarely associated with systemic disease, and not a threat to vision. It is occasionally seen in association with seronegative arthropathies, such as Reiter's syndrome, enteropathic arthritis and vasculitic diseases such as erythema multiforma and erythema nodosum. It may also be a manifestation of gout.

Clinical features

Patients complain of redness and irritation of the affected eye and note a burning, irritating ocular

▌ **Table 19.6** Scleral disease-selective investigations

Test	Episcleritis	Scleritis
Blood	ANA, IgE Uric acid, ACE HLA-B27	FBC, ESR, ANA, ANCA, ACE LFTs, calcium HLA-B27
Serology	Syphilis	Syphilis, *Lyme borrelia*, HZV, HSV, toxoplasmosis
Microbiology		Viral, bacterial, (mycobacterial), fungal cultures
Skin tests	Immediate hypersensitivity (allergy) tests	Mantoux, Kveim
Radiology	CXR, sacro-iliac joints	CXR, sacro-iliac joints, B scan, CT/MRI — eye + other organs
Biopsy	Episclera	Episclera, mucosa skin and other involved organs

ANA, antinuclear antibody; ACE, angiotensin-converting enzyme; CXR, chest X-ray; FBC, full blood count; ESR, erythrocyte sedimentation rate, ANCA, antineutrophil cytoplasmic antibody; LFT, liver function test; HZV, herpes zoster virus; HSV, herpes simplex virus.

discomfort, photophobia, and watering. There is no pain. Vasodilatation of the superficial episcleral vessels and oedema of the episclera are the cardinal signs of episcleral inflammation. The globe is not tender to palpation and vision is not affected. Keratitis, uveitis, and other intraocular inflammation are absent. Vision is normal.

Investigations are usually not necessary in patients with episcleritis as the majority of patients clearly have idiopathic disease on clinical assessment (Table 19.6).

Immunopathogenesis

Episcleritis may be produced by a variety of immune and non-immune mechanisms. Immune mechanisms may involve acute hypersensitivity responses (type I hypersensitivity) mediated by IgE-mediated degranulation of mucosal mast cells. Immune complex-mediated reactions (type III hypersensitivity) may occur in vasculitic diseases involving the episclera and delayed type hypersensitivity (type IV) reactions are seen in granulomatous diseases such as sarcoidosis, tuberculosis, and syphilis.

Management

Episcleritis is evanescent in many patients and may not require any therapy. It responds rapidly to local anti-inflammatory therapy in the vast majority of patients who require treatment. Patients who require systemic treatment for episcleritis should be assessed critically as episcleritis is often not the correct diagnosis in such patients.

Scleritis

Introduction

Scleritis is a chronic, severe, destructive inflammation of the sclera and is usually profoundly symptomatic, except for scleromalacia perforans which is a rare but well-recognized asymptomatic form of severe scleritis seen only in patients with severe rheumatoid arthritis. Scleritis is classified clinically into anterior and posterior types, with anterior scleritis further subclassified into diffuse, nodular, and necrotizing forms.

Clinical features

The disease occurs in all age groups and is most common in the fourth to sixth decades. There is a variable female preponderance of patients with scleritis with a female to male ratio of about 1.5:1.

Scleritis most commonly involves the anterior sclera (85–90%), but may also involve the posterior sclera, either in isolation or as spread from the anterior sclera. Up to 50% of patients with scleritis develop bilateral disease. Bilateral scleritis occurs nearly twice as frequently in patients with systemic disease.

The hallmark of scleritis is pain, and its severity, characteristic boring nature, facial radiation, and nocturnal worsening have been recognized since the earliest descriptions of the disease. Patients may also note other symptoms including: ocular redness, photophobia, lacrimation, and epiphoria. Corneal or posterior segment involvement may result in a change in vision.

The essential sign of scleritis is scleral oedema and this is usually accompanied by intense injection and tenderness of the globe. Careful ocular examination

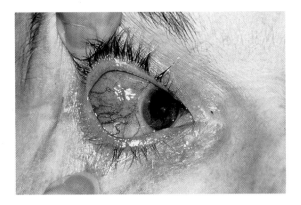

▌Fig. 19.6 Nodular scleritis.

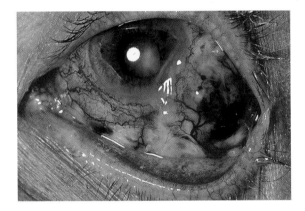

▌Fig. 19.7 Scleromalacia perforans.

reveals maximal dilatation of the deep episcleral vascular plexus and the presence of underlying scleral oedema which allow the diagnosis of scleritis to be made. Its severity is graded by the presence of additional signs such as scleral nodules (Fig. 19.6) or scleral necrosis (Fig. 19.7).

Immunopathogenesis

Histologically, the changes of anterior and posterior scleritis are identical and include a proliferative inflammatory cell infiltrate composed principally of T cells, plasma cells, macrophages, and occasionally granulomas. Associated with this cellular response, fibrinoid necrosis, and fibrin deposition are usually evident. The histopathological features of scleritis are those of a chronic granulomatous inflammation. Granulomatous inflammation adjacent to or involving scleral blood vessels may represent a cell-mediated immune response to local antigens or immune complex deposition producing a localized vasculitis. Episcleral biopsies in patients with active scleritis

reveal a vasculitis, which is believed to be the basic pathological lesion in most types of scleritis.

Scleritis may result from a variety of immune and a non-immune mechanisms. Immunopathological studies of available ocular tissue, have revealed evidence of local immune complex deposition and cell-mediated immunity in scleritis lesions. Other studies have documented a spectrum of systemic immunological abnormalities in patients with scleritis. Evidence from our laboratory suggests a specific immune response may be directed towards scleral antigens in some patients.

Management

The initial step in the management of patients with scleritis is to make the correct diagnosis. This is based on a careful history, detailed examination, and appropriate investigations. The aims of investigation of the patient with scleritis are to evaluate the severity and extent of the scleritis and to exclude the presence of an associated systemic disease or infiltrative process. It is essential for associated systemic disease to be diagnosed both clinically and with laboratory investigations, as it is well recognized that scleritis may be the initial presentation of a potentially fatal systemic illness, such as Wegener's granulomatosis.

Approximately 50% of patients with scleritis have an associated systemic disease. The clinician must therefore carefully exclude associated disease by clinical assessment and appropriate selective further investigation. A complete medical history, comprehensive ocular examination and a careful review of systems particularly directed towards symptoms of clinical entities known to be associated with scleritis are the essential first step in the investigation and management of the patient with scleritis. Investigations are selected on the results of the clinical assessment to rule out specific disease entities (Table 19.6).

The treatment of scleritis always requires systemic therapy and must be individualized according to the severity of the patients disease, response to treatment, side-effects, and the presence of associated disease.

High-dose systemic corticosteroids are an effective form of therapy in patients with scleritis. Unfortunately, this form of therapy is often associated with unacceptable side-effects and is therefore not always able to induce a remission in patients with severe scleritis. Common complications of corticosteroids may severely limit the usefulness of this drug in individual patients. Corticosteroids may be given orally on a daily or alternate day basis, or as intermittent intravenous or oral pulse doses. High-dose intravenous methylprednisolone has proved both safe and effective in bringing about remission in patients with scleritis. Pulse methylprednisolone therapy has advantages similar to those of alternate day oral corticosteroids in reducing the side-effects of corticosteroids.

Patients whose scleritis is not controlled with corticosteroids require additional immunosuppressive therapy. The decision to use such potent and potentially hazardous drugs should only be taken after careful consultation and consideration. In particular, the risk of permanent visual loss must be balanced against the short-term and long-term risks of immunosuppressive therapy in each patient. A number of cytotoxic drugs have been shown to be effective in treating ocular inflammatory disease including: azathioprine, cyclophosphamide, chlorambucil, methotrexate, and cyclosporin A. Azathioprine, cyclophosphamide, and cyclosporin A are the drugs most frequently used as additional immunosuppressive agents in the treatment of scleritis. Azathioprine is useful as an adjunct in the treatment of scleritis and allows the use of low-dose corticosteriods while still maintaining disease remission. Cyclophosphamide is generally considered to be the most effective drug for the treatment of severe scleritis. Cyclophosphamide may be used as a single daily oral dosage (2–3 mg/kg per day) or as intravenous pulse therapy. The long-term complications of cyclophosphamide, particularly infertility and oncogenesis, can be decreased to a certain extent by limiting duration of therapy to 6–12 months, which tends to be the duration of therapy in patients with scleritis.

Uveitis

Introduction

Inflammation of the uvea, the middle vascular coat of the eye is a relatively common ocular disease that may occur in isolation or as the first indication of a serious underlying systemic disease. Uveitis may involve the iris (iritis) and ciliary body (iridocyclitis), choroid (chorioiditis) and/or retina (retinochoroiditis). Uveitis has been classified in many ways, none of which are entirely satisfactory. Currently, an anatomical classification dividing uveitis into anterior, intermediate, posterior, and pan uveitis is used. Uveitis lasting less than 3 months is designated acute and longer duration disease is classified as chronic.

Immunological mechanisms and infection underlie the pathogenesis of many types of uveitis. There are a large number of potential causes for uveitis and a specific cause can be found in about 50% of patients with uveitis. The common aetiological agents and associated diseases are summarized in Tables 19.7 and 19.8.

Acute anterior uveitis

Introduction

Acute (AU) is a common ocular disease characterized by inflammation of the iris and ciliary body. There are a large number of diseases associated with acute AU and these are outlined in Fig. 19.9. In the majority of patients presenting with an acute attack of AU the only clues to the pathogenesis of this disease are its close association with the genetic marker HLA-B27 and the likely triggering role of a variety of Gram-negative bacteria. HLA-B27 acute AU appears to be a distinct clinical entity frequently associated with the seronegative arthropathies, such as ankylosing spondylitis and Reiter's syndrome. Recent advances in our understanding of the structure and function of class I HLA molecules has revealed their fundamental function in antigen presentation and this has led to a revaluation of their role in disease predisposition.

Clinical features

Acute AU presents with the onset of pain, redness, and photophobia over a period of hours to several days. Patients with recurrent attacks can usually recognize the prodrome of their attacks prior to the onset of clinical signs of uveitis. The signs consist of flare (increased protein concentration within the aqueous resulting in a visible light column) and cells within the anterior chamber (Fig. 19.8). There is often cellular infiltration in the anterior vitreous as well (iridocyclitis).

There may be other signs depending on the precise aetiology of the AU (e.g. corneal scarring in patients with herpetic disease) and the presence of complications such as elevated intraocular pressure, cataract, and synechiae (abnormal adhesions between the iris and other intraocular structures)

Patients with chronic AU present in an insidious manner with floaters and a change in vision. Chronic

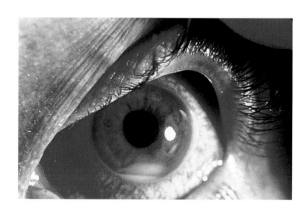

▌**Fig. 19.8**　Acute uveitis with hypopyon.

■ **Table 19.7** Ocular and laboratory features of common systemic, immune, and rheumatic diseases

Disease	Ocular manifestations	Laboratory features
Ankylosing spondylitis	Acute anterior uveitis	HLA-B27
		XR–sacro-ileitis
Reiter's syndrome	Conjunctivitis, anterior uveitis	HLA-B27
Psoriatic arthritis	Keratitis	XR-sacro-ileitis
Enteropathic arthritis	Recurrent anterior uveitis	HLA-B27
		Histopathology
Juvenile chronic arthritis	Recurrent anterior uveitis (males)	HLA-B27-
		XR–sacroileitis
	Chronic anterior uveitis and keratopathy (females)	HLA-DR5
		XR-changes
Rheumatoid arthritis	Keratoconjunctivitis sicca	↑RF, ↑/ESR
	Scleritis	↑CIC
	Scleromalacia perforans	HLA-DR4
Sjögren's syndrome	Keratoconjunctivitis sicca	RF, ↑CIC
	Scleritis	ANA, SS-A, SS-B
		HLA DR3
Systemic lupus erythematosus	Keratoconjunctivitis	ANA, DNA binding
	Scleritis	↑CIC
	Retinal vasculitis	HLA-DR3
	Cotton wool spots	
Behçet's syndrome	Conjunctivitis	↑Acute phase reactants
	Anterior uveitis	
	Retinal vasculitis	HLA-Bw51
	Retinochoroiditis	↑CIC
	Optic papilitis	
	Ophthalmoplegia	
Giant cell arteritis	Ischaemic optic neuritis	↑ESR
	Central retinal artery occlusion	Acute phase reactants
Vogt–Koyanagi–Harada syndrome	Retinal vasculitis	
	Retinal vasculitis	HLA
	Uveitis	CSF abnormalities
	Retinal detachment	

ANA, antinuclear antibody; CIC, circulating immune complexes; ESR, erythrocyte sedimentation rate; RF, rheumatoid factor; SS-A, SS-B, antibodies to nuclear antigens SSA, SSB; HLA, human leucocyte antigen.

uveitis such as that associated with juvenile chronic arthritis, may be asymptomatic. Patients with chronic AU often develop complications, such as cataract and glaucoma, as a result of their uveitis.

Immunopathogenesis

Acute AU may occur as a distinct clinical entity or in conjunction with the group of rheumatic diseases that are closely linked with HLA-B27. The strongest known association of disease with the HLA-B27 antigen is ankylosing spondylitis, in which more than 90% of patients are HLA-B27 positive. The next strongest associations are Reiter's syndrome (60%) and idiopathic acute AU with 19–88% of patients having this HLA phenotype.

Several hypotheses have been advanced to explain the association between acute AU and the HLA-B27 molecule. These hypotheses are similar to those that have been proposed for the association between the HLA-B27 antigen and rheumatic diseases, and have been the subject of several recent reviews. The basic tenant of these hypotheses has been that the HLA-B27 molecule is directly involved in the pathogenesis of uveitis and that this molecule plays a critical part in the interaction between some microbial initiating factor that leads to the development of uveal inflammation.

Aetiology and diagnosis

The aetiological diagnosis of acute AU remains a difficult and often frustrating endeavour. The vast majority of associated diseases or causes of AU can be ascertained from a careful history and physical examination (syndrome recognition, e.g. ankylosing spondylitis, reactive uveitis), supported by a small number of serological (to exclude infectious diseases, e.g. syphilis, *Lyme borreliosis*) and radiological investigations (e.g. chest X-ray for sarcoidosis and sacro-iliac joints for sacro-ileitis) (see Table 19.7).

Not all patients with uveitis require investigation. AU is a benign disease which responds readily to treatment with topical steroids and mydriatics in the vast majority of patients. However, patients with recurrent, bilateral, chronic, granulomatous, or refractory AU should be investigated.

HLA-B27 typing may be of value in the appraisal of patients with acute AU and may help in planning therapy and evaluating prognosis. This is based on the observed differences in the clinical features, associated diseases, and complications seen in patients with HLA-B27 acute AU. Such patients tend to have recurrent, unilateral disease with less severe and less frequent complications than there HLA-B27 negative counterparts. Male patients with HLA-B27 acute AU often have associated rheumatic diseases that require investigation and therapy. In the majority of such patients uveitis will respond to topical therapy with corticosteroids and cycloplegics, and the disease will run a relatively short clinical course. In contrast patients with HLA-B27 negative acute AU will more often have severe disease that may require systemic therapy. Thus knowledge of the subjects HLA-B27 status may aid in the diagnostic examination, treatment, and prognosis of patients with acute AU.

Treatment

The vast majority of patients with acute AU respond to treatment with topical steroids and mydriatics. Peribulbar corticosteroid treatment may be required in severe treatment refractory cases. Systemic treatment should be avoided in the vast majority of patients, especially those with uniocular disease. Systemic corticosteroid treatment is usually reserved for patients with chronic bilateral disease and may be necessary when vision in the better eye is reduced below 6/12 from an inflammatory mediated intraocular complication such as macular oedema.

Intermediate uveitis and pars planitis

Introduction

Intermediate uveitis and pars planitis are terms used to define a common clinical syndrome of chronic low-grade inflammation of the uveal tract whose primary focus is the peripheral retina and pars plana region of the eye. It is usually bilateral, occurs in all age groups and its aetiology is unknown. The terms intermediate uveitis and pars planitis can be considered interchangeable for the purposes of this discussion as they each describe a similar disease.

Aetiology

Intermediate uveitis is by definition idiopathic in nature. The clinical picture of intermediate uveitis can be closely mimicked by multiple sclerosis, sarcoidosis, syphilis, and Lyme disease. Intraocular lymphoma is well recognized as producing the signs and symptoms of intermediate uveitis and must always be considered in the differential diagnosis. Lymphoma may originate in the eye or may present in patients with previously diagnosed systemic lymphoma. B-cell lymphomas are the predominant type.

In patients with unilateral intermediate uveitis, there are a number of ocular syndromes such as ocular toxocariasis and Coat's disease which also should be considered. They are recognized by the ophthalmologist by their characteristic clinical pictures.

Clinical features

Intermediate uveitis often has a vague and poorly defined onset with floaters and disturbance of vision. The visual acuity is usually normal or slightly reduced. There may be mild AU. There is a mild to severe vitreous infiltrate of cells which is responsible for many of the symptoms. Some patients have a collection of inflammatory cells and fibroglial tissue overlying the pars plana of the eye termed a 'snowbank'. In these patients the term pars planitis is used and this subset of patients may develop retinal complications such as retinal detachments, related to the snowbank.

There is commonly diffuse retinal oedema, mild optic disc swelling, and macular oedema. Macular oedema is the common cause of poor vision and the usual indication for aggressive treatment. It is axiomatic that in patients with intermediate uveitis there are no focal retinal or choroidal lesions.

Pathology

Pathological studies of eyes with intermediate uveitis are based on specimens removed for end-stage ocular disease and have revealed features of chronic non-granulamatous inflammation centred on retinal blood vessels, the peripheral retina, choroid, and ciliary body. There is a perplexing preponderance of retinal inflammation in this disease which is classified clinically as a uveitis. The vitreous cells consist of aggregates of mononuclear inflammatory cells and giant cells. Snowbanks consist of organized, vascularized fibroglial tissue with a mononuclear cell infiltrate. Immunopathological studies have revealed that the infiltrate is predominantly of helper T cells with some B cells and macrophages. There are no consistent systemic immunological abnormalities in patients with intermediate uveitis.

Treatment

The vast majority of patients with intermediate uveitis do not require treatment. The usual indications for therapy are the presence of vision threatening complications of the persistent inflammation with reduction of vision below 6/12, this is usually due to the presence of macular oedema. Other complications which can affect vision include vitreous opacification, cataract, retinal neovascularization, glaucoma, and retinal detachment. These complications do not necessarily mean that aggressive medical therapy is required. Treatment must be individualized and carefully considered in conjunction with the ophthalmologist.

Many patients do well with topical and peribulbar corticosteroid treatment. Systemic treatment should be avoided in the vast majority of patients, especially those with uniocular disease. Systemic treatment is usually reserved for patients with bilateral disease and may be necessary when vision in the better eye is reduced below 6/12 from an inflammatory mediated intraocular complication, such as macular oedema.

Corticosteroids remain the preferred initial form of treatment. Owing to the chronic nature of intermediate uveitis, many corticosteroid-treated patients will require an additional agent and cyclosporin A is the logical second agent in most patients. Low-dose systemic steroids and cyclosporin A are usually well tolerated.

A small number of patients may require additional treatment including ocular surgery, such as cryotherapy or vitrectomy, or additional chemotherapy such as azathioprine or methotrexate.

Posterior uveitis

There are a large number of diseases that cause or are associated with posterior uveitis as outlined in

▮ **Table 19.8** Aetiology of uveitis

Primary disease	Anterior uveitis	Posterior and panuveitis
Infection	Herpes simplex Herpes zoster Herpes simplex Syphilis Tuberculosis Leprosy Onchocerciasis	Cytomegalovirus Herpes zoster Syphilis Tuberculosis Toxoplasmosis Toxocariasis Candidiasis Crytococcosis Histoplasmosis
Rheumatic disease	Ankylosing spondylitis Reiter's syndrome Juvenile chronic arthritis Behçet's syndrome	Behçet's syndrome
Immune ocular disorders	Phacogenic uveitis	Sympathetic ophthalmia
Trauma	Trauma/surgery	Trauma/surgery Sympathetic ophthalmia
Idiopathic	Fuchs' heterochromic cyclitis	Intermediate uveitis
Systemic diseases	Sarcoidosis Inflammatory bowel disease	Sarcoidosis Vogt–Koyanagi–Harada syndrome Multiple sclerosis

Table 19.8. The vast majority of cases remain idiopathic and are called endogenous uveitis.

Clinical features

Posterior uveitis may present with a fulminant picture of acute visual loss or with a more insidious onset of blurred vision, floaters, and decreased visual acuity. Acute choroidal and retinal lesions are pale and ill defined and there is often overlying inflammatory haze in the vitreous which results in a poor view of the lesions.

Immunopathogenesis

Humoral and cell-mediated immune mechanisms are thought to be involved in the pathogenesis of many forms of uveitis. Immune complexes have been detected in serum and aqueous humor in a variety of forms of uveitis, including Behçet's syndrome, sarcoidosis, sympathetic ophthalmia (SO), lens-induced or phacogenic uveitis, and idiopathic uveitis. Autoantibodies to a variety of uveal and retinal antigens (e.g. retinal S antigen) have also been described in patients with endogenous uveitis, indicating that antibody-mediated or antibody-dependent cellular cytotoxic mechanisms may be involved. Similarly, T-cell-mediated immune responses to retinal and uveal antigens are believed to play an important part in the pathogenesis of endogenous uveitis.

Uveal damage due to a penetrating injury or surgical wound involving the ciliary body may lead to the development of a granulomatous uveitis or sympathetic uveitis in the opposite eye within a few weeks or months. The pathogenetic mechanism in sympathetic ophthalmia is believed to involve a cell-mediated immune response to uveal antigens, possibly related to pigmented epithelial cells. Similarly, lens damage results in release of uveitogenic antigens with subsequent antibody and immune complex formation producing a chronic form of uveitis.

Treatment

Approximately 50% of patients with uveitis have a recognizable associated systemic disease or infection (Table 19.8). The clinician must therefore carefully exclude associated disease by clinical assessment and appropriate selective further investigation. A complete medical history, comprehensive ocular examination, and a careful review of systems particularly directed towards symptoms of clinical entities known to be associated with uveitis are the essential first step in the investigation and management of such patients.

The treatment of severe bilateral endogenous uveitis often requires systemic therapy and must be individualized according to the severity of the patients disease, response to treatment, side-effects, and the presence of associated disease.

High-dose systemic corticosteroids are an effective form of therapy in patients with severe bilateral posterior uveitis. Unfortunately, this form of therapy is often associated with unacceptable side-effects and is therefore not always able to induce a remission in patients with severe uveitis. Common complications of corticosteroids may severely limit the usefulness of this drug in individual patients. Corticosteroids may be given orally on a daily or alternate day basis, or as intermittent intravenous or oral pulse doses. High-dose intravenous methylprednisolone has proved both safe and effective in bringing about remission in patients with uveitis. Pulse methylprednisolone therapy has advantages similar to those of alternate day oral corticosteroids in reducing the side-effects of corticosteroids.

Patients whose uveitis is not controlled with corticosteroids require additional immunosuppressive therapy. The decision to use such potent and potentially hazardous drugs should only be taken after careful consultation and consideration. In particular, the risk of permanent visual loss must be balanced against the short-term and long-term risks of immunosuppressive therapy in each patient. A number of cytotoxic drugs have been shown to be effective in treating ocular inflammatory disease including: azathioprine, cyclophosphamide, chlorambucil, methotrexate, and cyclosporin A. Azathioprine, cyclophosphamide, and cyclosporin A are the drugs most frequently used as additional immunosuppressive agents in the treatment of uveitis. Azathioprine is useful as an adjunct in the treatment of uveitis and allows the use of low-dose corticosteroids while still maintaining disease remission. Cyclosporin A is generally considered to be the most effective drug for the treatment of severe posterior uveitis. This drug is usually combined with administration of corticosteroids. Cyclosporin A is commenced at a dose of 5–10 mg/kg per day and the dosage is slowly reduced after the disease is controlled to a maintenance dose of 2 mg/kg/per day. Potential side-effects of cyclosporin A, such as hypertension, interstitial nephritis and gingival hypertrophy can be minimized by careful monitoring and appropriate dose modification.

Sarcoidosis

Introduction

The frequency of the ophthalmic manifestations of sarcoidosis varies widely in different populations. The selection bias of patients and the thoroughness of ocular examination, undoubtedly affect the frequency figures for ocular manifestations in this disease.

In most large series the incidence of sarcoidosis as an aetiological diagnosis in uveitis is small, although in one Japanese study it was the most common diagnosis, occurring in 17% of cases of endogenous uveitis. In two British studies sarcoidosis occurred in 2 and 7% of patients with uveitis. This contrasts sharply with a study in North Carolina, USA, in which the frequency of sarcoid uveitis was 29%.

Clinical manifestations

Sarcoidosis has protean ocular manifestations related to its ability to mimic the clinical picture of many other ocular diseases. Sarcoidosis may involve virtually any part of the visual system and present with an acute or chronic clinical picture. Orbital and lacrimal gland lesions are well recognized as are scleral and episcleral involvement. Intraocular inflammation is the commonest form of ocular involvement. Neuro-ophthalmological disease is common and may present in many ways which are discussed elsewhere in this text (see Chapter 17).

Sarcoid-related uveitis may mimic any clinical uveitic entity. The commonest patterns of clinical disease are AU, particularly chronic indolent bilateral AU. Pan uveitis, intermediate uveitis, chorioiditis, and retinal vasculitis are all common. Retinal vasculitis may produce characteristic clinical signs such as 'candle wax drippings' along retinal veins. There are no pathognomonic ocular signs for sarcoidosis and it should be carefully considered in the differential diagnosis of all patients with uveitis.

Immunological features

The major immunological abnormalities detected in patients with systemic sarcoidosis are summarized elsewhere. Although many immunological abnormalities have been described in such patients, a clear-cut immunopathogenesis has not emerged. Several immunological findings reflect decreased T-cell function, including: anergy, decreased *in vitro* mitogen and antigen responses and a peripheral blood T-cell lymphopenia predominantly a lower proportion of helper T cells. The relatively high number of suppressor T cells in the peripheral blood of patients with sarcoidosis may explain the observed anergy and decreased lymphocyte transformation.

Investigation and management

In patients presenting with clinically isolated uveitis, a chest X-ray is arguably the best screening investigation for patients with suspected sarcoidosis. An abnormal chest X-ray clearly requires further investigation, while in an otherwise clinically normal patient, a normal X-ray largely rules out the need for extensive investigation as their results are unlikely to alter the patient's management.

Uveitis complicating sarcoidosis is treated on its merits. AU tends to be chronic and resistant to local therapy and may require systemic steroid therapy in some patients. Posterior uveitis and retinal vasculitis may require no therapy or aggressive systemic treatment depending on the degree of threat to vision. In patients with sarcoidosis, management is individualized according to the severity of ocular involvement.

Behçet's syndrome

Introduction

The triple symptom complex comprising recurrent mouth ulceration with genital ulceration and relapsing uveitis is named after Hulushi Behçet, Professor of Dermatology at Istanbul University, who described this entity in 1937. This systemic vasculitis of unknown aetiology is characterized by the triad of oral ulceration, genital ulceration, and uveitis. Ocular manifestations of this disease tend to produce a typical clinical picture and follow a progressively deteriorating clinical course. It is the ophthalmologist who often makes the diagnosis of Behçet's syndrome as it is a clinical diagnosis with no specific diagnostic feature or laboratory test and the ocular signs make the diagnosis in most patients.

The syndrome is most frequently observed in Greece, Turkey, Cyprus, the Middle East, and Japan. Incidence varies from a high of 1 in 10 000 in the population of Japan to 0.6 per 100 000 in England. The peak age of onset of the disease is in the third decade. Men are affected twice as often as women except for erythema nodosum and genital ulceration which are more common in women.

Immunopathogenesis

Vasculitis primarily affecting the venous side of the circulation is a basic lesion in patients with Behçet's syndrome. Small-to medium-sized vessels show lymphocyte infiltration together with macrophages, polymorphs, and plasma cells, with proliferation of the endothelium and occasional fibrinoid necrosis. The lesions are widespread and account for the protean manifestations of the disease.

Despite extensive research the aetiology of this disease remains unknown.

Evidence has accumulated to implicate immune mechanisms in the pathogenesis of Behçet's syndrome. This includes the presence of: polyclonal hypergammaglobulinaemia, mucosal autoantibodies, immune complexes, and cell-mediated immunity to mucosal antigens

HLA studies

The regional differences in the frequency of Behçet's syndrome is reflected in their associations with specific HLA antigens. The initial observation of a strong association with HLA-B5 was made in Japan in 1975. It is now known that the B5 antigen can be split into two, Bw51 and Bw52, antigens. It is the Bw51 antigen that is increased in patients with BS.

An immunogenetic basis for the tissue involvement in Behçet's syndrome has been claimed based on the observation that HLA-B51 was increased in patients with ocular disease, HLA-B27 with arthritic involvement and HLA-B12 with mucocutaneous Behçet's syndrome. This pattern of tissue distribution involving the HLA-B27 and HLA-B12 antigens has not been found in non-British countries, in which Behçet's syndrome is more prevalent and awaits confirmation.

Ocular features

Ocular disease dominates the clinical picture in most patients with Behçet's syndrome in whom uveitis and retinal vasculitis are the predominate ocular manifestations. Behçet's syndrome is more frequent in men and is more progressive with a higher morbidity. Episcleritis, conjunctivitis, keratitis, papilloedema, optic atrophy, and neurophthalmological involvement also occur but with far less frequency than uveitis.

The uveitis affects the posterior segment predominantly and produces a characteristic occlusive retinal vasculitis and retinitis which tends to progress in a stuttering fashion destroying more retina with each episode of inflammation. The retinal periphery is usually destroyed initially, but patients may present with florid retinitis and vasculitis involving the posterior pole or with major retinal vein obstruction. Attacks may be fulminant in nature and patients can resent with profound visual loss, hypopyon, and pan uveitis within 24 h of the onset of symptoms.

All patients with ocular or systemic manifestations suggestive of Behçet's syndrome require careful clinical assessment. There appears clinically to be an ocular form fruste of Behçet's syndrome which behaves clinically in a similar manner but lacks sufficient criteria to establish the diagnosis. Despite aggressive treatment the course of ocular disease in Behçet's syndrome tends to be progressive with macular involvement, optic atrophy, and irreversible blindness being frequent.

Management

The treatment of Behçet's syndrome is difficult due to the variable nature of the disease with relapses and remissions, and its poor long-term prognosis for vision. Many different treatments have been tried with varying success, including corticosteroids, alkylating agents, transfer factor, levamisole, fibrinolytic agents, and cyclosporin A.

A controlled trial has recently verified the efficacy of cyclosporin A in the treatment of uveitis associated with Behçet's syndrome.

Ocular Behçet's syndrome requires aggressive treatment to delay progress of the disease. Uniocular disease should be treated with local and oral steroids. There is evidence that cyclosporin and azathioprine may retard progress of ocular disease in patients with Behçet's syndrome and therefore are used in patients with uniocular disease in an attempt to decrease second eye involvement. Bilateral disease requires aggressive immunosuppression with cyclosporin A and oral steroids to control ocular inflammation. Flare-ups of retinitis and uveitis are treated by increased doses of steroids or pulsed intravenous methylprednisolone if acute visual loss has occurred. The persistent nature of Behçet's syndrome requires many years of therapy. Careful monitoring of the patient is critical. It is essential that only potentially reversible ocular disease is treated.

Sympathetic ophthalmia

Introduction

SO is a striking example of an immunological-mediated ocular disease. After injury to the uveal tract of one eye from penetrating injury or surgery, bilateral uveitis develops. Its onset has never been documented prior to 10 days from the time of ocular injury and its onset is most frequent in the 6 months following injury. Rarely, it may occur many years later. SO is a clinical diagnosis and presents a readily recognizable clinical picture of pan uveitis following ocular penetrating trauma.

Clinical features

Patients with SO usually present with visual loss in the uninjured eye and pan uveitis associated with a range of retinal changes including: multiple small discrete chorioretinal lesions (Dalen Fuchs nodules), disc swelling, and retinal detachment. A similar uveitis will be present in the injured eye if it is still present. If the injured eye is blind, removal of this eye will allow histological confirmation of the diagnosis in problematic cases. In general, removal of the injured eye is not indicated in the management of SO as it does not alter the outcome of the disease.

Immunology

Two theories have been proposed to explain the pathogenesis of this rare syndrome, one based on an immune response to ocular antigen and the other related to infection. Most evidence favours the first theory, although a viral aetiology cannot be disregarded.

The immune theory of SO implicated a hypersensitivity reaction to uveal melanin as the basic pathogenic mechanisms in SO. The role of uveal-specific antibodies in SO remains controversial.

Most evidence supports the concept that the antigens involved in SO are derived from either the pigment epithelium or retina. Whether antibody- or cell-mediated immune responses to these antigens are involved in the pathogenesis of SO or represent an epiphenomenon secondary to tissue damage and release of ocular antigens is unknown. Experimental evidence in humans and animals suggests that cell-mediated effector mechanisms are involved in the pathogenesis of SO, which may have a predilection to occur in certain genetically predisposed individuals.

Management

The diagnosis of SO is clinical and must be considered in the differential diagnosis of uveitis following trauma or surgery. As it is a serious threat to vision, treatment involves systemic corticosteroids in the first instance. The majority of patients will respond to this treatment and can then be maintained in remission on a low oral dose. Some patients require additional immunosuppressive therapy and cyclosporin A is the logical drug based on the immunopathology of SO. In patients where cyclosporin therapy is contraindicated or where side-effects force the cessation of treatment, other drugs such as azathioprine or even cyclophosphamide may be indicated.

Lens-induced uveitis

Lens-induced uveitis is rare and can occur following ocular trauma, cataract surgery, and in patients with advanced cataracts. In patients with an advanced cataract, uveitis, glaucoma, and characteristic keratic precipitates, the diagnosis is straightforward. In complex cases, the distinction between lens-induced inflammation and SO is histological rather than clinical and of little significance in terms of patient management as both diseases are managed the same way. There is evidence to suggest that phacoanaphylactic lens-induced uveitis may be an immune complex-mediated disease.

Vogt Koyangi Harada syndrome (VKHS)

Introduction

VKHS is a specific bilateral inflammation of the eye characterized by a granulomatous uveitis associated with pigmentary disturbances, such as alopecia, vitiligo, and poliosis (whitening of the eye lashes). It is prevalent in Japanese and rarely seen in Caucasians. The cause is unknown, although an autoimmune mechanism, possibly related to the melanocyte, is postulated and believed to be similar to that involved in the pathogenesis of SO.

Clinical features

VKHS is a chronic bilateral pan uveitis which presents as a recognizable and evolving pattern of clinical symptoms and signs. The clinical features are usually divided into three phases (neurological, ocular, and cutaneous) with the ocular manifestations and phase of the illness being dominant.

The neurological symptoms and signs vary from subclinical to severe. Patients may present with a mild meningitic illness characterized by headache and neck stiffness associated with sensory neural hearing loss and hyperacusis. There is an elevated protein and a low-grade lymphocyctic pleocytosis in the cerebrospinal fluid (CSF).

Ocular disease usually manifests as a rapidly evolving severe pan uveitis associated with sluggish pupillary responses, characteristic deep whitish choroidal lesions, exudative retinal detachments, and disc swelling. Ocular disease is often severe and chronic and may result in severe permanent visual loss as a result of retinal detachment, macular changes, or optic neuropathy.

The cutaneous manifestations of vitiligo, alopecia, and poliosis tend to occur late in the course of VKHS and are uncommon.

Immunopathogensis

A number of studies have reported ocular-specific antibodies in patients with VKHS.

Evidence of cell-mediated immunity in VKHS has been provided by findings of cutaneous hypersensitivity to bovine uveal pigment, lymphocyte transformation studies to bovine uveal pigment and human uvea, and macrophage migration inhibition studies.

Lymphocyte-mediated cytotoxicity to a melanoma cell line realized cytotoxicity in eight of 28 patients with VKHS, when compared with patients with other forms of uveitis and controls. Electron microscopic studies revealed close adherence between the patient's lymphocytes and target cells, suggesting that melanocyte surface antigens are induced in the reaction. Monkeys injected with the CSF from a patient with the VKHS developed vitiligo.

Management

VKHS is a severe threat to vision and requires high-dose corticosteroid therapy. VKHS is exquisitely sensitive to steroids and there is often a profound symptomatic response within 24 h. The precise starting dose of corticosteroids has been much debated in the literature and the Japanese who have a vast clinical experience with this disease prefer high doses of oral prednisolone (200–300 mg/day) over other regimens to control the disease. Patients require long-term steroid therapy (at least 9–12 months) and therefore a steroid sparing agent such as azathioprine or cyclosporin A is often necessary. Patients may also require additional treatment with local steroids to control AU.

Retinal vasculitis (RV)

Introduction

RV refers to inflammation of the retinal vessels and may involve arteries, veins, or capillaries. Retinal arteritis is a rare condition occurring in diseases such as syphilis and polyarteritis nodosum. In contrast, retinal capillary involvement by vasculitis is common and is present to some degree in most cases of uveitis. Inflammatory involvement of retinal veins (periphlebitis) comprises the vast majority of cases diagnosed as RV.

Clinical features

RV is diagnosed on the basis of a combination of ocular and systemic clinical features and supported by typical fluorescein angiographic findings. The presenting symptoms are variable and depend largely on the stage of the disease. Patients are usually young (<40 years), and complain of ocular discomfort, blurred vision, floaters, veiling, or sudden loss of vision.

The clinical signs of RV, the features of which are summarized in Table 19.9, comparing the pathological features of RV with the associated clinical symptoms and signs during the early, severe, and late stages of the disease. Fluorescein angiography in patients with RV reveals focal areas of leakage in the vein walls. Other changes include focal venous dilation, narrowing, and occlusion. Retinal oedema is common and areas of capillary closure, neovascularization, and macular oedema may also be present.

RV is associated with a large number of ocular and systemic diseases. The majority of cases of RV, are idiopathic and careful clinical and laboratory investigations do not reveal a definable aetiology. A careful review of systems and selective investigations are the most critical steps to find an associated or underlying systemic disease. Diseases reported in association with RV are summarized in Table 19.10.

Immunopathogensis

Autoimmunity probably occurs in various forms of RV. The retina is involved in several systemic auto-

∎ **Table 19.9**   Clinical and pathological stages in retinal vasculitis

Stage		Pathology	Symptoms	Signs
1	Early	Vein wall infiltration lymphocytes plasma cells Fibrinoid necrosis	Asymptomatic Discomfort Blurred vision	Patchy narrowing or straightening Dark blood column Vein wall narrowing
2	Severe	Hyalinization Endothelial cell proliferation Venous sheathing	Floaters Veiling	Perivascular cuff Local dilation and tortuosity Vitreous cells
3	Late	Venous occlusion Neovascularization Haemorrhages Exudates	Vision loss	Venous occlusion Haemorrhages Neovascularization Glaucoma Cataract Retinal detachment

∎ Table 19.10 Retinal vascultis — disease associations

Associated with uveitis

Infections Cytomegalovirus
            Tuberculosis
            Syphilis
            Infectious mononucleosis
            Toxoplasmosis
Pars planitis
Behçet's syndrome
Sarcoidosis
Sympathetic ophthalmia

Associated with systemic disease

Infections Cytomegalovirus
            Syphilis
            Streptococosis
            Brucellosis
            Herpes zoster
            Amoebiasis
            Rickettsiosis
Demyelinating disease: multiple sclerosis
Hodgkin's disease
Glomerulonephritis

Associated with systemic vasculitis

Behçet's syndrome
Giant cell arteritis
Polyarteritis nodosa
Systemic lupus erythematosus
Wegener's granulomatosis
Takayasu–Omnishi syndrome

immune diseases in which the basic pathology is a vasculitis. RV of veins for example is the basic histopathological lesion of Behçet's syndrome. RV is also frequent in polyarteritis nodosa, giant cell arteritis and less frequent in systemic lupus erythomatosus. The clinical similarity between RV in this group of diseases, uveitis, and the experimental Arthus type reaction produced in rabbits, suggests that immune complexes may be involved in the pathogenesis of RV in humans.

The role of immune complexes in RV and their possible association with organ-specific autoantibodies has been extensively investigated. Retinal antibodies were present in 70% of all patients with RV. An interesting relationship between circulating immune complex (CIC), retinal antibodies, and the nature and severity of disease has been noted. Severe retinal disease occurred in patients with CIC who did not have circulating retinal antibodies. Patients with RV and SID had mild to moderate RV with both CIC and retinal autoantibodies present in the circulation. These results suggests that the formation of CIC containing

idiotypic antibody may be a compensatory mechanism to the development of antiretinal autoimmunity and that patients may under- or over-compensate in trying to maintain a balance between immune complex-mediated disease and retinal autoimmunity.

Management

Modern treatment approaches have been based on the presumed immunological basis of the disease and there are several reports of the efficacy of corticosteroids and alkylating agents. However, there have been no controlled trials of therapy for idiopathic RV. The treatment of RV depends on the extent and severity of the condition. An approach to the treatment of RV is outlined in Fig. 19.9. Only patients with severe bilateral, sight-threatening disease require systemic immunosuppression. Recent studies on the use of cyclosporin A in ocular inflammatory disease suggest that it is an extremely useful drug in patients with RV.

Opportunistic infections and the eye

The advent of the acquired immune deficiency syndrome (AIDS) pandemic and the widespread use of corticosteroids and cytotoxic drugs for the treatment of malignancy, autoimmune disorders, and prevention of graft rejection have resulted in an increased frequency opportunistic infections of the eye. Micro-organisms commonly associated with ocular infections in the immunocompromised host are listed in Table 19.11. A comprehensive review of the ocular manifestations of HIV infection and AIDS is beyond the scope of this review and the reader is referred elsewhere for further

∎ Table 19.11 Opportunistic infections of the eye

Viruses	Cytomegalovirus, HIV
	Herpes simplex virus
	Herpes zoster virus
	Human herpesvirus-6
Fungi	*Candida albicans*
	Aspergillus
	Crytococcus neoformans
	Mucor
Bacteria	*Nocardia*
	Mycobacterium
Protozoa	*Toxoplasma gondii*
	Microsporidia
	Pneumocystis carinii

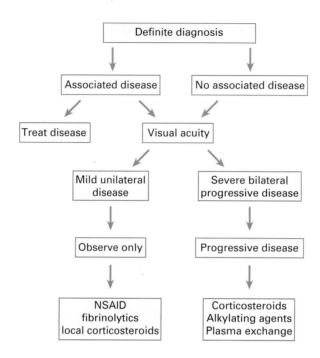

∎ **Fig. 19.9** Protocol for the treatment of patients with retinal vasculitis. NSAIDs, non-steroidal anti-inflammatory drugs.

∎ **Table 19.12** Ocular features of HIV infection

Structure	Manifestation	Stage of disease
Eyelids	Seborrhoeic blepharitis	Intermediate
	Molluscum contagiosum	Intermediate
	Herpes zoster	Intermediate
	Kaposi's sarcoma	Late
Conjunctiva	Sicca syndrome	Early
	Kaposi's sarcoma	Late
	Conjunctivitis,	Early
	Reiter's syndrome	Intermediate
Cornea	Herpes simplex keratitis	Intermediate
	Microsporidia	Late
Uvea	Iritis, Reiter's syndrome	Intermediate
Retina	HIV microvaculopathy	Early
	Cytomegalovirus retinitis	Late
	Retinal vasculitis	Early
	Acute retinal necrosis	Late
Optic nerve	Optic neuritis	Intermediate
	Papilloedema (lymphoma, cryptococcus, toxoplasmosis)	Late

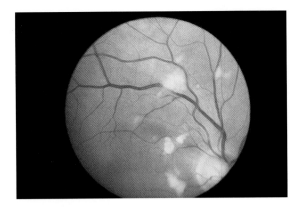

▮ **Fig. 19.10**　HIV retinopathy.

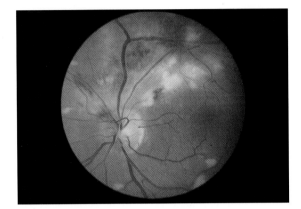

▮ **Fig. 19.11**　Cytomegalovirus retinopathy.

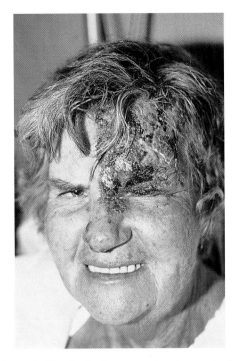

▮ **Fig. 19.12**　Varicella zoster involvement of the ophthalamic divisions of the trigeminal nerve.

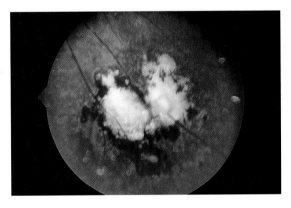

▮ **Fig. 19.13**　Toxoplasma retinochoroiditis.

information on this subject. The ocular manifestations of HIV are summarized in Table 19.12.

Opportunistic infections most frequently involve the cornea, uvea, and retina. The herpesviruses, especially cytomegalovirus, are a frequent cause of severe retinitis in immunosuppressed patients (Figs 19.10 and 19.11). Such infection results in a characteristic fundus appearance of creamy white full thickness retinal opacification associated with retinal haemorrhages. There is minimal inflammation in the vitreous or anterior chamber of the eye. Peripheral areas of retinitis may be asymptomatic initially. Cytomegalovirus retinitis is slowly progressive in nearly all patients without treatment. Herpes simplex and herpes zoster (Fig. 19.12) retinitis have similar but clinically distinct patterns of retinal infection.

Fungal endophthalmitis is increasingly recognized as a serious ocular complication in immunosuppressed patients. Infection is usually associated with the use of intravenous injections, either therapeutically or associated with intravenous drug abuse.

Ocular examination reveals an area of focal retinochoroiditis associated with overlying vitreous opacities which may develop the appearance of 'snowballs' within the vitreous. *Toxoplasma gondii* may lie dormant within the retina following congenital infection or there may be ocular involvement from newly acquired infection. Immunosuppression may then lead to severe retinochoroiditis (Fig. 19.13). Nocardia is a common infection in immunocompromised hosts and the eye is secondarily infected in about 3% of such individuals, with choroidal abscess formation and papillitis.

The approach to the management of ocular infection in the immunocompromised host requires rapid intervention and early definitive diagnosis. Immunosuppressive agents should be withdrawn if possible and treatment with the appropriate antimicrobial agent instituted. Even with these measures there is often considerable morbidity.

Further reading

Abi-Hanna, D. and Wakefield, D. (1988). HLA antigens in ocular tissue. *Transplantation*, **45**, 610–13.

Aziz, K., Markovic, B., and McCluskey, P. J., (1993). A study of cytokines in minor salivary glands in Sjögrens syndrome. *Australian New Zealand Journal of Medicine*, p. 549.

Francis, I. C., McCluskey, P. J., Walls, R. S., Wakefield, D., and Brewer, J. M. (1990). Ocular cicatricial pemphigoid. *Australian New Zealand Journal of Ophthalmology*, **18**, 143–50.

Jabs, D. A., Green, R. W., Fox, R., *et al.* (1989). Ocular manifestations of the acquired immune deficiency syndrome. *Ophthalmology*, **96**, 1092–9.

McCluskey, P. J. and Wakefield, D. (1985). Ocular involvement in the acquired immune deficiency syndrome (AIDS). *Australian Journal of Ophthalmology*, **13**, 293–8.

McCluskey, P. and Wakefield, D. (1988). Current concepts in the management of scleritis. *Australian Journal of Ophthalmology*, **165**, 169–76.

McCluskey, P. J., Wakefield, and D., Penny, R. (1985). Scleritis and the spectrum of inflammatory eye disease. *Australian Journal of Ophthalmology*, **13**, 159–64.

McCluskey, P. and Wakefield, D. (1991). Cytomegalovirus retinopathy and the acquired immune deficiency syndrome (AIDS): Results of treatment with ganciclovir. *Australian New Zealand Journal Ophthalmology*.

Nussenblatt, R. B. and Palestine, A. G. (1989). *Uveitis: fundamentals and clinical practice*. Year Book Medical Publishers, Chicago.

Wakefield, D. and McCluskey, P. (1992). Cyclosporin therapy in inflammatory eye disease. *Ocular Pharmacology*.

Wakefield, D. and Penny, R. (1985). Uveitis. In *Immunology Illustrated*, (ed. D. Nelson and J. V. Wells), pp. 348–59. Williams & Wilkins, Adis pty, Sydney, Baltimore, London.

Wakefield, D., Wright, J., and Penny, R. (1983). HLA antigens in uveitis. *Human Immunology*, **7**, 89–93.

Wakefield, D., Easter, J., and Penny, R. (1986a). Immunological abnormalities in patients with untreated retinal vasculitis. *British Journal of Ophthalmology*, **70**, 260–4.

Wakefield, D., Dunlop, I., McCluskey, P., and Penny, R. (1986b). Uveitis: aetiology and disease associations in an Australian population. *Australian New Zealand Journal of Ophthalmology*, **14**, 181–7.

Wakefield, D., Montanaro, A., and McCluskey, P. J. (1991). Anterior uveitis and HLA B27. *Survey of Ophthalmology*, **36**, 223–32.

Wakefield, D., McCluskey, P. J., and Penny, R. (1986c). Pulse methylprednisolone in severe inflammatory eye disease. *Archives of Ophthalmology*, **104**, 847–51.

<u>20</u> Blood

K. Cheney

Introduction

Immunohaematology is concerned with all aspects of blood transfusion and the investigation, diagnosis and management of diseases that result from interactions between antibodies and the antigens of haemopoietic cells. The targets for such interactions are usually mature, circulating cells and the consequences are those of haemolytic anaemia, thrombocytopenia, and neutropenia. Occasionally, marrow progenitor cells are also affected with resulting aplasia of a specific cell series or inhibition of full cell maturation.

The antigens of haemopoietic cells

Karl Landsteiner described the first blood group system in 1901. The MN and P systems were discovered in 1926 and the Rh complexes in 1939–40. By 1951, nine of the major blood group systems (ABO, MN, P, Rh, Lutheran, Kell, Lewis, Duffy, and Kidd) had been identified. Today more than 600 red cell antigens have been allocated to 22 blood group systems and seven antigen collections. Others of high or low frequency (public and private antigens) are known but are yet independent of any of the known systems or collections. Antigens included in a system are those produced at alleles that are so closely linked that crossing-over between them is rare or does not occur. An antigen collection includes a group of antigens that are related phenotypically, biochemically or genetically but are not known to be alleles.

Red cell antigens have usually been recognized following the discovery of an anti-red cell antibody in the serum a multiparous woman or a multi-transfused patient. Inevitably, the investigation of such sera disclosed the existence of antibodies directed against the antigens of other haemopoietic cells. Some such as the human leucocyte class I antigens (HLA) were found to be expressed on virtually all nucleated cells, leuco-

cytes, platelets, and red cells. Other appeared to be restricted to either platelets or neutrophils.

As the number of haemopoietic antigens increased so did the confusion surrounding their identity and classification. In 1990 the International Society of Blood Transfusion (ISBT) recommended the introduction of a modified nomenclature for red cell antigens wherein a number and symbol is assigned to each of the known systems and collections. Particular antigens within a system are further identified by the system symbol and a sequential number indicating its order of discovery within a system. For example the system symbol for the Kell group is Kel and its ISBT number of 006. The antigen first discovered in this system, K, is identified as Kel 1, 00601; k is Kel 2, 00602 and so on. Table 20.1 lists the presently recognized blood group systems and collections. Table 20.2 illustrates the identification of antigens within two of the systems, MNS and Kell, by symbol and number.

A revised system has also been introduced for the classification of platelet antigens. Platelet specific antigen systems are now known as human platelet antigen (HPA) and they are numbered chronologically in order of the date of their publication. In contrast to many of the complex red cell systems, the platelet systems are relatively simple and they all appear to be bi-allelic. Table 20.3 lists the HPA systems, the antigens in each and their former designations. The table does not include alloantigens shared with other cells such as the glycoconjugate antigens of the A, BH, Le, I, and P blood group systems or the highly polymorphous HLA class I antigens. Most platelet antigens have been localized to specific platelet glycoproteins or glycoprotein complexes and this, too, is included in Table 20.3.

Neutrophil-specific antigens have been classified in a similar scheme. They are grouped into NA, NB, NC, ND, and NE systems. With the exception of the NA antigens, they, too, appear to be biallelic. Their shared antigens include those of the I and P blood group

∎ **Table 20.1** Blood group systems and antigen collections

Conventional name	ISBT symbol	ISBT number
Blood group systems		
ABO	ABO	001
MNSs	MNS	002
P	P1	003
Rh	RH	004
Lutheran	LU	005
Kell	KEL	006
Lewis	LE	007
Duffy	FY	008
Kidd	JK	009
Diego	DI	010
Cartwright	YT	011
Xg	XG	012
Scianna	SC	013
Dombrock	DO	014
Colton	CO	015
LW	LW	016
Chido/Rogers	CH/RG	017
H	H	018
Kx	XK	019
Gerbich	GE	020
Cromer	CROMER	021
Knops	KN	022
Antigen collections		
Indian	IN	203
Cost	COST	205
Ii	I	207
Er	ER	208
P$_k$, LKE	GLOBO	209
(Lewis-like: Le^c, Le^d)	210	
Wright	WR	211

International Society of Blood Transfusion, ISBT.

systems and HLA class I antigens. Less is known about their membrane localization, but some, including NA, NC, and ND are present on the neutrophil immunoglobulin (Ig) G receptor FcRIII.

Haemopoietic antigens are inherited to according to Mendelian principles. They appear early in fetal life. For example, the ABH red cell antigens are present by 5–6 weeks' gestation and most others can be detected by 12 weeks. Despite this, many are not fully developed at birth and some such as the ABH, Lewis, and I antigens may not achieve their full adult expression for 2 years or longer. By contrast the antigens of the Rh, MNS, Kell, Duffy, and Kidd systems are fully expressed on cord cells.

The distribution of haemopoietic antigens is also quite variable. Antigens of the Rh, Duffy, Kell, and Kidd systems are restricted to red blood cells, but the ABH antigens are present on many body cells including all endothelial and epithelial cells (except those of the central nervous system), platelets, and lymphocytes. They are also found in plasma and body secretions. Contrary to earlier opinion many of the so-called platelet-specific antigens have now been demonstrated on other cells and tissues. In particular the HPA-1 and HPA-4 antigens have been found on endothelial cells, smooth muscle, and fibroblasts and those of the HPA-5 system on activated T lymphocytes and endothelial cells.

The expression of different antigens is also quite variable. It has been calculated that there are between 1.0 and 2.0 × 10^6 sites for the A, B, and H antigens on each, adult erythrocyte, 1.0–3.0 × 10^4 for D, Fy^a and Jk^a antigens but only 5 × 10^3 for K and Le^a antigens. Individuals who are homozygous for an allele can express many more antigen sites than heterozygotes, an effect known as 'dosage'. This may influence the strength of a reaction with a specific antibody but dosage is affected by factors other than zygosity.

These include haplotype pairing, gene interaction, the activity of regulator genes and, in some instances, variation as an inherited trait.

Antibodies directed against haemopoietic cells

The significance of any haemopoietic antigen system depends on the frequency with which antibodies appear and their essential characteristics, that is, whether they are IgM, IgA, or IgG, their IgG subclass and their ability to fix complement to cell surfaces. In turn these features determine an antibody's capacity to cause cell destruction, the method of such destruction, and whether the antibody is able to cross the placenta and cause disease in the fetus and newborn. IgM antibodies cannot cross the placenta while all four subclasses of IgG are able to do so.

The response of any individual to a particular antigen is influenced by many factors. These include the immunogenicity of the antigen itself, details of its introduction into the host, and host factors.

The immunogenicity of an antigen is determined by its size, shape, biochemical composition, complexity, and charge. Molecular shape and charge have emerged as the most important factors and with this, complex biochemical compounds and especially those containing proteins or protein–carbohydrate combinations are highly immunogenic. Other factors relating to the antigen itself are the dose received, its frequency, route

∎ **Table 20.2** Revised terminology for selected blood group antigens – examples

ISBT blood group system	Common antigens	ISBT symbol	Numerical designation
MNS	M	MNS1	00201
	N	MNS2	00202
	S	MNS3	00203
	s	MNS4	00204
	U	MNS5	00205
KEL	K	KEL1	00601
	k	KEL2	00602
	Kp^a	KEL3	00603
	Kp^b	KEL4	00604
	Ku	KEL5	00605
	Js^a	KEL6	00606
	Js^b	KEL7	00607

ISBT, International Society of Blood Transfusion.

of administration (i.e. intravenous, intradermal, subcutaneous, intramuscular, intraperitoneal), and its survival in the circulation. Host factors influencing the response are age, nutritional status, prior exposure to the antigen, and the activity of the hosts' own immune system.

Antibodies reacting with haemopoietic cells are of four types. They may be:

(1) naturally occurring antibodies;
(2) alloantibodies;
(3) autoantibodies;
(4) antibodies directed against bound or induced antigens (drug-dependent antibodies).

Naturally occurring antibodies

An antibody is naturally occurring if it is found in an individual who has never been transfused, pregnant or injected with a product containing the antigen. Anti-A and anti-B are the only naturally occurring antibodies that are found in virtually all individuals who lack the corresponding antigens, but such antibodies have occasionally been found in association with other blood group systems including Lewis, I, P, MNSs, Rh, Kell, and Lutheran. About 1% of normal blood donors show weak anti-HLA, naturally occurring antibodies. It is likely that naturally occurring anti-A and anti-B develop in response to environmental substances that are antigenically identical with or similar to red cell antigens, but this is a doubtful explanation for the presence of others. It has been suggested the latter are produced by an immune system triggered into action by a non-specific stimulus such as a virus. This is a doubt-

ful explanation for the production of potent naturally occurring antibodies.

Alloantibodies

These are produced in response to an antigen introduced from one individual into a second individual of the same species who lacks the antigen, e.g. the introduction of the D antigen into a D-negative person. Early, primary immunization elicits an IgM antibody response with a switch to IgG production later and, in the majority of subjects, IgG soon predominates. However, in a minority of individuals a significant IgM component can persist, particularly in response to Rh, K, Fy^a, and Jk^a antigens.

The immune response to A and B antigens needs separate mention. All individuals of groups A, B, and O should be regarded as already immunized. Further exposure to A or B antigens is likely to produce significant quantitative and qualitative changes in their anti-A and anti-B antibody levels. The immune anti-A and anti-B developed in group B and A subjects, respectively, remains predominantly IgM but group O individuals may produce a predominantly IgG antibody. This can readily cross the placenta.

Autoantibodies

An autoantibody is one that reacts with an individuals own cells. Why antibodies should develop against self antigen is not clear but suggested mechanisms include subtle, structural alterations to antigens that are then perceived as non-self; the production of an antibody that cross-reacts with particular antigens and failure of the immune system to recognize self antigen. Red cell autoantibodies may show a specificity to particular antigens but often this appears to be lacking. In these circumstances it is assumed that the antibody is directed at membrane components unrelated to blood group antigens or to an antigen common to all but a very few individuals.

Autoantibodies are classified as 'warm' or 'cold' depending on their thermal behaviour and harmful or harmless depending on their propensity to cause cell destruction. Cold antibodies are usually IgM. Their capacity to cause cell destruction depends largely on their ability to fix complement. The capacity of IgG antibodies to promote cell destruction depends on their subclass and, with this, their capacity to fix complement and to bind to specific macrophage receptors.

Drug-induced antibodies (antibodies against bound or induced antigens)

At least three mechanisms may operate to induce as a drug-dependent antibody: a high-affinity hapten mechanism; a ternary complex with low-affinity hapten mechanism; and the induction of autoantibodies.

High-affinity hapten mechanism

In this mechanism a drug such as penicillin binds firmly to cell membrane proteins. When an antibody forms against the drug, the drug-coated cells are destroyed.

Ternary complex (low-affinity hapten) mechanism

An original proposal suggested that when drug–antidrug complexes formed, they became secondarily attached to cell membranes, complement was activated, and the cells were destroyed. The cells are an 'innocent bystander' in this process. Newer concepts suggest that cell injury is more likely to be the result of a cooperative interaction between a drug or one of its metabolites, a drug binding site on a target cell membrane and an antibody, this resulting in the formation of a ternary complex. The drug is not firmly bound. When an antibody is formed it binds through its Fab domain to a compound antigen consisting of loosely bound drug and an antigen intrinsic to the cell membrane. Drug-dependent antibodies of this type may show specificity for specific antigens on red cells, platelets, or neutrophils if these form part of the drug-binding site on the target cell. If the participating antigen is lacking the antibody will not react even in the presence of the drug. The antibodies may be either IgM or IgG but in either case cell destruction is mediated by complement-induced intravascular lysis. The drugs most commonly implicated on this type of process are quinine, quinidine, and stibophen.

Autoantibody induction

Several drugs including α-methyldopa, L-dopa, mefenamic acid, and teniposide induce the formation of antibodies indistinguishable from the warm antibodies of autoimmune haemolytic anaemia. The presence of the drug is not necessary for the action of the antibody.

Suggested mechanisms for the production of such autoantibodies include: drug-induced alterations to membrane components with the creation of new epitopes recognized as foreign; drug-induced aggregation of IgG molecules with their subsequent adsorption to cell membranes; drug-induced modification of the immune system, possibly enhanced helper T-cell function or inhibition of suppressor T-cell function, leading to unregulated antibody formation.

It should be noted that some drugs such as the cephalosporins can promote the non-specific adsorption of plasma proteins to cell surfaces. This may result in a positive antiglobulin test but there is no associated cell destruction.

Mechanisms of cell destruction

The mechanisms of immune-mediated cell damage are best illustrated by reference to red cell destruction. This is influenced by many factors including the nature of the antibody itself — IgM, IgA, IgG, and IgG subclass — the concentration of antigen sites, complement, and macrophage activity. Cell destruction may be intravascular or extravascular.

In the presence of a potent complement-fixing antibody and a large number of antigen sites, the complement cascade may proceed to its full amplification with the formation of the destructive C5b, 6, 7, 8, 9 terminal attack complex. This inserts itself into the plasma membrane with resulting intravascular cell lysis. This is seen it its most fulminant form in ABO incompatible blood transfusions.

Extravascular lysis occurs when red cells are coated with either IgG, sublytic amounts of complement components, or both. The abnormal protein coatings acts as a signal to macrophages of the reticuloendothelial system especially those in the spleen and liver. Macrophages have two receptors for fragments of C3 and C4 complement components and three classes of IgG Fc receptors. The latter differ in their specific binding of IgG subclasses and this parallels the capacity of the subclasses to bind complement. IgG1 and IgG3 are readily recognized by the IgG Fc receptors and they both bind complement efficiently. IgG4 does not appear to bind complement or to be recognized by macrophages. IgG2 occupies an intermediate position in both contexts. These differences in macrophage binding and complement fixing explain variations in the severity of haemolysis induced by different IgG subclasses and the fact that a positive direct antiglobulin test due to bound antibody is not necessarily associated with any demonstrable haemolysis.

Once a coated cell is bound, the macrophages attempt to remove the abnormal protein; the cells are subjected to destruction by immune phagocytosis. During this process some of the bound cells, now membrane depleted, become detached and re-enter the circulation often as spherocytes. These are then exposed to either mechanical destruction in the circulation or more importantly premature death in the adverse metabolic and osmotic environment of the splenic sinusoids.

Red cell antibodies

As mentioned earlier the clinical significance of any particular blood group system depends on the frequency with which antibodies appear and their essential characteristics. Most IgG blood group antibodies belong to the subclasses IgG1 and IgG3 or more often a mixture of the two. IgG2 and IgG4 antibodies do occur but are much less frequent. Molecules of all four subclasses can cross the placenta.

Red cell antibodies may be:

(1) naturally occurring;

(2) alloimmune;

(3) autoimmune;

(4) antibodies against bound or induced antigens — drug-dependent antibodies.

These have been discussed in general terms above.

Clinical associations of red cell antibodies

Apart from their paramount importance in routine transfusion practice, red cell antibodies are responsible for a range of clinical disorders which share the common denominator of abnormal red cell destruction. The immune-mediated, haemolytic anaemias include:

(1) haemolytic transfusion reactions;

(2) haemolytic disease of the newborn (HDN);

(3) autoimmune haemolytic anaemia (AIHA);

(4) drug-related immunological destruction of red cells.

Haemolytic transfusion reactions

Haemolytic transfusion reactions may be immediate or delayed in onset and they may be associated with either intravascular or extravascular destruction of red cells.

Immediate intravascular haemolysis

The most severe dramatic and life-threatening complication is an immediate, acute haemolytic reaction resulting in intravascular destruction of transfused red cells by an antibody in the patient's plasma (major incompatability). Less often an antibody passively transfused in donor plasma may have a similar effect either on the recipients own cells (minor incompatability) or on other donor red cells transfused to the same patient (interdonor incompatability). Severe reactions may occur in the latter situations but are more likely when the antibody is in the recipient's plasma. In this case the antigen-carrying, transfused cells are immediately surrounded by full strength antibody under optimum conditions. In the other situations the transfused antibody is diluted in the patient's circulation and it is exposed to a large excess of antigen sites. In these circumstances full complement activation is less likely to ensue.

The antibodies most likely to be involved in severe, intravascular destruction are the naturally occurring IgM antibodies of the ABO system but others such as anti-Tj[a], anti-Vel and some examples of anti-Le[a] which act as haemolysins *in vitro* have also been incriminated.

Three factors contribute to the severity of ABO haemolytic transfusion reactions: the large number of A or B antigen sites on the red cells, the large number of antibody molecules in the plasma, and the ease with which IgM antibodies can initiate full activation of the complement cascade with the formation of the membrane–attack complex.

The biological systems activated in acute, severe intravascular haemolysis are complement, coagulation, and kinin. With activation of the complement system C3a and C5a are released into the plasma and act as powerful anaphylotoxins. They increase vascular permeability, dilate blood vessels and act to release the vasoactive amines, serotonin, and histamine. These cause fever, chills, hypotension, and shock. The release of thromboplastic material from haemolysed red cells and interactions between the complement activation and coagulation mechanisms together initiate disseminated intravascular coagulation. At the same time activated coagulation factor XII (Hageman factor) activates the kinin system with the production of bradykinin. This causes arteriolar dilation and increased capillary permeability. In turn, this may cause hypotension and the sympathetic nervous system is stimulated to increase levels of noradrenaline and other catecholamines. These are responsible vasconstriction in the kidney and other organs. The cumulative effect of these complex changes is to produce systemic hypotension, disseminated intravascular coagulation, renal vasoconstriction, the formation of renal intravascular thrombi, shock, renal failure, and sometimes death.

Clinical and laboratory features

The major symptoms are fever, chills, a burning sensation at the site of the infusion, chest pain, pain in the lower back and joints, restlessness, and dyspnoea. Patient's often express 'a feeling of impending doom' and such comments should be taken seriously if made during or shortly after a transfusion. Signs include fever, hypotension, shock, haemoglobinuria, oliguria, anuria, and excessive bleeding.

The clinical symptoms characteristic of a transfusion reaction involving intravascular destruction of cells may appear after a relatively small volume of blood has been transfused and certainly before a whole unit has been given. Severe reactions may occur after as little as 30 ml of blood but in general the consequences are more severe the larger the volume of blood infused. Because of this it is imperative that any transfusion be stopped immediately if signs and symptoms of a haemolytic reaction appear.

The investigation of a suspected haemolytic transfusion reaction must include immediate and serial documentation of the clinical signs and symptoms, general tests to confirm the occurrence of haemolysis and specific detailed serological investigation. As a preliminary to the latter it must be established that the right patient did receive the intended units. General tests include those for the presence of free haemoglobin or haemoglobin breakdown products in the patient's plasma, tests for haemoglobinuria, bilirubin and haptoglobulin estimations, and a reticulocyte count.

Serological investigation includes repeat ABO and Rh typing on pre- and post-transfusion samples from the patient, cells from the donor bag and the pilot tube: repeat of compatibility tests using patient pre- and post-transfusion samples; repeat antibody screens using patient pre- and post-transfusion serum, serum from the donor unit and a combination of patient pre-transfusion cells and serum from the donor unit, and direct antiglobulin tests on both the patient's post-transfusion cells and donor cells from the bag of blood.

Treatment of a haemolytic transfusion reaction must be directed to the control of hypotension and shock, control of disseminated intravascular coagulation, and the management of renal complications. It is far better to involve a nephrologist in the management of the latter earlier rather than later.

Extravascular destruction of cells

If a patient has an antibody that is unable to bind complement at all or only at relatively slow rates and if the patient is transfused with cells, incompatible with that antibody, red cell destruction and a transfusion reaction may occur. In these circumstances the destruction of the transfused cells is via the extravascular mechanism and, in general this is much slower than intravascular destruction. Accordingly, and in general, the reactions are less severe than those associated with intravascular cell destruction, and the consequences are not usually as serious.

The symptoms seen in this type of reaction are similar to those seen in reactions involving intravascular destruction but again they are usually less severe and they may not occur until some time after completion of the transfusion.

The two types of antibody that can cause extravascular red cell destruction are those which do not bind complement (e.g. Rh antibodies) and those which activate sublytic amounts of complement, such as antibodies of the Duffy and Kidd systems.

When intravascular haemolysis occurs there is immediate release of haemoglobin into the plasma. Depending on the severity of the process haemoglobinaemia may be readily apparent by naked-eye inspection of the plasma or its breakdown products may only be detected by spectroscopic examination. These may also be found in the urine shortly after an episode of acute intravascular haemolysis. Bilirubin levels will also rise as further breakdown products of haemoglobin are released. It might be expected that haemoglobinaemia and haemoglobinuria would be uncommon in the slower processes of extravascular destruction but it is not unusual for these to occur. The reasons are probably twofold and depend upon the intravascular rupture of severely damaged cells that have detached themselves from tissue-bound macrophages and the release of haemoglobin from red cells sequested in the spleen when the capacity of the spleen to process the haemoglobin is exceeded. To what extent lysis may be mediated by large lymphocytes carrying Fc receptors (K cells) as well as macrophages is unknown.

The investigation and management of haemolytic transfusion reactions of this type follows the same principles as those outlined for the more acute situations of intravascular haemolysis. The outcome is more uniformly favourable.

Delayed haemolytic transfusion reactions

Occasionally, the uneventful transfusion of apparently compatible blood is followed a few days later by a progressive fall in haemoglobin and the onset of jaundice. This can occur when a patient has had prior exposure to an antigen but has no demonstrable antibody in their serum at the time of the transfusion. The transfused cells provide a secondary immunogenic stimulus and a significant antibody response is produced while the transfused cells are still in the circulation. As the patient has both antigen and antibody present, *in vivo* red cell destruction follows.

The antibodies that cause delayed transfusion reactions mostly have the same specificities as those that cause immediate reactions, but commonly they are those of the Rh and Kidd systems.

As is to be expected many of the reactions are characterized by gradual and slow extravascular clearance of the red cells as the levels of antibody build up.

Fever, anaemia, and jaundice may occur any time between the third and fourteenth day after a transfusion, most commonly between the fifth and seventh days. Haemoglobinuria is uncommon but it can occur. Disseminated intravascular coagulation and renal failure are rare complications.

Diagnosis is usually suspected from the history of a recent transfusion and the onset of fever, jaundice, and anaemia. If a delayed reaction is recognized before all the transfused cells have been destroyed the direct, antiglobulin test will be positive, detecting transfused cells coated with antibody. If the reaction is investigated after all the transfused cells have been cleared the direct antiglobulin test will be negative but the presence of antibody in the patient's serum may be demonstrated by the indirect, antiglobulin test.

Haemolytic disease of the newborn

HDN occurs when an IgG antibody developed in a mother in response to a fetal antigen inherited from the father, crosses the placenta, reacts with the antigen-carrying fetal cells, and promotes their extravascular destruction. Any antigen in any blood group system that is capable of eliciting an IgG antibody response has the potential to initiate HDN, but the most common cause is ABO incompatibility. By contrast the most severe disease results from incompatibility with antigens of the Rh system and especially the D antigen. Only IgG antibodies can cross the placenta and cause HDN.

There are several reasons why ABO haemolytic disease is usually mild compared with Rh disease. Rh antigens are found only on red blood cells, are well developed before birth and are fully expressed on cord cells. Rh antibodies are therefore concentrated on the red cell surface and are also usually of the more active IgG1 and IgG3 subclasses. By contrast the ABH antigens are widely distributed throughout the body, and they are relatively poorly developed on red blood cells at birth. Thus only a fraction of the antibody is available to combine with the corresponding A or B antigens and the antibody itself is often partly of the inert IgG2 subclass.

ABO haemolytic disease often occurs in a first pregnancy and it is more likely to affect infants born of group O mothers. This relates to the fact that virtually all adults have naturally occurring anti-A or anti-B antibodies if they lack the corresponding antigens. The mechanism for the production of these particular antibodies, albeit IgM in the first instance, is already in place. When further antibody production is stimulated by fetal A or B antigens this is likely to remain IgM in group A or B subjects but those who are group O are likely to produce significant amounts of IgG. HDN due to ABO does not tend to become more severe with succeeding pregnancies.

With Rh disease pregnancy usually provides the first exposure of an Rh-negative woman to foreign Rh antigens, although in a few individuals an earlier transfusion or an intramuscular injection of D-positive cells may have been the initiating event. In most instances the response to primary immunization is slow and weak with the production of an IgM antibody. The infant is spared. Second and subsequent pregnancies with a D-positive fetus usually cause a rapid response with the production of an IgG antibody. Rh haemolytic disease usually becomes more severe with succeeding affected pregnancies.

HDN presents a wide spectrum of severity. In some, despite a positive direct antiglobulin test there are no signs of cell destruction. In others the only evidence of disease is the early onset of jaundice and a more rapid postnatal decline in haemoglobin than is usual. More severely affected infants may develop jaundice rapidly and to toxic bilirubin levels. Unless this is promptly treated by exchange transfusion kernicterus may result with yellow staining of the basal ganglia and permanent brain damage. Those who survive show clinical disorders varying from choreoathetosis and spasticity to high-frequency deafness. The most severely affected infants develop a profound anaemia and they may die *in utero* with hydrops fetalis from about the eighteenth week of gestation onwards. In this syndrome there is ascites, generalized oedema, gross hepatosplenomegaly, and heart enlargement. It is frequently associated with disseminated intravascular coagulation, widespread pulmonary haemorrhages, and subarachnoid haemorrhage.

If HND is suspected at birth the appropriate serological studies must be initiated to confirm the diagnosis and establish the exact cause and the infant's progress must be monitored by serial bilirubin and haemoglobin estimations.

If the birth of a severely affected infant is anticipated from the obstetric history or the results of routine antenatal serology, other procedures can be helpful in predicting severity more accurately and thus the need for early intervention. These include cell-mediated maternal antibody function assays which better predict the potential of an antibody to produce severe disease; amniotic fluid spectrophotometry, an accurate measure of amniotic fluid bilirubin; perinatal ultrasonography to assess placental and hepatic size and the presence or absence of ascites, oedema, or other effusions, i.e. hydrops; and percutaneous umbilical blood sampling. The latter is the most useful as it allows measurement of all blood parameters that would be measured after birth.

In severe disease an attempt can be made to reduce the level of maternal antibody by intensive plasma exchange or the use of intravenous γ-globulin. Management of the fetus may include induced, early delivery and intrauterine transfusion by either the intraperitonal route or direct intravascular transfusion into the umbilical vein under ultrasound guidance.

Postnatal management may include exchange transfusions or other measures to reduce damaging levels of indirect-reacting bilirubin. These include phototherapy and the use of phenobarbital to enhance the formation of bilirubin conjugating enzymes.

There is no doubt that the most important factor in reducing the incidence of Rh haemolytic disease has been the use of anti-D immunoglobulin. This is given to all Rh(D)-negative women who deliver a D-positive baby, who have miscarriages or termination of pregnancy, ectopic pregnancies, placental haemorrhages, or obstetric procedures likely to allow D-positive fetal cells to enter the maternal circulation. This has greatly reduced the incidence of severe D-HDN. However, the small incidence of severely affected infants from other potent antibodies such as anti-c and anti-Kell will remain.

Autoimmune haemolytic anaemia

AIHA may be associated with antibodies that react optimally at 37°C, the so-called warm autoimmune haemolytic anaemia (WAHA), or those that react optimally at 0–5°C but capable of reacting at temperatures achieved in the peripheral circulation, with resulting cold autoimmune haemolytic anaemia. The cold autoimmune haemolytic anaemia (CAHA) group includes cold haemagglutinin disease and paroxysmal cold haemoglobinuria (PCH). Any of the AIHAs may be primary, or secondary to some other underlying disease. However, the distinction is not absolute and many cases of primary disease prove to be secondary later. So, too, a few rare cases show features of disease caused by both warm and cold antibodies. These are usually associated with systemic lupus erythematosus (SLE).

Warm autoimmune haemolytic anaemia

The aetiology is unknown. The antibodies are usually of IgG class but they may be IgM or IgA. The IgG antibodies may bind complement and so the red cells of a high proportion of patients are coated with both antibody and C3 and C4 components. These coated cells are exposed to extravascular destruction in the macrophages of the liver and spleen. The antibodies may show some specificity to defined red cell antigens but often they appear to bind to membrane components unrelated to these and common to all normal red cells.

Many cases are idiopathic but a significant number are associated with lymphoproliferative disorders, collagen diseases, immune deficiency syndromes, infections and drugs, e.g. α methyldopa. WAHA is highly variable in onset, clinical characteristics, and course. Common presenting complaints are those referable to the anaemia itself or jaundice. Symptoms are usually slow in onset extending over weeks or months but the onset may be abrupt with rapidly developing, severe anaemia and jaundice. In secondary cases the haemolytic anaemia may be overshadowed by the symptoms and signs of the underlying disease.

Routine haematological studies will establish the diagnosis of haemolytic anaemia, but the diagnosis of its immune basis will depend on the demonstration of immunoglobulin and/or complement bound to the patient's red cells. Further studies are required to establish the serological characteristics of the antibody and to determine as far as is possible whether the disease is primary or secondary.

Therapy is directed to the control of the underlying disease in secondary cases and the management of the haemolytic process itself. Transfusion may be necessary in patients with severe anaemia but it is often difficult to obtain fully compatible blood and the transfused cells themselves are often rapidly destroyed. Other treatment modalities have included glucocorticoids immunosuppressive drugs, plasma exchange, high-dose intravenous γ-globulin, and splenectomy.

The course of the disease is unpredictable and it is often punctuated with relapses and remissions. The prognosis in secondary cases is largely dependent on the course of the underlying disease.

Cold autoimmune haemolytic anaemia

CAHA may also be idiopathic or secondary. The most common settings for the secondary forms are:

1. An acute self-limiting haemolytic process occurring principally in adolescents and young adults and often as a complication of *Mycoplasma* pneumonia or infectious mononucleosis.

2. A chronic disorder occurring in older patients with a known lymphoproliferative disorder. Idiopathic chronic cold haemagglutinin disease with no identifiable underlying disease at presentation usually occurs after age 50, but a proportion of these cases gradually develop a lymphoproliferative disease. The distinction between primary and secondary chronic disease is often blurred.

The antibodies are of IgM class and unlike those of WAHA they show well defined specificity, usually anti-1 but occasionally anti-i or anti-Pr. Their thermal characteristics are such that they bind to red cells and fix complement in the peripheral circulation where temperatures fall below 32°C. When the cells return to the warmer, central circulationantibody dissociates leaving the cells coated with complement. Complement activation may proceed to intravascular lysis.

The clinical picture may be that of a chronic haemolytic anaemia with or without jaundice or episodic acute haemolysis with haemoglobinuria induced by chilling. Acrocyanosis and other cold-mediated vaso-occlusive phenomena affecting fingers, toes, nose, and ears associated with red cell agglutination and sludging may be prominent. Combinations of these features are common.

Diagnosis is established by the appropriate haematological and serological studies. Other than the treatment of any underlying associated disorder the mainstay of management is avoidance of cold. This alone is effective in many patients. Chlorambucil and cyclophosphamide have proven helpful in some difficult cases but responses to glucocorticoids and splenectomy have been disappointing. The post-infectious form of the disorder is typically self-limiting and the idiopathic type often follows a relatively benign course with long survival. The prognosis in secondary cases depends largely on the underlying condition.

Paroxysmal cold haemoglobinuria

PCH is a rare disorder caused by the presence of an unusual, cold-reactive, biphasic, complement fixing IgG antibody, the Donath–Landsteiner antibody. Classically, the antibody has anti-P specificity but occasionally it may be anti-p. In the past PCH was commonly associated with syphilis but this is now unusual. Present cases are mostly idiopathic or secondary to viral infections. The antibody combines with the antigen at reduced temperatures and causes complement to be irreversibly bound. On warming the antibody dissociates from the cells but they are rapidly lysed by propagation of the complement terminal attack complex.

The disease is characterized by episodes of acute, massive, haemolysis following exposure to cold. This may happen within a few minutes or a few hours after exposure and it is accompanied by shaking chills, high fever, back and leg pain, and abdominal cramps. Raynaud's phenomenon and cold urticaria may be present at the time of an attack.

The laboratory features are those of an acute, intravascular haemolysis with haemoglobinaemia and haemoglobinuria. Definitive diagnosis depends on a positive, biphasic, cold–warm, Donath–Landsteiner test.

Other than the avoidance of cold there is no specific therapy. In those rare cases secondary to syphilis, effective treatment of the latter may stem the process. Post-infectious forms terminate spontaneously within a few days or weeks but chronic forms of the disease may persist for years. The prognosis of these depends to a large extent on the nature and course of any associated underlying disease.

Drug-related immunological destruction of red cells

The three general mechanisms of drug-mediated immunological damage to red cells have been outlined earlier, together with the fact that some drugs can promote a positive direct antiglobulin test without actual cell injury by inducing a non-specific adsorption of plasma proteins. The antibodies may be either IgG or IgM. Both may fix complement.

The clinical picture is quite variable, the severity of symptoms depending largely on the rate of haemolysis. In turn this depends to some extent on the antibody class and whether or not significant amounts of complement are fixed and whether this will proceed to the formation of the terminal attack complex. In general, patients with the high-affinity hapten (e.g. penicillin) and autoimmune (e.g. α-methyldopa) types show mild to moderate haemolysis with an insidious onset of symptoms over days or weeks. By contrast, where haemolysis is mediated by the ternary complex mechanism even a single dose of the drug may induce acute, severe intravascular haemolysis with haemoglobinaemia and haemoglobinuria.

The laboratory findings are similar to those of spontaneously occurring WAHA. A careful history of drug exposure should be obtained in all patients with haemolytic anaemia or a positive direct antiglobulin test. The prognosis is generally good but renal failure or death have been recorded usually in association with exceptionally severe haemolysis induced by the ternary complex mechanism. Treatment is to discontinue the offending drug and transfusion of red cells if clinically indicated.

The HLA system, platelet and granulocyte antigens, and antibodies

The HLA system: antigens and antibodies

HLA antigens

The HLA system comprises a large number of genes located on the short arm of chromosome 6. It is intensely polymorphic and with the large number of alleles known to exist at the various loci, the number of potential haplotypes is bewildering. The genes are co-dominant: the antigens they encode are transmembrane glycoproteins.

The HLA genes have been divided into three classes, the class I, II, and III genes. Class I genes include the HLA-A, -B, and -C genes which encode for class I molecules on which HLA-A, -B, and -C antigens are expressed; class II genes encode for class II molecules on which the HLA-DP, -DQ and -DR antigens are expressed; and class III genes which code for some complement components (C2, C4a, C4b, and Bf), tumour necrosis factor and other products not directly related to the HLA system. For more information see section on HLA, Chapter 32.

Class I antigens are expressed on all nucleated cells except spermatozoa and placental trophoblasts. They are present on platelets and some are found on red cells. A28 and B7 are expressed most strongly on the latter followed by B8 and B17 but A10, A9, B12, and B15 may also be expressed. Soluble class I antigens, may be present in plasma. Class II antigens are much more restricted in distribution being found only on B

lymphocytes, activated T lymphocytes, monocytes, and epidermal cells.

HLA antibodies

HLA antibodies are usually induced by pregnancy or transfusion but they may be naturally occurring. About 1% of normal blood donors have a weak anti-HLA antibody, commonly anti-B8, in the absence of any known stimulus. Those formed as a result of pregnancy are more likely to be anti-HLA-B than anti-HLA-A. Because of their exposure to a wide range of antigens the incidence of HLA antibodies is very high in individuals who have had multiple transfusions but it is still high in those who have been exposed to the blood of a single donor only. They are present in virtually all subjects who have had a massive transfusion. The incidence of HLA antibodies following transfusion can be substantially reduced by using leucocyte-depleted blood.

Characteristically, HLA antibodies are IgG, fix complement, and have cytotoxic properties. Like most granulocyte-reactive IgG antibodies, they are leucoagglutinins.

Platelet antigens and antibodies

Platelet antigens

Many different types of alloantigens are present on platelets. Some, such as the glycoconjugate antigens of the ABH, Le, I, and P blood group systems and the highly polymorphous HLA class I (A, B, C) glycoproteins are shared with other blood cells and tissues. Others have been considered specific for platelets but there is evidence to suggest that many of these are not as unique as was once thought.

Many platelet antigens have been described under different names and in an attempt to reduce the confusion that this has created a new nomenclature has been proposed for platelet alloantigens. Platelet specific alloantigen systems are now called HPA (human platelet antigen) and the different systems are numbered chronologically in order of the date of publication of their description. All of the HPA systems discovered to date appear to be biallelic. The high-frequency allele of a system is designated with the letter 'a' and its low frequency counterpart with the letter 'b'. Most platelet-specific antigens have been localized to specific platelet glycoproteins (GP) or GP complexes, many in the GPs of the GP 11b/111a complex. Table 20.3 provides a current classification of platelet antigens together with their earlier designations and their GP associations.

Many of the platelet alloantigens previously considered platelet specific have now been found in other

▌ **Table 20.3**   Platelet antigen systems

Antigen system	Antigens	Other names	Glycoprotein location
HPA-1	HPA-1a	Zw^a, Pl^{a1}	GPIIIa
	HPA-1b	Zw^b, Pl^{a2}	
HPA-2	HPA-2a	Kob	GPIb
	HPA-2b	Ko^a, Sb^a	
HPA-3	HPA-3a	Bak^a, Lek^a	GPIIb
	HPA-3b	Bak^b	
HPA-4	HPA-4a	Pen^a, Yuk^b	GPIIIa
	HPA4b	Pen^b, Yak^a	
HPA-5	HPA-5a	Br, b, Zav^b	GPIa
	HPA-5b	Br^a, Zav^a, Hc^a	

cells and tissues. The antigens of the HPA-1 and HPA-4 systems have been demonstrated on endothelial cells, smooth muscle cells and fibroblasts and those of the HPA-5 system on activated T lymphocytes and endothelial cells. HPA-2 and HPA-3 antigens still appear to be restricted to platelets.

The broader tissue distribution of platelet antigens is potentially of great significance as it suggests that antibodies directed against such antigens may not only react with and destroy platelets but other cells as well including vascular endothelium. Purpura, a characteristic sign of immune-mediated thrombocytopenia, may thus result from direct vessel wall damage by platelet antibodies as well as the thrombocytopenia itself.

Population studies have shown that phenotype and genotype frequencies of some antigens vary considerably between different ethnic groups.

Platelet antibodies

The mechanisms underlying the production of platelet antibodies are the same as those responsible for the production of the corresponding red cell alloantibodies, autoantibodies and drug-dependent antibodies.

Alloantibodies may arise following exposure to foreign platelet antigens through transfusion or pregnancy. Many react only with HLA antigens but others are directed to platelet-specific antigens. Autoantibody production may be stimulated by subtle changes to platelet structure so that to render them antigenic or an infective agent may result in the formation of an antibody which cross-reacts with a platelet surface constituent. In other instances there may be an inappropriate production of antibody in association with other immune responses. Mechanisms suggested as responsible for drug-induced immune thrombocytopenia include a drug hapten process (e.g. penicillin), the adsorption of immune complexes to the platelet membrane (e.g. heparin–antiheparin antibody complex), reversible, drug-induced structural changes to the platelet membrane with the creation of a neoantigen recognized as foreign and finally true autoantibody formation with such antibodies acting independently of the drug. Gold salts and α-methyldopa provide examples of the latter process.

Clinical associations of platelet antibodies

Platelet antibodies may have some association with non-specific febrile transfusion reactions but their major clinical associations are:

(1) neonatal alloimmune thrombocytopenia;

(2) post transfusion purpura;

(3) autoimmune thrombocytopenia;

(4) drug-induced immune thrombocytopenia.

Neonatal alloimmune thrombocytopenia

This disorder is the platelet counterpart of HDN. It follows maternal alloimmunization to fetal platelet antigens inherited from the father and the transplacental passage of an IgG alloantibody which reacts with the fetal platelets. In most cases, the antibody is directed against the HPA-Ia (PL^{A1}) antigen but other platelet-specific antigens, have been incriminated in a few cases. Rarely, maternal immunization to HLA determinants has been implicated. Immune-mediated neonatal thrombocytopenia may also be caused by the transplacental passage of maternal IgG platelet autoantibodies.

First-born children are often affected and there is a high rate of recurrence in subsequent pregnancies. In most cases pregnancy and delivery are uneventful but widespread purpura and other haemorrhagic symptoms appear within a few hours of birth. However, life-threatening CNS haemorrhage, a well recognized complication, may occur *in utero*, during delivery or postnatally. This may result in the formation of porencephalic cysts, hydrocephalus, and other serious cerebral and spinal cord lesions.

Diagnosis may be inferred from the clinical presentation, especially if there have been previously affected infants, but other causes of neonatal thrombocytopenia need to be excluded. These include inherited thrombocytopenic disorders, maternal immune thrombocytopenia, maternal drug ingestion, infection, and disseminated intravascular coagulation. Definitive diagnosis depends on the serological demonstration of a maternal IgG antibody which reacts with the paternal platelets.

The disease is self-limiting. The platelet count may show a significant improvement in 2–3 days, often within 2–3 weeks but occasionally not for some months. Where active intervention is indicated the treatment of choice is the transfusion of compatible platelets (usually HPA-1a negative) and these are most readily available from the mother. Other treatment regimens have included glucocorticoids, exchange transfusion, and intravenous γ-globulin. The latter may prove to be the treatment of choice in many cases.

Management of subsequent pregnancies is difficult. Caesarean section has been advocated as well as the administration of glucocorticoids to the mother for several weeks prior to delivery. In a few cases where prenatal fetal blood sampling has indicated severe disease, the transfusion of washed maternal platelets via the umbilical vein has been successful.

Post-transfusion purpura

This perplexing acute, severe, thrombocytopenia occurs approximately 1 week after a transfusion, in association with the presence of platelet alloantibodies. The antibodies have been shown to be specific for at least five different platelet antigens but like those responsible for alloimmune neonatal thrombocytopenia, the vast majority are anti-HPA-1a (anti-PL^{A1}). Most patients are women who have probably been pre-immunized against platelet antigens through pregnancy. Platelets obtained from patients when they have recovered invariably type antigen negative for the alloantibody present during the acute phase.

There is no proven explanation for these seemingly anomalous results. The various suggestions have included: (i) the production of a second antibody in parallel with anti-HPA-1a, which cross-reacts with HPA-1a negative platelets; (ii) an immune complex formed between the antibody stimulated by the transfused HPA-1a antigen and the antigen itself attaches to high-affinity sites on the platelet membrane; and (iii) the platelet-specific antigen contained in the provocative transfusion binds to the autologous antigen-negative platelets and in so doing primes them for destruction by the alloantibody.

The clinical symptoms at the onset of the thrombocytopenia include fever, chills, hypotension or hypertension, and bronchospasm. Severe haemorrhagic manifestations (including intracranial haemorrhage) may be prominent.

The diagnosis may be confidently made when a previously haematologically normal person develops a profound thrombocytopenia with a platelet-specific alloantibody (notably HPA-1a) a few days after transfusion. The appropriate serological tests are necessary to prove the existence and specificity of the suspected alloantibody.

Compatible platelets are ineffective as a means of treatment: presumably they are destroyed as well. Plasma exchange may lead to dramatic improvement by removing antibodies, immune complexes, and transfused antigens. However, as intravenous γ-globulin seems to be effective this is likely to become the treatment of choice.

Autoimmune thrombocytopenia

Idiopathic thrombocytopenic purpura (ITP) is divided into at least two distinct entities designated acute and chronic, based largely on their clinical presentation and the duration of the disease.

Acute ITP (post-infectious thrombocytopenia)

This is predominantly a disease of children and is characterized by the abrupt onset of thrombocytopenia some 7–21 days after an infection (usually viral), and in most cases spontaneous recovery occurs within 1–3 months.

The fact that acute ITP is usually preceded by a viral illness suggests a close aetiological relationship between the two but this is not completely understood. Suggested mechanisms have included: (i) immune complexes whose antigenic component derives from the infecting agent bind to platelet Fc receptors and promote their destruction; (ii) that the infectious agent alters the platelet structure so as to cause autologous platelets to become antigenic; (iii) antibodies formed against the infecting virus cross-react with a surface constituent of platelets; and (iv) the immune response against the infecting organism might be accompanied by the inappropriate production of a platelet-specific autoantibody. In the latter context it can be said that while elevated levels of platelet-associated immunoglobulin have been demonstrated frequently in cases of acute ITP, tests for antibody in plasma have generally been negative or inconclusive.

Preceding infections are usually of viral origin but acute ITP may follow vaccination with live vaccines. Cardinal symptoms are petechial haemorrhages, purpura, and other haemorrhagic manifestations. In the more severe cases these include epistaxis, bleeding from the gums, and gastrointestinal and urinary tracts. The onset may be abrupt with the appearance of symptoms and signs over a few hours. More often petechiae have been present for a few days before help is sought.

The clinical picture and routine haematological studies are usually so typical that the diagnosis is obvious. Acute leukaemia is readily excluded by other features of the blood film and bone marrow examination while the haemolytic–uraemic syndrome and thrombotic thrombocytopenic purpura are readily excluded by the absence of haemolysis and microangiopathic red cell changes.

Most patients recover regardless of treatment, but a few progress to a state of chronic thrombocytopenia. The options for treatment are essentially glucocorticoids or intravenous γ-globulin. Immunosuppressive therapy has been used in children with more prolonged thrombocytopenia but it is doubtful whether this can be justified because of the uncertainty about its long term-side effects and the acknowledged effectiveness of intravenous gammaglobulin.

Chronic ITP (autoimmune thrombocytopenia)

This is primarily a disease of adults and it rarely resolves spontaneously. There is rarely a history of preceding infection. Patients generally feel well and typically the disease begins insidiously with petechiae and other minor bleeding manifestations. A bruising tendency, recurrent epistaxis, or menorrhagia may have been present for months or years before a diagnosis is made.

Autoantibodies can be demonstrated in most patients with chronic ITP. The antibodies are mostly of IgG and IgM classes but they may be IgA in some cases. Increased levels of surface bound complement may be present. The preferred targets for such antibodies are epitopes on GPIIb and/or IIIa.

Diagnosis is made on the clinical history, the blood picture, the bone marrow examination demonstrating normal or increased numbers of megakaryocytes and the absence of other pathology, the demonstration of autoantibodies and the exclusion of other conditions causing secondary, chronic, thrombocytopenic purpura. The latter include chronic lymphoproliferative diseases, Hodgkin's disease, other autoimmune diseases such as SLE and rheumatoid arthritis, a range of organ specific autoimmune diseases, autoimmune haemolytic anaemia, and the acquired immune deficiency syndrome. Drug-induced immune thrombocytopenia must also be considered.

The mainstays of treatment have been glucocorticoids, and splenectomy if a satisfactory response to the former was not achieved or maintained. Intravenous γ-globulin has been tried but is very expensive and the benefits appear to be short-term only. Immunosuppressive therapy has been tried in patients who have not responded to glucocorticoids or splenectomy with some success but the possible benefits have to be weighed against the risks of infection and induced malignancy. Other measures have included intravenous anti-Rh immunoglobulin and plasmapheresis. The latter is only appropriate for patients with life-threatening haemorrhage unresponsive to other measures.

About 10% of adults with chronic ITP recover spontaneously usually those with severe thrombocytopenia of more acute onset. These may be individuals with acute ITP of the type seen in children or examples of unrecognized drug sensitivity. In any individual case the prognosis must be guarded but many patients live long lives relatively untroubled by their thrombocytopenia.

Drug-induced immune thrombocytopenia

Numerous drugs have been reported to cause immunological thrombocytopenia. In many instances the relationship may be coincidental or the thrombocytopenia may have been induced by suppression of platelet production rather than an immune mechanism. However, there is convincing evidence that many drugs can precipitate thrombocytopenia by one or other of the immunological mechanisms outlined earlier.

The greatest number of cases have been described in relation to quinine, quinidine, sedormid, gold salts, aspirin, and heparin, although the latter may cause thrombocytopenia by non-immunological mechanisms as well. Occasional cases have apparently been triggered by foodstuffs.

Up to 5% of persons treated with gold salts develop purpura and thrombocytopenia. The mechanism appears to be the induction of true autoantibodies. The incidence is much less with the other drugs listed above and it is quite unpredictable. Some drug-dependent antibodies have been shown to bind to epitopes on the GP complexes GPIb/IX and GPIIb/IIIa.

Ingestion of a drug to which a patient is sensitive is sometimes followed within minutes by a warm sensation, flushing, and later a chill with the appearance of petechiae, purpura, haemorrhagic bullae of the oral mucosa and haemorrhage from the gastrointestinal and urinary tracts some hours later.

A careful drug history is of the utmost importance in diagnosis and in addition to enquiries about conventional medications the patient must be asked about the ingestion of patent remedies, soft drinks, mixers, and aperitifs that may contain quinine. Definitive diagnosis depends on the demonstration of an antibody by one or other immunological technique using mixtures of the patient's serum or plasma, normal platelets, and the offending drug. Direct *in vivo* challenge with a suspected drug is exceptionally hazardous and cannot be condoned under any circumstances.

If a drug-induced antibody is suspected to be the cause of a thrombocytopenia the drug should be stopped immediately and another drug with comparable pharmacological actions introduced in its place. Steroids have limited value, but some critically ill patients have benefited from plasma exchange, the infusion of drug-specific antibodies and intravenous γ-globulin.

Recovery usually occurs within a few days of ceasing the offending drug, but patients with gold sensitivity may remain thrombocytopenic for many months because of the slow turnover of the drug. Once induced, sensitivity to drugs causing immunological thrombocytopenia persists indefinitely.

Neutrophil antigens and antibodies

Neutrophil antigens

There are many features common to neutrophil and platelet antigens. Neutrophil antigens were identified using sera containing leucoagglutinins obtained from subjects immunized through pregnancy or transfusion or with autoimmune agranulocytosis. Common antigens shared with other blood or tissue cells are the glycoconjugate antigens of the blood group 1 and P systems and the GP HLA -class I (ABC) antigens. Some are common to neutrophils, lymphocytes and monocytes only. The latter are the antigens of the 9 system (identical to those of the monocyte HMA-1

system) Cnd[a] and Mart[a]. Antigens specific for neutrophils have been classified into NA, NB, NC, ND, and NE systems. Like their platelet counterparts, with the exception of the NA antigens, they appear to be 'bi-allelic' and they show significant differences in phenotypic and genotypic expression between different ethnic groups.

The neutrophil specific antigens NA1 and NA2 are located on the Fc γ receptor III (FcRIII) GP. The exact location of the others is yet to be defined.

Granulocyte cytoplasmic antigens also exist and the associated antibodies (antineutrophil cytoplasmic autoantibodies) have been shown to be present in a spectrum of diseases including Wegener's granulomatosis, necrotizing vasculitis, idiopathic crescentic glomerulonephritis, and Churg–Strauss syndrome.

Neutrophil antibodies

Antibodies reacting with neutrophils may be alloimmune, autoimmune, or drug-induced. The underlying mechanisms are the same as those described for the production of red cell and platelet antibodies.

Granulocyte agglutinins are usually IgG, although mixtures of IgG, IgM, and IgA have been reported. This contrasts with red cell antibodies that cause direct agglutination. These are usually IgM. Granulocyte cytotoxins are usually IgM but occasionally they may be IgG.

Clinical associations of neutrophil antibodies

Those of prime importance are:

(1) transfusion-related acute lung injury (TRALI);

(2) neonatal alloimmune thrombocytopenia;

(3) autoimmune neutropenia of infancy;

(4) autoimmune neutropenia in adults.

Transfusion-related acute lung injury

TRALI, a dramatic complication of transfusion, is second only to haemolytic reactions as a cause of transfusion associated deaths. Most cases have followed the infusion of whole blood or plasma containing alloantibodies reactive with the recipients leucocytes but in others the reaction has involved transfused leucocytes and an antibody in the plasma of a sensitized recipient. The antibodies involved have been anti-NA1, -NA2, -NB1, and anti-HLA. Donors implicated in TRALI reactions are typically multiparous women and persons with a history of multiple blood transfusions.

The condition results from an intravascular reaction between neutrophils (or leucocytes in general) and the antibodies with resulting complement activation and massive sequestration of the cells in the lung. These processes and the release of proteases, superoxides, and cytokines from activated neutrophils lead to acute lung injury.

Symptoms and signs may appear within minutes of starting a transfusion and they include nausea, vomiting, cough with serosanguineous sputum, dyspnoea and cyanosis, tachycardia, hypotension, and hypoxia. X-rays shows diffuse, mottled, pulmonary infiltrates.

Treatment is difficult and involves intensive respiratory and circulatory support, corticosteroids and prophylactic antibiotics.

Neonatal alloimmune neutropenia

Neonatal alloimmune neutropenia is a rare but important disease resulting from maternal alloimmunization to specific antigens on fetal granulocytes. It can occur in a first pregnancy. The clinical course is variable; some children have no infections but others have frequent skin and respiratory infections or sepsis caused by Gram-positive organisms.

The blood shows a selective neutropenia and, often, a compensatory monocytosis. The marrow is either normal or shows a 'maturation arrest' of myeloid development. Proof of the diagnosis rests on the demonstration of granulocyte specific alloantibodies in the maternal serum. The granulocytopenia persists for 2–4 months if untreated. Therapy includes the use of antibiotics prophylactically, plasma exchange and high-dose intravenous γ-globulin.

Autoimmune neutropenia of infancy (chronic idiopathic neutropenia of infancy)

This disorder is uncommon but not rare. It usually appears between 6 months and 2 years of age without any apparent cause (although a preceding infection is not unusual) and resolves spontaneously in 6 months to 3 years. Serological studies often demonstrate neutrophil bound immunoglobulin and the serum may contain neutrophil antibodies. In contrast to the adult counterpart of this disease these autoantibodies often show specificity, most commonly anti-NA1. The blood and marrow appearances are the same as those found in the neonatal disorder. Many patients appear to be unaffected by the neutropenia; others do suffer recurrent infections of mild to moderate severity. Overwhelming infection is rare. Most infections can be controlled with routine antibiotic therapy but occasionally intravenous γ-globulin may be indicated for additional support.

In some circumstances a chronic neutropenia in infancy and childhood may be secondary to other immunological or haematological disorders.

Autoimmune neutropenia in adults

Although primary autoimmune neutropenia has been described in adults, it has usually been associated with other autoimmune disorders or haematological malignancies especially lymphoproliferative diseases. Antibodies to granulocyte antigens have been found in some patients and circulating immune complexes in others. The antibodies have been auto-anti-NA1,-ND1, and-NE1. Severe infections are uncommon and active treatment of the neutropenia is rarely required.

Drug-induced immune granulocytopenia

The underlying mechanisms are the same as those responsible for the production of drug-induced immune destruction of red cells and platelets. The antibodies are directed to mature granulocytes but some may react with progenitor cells and cause pure white cell aplasia. Management includes withdrawal of the offending drug and appropriate treatment of any intercurrent infections.

Miscellaneous conditions

Reactions to transfused proteins

After febrile reactions, urticarial reactions are the most common untoward response to transfusion. They are usually mild and respond to antihistamines or steroids. At the opposite extreme the severest reaction is anaphylactic shock. The cause may be unknown but some cases are due to a reaction between transfused IgA and class-specific anti-IgA. It was thought that the reactions were due to the release of complement components but it seems now leukotrienes may play an important part. They are extremely potent bronchoconstrictors and vasoconstrictors and exceedingly active in promoting plasma leakage. Management is that of an acute anaphylactic reaction.

Refractoriness to transfused platelets

Patients undergoing long-term platelet support develop refractoriness to transfused platelets. An important component of this may be the development of HLA-specific antibodies. The prime stimulant for the production of these appears to be leucocyte contamination of the platelet concentrates. Refractoriness may be prevented or its onset delayed by the use of leukocyte depleted products in those needing long-term platelet support. Improved platelet survival may be achieved in many immunized patients by the use of HLA-A, B matched donors. Class II antigens are poorly expressed on platelets and compatibility is not necessary for effective platelet support.

<u>21</u> Nervous system

D. W. Schultz and J. D. Sedgwick

Introduction

The nervous system was once thought to be an immunologically privileged site, protected from systemic immune responses. It is now recognized that immune responses can significantly affect the nervous system. A number of neurological disorders already have a confirmed immunological pathogenesis, such as myasthenia gravis (MG). In other conditions, such as the recently recognized multifocal motor neuropathy (MMN), autoantibodies are frequently identified and are suspected to be vital to the development of the disease, although the pathogenesis is yet to be clarified.

This chapter begins with a brief overview of nervous–immune system interactions and immunopathological mechanisms of relevance to autoimmune disease of the nervous system. Conditions identified or strongly suspected of having an immunological pathogenesis, with sole or predominant neurological manifestations, are examined subsequently.

Nervous–immune system interactions and development of autoimmunity

1. The nervous system is immunologically different.
2. Antigen escape from the nervous system.
3. T-cell blasts non-specifically cross into the central (CNS)/peripheral (PNS) nervous systems.
4. Major histocompatibility complex (MHC) expression and antigen recognition in the nervous system.
5. Tissue damage by T cells and the role of antibody.
6. Triggering autoimmunity in the nervous system.

Polyneuropathies

1. Guillain–Barré syndrome (GBS).
2. Chronic relapsing polyneuropathy.
3. Multifocal motor neuropathy (MMN).
4. Plexopathies.
5. Paraproteinaemic neuropathy.

CNS demyelination

1. Multiple sclerosis (MS).
2. Acute disseminated/haemorrhagic encephalomyelitis.
3. Subacute sclerosing panencephalitis (SSPE).

Neuromuscular disorders

1. Myasthenia gravis (MG)
2. Lambert–Eaton syndrome (LES).

Spinal disorders

1. Tropical spastic paraparesis (TSP).
2. Stiff-man syndrome (SMS).

Paraneoplastic syndromes

1. Cerebellar degeneration.
2. Encephalomyelitis.
3. Opsoclonus–myoclonus.

Nervous–immune system interactions and development of autoimmunity

Introduction

There is substantial indirect evidence that the immune system very effectively patrols the central (CNS) and peripheral (PNS) nervous systems. In particular, the emergence of a variety of viral infections of, or in association with, the nervous system during periods of immune suppression which otherwise are uncommon, imply the normal presence of an immune system that is controlling the spread of such infections. A good example is the relatively high incidence of progressive multifocal leucoencephalopathy (PML) in immune-suppressed patients, particularly those with acquired immune deficiency syndrome (AIDS). The agent causing this disease, the JC virus, is thought to exist in latent form in CNS oligodendrocytes in many people, most of whom will never suffer PML. Another more common example is herpes simplex virus type 1 which also resides in a latent form in the trigeminal ganglion. Reactivation of this virus (producing cold sores for example) tends to correlate with stressful events which may induce some level of immune suppression.

The nervous system is immunologically different

Until recently, the way in which the immune system carried out this immune surveillance role was unclear. Additionally, the pathways leading to development of autoimmune responses in the CNS and PNS were enigmatic as, at least in principle, a variety of features made development of immune responses generally, potentially hard to generate within the CNS or PNS. First, unlike most other tissues, there is no dedicated lymphatic drainage from nervous tissue to enable the immune system to detect the presence of antigen. Second, the normal CNS and PNS is, in most places, 'encapsulated' within the blood–brain (BBB) or blood–nerve (BNB) barrier, formed by specialized endothelium whose basement membrane is in contact

with glial cells of these tissues (astrocytes in the CNS, for example). As a consequence, the CNS and PNS contain few blood-derived leucocytes (T cells in particular) which are unable to bypass these barriers. Third, MHC expression required for T cell recognition of peptide antigen is absent or at very low level (particularly MHC class II expression) and finally, highly efficient dendritic antigen-presenting cells (APC) are not found (Table 21.1). It is now apparent that all these 'deficiencies' are relative and mechanisms or routes of contact with the immune system exist and operate, for the most part, quite efficiently. These have been labelled as 'compensatory mechanisms' in Table 21.1.

Antigen escape from the nervous system

The first compensatory mechanism is the movement of soluble antigen from the nervous system by other than lymphatic drainage. Unlike the latter mechanism, that involves the capture of antigen by APC within tissues which traffic via afferent lymphatics to lymph nodes (LN) to stimulate antigen-specific T-cell populations, movement of antigen out of the nervous system is a more passive process. In the CNS (Fig. 21.1), the main route of antigen escape is via the olfactory nerve with antigen dripping on to the cribriform plate that is drained by the deep cervical LN. In experimental systems involving infection of animals with neurotropic viruses, it is these LN that become enlarged and where the highest frequency of viral antigen-specific T cells can be found. Additionally, the majority of antibody produced in response to soluble antigen instilled in the CNS (within ventricles for example), is dependent on this same route of exposure to the immune system. There is also movement of cerebrospinal fluid-associated antigen via the arachnoid

▮ **Table 21.1** Immune deficiencies of nervous system tissues

Property	Other tissues (e.g. skin)	Normal CNS/PNS	Compensatory mechanisms
Lymphatic drainage	Present	Absent	†Antigen escape via olfactory nerve and deep cervical LN drainage
Blood–tissue barrier	Mostly absent	Present	Traffic of T blasts
Leucocytes	Present	*Very few	Traffic of T blasts
MHC expression	MHC class I and II	Minimal	Inducible
Dendritic APC	Present — e.g. Langerhans cells	*Absent	Perivascular macrophages

*The CNS and probably also the PNS contain a resident population of macrophage-like cells with a dendritiform morphology, called microglia. Strictly speaking therefore, these can be thought of as resident leucocytes of these tissues. However, in many ways they are quite different to blood-derived cells of the monocyte/macrophage lineage and their role as APC within the CNS is in some doubt.

†Demonstrated for the CNS but similar antigen leakage to LN is likely also from peripheral nerve.

PNS, peripheral nervous system; LN, lymph node; APC, antigen-presenting cell.

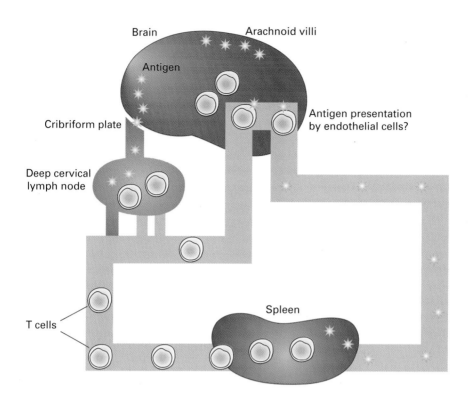

∎ Fig. 21.1 Antigen drainage from the CNS.

villi to the blood and thence to the spleen, although this route is probably a less important one. Finally, there is the possibility that some antigen within the nervous system may be transported in a retrograde manner back via the vascular endothelium to be presented to T cells in the vessel lumen. There is little evidence this latter mode of antigen transport is of importance for recognition of CNS/PNS-associated autoantigen by MHC class II-restricted CD4+ T cells. Nevertheless, it is likely to occur for some viral antigens are presented to MHC class I-restricted cytotoxic CD8+ T cells (CTL) by the constitutively MHC class I+ vascular endothelial cells.

At least with respect to the CNS, it should be stressed that this route of antigen release does not appear to operate for particulate antigens, particularly cells. First, there is no evidence for any substantial level of leucocyte movement out of nervous tissue. Second, implantation of cells or tissues allogeneic to the host, are rejected relatively slowly. It is only when the same cells or tissues are transplanted concomi-

tantly *outside* the CNS, that rejection occurs rapidly, suggesting that once the immune system outside the CNS knows about an antigen, that same antigen *within* the CNS becomes very visible. The explanation for this apparent paradox can be explained by the traffic of activated T cells into neural tissue.

T cell blasts non-specifically cross into the CNS/PNS

In 1986, Wekerle and colleagues suggested that activated T cells were capable of crossing the BBB and entering the CNS and most importantly, that this process was a non-specific one not requiring antigen recognition for extravasation to take place. Subsequent studies by, among others, Hickey and colleagues, showed that this was indeed what happened when CD4+ T-cell blasts were injected into experimental animals. That is, activated CD4+ T cells specific for the CNS myelin protein, myelin basic protein (MBP) as well as CD4+ T cells specific for a control antigen not found in the CNS, both traversed the intact BBB and entered the CNS in similar numbers and with a similar tempo. Notably, the former were found to remain for longer periods in the CNS suggesting some recognition process had occurred. Resting CD4+ T cells were unable to pass through the BBB. The ability of T-cell blasts to extravasate in this way is probably related to heightened expression of certain adhesion molecules (VLA-4 for example) by activated T cells as well as cell surface enzymes that can break down the endothelial basement membrane. This capacity of T-cell blasts to cross into the CNS and PNS explains the result mentioned above, of rapid rejection of allogeneic tissue in the CNS only after parallel peripheral transplantation, as the latter would lead to priming of specific T cells which then may enter the CNS and attack the same allogeneic tissue within it. Similarly, normal T cell surveillance of the CNS and PNS may occur in this way following T cell activation in the periphery, for example to a common viral infection. In most cases, because of the existence of the BBB and BNB, blood-borne pathogens are excluded from nervous tissue (unless of course, infection of vascular endothelial cells themselves occurs); however, activated T cells can check the infectious status of the CNS or PNS.

MHC expression and antigen recognition in the nervous system

The low level expression of products of the MHC class I and II genes in nervous system tissue was first reported in the late 1970s and early 1980s and included the observation by Hart and Fabre in 1981, that most tissues but not the CNS, contained constitutively MHC class II dendritic leucocyte APC. Figure 21.2 shows a typical staining for MHC class II (blue) in normal spinal cord from two different rat strains, the Lewis (a) and the Brown Norway (b). The sections are co-stained (brown) using antibodies against MHC class I and the transferrin receptor to reveal the vasculature, as both of these molecules are expressed constitutively by CNS and PNS vascular endothelial cells. The notable result is that MHC class II staining in both cases is sparse, although in the Brown Norway, there are a number of cells both in the parenchyma and others more closely associated with vessels, that are MHC class II+. The Brown Norway strain is in fact rather unusual as most others are more like the Lewis strain with little detectable MHC class II expression under normal conditions. The cells in the parenchyma of the Brown Norway spinal cord expressing MHC class II, are microglia.

In the human, there are a number of reports indicating greater constitutive MHC class I and II, usually on microglia of the CNS, in ostensibly 'normal' tissue.

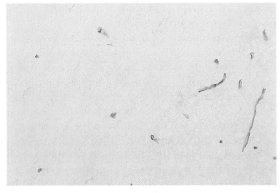

(a)

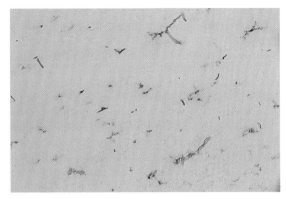

(b)

▮ **Fig. 21.2** Constitutive major histocompatibility complex (MHC) class II expression in the rodent CNS is strain dependent. Horizontal sections of thoracic spinal cord from normal Lewis (a) and Brown Norway (b) rats. The brown staining reveals vessels and blue staining shows MHC class II positive cells. Vessels are in focus while some MHC class II+ cells are out of plane.

However, there are uncertainties whether such expression is really a feature of the 'normal' CNS as it is generally difficult to get very fresh, normal tissue to examine. Microglia are a highly reactive cell population upregulating MHC expression in response to a variety of non-immunological stimuli, particularly neuronal damage. It is possible that MHC expression on microglia, for example in a fresh biopsy specimen, may have resulted from some other underlying pathology or in the case of samples taken post mortem, as a result of ischaemia, the latter known to lead to rapid MHC class II upregulation on microglia in experimental model systems. In general, it is probably fair to say that MHC expression on cells within the normal CNS and PNS is likely to vary from one individual to another (cf. Fig. 21.2) but at best is minimal and on some cells (see below) is absent.

Despite the dearth of MHC-expressing cells, particularly MHC class II in normal nervous tissue, it had been apparent for many years from observations of a variety of clinical conditions, that inflammatory responses could develop in these sites. Subsequently, the description of models of experimental autoimmune inflammation of the CNS and PNS, like experimental autoimmune encephalomyelitis (EAE) and experimental autoimmune neuritis (EAN), respectively, which could be transferred passively to naive animals by autoantigen-specific MHC class II-restricted CD4 T-cell lines and clones, provided unequivocal evidence that antigen in the context of the MHC class II molecule, was being recognized somewhere in the target organ. But how did this happen when MHC class II was supposedly not present in the normal CNS or PNS into which the activated T cells entered?

The main driving force behind the search for the APC of the CNS or PNS, probably lay in the widespread availability in the early to mid-1980s of MHC class I and II specific monoclonal antibodies to detect expression, particularly at the immunohistological level. It soon became clear that after inflammation had developed in the CNS or PNS, whether in a clinical condition like MS or GBS, or in experimental models of autoimmunity (for example EAE) or viral encephalitls such as that induced in mice by Theiler's virus, MHC expression was substantially upregulated. Also a number of studies were published showing that mixed glial cultures or astrocytes derived from the neonatal rodent CNS, could be induced to express MHC class II *in vitro* by treatment with interferon (IFN)-γ. Moreover, Fontana and colleagues showed in 1984, that such astrocyte cultures could also function as APC, processing and presenting autoantigen (MBP) to encephalitogenic CD4 T cells. This description of astrocyte function *in vitro* resulted, perhaps not surprisingly, in the search for astrocyte MHC class II expression *in vivo* and such expression was recorded in many studies. With few exceptions, the data recording astrocyte MHC class II expression *in vivo* have not stood the test of time. Also in the mid-1980s, a few voices in the wilderness, which included those of Hickey, Vass and Lassmann, Matsumoto, and Cuzner, reported that MHC class II expression in both MS as well as in experimental animal models, was not on astrocytes, but rather on a parenchymal dendritiform cell of the CNS — the microglia. Indeed, it is now known that MHC class II expression on astrocytes *in vivo* is a relatively rare event, although they can express MHC class I more readily, so there may be a role for them in interactions with CD8 T cells.

So are MHC class II expressing microglia the APC of the CNS and what about antigen recognition by T cells in the PNS? Evidence accumulated over the past 4–5 years and particularly from *in vivo* studies indicates that the most important APC in the CNS and probably also the PNS, is probably *not* microglia but rather, a population of cells called perivascular cells or perivascular macrophages (Fig. 21.3). These cells lie outside the parenchyma proper, are blood derived, turning over in weeks to months and may express MHC class II constitutively. In contrast, microglia, at least of the CNS, lie within the glial limitans, are a stable population with little evidence for replacement from blood-derived precursor cells, and although readily inducible for MHC expression, do not necessarily express it constitutively. It is uncertain whether the PNS contains a population equivalent to microglia but perivascular cells have been demonstrated. Recent studies by Ford and Sedgwick using fleshly isolated adult microglia versus other CNS-derived macrophage populations which may include perivascular cells, indicate that MHC class II expressing microglia are not particularly efficient APC in comparison with the latter CNS macrophage populations. There is no real evidence that any resident or even transient macrophage population in the CNS or PNS are equivalent to the leucocyte dendritic cell known to be highly efficient in stimulation of both primary and secondary T-cell responses.

As Fig. 21.3 illustrates, it seems likely therefore, that CD4 T cells activated in the periphery pass nonspecifically through the BBB or BNB and see antigen again on perivascular macrophages in the perivascular compartment. Further activation at this stage may stimulate effector mechanisms, including cytokine production particularly tumour necrosis factor, by the T cells. This leads to vascular damage or alterations in permeability, enabling other cells as well as antibody to gain access to the tissue. It is presumed that those T cells which fail to see antigen after crossing into the perivascular compartment, either leave again to search for antigen in another tissue, or die *in situ*.

Tissue damage by T cells and the role of antibody

In the elicitation of disease, it is not the microglia, astrocytes, or perivascular cells that are the important target cells but rather myelinating cells (oligodendrocytes of the CNS and Schwann cells of the PNS) and of course, nerve cells (Fig. 21.3). Like astrocytes, there is little evidence for MHC class II expression on oligodendrocytes and neurons of the CNS and so damage to these cells is unlikely to be mediated directly via CD4 T cells recognizing antigen on them and killing them.

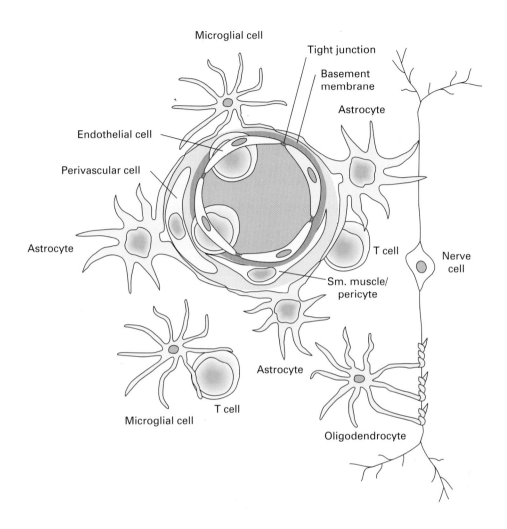

∎ **Fig. 21.3**   T-cell extravasation and interaction with antigen-presenting cells in the CNS.

Cytokines may be more relevant here when one considers the T cell in isolation. There is nevertheless, good evidence both in humans and in experimental animals, for Schwann cell MHC class II expression *in vivo*; so in principle, these cells could serve as direct targets of T cells in demyelinating diseases of the PNS. In general, however, it seems likely the processes of demyelination are dependent on the combined effects of T-cell-mediated breakdown of the BBB/BNB and antibody-dependent demyelination (probably also involving macrophages phagocytosing opsonized cells or myelin), the latter proceeding only after T cells alter

the vasculature sufficiently that myelin/oligodendrocyte/Schwann cell-reactive antibody can gain access to the tissue. Studies by Linington and Wekerle have provided good experimental evidence in the EAE model for CNS demyelination if these two arms of the immune responses are combined but not if applied separately.

A number of neurological diseases discussed below seem to be mediated primarily by antibody and MG is a clear example where antibody is the final 'effector' of disease, not T cells. Of course T cells will most likely be involved in the T–B-cell interactions required for generation of a high affinity, switched humoral response but otherwise are thought not to be integral to the disease process. For diseases of the CNS and PNS (for example paraneoplastic disorders of the CNS), but not MG, this presents something of a quandary as it is unclear exactly how antibody gains access to the tissue in the absence of an obvious inflammatory response (for example as seen in MS). There are two possibilities. First, that the BBB/BNB is not as tight in those individuals who get these conditions, allowing antibody to pass into the tissue from the blood. Second, that plasma cells or activated B cells, like activated T cells, can cross the BBB or BNB. The presence of oligoclonal bands in some of these conditions argues strongly for the production of antibody by cells residing within the tissue but it is still to be resolved whether such cells may access the CNS or PNS through an intact barrier.

Triggering autoimmunity in the nervous system

Theories must take account of the association between infection/geographic distribution and autoimmune disease onset or incidence on the background of a permissive genetic predisposition. Triggering mechanisms could include cross-reactive stimulation of specific autoreactive T/B cells (molecular mimicry) or a more non-specific T/B cell activation (superantigen-type stimulation?). It also seems likely that the propensity of one individual versus another, to progress on to the production of a tissue-damaging immune response after receiving the 'trigger' (such as a viral infection) lies in their ability or otherwise to regulate the emerging response properly. Recent experimental evidence has provided good evidence that normally healthy animal strains can develop a range of tissue-specific autoimmune diseases simply by manipulating the immune response, for example by removing certain CD4+ T-cell subpopulations that are believed normally to prevent self-reactive T- and B-cell responses from escalating uncontrollably. It is not known whether similar mechanisms control susceptibility to autoimmune disease in humans.

Polyneuropathies

Guillain–Barré syndrome

Definition

GBS is an acute inflammatory, rapidly progressive, predominantly motor, peripheral neuropathy, often preceded by a mild infection which is believed to result in an autoimmune reaction directed against myelin. In the more severe cases, plasmapheresis or intravenous γ-globulin is administered with proven beneficial effects. While respiratory failure and death can result in severe cases, the majority of patients make a good recovery, although some are left with residual weakness.

Introduction

A report on acute ascending paralysis resulting in respiratory failure and death was published by Landry (1859). Subsequently in 1916, Guillain, Barré (and Strohl) described the clinical features and characteristic CSF findings of GBS.

Epidemiology

The incidence is estimated to be ~ 1 per 100 000, being slightly higher in females. It occurs at all ages, in all countries, and is not seasonal. In more than half the patients there is a history of a recent (prior 3 weeks) upper respiratory or gastrointestinal infection and identified viral exanthems, cytomegalovirus, Epstein–Barr virus, human immunodeficiency virus 1, *Mycoplasma pneumoniae*, *Campylobacter jejuni*, and Lyme disease. The 1976 swine influenza vaccination programme in the USA resulted in an increased incidence of GBS. Anaesthetics, surgical procedures, and lymphoma have also been linked to some cases.

Pathogenesis

The animal model, experimental autoimmune neuritis (EAN), described by Waksman and Adams in 1955 was first produced in rabbits after subcutaneous injection with sciatic nerve emulsified in Freund's complete adjuvant. Acute paralysis was observed and focal areas of myelin loss in peripheral nerve was discovered pathologically. This model provided direction for investigation of GBS as an immunopathological condition, thought to involve early T-cell disruption of the BNB allowing entry of myelin-reactive antibody and subsequently, macrophages which in combination, demyelinate peripheral nerve axons. However, the exact pathogenesis of GBS has not been elucidated.

Pathology

The pathological hallmark of GBS is demyelination involving the PNS. This results in conduction block (Fig. 21.4), there being an inability to transmit impulses across the demyelinated segment of axon. This is often widely disseminated and can involve spinal roots and nerves, dorsal root ganglia, plexuses, peripheral and cranial nerves (3–12), and sympathetic trunks and ganglia.

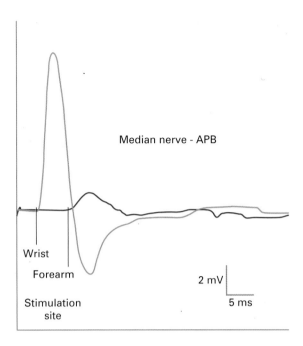

Median nerve - APB

Wrist

Forearm

2 mV

5 ms

Stimulation
site

▌**Fig. 21.4** Nerve conduction block. The compound muscle action potential amplitude drops by 90%, the negative peak area by 86%, and the change in duration is 14%. (Adapted from Chaudhry, V., *et al*. (1993). Multifocal motor neuropathy: response to human immune globulin. *Ann. Neurol.* **33**, 237–42.)

In actively demyelinating lesions, perivascular lymphocytic infiltrates are seen with invasion of apparently normal myelinated fibres by macrophages and subsequent phagocytosis of myelin (Fig. 21.5). Myelin-reactive antibody probably is also involved in the demyelinating process. There is extensive MHC class II expression on inflammatory macrophages and some T cells and Schwann cells can also upregulate MHC class II, unlike oligodendrocytes of the CNS. In EAN, the earliest change is the presence of endoneurial and subperineurial oedema in the *apparent* absence of cellular infiltration, although a few specific T cells are almost certainly present. This has yet to be described in GBS patients probably because progression past such early events has occurred at first presentation. Resolution is heralded by Schwann cell proliferation. In most cases, there is also some axonal loss, possibly due to an immune-mediated bystander effect. Elevated levels of antibodies to the ganglioside GQ1b have been demonstrated recently, in patients with the Miller–Fisher variant of GBS.

Clinical features

The severity of GBS varies greatly, ranging from minimal distal weakness to quadriplegia, bulbar paralysis, and respiratory failure. By definition, it peaks in less than 4 weeks, although the majority reach their nadir within 2 weeks. Approximately half notice a sensory disturbance, while the remainder present with motor complaints. In the majority, weakness progresses to a variable extent from the lower limbs to the trunk, arms, and cranial muscles. Facial and, to a lesser extent, bulbar weakness are the commonest cranial manifestations. Atrophy does not usually develop, but areflexia is characteristic. Sensation is affected in the majority, although usually to a lesser degree than the motor involvement. Pain of involved muscles, especially proximal ones, is often a feature, and occasionally requires narcotics for relief. Autonomic disturbances are frequently overlooked, but include tachyarrhythmias, labile blood pressure, diaphoresis or impairment of sweating, and sphincter disturbances. Up to one-third require a period of artificial ventilation, and all patients should have frequent forced vital capacities (FVC) to detect impend-

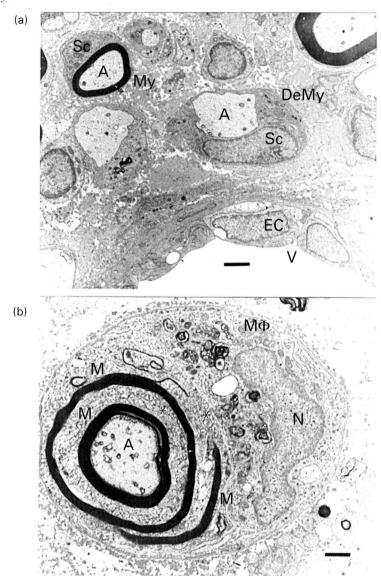

▮ Fig. 21.5 Peripheral nerve demyelination. (a) Perivenous demyelination in experimental autoimmune neuritis in the peripheral nerve of rat. Plate shows both demyelinated (DeMy) and myelinated (My) axons (A) while retaining an intact Schwann cell (SC). The area of demyelination is in close apposition to a vessel (V). Endothelial cells (EC) are indicated. Bar = 5 μm. (b) Stripping of myelin (M) from the axon (A) by a macrophage (M$\emptyset$) in acute GBS. *Vesiculating myelin. The macrophage nucleus (N) is prominent. Tissue from sural nerve biopsy. Bar = 2 μm. M = Myelin. (Both plates kindly provided by Professor John Pollard, Department of Medicine (Neurology), University of Sydney and Royal Prince Alfred Hospital).

ing respiratory failure, with elective intubation to be strongly considered if the vital capacity falls to about 15 ml/kg. Clinical variants of the disease include predominant sensory or autonomic involvement, lower bulbar involvement (termed polyneuritis cranialis), and the Miller–Fisher syndrome, which is characterized by the combination of ophthalmoplegia, ataxia, and areflexia.

Diagnosis

The diagnosis remains essentially a clinical one, although supportive evidence on electromyography

▌ **Table 21.2** Diagnostic criteria for Guillain–Barré syndrome

Features required
   Absence of other identifiable cause
   Progressive motor weakness of one or more limbs
   Areflexia

Features strongly supportive
   Clinical
      Progression less than 4 weeks
      Cranial nerve involvement
      Relative symmetry
      Onset of recovery after a variable plateau phase
      Autonomic involvement
      Absence of fever at onset
      Cranial nerve involvement
      Mild sensory symptoms and signs
   Cerebrospinal fluid
      Raised total protein level after the first week
      Cells less than 10 mononuclear cells per mm^3
   Electrodiagnostic features
      Slowing of conduction

Features casting doubt on the diagnosis
   Marked persistent asymmetry of the weakness
   Persistent bladder or bowel dysfunction
   Sharp sensory level
   Bladder or bowel dysfunction at onset
   More than 50 mononuclear cells per mm^3 in CSF
   Presence of polymorphonuclear cells in the CSF

(EMG) and in CSF is usually present. Diagnostic criteria have been devised, and are listed in Table 21.2.

The characteristic CSF finding in GBS is a high protein count with a normal cell count, termed 'albuminocytological dissociation' by Guillain, Barré, and Strohl. However, this finding is time dependent and protein is often normal in the first week, and occasionally the cell count is raised.

Nerve conduction studies are more useful in confirming the diagnosis: decreased conduction velocity, a decrease in the compound muscle action potential (CMAP) with more proximal stimulation (termed 'conduction block' — see Fig. 21.4), dispersion of the CMAP, and absent or prolonged F waves.

Treatment

General supportive care, with attention to pressure areas, close monitoring of respiratory function and blood pressure, and adequate pain relief is required. Artificial ventilation should be instituted if the forced vital capacity falls below 12–15 ml per kg, or the arterial PO_2 falls below 70 mmHg. In mild cases,

no specific immunomodulation may be required. However, if there is progressive weakness with debility or respiratory compromise, specific therapy with either plasmapheresis or intravenous γ-globulin is indicated. More than 3 weeks after symptom onset, these therapies have little value.

Plasmapheresis, with 3–5 alternate day exchanges, results in earlier improvement, significantly less rates of artificial ventilation, and a reduced time to independent mobility. Recently, the efficacy of intravenous γ-globulin over plasmapheresis was demonstrated with greater functional improvement, less complications, and less time requiring artificial ventilation.

In the past, steroids have not been shown to be beneficial in the treatment of GBS, but recently there has been renewed interest in their potential use. Nerve growth factors may prove to be useful in the future.

Prognosis

Remyelination is an efficient process which is usually completed within 6 months. However, if there has been significant axonal degeneration, improvement may continue for up to 2 years after the illness. While the majority of patients make a complete or nearly complete recovery, up to 5% die being at risk of cardiac arrhythmias and adult respiratory distress syndrome (ARDS) in the early stages, and pulmonary emboli or sepsis later. About 15% are left with a significant functional deficit.

Chronic inflammatory demyelinating polyradiculoneuropathy

Definition

Chronic inflammatory demyelinating polyradiculoneuropathy (CIDP) is very similar to GBS, being a symmetrical polyradiculoneuropathy with evidence of demyelination, electrophysiologically and histologically. However, it runs either a progressive or relapsing course, and is distinguished by being steroid responsive.

Introduction

The incidence of this condition is not known exactly, but seems to be about two to five per 100 000. Males appear to be affected more than females, and patients with the relapsing form of the disease are significantly younger than those in the progressive group.

Pathogenesis

Chronic or relapsing EAN, produced by sensitizing animals to peripheral myelin or myelin proteins is the experimental model of CIDP. This can be induced by giving larger doses of myelin than that used to induce EAN, by giving repeated sensitizing injections or most commonly, by injecting immunosuppressed animals, for example after low-dose cyclosporin A treatment. There is evidence of a possible genetic susceptibility to this condition, with increased frequencies of HLA-A1, -B8, -A3, -DR2, -DR3, and -Dw3 reported.

Pathology

As with GBS, the histological features are those of an inflammatory, predominantly proximal demyelinating neuropathy.

Clinical features

CIDP tends to have a more insidious onset, and slower course than GBS, often being subclassified into either a relapsing, or the less common progressive form, the latter accounting for approximately one-third of cases. Occasionally, the presentation is acute, and the distinction between GBS and CIDP cannot be made until a relapse occurs or the illness continues to progress beyond 4 weeks.

The symptoms and signs are usually those of a mixed sensorimotor polyneuropathy, although occasionally, patients present with pure motor or sensory syndromes. Proximal weakness is frequently present, with weakness of neck flexors distinguishing it from most other neuropathies, but cranial nerve abnormalities are less frequent.

The diagnosis of CIDP is based upon clinical, laboratory, pathological, and electrophysiological evidence.

The essential features required are the presence of a relapsing or progressive usually sensorimotor polyneuropathy developing over at least 2 months, with hypo- or areflexia, nerve conduction evidence of predominant demyelination, pathological evidence of demyelination and remyelination and commonly, CSF albuminocytological dissociation. Unlike GBS, a nerve biopsy (usually the sural) is often required to confirm the diagnosis, and exclude other causes of neuropathy.

Treatment and prognosis

Steroid therapy has been shown to be beneficial in the treatment of CIDP, in contrast to GBS. The usual dose is about 50–75 mg for approximately 4 weeks, with gradually reduced doses thereafter. For more prolonged therapy, azathioprine may be added as a steroid sparing agent. Plasmapheresis and high-dose intravenous γ-globulin has been reported to be efficacious in some patients. Following treatment, many patients improve within 2–4 weeks. In long-term follow-up studies, the majority (60–70%) of patients made a good or full recovery.

❚ **Table 21.3** Proposed diagnostic criteria for chronic inflammatory demyelinating polyradiculoneuropathy

---

Clinical features (all present)
  Symmetrical proximal and distal weakness
  Fluctuating, steady or progressive course > 2
    months
  Hypo- or areflexia

Laboratory features (at least two present)
  Raised CSF protein
  Nerve conduction evidence of demyelination
  Nerve biopsy evidence of demyelination
    ± remyelination

Exclusion of other causes of neuropathy
  Inherited
  Drugs/toxin-related
  Association with paraprotein/lymphoproliferative
    disorders/other systemic disorders

Multifocal motor neuropathy

Definition

This is a recently recognized disorder, characterized by multifocal conduction block principally affecting motor nerves, in which the immune attack is directed against the myelin of motor axons. The presence of antiganglioside antibodies and response to immunoglobulin favours an immunological pathogenesis, although this has not been clearly elucidated.

Introduction

This is a chronic neuropathy with multifocal motor conduction block. The presence of high concentrations of IgG and IgM antibodies to ganglioside monosialac acid (GM_1) was found in two patients with a pure motor disorder, leading to the association of MMN and some other motor syndromes with these antibodies. It occurs most commonly in young and middle-aged adults, but has also been reported in children and the elderly. Males seem to be affected predominantly.

Pathogenesis

The conduction block is confined to motor axons and it has been suggested that there may be a difference in the antigenic properties of the components of myelin enveloping motor and sensory axons. Targets could include gangliosides such as GM_1, GQIb, and antisialo antibodies. These are acidic glycolipids located in the membrane of neurons, on the axolemma, and to a smaller extent on myelin. Elevated concentrations of anti-GM_1 antibodies are found in up to 84% of patients with MMN. However, they are not specific for this condition, being found in 23% of patients with motor neuron disease (MND) as well as in a number of other conditions, suggesting that antibody production could potentially be an epiphenomenon secondary to myelin damage. Thus, the part of ganglioside antibody in the pathogenesis of MMN is unclear.

Pathology

Biopsies of motor nerves have been reported to demonstrate evidence of demyelination, with onion-bulb formations containing demyelinated and thinly remyelinated axons. Inflammatory cells are absent. Surprisingly, sural nerve pathology may be abnormal with loss of myelinated axons and perivascular lymphocytic inflammation reported in some despite normal sural nerve sensory conduction. This indicates that sensory nerves are involved, despite the lack of sensory and electrophysiological abnormalities.

Clinical features

Patients characteristically present with progressive weakness and muscular atrophy, accompanied by cramps and occasionally minor sensory symptoms. The disease usually begins and remains more prominent in the upper limbs. Examination reveals a combination of muscle atrophy, often accompanied by fasciculations. Reflexes may be preserved or absent. Sensory abnormalities are typically absent or minor.

Treatment and prognosis

Steroids, plasmapheresis, azathioprine, and oral cyclophosphamide have had disappointing results in this condition; however, a number of patients responded to intravenous cyclophosphamide, the reduction in anti-GM$_1$ antibodies paralleling clinical improvement. Intravenous immunoglobulin in a placebo-controlled trial produced a significant improvement in muscle strength, although disability was not altered.

The course is usually slowly progressive, patients remaining functional for many years. Best results have been seen in those patients receiving intravenous immunoglobulin early in the course of the condition.

Plexopathies

Definition

The brachial and lumbosacral plexuses occasionally are affected by a process believed to be immunologically mediated, with the resultant development of pain and patchy weakness and to a lesser extent sensory

changes. Recovery is the rule, although this is not always complete.

Introduction

First noticed when serum therapy became popular in the early part of the twentieth century to treat or prevent infectious diseases. Infections have also been linked to plexopathies for many years. However, it was only recently that abnormalities in immune responses were detected in affected individuals.

Epidemiology

The annual incidence of brachial plexopathy (BP) is estimated to be 1–2/100 000, all ages being affected. Young to middle-aged adults are particularly susceptible, and males tend to be affected more commonly. Recurrence occurs in about 5%, but tends to be less severe. Lumbosacral plexopathy (LSP) occurs less frequently, although the axact incidence is uncertain.

Pathogenesis

A number of viral infections have been implicated in the genesis of BP and to a lesser extent LSP, including influenza, infectious mononucleosis, cytomegalovirus, coxsackie B, poliomyelitis, and acute infectious hepatitis. Other infectious agents reported in association with BP are typhoid, typhus, tuberculosis, and toxoplasmosis. Serum and vaccine therapies including those used for tetanus, smallpox, polio, and triple antigen injections may also produce the syndrome. Patients with systemic disorders such, as serum sickness, rheumatoid arthritis, systemic lupus erythematosus, ankylosing spondylitis, and polyarteritis nodosa may also develop plexopathies.

T cells are thought to be activated against sections of the plexus to produce the neuropathy, possibly secondary to activation by an infectious agent (see GBS). An immunological basis is supported by the presence of a blastogenic lymphocytic response to fresh autopsy extracts of human nerves, using lymphocytes obtained from patients with BP. The antigenic component within the plexuses has yet to be elucidated.

Pathology

In the few reports of histological findings in cases of BP, mononuclear infiltrates were seen around endoneurial vessels, and onion-bulb formation was evident around demyelinated axons.

Clinical features

Pain is usually the initial symptom, around the shoulder most commonly in BP, although it may extend to the neck, into the pectorals or down the arm. This is followed within 2–4 weeks by arm weakness, which is often diffuse and incomplete. Shoulder girdle muscles are particularly affected. Reflexes may be depressed or absent depending on the distribution of the neuropathy. Sensory loss is usually less severe than the motor findings. In up to 5% of cases the facial, phrenic, or accessory nerves may be involved.

In LSP, pain is present in the anterior thigh in upper plexus lesions, and in the buttock and posterior thigh in lower plexopathies. Weakness occurs within 3 weeks, initially progressing before eventually slowly recovering. As with BP, sensory findings are less marked.

Diagnosis

In the early stages where pain is the main feature, local joint problems are often suspected. The diagnosis becomes more apparent following the development of weakness. If doubt exists, a cervical magnetic resonance imaging (MRI) or myelogram should be performed. The presence of reduced sensory nerve action potentials (SNAPs) from a peripherally affected nerve is helpful in excluding a radicular or more proximal lesion. EMG is helpful in characterizing the muscles involved.

Treatment and prognosis

Steroids are often used in the acute stages to ease the pain; however, there is no evidence they speed recovery or alter the eventual outcome. Physiotherapy helps to preserve limb function.

The majority (90%) of patients with BP make a full recovery within 3 years, although upper plexus lesions appear to have a more favourable outcome. Recurrence occurs in about 5%. Prognosis tends to be less favourable for LSP, although most achieve a significant degree of recovery.

Paraproteinaemic neuropathy

Definition

Monoclonal immunoglobulins may be associated with a peripheral neuropathy either as part of the systemic manifestation of a paraproteinaemia, or as the sole feature. Benign monoclonal gammopathy, multiple myeloma, plasmocytoma, Waldenström's macroglobulinaemia, cold agglutinin disease, cryoglobulinaemia, lymphoma, and primary amyloidosis may all be associated with the condition. With osteosclerotic myeloma, in addition to the sclerotic bone lesions there is polyneuropathy, organomegaly, endocrinopathy, monoclonal protein, and skin changes (termed POEMS syndrome).

Only the benign gammopathies will be considered in this section.

Introduction

Only in the last two decades, has the clear association between paraproteins and neuropathy emerged. Approximately one-third of all patients with a benign monoclonal gammopathy eventually develop a systemic B-cell disorder, most commonly multiple myeloma, indicating that all patients with a presumed benign gammopathy should be followed. The term monoclonal gammopathy of uncertain significance (MGUS) is now favoured. Of the neuropathies associated with paraproteins, IgM is the commonest (about 50%), followed by IgG and IgA. The peak incidence is in the sixth or seventh decade. Males are far more commonly affected in IgM neuropathy, whereas the male–female ratio is approximately equal in IgG cases. There have been too few cases of IgA neuropathy reported to enable accurate characterization.

Pathogenesis

Some IgM paraproteins appear to react with myelin-associated glycoprotein (MAG), accounting for 50% of IgM paraproteins occurring with sensorimotor neuropathy. Another group of IgM paraproteins react with GMI ganglioside. There are several potential antigens in the peripheral nerve capable of binding MAG antibodies. These antibodies are evident in purely motor disorders such as multifocal motor neuropathy (see previous section) as well as sensorimotor neuropathies, and occasionally coexist with anti-MAG antibodies as a biclonal gammopathy. Possibly, immunoglobulin deposition produces demyelination and prevents remyelination. The reactivity of IgG and IgA paraproteins with defined neural antigens (neurofilament proteins) has yet to be identified.

Pathology

The commonest pathological finding is chronic demyelination with secondary axonal loss, although occasionally the changes are predominantly those of an axonopathy. Deposition of IgM may be demonstrable by immunohistochemistry on remaining myelin sheaths. This deposition of IgM paraproteins is felt to produce the almost pathognomonic pathological appearance of widely spaced myelin. Complement components have been identified, suggesting demyelination may be complement mediated. Focal areas of hypermyelination, called tomacula may also be seen in areas.

Clinical features

As with most peripheral neuropathies, the pattern is of a distal and symmetric sensorimotor neuropathy, affecting the lower limbs especially. Cranial nerves are not affected. Paraesthesias are common, and pain is present in about one-third.

In benign monoclonal gammopathies, the paraprotein concentration is usually less than 3 g/dl and suppression of other immunoglobulin classes is not present. Plasma cells make up less than 5% of the bone marrow, unlike malignant conditions, and there are no lytic lesions. Cryoglobulins and cold agglutinins should be sought. A skeletal survey should be performed to exclude POEMS syndrome, as radiotherapy to the sclerotic lesions often produces a good recovery of the polyneuropathy in this condition. Nerve conduction studies typically reveal a significantly reduced conduction velocity, and absent or reduced sensory nerve action potentials. An elevated protein level is usually found in the CSF.

Paraproteinaemic neuropathy differs from CIDP by the presence of a monoclonal paraprotein, being progressive rather than relapsing, and typically having prominent sensory features.

Treatment and prognosis

In most patients, the course is usually slowly progressive and requires no treatment. Occasionally, the neuropathy follows a relapsing and remitting course. Prednisolone is usually tried initially. The response to treatment is less favourable for those with the commoner IgM neuropathy. Approximately one-third of patients with 'benign monoclonal gammopathies' ultimately develop a related malignant condition, and so all patients should be followed indefinitely.

CNS demyelination

Multiple sclerosis

Definition

MS is a highly variable condition characterized by episodes of white matter dysfunction due to the development of plaques of demyelination, usually interspersed between periods of clinical stability. Disability develops as a result of the cumulative dysfunction from multiple attacks, or from progressive disease. The clinical diagnosis is dependent upon the history of two episodes of focal neurological dysfunction involving more than one region of the CNS at different times.

Introduction

Charcot described the features of MS in 1868. Since that time, numerous theories as to the aetiology and pathogenesis of this condition have been proposed. Viral and other infections, toxins, nutritional deficiencies and excesses, vascular occlusions, and biochemical defects have all been proposed at various stages. Following the studies of EAE in the 1950s, an immunological pathogenesis was proposed. An autoimmune reaction directed against myelin proteins is now the favoured mechanism, although the trigger has not been identified.

Epidemiology

MS has a prevalence of about 1/1000, with regions further from the equator having a greater incidence of the disease. It is the most common disabling neurological condition affecting young Caucasians. The 'protective' effect from being African, Asian, or West Indian was shown to be lost in the first generation of immigrants to the UK from these regions; their rates of MS were equivalent to those of indigenous peoples in cities of the UK, suggesting environmental factors play a major part in the genesis of demyelination.

Genetic factors

MS is predominantly a disease of Caucasians and is rare in other races. However, these racial tendencies are modified by geographical location. Concordance in identical twins may be as high as 70% and 15% of those with MS have an affected relative. Females are afflicted at a rate approaching 2:1 compared with males. Associations with major histocompatibility antigens have been reported, including A3, B7, DR2, DQwl, DQB1, and DQA1, the strongest being with DR2, which carries a relative risk of 2.5. In families the diseases does not always segregate with the HLA haplotype. MS-associated haplotype DRB1*1501, DQB1*0602, DQA1*0102 is present in 30–50% of cases.

Examination of T-cell receptors in MS reveals that certain rearrangements confer an increased risk.

Pathogenesis

Epidemiological/twin studies (see above) implicate a role for environmental factors in triggering the disease. Viral infections have been shown in a prospective study to be a risk factor for attacks of MS, although the link between onset of MS and recent infection with a variety of infectious agents is not as strong as is seen with GBS. Otherwise, there is no definite correlation between trauma or other events and exacerbations, with the possible exception of electrical injury. Pregnancy also has inconsistent effects on the course of the disease, patients possibly improving during the pregnancy, but being at increased risk of exacerbations in the first few months post-partum. Heightened familial susceptibility and association with certain MHC haplotypes, is strongly suggestive of an immunological basis to MS.

A simplistic encompassing view of the pathogenesis of MS is that in patients with an inherent genetic susceptibility, a viral (or other?) infection precipitates an autoimmune response that ultimately results in predominantly CNS demyelination. The immunopathogenesis of MS can be described along very similar lines to those outlined for GBS where, based on model systems like EAE which share some of the pathological features of MS, early T-cell disruption of the BBB enables entry of myelin-reactive antibody and subsequently macrophages, which in combination and possibly with an involvement of complement, demyelinate CNS axons. As with GBS, the exact pathogenesis of MS has not been elucidated. It still is unclear whether infection somehow precipitates an autoimmune response which is directly responsible for myelin destruction or rather, that the inflammation and demyelination is the result of a normal immune response towards an infectious agent within the CNS. Both aetiological pathways have been reproduced experimentally, the former for example demonstrated by Watanabe, Wege, and ter Meulen, where MBP-reactive T cells were recovered from rats infected only with a neurotropic form of the murine hepatitis virus but not injected with the myelin antigens or adjuvants normally required to induce MBP-reactive T cells.

Pathology

Early events are thought to involve BBB disruption and vascular permeability changes which can be viewed most readily by MRI, particularly in combination with gadolinium enhancement. Plaques of demyelination, ranging from less than a millimetre to several centimetres in diameter are present throughout the white matter of the brain and spinal cord. Periventricular localization is characteristic.

The histological appearance is dependent on the age of the lesion. In the early stages of plaque formation, T cells and macrophages adhere to the endothelium in the brain and migrate into the nervous tissue to form infiltrates. There is increased expression of MHC class II on microglia. A small proportion of T cells display markers of activation, e.g. interleukin (IL) 2 receptor. At a later stage CD4+ T cells are found in the centre of the plaque while CD8+ T cells are at the periphery. The meaning of this distribution is unclear. Acute lesions exhibit demyelination in a pre-

dominantly perivenous distribution, with associated perivascular infiltration by mononuclear cells and lymphocytes, and macrophages may be seen attached to and removing, myelin. Oligodendrocytes are damaged and astrocytes proliferate. Eventually, plaques are characterized by relatively acellular fibrous and glial areas with bare axons, depleted oligodendrocytes, astrocytic overgrowth and with sparse inflammatory cells. The oligodendrocytes responsible for remyelination appear to be previously undifferentiated immature oligodendrocytes, rather than surviving mature cells.

Clinical features

Patients may either have progressive neurological decline and disability, or may follow a relapsing–remitting course with episodes of neurological dysfunction from which partial or complete recovery is achieved. The clinical manifestations of MS are protean, commoner presentations being optic neuritis, hemisensory or hemiparetic syndromes, disturbances of co-ordination, or cord syndromes. Spinal cord involvement results in sphincteric disturbances and a mixture of motor and sensory signs. Brainstem involvement can result in a plethora of symptoms and signs, including vertigo, diplopia due to gaze palsies, vomiting, facial paralysis, and long tract signs. An internuclear ophthalmoplegia (nystagmus in the abducting eye, and incomplete adduction of the adducting eye) is almost pathognomonic of MS, especially in patients under the age of 50, being produced by a lesion of the medial longitudinal fasciculus.

Optic neuritis is the initial manifestation in 25% of patients. Approximately 75% of all females with an episode of optic neuritis will eventually develop manifestations of MS, while the frequency in males is only about 34%. Symptoms of MS are often worse in hot weather, or following hot showers or baths. Other less commonly recognized manifestations include Lhermitte's phenomenon, deafness, tinnitus, myokymia, trigeminal neuralgia, pain syndromes, and seizures. A variety of neuropsychiatric disturbances are possible, including euphoria, depression, confusion, and dementia. Approximately 50% of patients have manifestations indicating multiple sites of involvement, while one-third have a spinal form. The remainder have predominantly cerebellar or amaurotic manifestations. Occasionally, patients present with a malignant form of MS which rapidly evolves over a few weeks until they eventually succumb.

Diagnosis

For many years, the diagnosis of MS relied purely on clinical findings. The currently accepted criteria, prepared by Poser and colleagues (1983; Table 21.4),

∎ **Table 21.4** Diagnostic criteria for multiple sclerosis

Category	Attacks (>24 h)	Clinical evidence	Paraclinical evidence (MRI, evoked responses)	Oligoclonal bands/raised IgG levels
A. Clinically definite (CD)				
CDMS A1	2	2		
CDMS A2	2	1	and 1	
B. Laboratory supported definite (LSD)				
LSDMS B1	2	1	or 1	+
LSDMS B2	1	2		+
LSDMS B3	1	1	and 1	+
C. Clinically probable (CP)				
CPMS C1	2	1		
CPMS C2	1	2		
CPMS C3	1	1	and 1	
D. Laboratory supported probable (LPS)				
LSPMS D1	2			+

Adapted from Poser *et al.* (1983). *Ann. Neurol.* **13**, 227–231.

takes into account laboratory and radiological studies, from which four broad categories are derived. These are used mainly for research purposes, a simpler clinical classification being relapsing–remitting, primary progressive, or secondarily progressive disease.

Visual evoked responses (VERs) can detect evidence of current or previous ocular nerve involvement, which often is subclinical, and is especially useful for example in patients who present with an episode of transverse myelitis in providing evidence of demyelination in an area remote to the cord, thereby fulfilling the diagnostic criteria. Auditory and somatosensory evoked responses can also provide indirect evidence of occult demyelination.

Examination of the CSF can provide additional evidence of MS, approximately 40% having a mild mononuclear pleocytosis, a similar number having an elevated protein, while the majority have increased levels of IgG and/or oligoclonal bands (only supportive of MS if they are not present in the blood). The presence of oligoclonal bands in the first attack of MS is believed to be predictive of the chronic-relapsing form of the condition.

The advent of MRI has finally provided a radiological method to assist in confirming the diagnosis, and often is the only investigation undertaken (Fig. 21.6). White matter changes are sought, especially in the periventricular and corpus callosum regions of the brain. These changes are not specific, however, especially in older patients, with cerebrovascular disease being the principal differential diagnosis radiologically. Enhancement following gadolinium is suggestive of active disease. It is also important to note that during recent IFNβ trials (see below), reduction in the size and frequency of lesions as detected by MRI, was substantially more spectacular than the improvement in disability score over time. In light of this, it is worth considering exactly what the appearance of MRI detectable lesions means for diagnosis.

Treatment

The treatment of MS is still controversial. In recent years, there has been increasing evidence supporting the use of high-dose corticosteroids in acute exacerbations of MS. Steroids are believed to produce an improvement in symptoms by reducing inflammation and oedema associated with new lesions. Patients with acute optic neuritis, which is often the initial presentation of MS, had a significantly lower incidence of the subsequent development of MS when treated with a 3-day course of high-dose (1 gram) intravenous methylprednisolone. However, the effects of steroids are transient and their effectiveness often is diminished with repeated use. Therefore, steroids should be used judiciously, being reserved for definite relapses producing a significant functional impairment. Rare

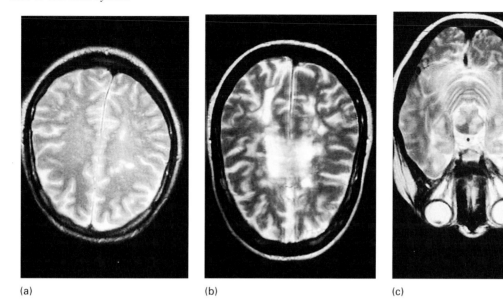

(a)   (b)   (c)

▮ **Fig. 21.6**   MRI of lesions present in MS.

(a) T2 weighted transverse image taken through white matter just above the bodies of the bodies of the lateral ventricles. Several small white matter lesions are present on the right. The largest is ovoid with a transverse long axis, a feature suggesting demyelination

(b) T2 transverse image at the level of the lateral ventricles. This patient had a ten-year history of multiple sclerosis. In addition to multiple large plaques of demyelination there is atrophy, a common finding in longstanding multiple sclerosis.

(c) The same patient has several large plaques within the pons illustrating the frequent occurrence of brainstem disease in chronic M.S.

patients appear to be steroid dependent, benefiting from long-term steroid therapy. However, overall, steroids have not been demonstrated to alter the natural history of the disease.

Other immunosuppressants have proven to be disappointing in altering the course of MS. Azathioprine (2 mg/kg) has been shown to produce modest effects in reducing relapses and slowing progression, and deserves consideration in rapidly progressive cases. Other agents such as cyclophosphamide, cyclosporin, anti-T-cell (CD3) antibody, and copolymer 1 have produced minor if any beneficial effects. Anti-CD4 treatment trials are underway currently.

The most exciting advance in the treatment of MS has been the recent report of beneficial effects of a recombinant, non-glycosylated form of IFNβ. This agent has known immunomodulatory actions including inhibition of IFNγ-induced MHC class II upregulation on the surface of APCs. In a 1987 study IFNγ was shown to increase attacks of MS. Although there were significant reductions in exacerbation rates, the severity of exacerbations and accumulation of MRI abnormalities, there was no discernible benefit on disability

after 2 years. Ongoing studies with an alternative (glycosylated) form of IFNβ look promising and hopefully will clarify the role of this agent in reducing the incidence of relapsing–remitting disease, as well as assess its effect in patients with progressive forms of MS.

Symptomatic management is an important aspect of the management of these patients. Spasticity may be improved with baclofen, administered orally or occasionally via a subcutaneous infusion or intrathecally. Neurogenic bladder disorders are a frequent problem, especially in those with spinal involvement, but can be improved with bladder retraining, anticholinergics, or intermittent catheterization.

Prognosis

Factors associated with reduced survival rates and a shorter period to advanced disability include being male, older age at onset, progressive course from onset, and having cerebellar symptoms at onset. Relapses tend to reduce in frequency with time, being highest in younger patients. The average relapse rate is about 0.4 attacks per year; however, there is a wide variation. Approximately 14% have a progressive form of the disease from onset. In one study with a mean follow-up of 9 years, 30% became secondarily progressive, while a similar number remained in a relapse-free state. A multivariate analysis demonstrated that the shorter the length of the first remission, the more likely a poor outcome will ensue. Other studies suggest the majority of patients with relapsing–remitting MS eventually develop progressive disease.

At 15 years from disease onset, 10% are wheelchair bound, and a further 50% need a walking stick or frame.

Acute disseminated/haemorrhagic encephalomyelitis

Definition

The term acute disseminated encephalomyelitis (ADEM) encompasses a range of disease states including postinfectious, postexanthem, and postvaccinal encephalomyelitis, in which there is an acute demyelinating illness following an infection or vaccination. Acute necrotizing haemorrhagic encephalomyelitis (ANHEM) is a fulminant disorder characterized by demyelination and necrosis and is most likely a related condition.

Introduction

Neurological sequelae after vaccines were first noted in the nineteenth century with rabies and smallpox vaccines, some patients developing paralysis. The first major outbreak of postvaccinal ADEM was in 1922 in association with smallpox vaccinations.

Epidemiology

The incidence of ADEM following smallpox infection was about 0.3%, and for other exanthems such as measles, chickenpox, and rubella it is 0.2% or less. With the earlier rabies vaccines derived from nervous tissue the incidence was also about 0.2%. The incidence of ANHEM is uncertain; however, young adults are affected most frequently.

Pathogenesis

Encephalomyelitis has been reported to occur in association with a variety of infections including measles, rubella, smallpox, chickenpox, mumps, mycoplasma, and influenza. Vaccinations which have been complicated by ADEM include rabies, smallpox, and tetanus antitoxin. Original rabies vaccines derived from virus grown in rabbit brain tissue were associated with high rates of ADEM. The development of alternative vaccines which do not contain nervous tissue appears to have eliminated this complication.

EAE is the laboratory model of ADEM, a similar illness developing in animals 1–2 weeks following inoculation with brain tissue and adjuvants, due to a T-cell-mediated reaction against MBP and probably other myelin components.

Infective agents have never been recovered from the brains or CSF of affected patients, the disease presumably being an immune-mediated complication. In patients with postmeasles ADEM there is no antibody production against measles virus in the CSF, indicating the disease is not dependent on viral replication in the CNS; but there are T-cell proliferative responses to MBP in peripheral blood leucocytes providing evidence of a cell-mediated pathogenesis.

The vascular lesions of EAE can be converted to those seen in ANHEM by intravenous injection of meningococcal toxin, which produces a Shwartzman reaction.

Pathology

Demyelination is evident throughout the brain and spinal cord in ADEM, usually in close vicinity to small- and medium-sized veins, with lymphocytes and mononuclear cells also evident in these regions. The nerve cells and axons are largely unaffected.

Clinical features

The symptoms may develop while the patient has the rash, or up to 3 weeks following the infective illness, or after a vaccination. Typically, there is the acute onset of a febrile illness with altered conscious state, ranging from confusion and drowsiness to coma in the most severe cases. Associated headache, neck stiffness, and seizures are often present. If the cord is also involved, varying degrees of para- or quadriplegia may develop. In such cases, initially, there is a flaccid weakness with loss of reflexes but extensor plantars, loss of sphincteric control, and variable sensory loss. Increased tone and reflexes develop later. Rarely, choreoathetosis is seen.

Patients with ANHEM also invariably have a history of a preceding respiratory infection, and the presentation is clinically indistinguishable from ADEM.

The diagnosis remains essentially clinical unless a brain biopsy is undertaken. Lumbar puncture usually reveals a moderate lymphocytic pleocytosis in ADEM, while polymorphs may predominate in the CSF in ANHEM. Variable numbers of red cells may be seen in the latter condition, while the CSF protein is often increased in both disorders. White matter changes consistent with acute inflammation aid in making the diagnosis.

Treatment and prognosis

Controlled trials have not been performed but the use of steroids in ADEM and ANHEM is generally accepted as they have been shown to reduce the severity of complications. Plasmapheresis may be tried in those who continue to deteriorate despite steroids.

The outcome is often poor, the mortality rate being 30–50% in postvaccinal cases, and 10–20% in postinfectious cases. Survivors are often left with significant neurological deficits, such as retardation, epilepsy and behavioural disturbances. Full neurological recovery does occur in some cases. The prognosis is even worse in ANHEM, patients often dying within a few days of the onset.

Subacute sclerosing panencephalitis

Definition

Subacute sclerosing panencephalitis (SSPE) is an increasingly uncommon progressive and fatal disease produced by an immune response to persistent measles virus (MV) infection of the CNS. Previously known as *subacute inclusion body encephalitis* and *subacute sclerosing leucoencephalitis* they are now thought to be part of the spectrum of SSPE, being host-determined, phenotypically different expressions of the persistent infection of neurons by MV. The importance of the immune response was first appreciated in 1952 with the demonstration of an elevated level of immunoglobulin (Ig)G in the CSF of patients with SSPE. Elevated anti-MV antibody titres in the blood were reported in 1967 and subsequently, MV containing immune complexes in the walls of affected blood vessels was demonstrated.

Epidemiology

The disease characteristically affects children, rarely occurring after the age of 18, the mean age of onset being 11 years. There is usually a history of measles at a young age. With the extensive vaccination programme in many countries, the estimated incidence is now about one per million children per year. Males are affected two to three times more commonly than females.

Pathogenesis

The exact pathogenesis of this condition remains poorly understood. Normally, infection with MV produces an acute, limited disease, with occasional evidence of CNS involvement in the form of an encephalitis. It is speculated that in those who go on to develop SSPE, the antiviral immune response which develops is incapable of fully clearing the MV infection, which may become latent, failing to produce infectious viral particles. Infection is maintained by the intact replicative complex of MV within cells, with virus spreading to neighbouring cells by axonal transport through synaptic defts.

How MV infection within the CNS produces the disease is unclear. Possibly, cell death is a direct function of a lytic virus. Patients with SSPE have high titres of MV antibody in both serum and CSF, whereas those with natural MV infection have lower serum titres, and no antibody in the CSF. It is possible that either antibody or T-cell responses directed to the virus may participate in cellular destruction within the CNS, although T-cell targeting to neurons, the main host cell for the virus in the CNS, is difficult given the absence of constitutive or inducible MHC expression on this cell type.

Pathology

The disease involves both grey and white matter, although it usually spares the cerebellum. There is destruction of nerve cells and degeneration of medullated fibres with perivenous cuffing by lymphocytes and mononuclear cells typical of a viral infection. The pathological hallmark of SSPE is the presence of intranuclear and intracytoplasmic eosinophilic inclusions containing paramyxovirus nucleocapsids seen with the electron microscope. MV-specific fluorescence can also be demonstrated in the brain tissues of patients with SSPE.

Clinical features

The clinical features usually develop at about 7 years following the MV infection, which typically occurs at a young age. The deterioration is usually steadily progressive, with death occurring 12–36 months after the first symptoms. Personality change or a decline in school performance may be the initial manifestations, followed by a progressive intellectual deterioration in association with focal or generalized seizures, myoclonus, ataxia, muteness, and signs of spasticity.

The electroencephalogram (EEG) often has periodic bursts every 5–8 seconds of high-voltage slow-waves, followed by a relatively flat trace. There are elevated levels of MV antibody in the serum and CSF, not usually seen in natural measles infection. The CSF contains few or no cells; however, the protein is usually elevated, and there are IgG oligoclonal bands.

Biopsy may be undertaken where the diagnosis is uncertain, revealing the previously described pathological features, and helping to exclude other childhood dementing diseases, such as lipid storage disease and Schilder disease.

Treatment and prognosis

There is no effective therapy for SSPE as yet. Intrathecal IFNα is being investigated. Although there are rare reports of patients who have made a spontaneous recovery, almost all are dead within 3 years, some having a fulminant course over 3 months.

Prevention remains the best treatment, through immunization programmes.

Neuromuscular disorders

Myasthenia gravis

Definition

MG literally means muscle weakness with a grave prognosis. It is an autoimmune condition, principally caused by antibodies directed against the nicotinic acetylcholine receptors (AChR) of the neuromuscular junction. Clinically, MG is characterized by voluntary muscle fatiguable weakness of varying severity, with relapses and remissions.

Introduction

The first clinical description of the condition was by Thomas Willis in 1672 but the name myasthenia gravis was introduced in 1895 by Friedrich Jolly. The first reported case of thymectomy in MG was in 1911. John Simpson was the first to propose an immunological pathogenesis in 1960, suggesting there was an autoimmune attack on the motor end plate. At this time Arthur Strauss demonstrated the presence of antibodies against skeletal muscle, especially in patients with thymomas.

Epidemiology

The incidence is estimated to be about 2–4/100 000. Published prevalence rates vary from 0.5 to 14.2 per 100 000, with numbers increasing in the older age groups as a result of successful treatment. MG may present at any age; however, it is most common during adulthood, females outnumbering males, except in the older age groups where the rates are approximately equal. The peak age of onset for women is between 20 and 30 years.

Genetic factors

All races are affected by this disease. Three groups have been identified exhibiting certain MHC haplotype associations:

(1) a young group without thymoma — HLA-A1-B8 and -DR3;

(2) an older group without thymoma — HLA-B7 and -DR2;

(3) a group with thymoma but with no apparent HLA association.

In the Chinese, particularly those with ocular disease, there is an association with Bw46 and DR9.

Pathogenesis

Synaptic vesicles release ACh from the motor nerve terminal of the neuromuscular junction, which then binds to the receptor, resulting in a miniature end-plate potential. The importance of AChR antibodies in MG was found when Patrick and Lindstrom (1973) produced a generalized weakness in rabbits by injection of AChR protein from the electrical organ of the eel. The injected rabbits produced high levels of AChR antibodies and a myasthenic response to repetitive stimulation with improvement after administration of cholinesterase inhibitors. These antibodies were demonstrated subsequently in patients with MG. Antibodies act at AChRs by three main mechanisms (Fig. 21.7):

1. Binding to antigenic epitopes located on AChR subunits, producing a reduction in AChR numbers by cross-linking and increased receptor turnover.

2. Blockage of agonist binding or direct blockade of ion channel function.

3. End-plate destruction occurs, resulting in reduced miniature end-plate potential (MEPP) amplitudes. This is manifest clinically as weakness and fatiguability.

Patients with thymomas usually have antibodies to various components of striated muscle, such as actin, α-actinin, myosin, and titin. Recently, autoantibodies directed against the ryanodine receptor (RyR), a calcium release channel in the sarcoplasmic reticulum of striated muscle, have been identified. RyR antibodies are found in 50% of patients with a thymoma, and their presence correlates with a more severe form of MG.

Pathology

Thymic abnormalities are found in the majority of patients with MG, although in 70% of cases, this is only evident microscopically, showing changes of lymphoid follicular hyperplasia. Macroscopic hyperplasia is evident in 10%, while a similar proportion have a thymoma present, almost invariably benign. These tumours are especially seen in older males, and are separated into two types, one being composed predominantly of histiocytic cells and the other lym-

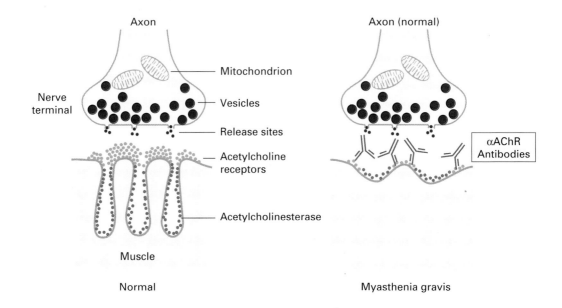

▌ Fig. 21.7 Normal and myasthenic neuromuscular junctions. AChR, acetylcholine receptor.

phocytic. Some cells within the thymus (myoid cells) have morphological and biochemical similarities with striated muscle, and can express epitopes of the main immunogenic region of the AChR, suggesting that they may act as a primary target in the immunopathogenesis of MG.

The muscle fibres, except for possible mild atrophic changes due to disuse, appear normal. Regenerating axons may be seen near the neuromuscular junction, indicating an active process of degeneration and repair of the junction in MG.

There is a reduction in the number of post-synaptic AChR to 30–50% of normal. Ultrastructually, the normal post-synaptic membrane is extensively folded, AChR being concentrated at the tips of the folds. This becomes distorted in MG, with flattening of the folds and widening of the synaptic cleft (Fig. 21.7). Cellular infiltration is unusual, whereas antibodies and complement components are typically present.

Clinical features

Myasthenia can mimic many neurological conditions. Presentation may be with mild ptosis alone, or in the most severe cases can affect virtually all muscles, with resultant severe debility and even respiratory failure. A subgroup of patients may have only ocular muscle involvement, with ptosis and diplopia in one or a number of directions. These patients often have a better prognosis, and if the disease remains localized to only these muscles after 2 years, it is unlikely the condition will spread to involve peripheral muscles. Pupillary changes are absent in MG, distinguishing it from other commoner causes of ptosis. Another distinguishing feature from a neuropathic aetiology is the typical involvement of muscles innervated by more than one cranial nerve. The presence of fatiguability usually provides the diagnosis as myasthenia.

Bulbar involvement is manifest through fatiguable, hypophonic and often nasal speech, and dysphagia, sometimes coexistent with nasal regurgitation of foods and fluids due to weakness of the soft palate. Fatigue of mastication is evident in some patients, characteristically, jaw opening being stronger than closure. Facial weakness if present is usually bilateral, and may easily be overlooked in a cursory examination, as the facial movements although weak, are symmetrical.

Fatigue is a frequent complaint among patients with many disorders. For the myasthenic, it usually means weakness of a group of muscles due to repetitive activity (e.g. hair-brushing). Depression is a concomitant of many chronic diseases, including MG. Unlike depression, fatigue due to myasthenia is worse towards the end of the day, and is often relieved by a 30 min rest.

With severe involvement, weakness is present all the time, and eventually, patients may develop a co-existent myopathy due to disuse. This is important to recognize, as this will not respond to increased treatment frequency or dosage.

Occasionally, respiratory muscle involvement predominates and the diagnosis is overlooked. Diaphragmatic weakness can produce orthopnoea, the effect of gravity on full inspiration being lost in the supine position. Initially, the respiratory pattern is rapid and shallow, however, as the muscles decompensate, carbon dioxide retention and respiratory failure ensues.

MG frequently improves during pregnancy, although occasionally it deteriorates. About 10% of newborns to myasthenic mothers have a transient myasthenic reaction due to the transplacental passage of AChR antibodies, manifest as weak crying and poor sucking. It usually resolves within a few weeks spontaneously; however, occasionally pyridostigmine or even plasma exchange and temporary ventilation are required.

Diagnosis

A history of intermittent weakness, diplopia, dysphagia, dysarthria, or fatigue in the absence of sensory symptoms should alert to the possibility of MG. The examination should include repetitive tests to reproduce the symptoms, such as prolonged upgaze to elicit ptosis, careful examination of extraocular movements, counting to 100 to highlight a dysarthria, and repeated strength testing of peripheral muscles. Clinical suspicion should then be confirmed using a Tensilon test and/or EMG.

If fatigue of muscle groups can confidently be demonstrated, the diagnosis should be confirmed with an edrophonium (Tensilon) test, preferably in a blinded fashion with a placebo control. Atropine is often administered first to counteract the peripheral cholinergic side-effects, followed by a small dose (1–2 mg) of Tensilon. If there is no definite improvement in the symptoms within a couple of minutes, a further 3 mg is administered, and then if necessary the remaining 5 mg of the ampoule.

EMG can assist in the diagnosis, with decreased amplitude of muscle action potentials (decrementing response) on repetitive stimulation at a rate of three per second, mimicking the clinical fatiguability seen. Tensilon reverses this response.

The majority of patients have detectable autoantibodies to AChR, being found in 85% of those with generalized myasthenia, and 60% of patients with the ocular form. Their presence strongly supports the diagnosis. The level does not correlate with the severity of the disease but can sometimes be used to follow the response to immunosuppressive therapy. False positive results only occur in rare patients with systemic impus erythematosus.

In all patients with MG, a thymoma or thymic enlargement should be sought with a computerized tomography (CT) scan of the chest. If discovered, in most cases the patient should have the thymus removed, preferably within the first 2 years after diagnosis, as this can lead to a permanent remission.

Hyperthyroidism may coexist with MG in up to 5% of patients, both conditions potentially producing an ophthalmoplegia. An important differential diagnosis is the Lambert–Eaton (LES). D-penicillamine may produce MG, usually restricted to the ocular muscles and associated with AChR antibodies. It usually remits without immunotherapy within a year but if still present after this period, should be treated as for acquired MG.

Treatment

Anticholinesterase inhibitors

The symptoms can often be controlled by increasing the levels of ACh. This is achieved by administering anticholinesterase inhibitors, such as neostigmine and pyridostigmine (Mestinon). Because of their short half-life, they often have to be given frequently, although long-acting preparations are now available. The majority of patients require between 30 and 120 mg every 4–6 h. Unfortunately, many patients experience dose-limiting side-effects, due to excessive stimulation of muscarinic receptors by ACh. These include nausea, diarrhoea, abdominal cramps, sweating, and excessive salivation.

If a patient on anticholinesterase inhibitors develops increasing weakness, it is important to establish if this is due to inadequate therapy or cholinergic blockade, which results from excessive medication. This is readily determined by performing a Tensilon test (as when diagnosing myasthenia). If the patient is under-dosed, there will be an improvement in their strength, whereas there is no change or a mild deterioration if they are 'overdosed'.

Thymectomy

This should be considered seriously in all patients, except those with purely ocular myasthenia, or only mild symptoms. There has never been a controlled trial of thymectomy but most reports indicate a beneficial effect which in some cases gives a complete remission. Those with a thymoma particularly benefit. The response is maximal by 3 years.

Immunosuppressants

Often the symptoms are inadequately controlled with anticholinesterase inhibitors alone, and immunosuppression is also required. Prednisolone is the agent of choice, usually at an initial dose of 50–75 mg daily. Remission or marked improvement occurs in 75% of patients treated with steroids, usually within 2 months. In 30% of patients, a transient deterioration may occur in the first 3 weeks following instigation of steroid therapy. In patients with severe weakness, especially with involvement of bulbar or respiratory muscles, therapy should therefore be instituted in a hospital setting.

Other immunosuppressants have been tried with variable success. Azathioprine is the most commonly employed, predominantly as a steroid sparing agent for those likely to be on long-term therapy. The usual starting dose is 50 mg daily, increasing to 150 or 200 mg if tolerated over a few weeks. Patients need to be monitored for any haematological or hepatic adverse effects. Cyclosporin and cyclophosphamide have also been used in some patients.

Plasmapheresis is usually reserved for acute and severe exacerbations, while treatment is stabilized with other agents, or while patients are prepared for thymectomy.

Improvement of MG following intravenous immunoglobulin has been reported. Improvement usually begins within 1 week and lasts for several weeks to at most a few months.

Drugs to be avoided because they may exacerbate myasthenic symptoms by compromising neuromuscular transmission include D-tubocurarine and pancuronium (used in anaesthesia), succinylcholine, aminoglycosides, local anaesthetics, beta blockers, quinine, quinidine, and procainamide.

Prognosis

Thirty years ago, 25% of patients with MG died from their condition. Now most can have their symptoms controlled and can expect to have an almost normal life expectancy. The risk of death is greatest during the first year after diagnosis. Remission is more likely to occur in the early rather than the later years of the condition. After about 7 years, the disease tends to stabilize in the majority, the risk of severe relapse being less.

Lambert–Eaton syndrome

Definition

LES is a rare autoimmune neuromuscular disorder in which there is an insufficient release of ACh with each nerve impulse at cholinergic neuromuscular and autonomic nerve terminals, producing muscular fatiguability and autonomic dysfunction. It is often associated with internal malignancies, but there is a primary form where no underlying malignancy is demonstrable.

Introduction

First described by Lambert and Eaton as defective neuromuscular conduction in association with malignancy in 1956, it was not until 25 years later that an autoimmune pathogenesis was outlined. The paraneoplastic form is commoner in males due to their higher incidence of smoking, whereas there is not such a clear sex difference in primary LES. The condition is seen in all age groups, but is most common in middle-aged and elderly patients. Approximately 50% of patients with LES are found to have cancer, although often this is not clinically apparent until months or even years later. Small-cell cancer is the commonest neoplasm identified; however, lymphoma, prostate, breast, renal cell, and other cancers have also been discovered in some patients.

Pathogenesis

Evidence has accumulated in recent years of the immunological nature of LES. Approximately one-third of patients developing LES have a predisposition to autoimmune diseases, with either a personal or family history of such conditions. Transmission of the syndrome to mice by injecting purified IgG from LES patients, as well as immune localization to the motor end-plates, provides direct evidence for the autoimmune nature of LES. End-plate potentials are dependent on the rapid entry of calcium during the arrival of the action potential. Antibody-mediated blockade of calcium entry into the nerve terminal results in the release of an insufficient ACh quantity with each nerve impulse, thus producing a failure of neuromuscular transmission.

The antigenic epitopes producing the antibody response are yet to be identified. Synaptotagmin, located in the membrane of synaptic vesicles has been postulated to be the antigen. Calcium-channel antibodies are found in paraneoplastic and primary forms of LES. The presence of similar channels in the membranes of small-cell cancer cells is believed to provide the stimulus for antibody production in these patients.

Pathology

Electron micrographs of normal motor terminals demonstrate parallel arrays of particles, believed to represent the voltage-gated calcium channels, the presumed site of attack by antibodies. Antibody attack reduces the number of these particles, producing the deficient ACh release at cholinergic neuromuscular junctions and autonomic nerve terminals. The lack of cellular infiltration at the neuromuscular junctions indicates that complement activation plays an insignificant part, unlike in MG.

Clinical features

The classical triad of LES is weakness, hyporeflexia, and autonomic dysfunction. The weakness has a different pattern to that usually seen in MG, ocular and bulbar muscles rarely being affected, weakness being most marked in the legs (especially proximally, usually symmetrically) and to a lesser extent the arms. Hip girdle weakness produces a waddling gait. Autonomic symptoms include erectile dysfunction, lack of sweating, and dry mouth. A rare presentation is unexplained apnoea or ventilatory failure following anaesthesia. The rapid progression of symptoms favours a paraneoplastic aetiology.

Diagnosis

Diagnosis is usually dependent on the clinical findings, absence of AChR antibodies and demonstration of malignancy in about 50%, and the demonstration of characteristic electrophysiological abnormalities. The CMAP is usually small, often being less than 10% of normal, and in response to slow repetitive stimulation (2 Hz) there is a decrementing response. The other characteristic feature is facilitation, whereby there is an increase in size of CMAP by at least 100% after 10 s voluntary contraction of the muscle or rapid (20–50 Hz) stimulation.

Antibodies directed against calcium channels are found in 50–60% of all patients with LES, both in the primary and paraneoplastic forms.

In view of the association with small-cell lung cancer, in addition to a chest X-ray, appropriate patients should probably have sputum cytology, CT chest, and bronchoscopy, which may need to be repeated at intervals if the suspicion of malignancy is high.

Treatment and prognosis

Although successful removal of a tumour may produce a remission, others may remain symptomatic. For those patients entering a remission, recurrent symptoms may herald a recurrence of the tumour.

Anticholinesterases are often of little benefit, unlike in MG, although they should still be tried and may be useful in conjunction with other agents. Of the drugs enhancing ACh release 3,4-diaminopyridine in doses ranging between 5 mg three times a day and 25 mg four times a day seems to be the most effective. Its potassium-channel blocking effect produces a prolongation of the action potential, and hence a prolongation of the activation of the voltage-gated calcium channels. The usefulness of other agents such as 4-aminopyridine and guanidine is tempered by side-effects.

The other line of treatment involves immunosuppression, e.g. prednisolone and azathioprine, although the response is not as quick as that seen in MG sufferers. Plasmapheresis or intravenous immunoglobulin may be used in the rare circumstances where respiratory or bulbar function is severely compromised. Thymectomy is of no benefit.

Agents, as listed in the section on MG, should be avoided which may interfere with neuromuscular transmission.

In patients with an underlying malignancy, their outcome is largely determined by the success of treating the neoplasm. The primary form of LES tends to follow a stable course, unlike the fluctuating profile seen in MG. Spontaneous remissions are rare.

Spinal disorders

Tropical spastic paraparesis

Definition

TSP is an insidious myelopathy predominantly affecting the lower limbs which develops during early to middle adulthood. In the majority of reported cases it is associated with antibodies directed against human T-cell leukaema virus type 1 (HTLV-1), which are believed to produce the syndrome.

Introduction

A number of patients in the tropics develop a fairly uniform clinical picture of progressive paraparesis. In 1985 HTLV-1 IgG antibodies were demonstrated in the sera of many of the patients in Martinique with TSP. Subsequently, the same antibodies were found in the sera of similar patients throughout the Caribbean, and also in south Japan, where the condition was originally termed HTLV-1-associated myelopathy (HAM).

Epidemiology

This condition is endemic in tropical and subtropical areas, especially the Caribbean, Japan, and the Pacific coast of Colombia, but cases have also been seen among migrants to non-endemic areas such as the UK. Recently, there have been reports of HTLV-1 infection in migrants from northern Iran, the Solomon Islands, and in Australian Aborigines, West African and South

African residents. The highest prevalence rate in the world is in Martinique, being 65.4 per 100 000. Based on data from Japan, the estimated lifetime risk of HTLV-1 carriers developing TSP is 0.25%, being highest in those acquiring the infection early in life. There is a higher HTLV-1 seroprevalence ratio in women which is about three times that of males.

Pathogenesis

The HTLV-1 virus is a retrovirus which can be transmitted in a number of ways, including intravenously, sexually, transplacentally, and in breast milk. Although some patients diagnosed with the condition have not had demonstrable antibodies to HTLV-1, this may be due to incorrect diagnosis, or inadequate specimen storage. While it is possible the disease is produced by direct viral invasion, an immunological mechanism is favoured, evidence for this including the presence of oligoclonal bands in the CSF, the presence of IL-2R-positive T lymphocytes in the CNS, high antibody titres to HTLV-1, and the efficacy of steroids in some cases. The way in which such an immune response may induce pathology is unknown but could parallel those outlined for GBS and MS (see above).

Pathology

The main features are those of a chronic meningomyelitis affecting all parts of the spinal cord, with focal demyelinative and necrotic changes, and perivascular and meningeal inflammatory infiltrates. The corticospinal tracts and posterior columns are particularly affected. There has been no demonstration of infection of the spinal cord neural cells.

Clinical features

The disease is characterized by the insidious onset of a progressive myelopathy, beginning between the third and sixth decades. Although the weakness may initially be unilateral, symmetrical spastic weakness eventually develops. Paraparesis is the major disabling feature, with weakness, increased tone and reflexes and extensor plantar responses. In up to 25% of cases, there may be evidence of radicular or peripheral nerve involvement, manifest by absent ankle jerks. Upper limb involvement is usually far less significant. Although paraesthesias are common, sensory signs are not usually prominent. Sphincteric and erectile dysfunction occurs in the majority, often at an early stage.

Other conditions produced by HTLV-1 include acute T-cell leukaemia (ATL), and the more recently reported polymyositis, characterized by slowly pro-gressive proximal muscle weakness with supportive EMG and muscle biopsy findings.

Diagnosis

The diagnosis of TSP is made by demonstrating HTLV-1 antibodies in the serum and CSF in a patient with the clinical features of TSP. Evidence of viral presence has been detected in some 'HTLV-I negative' patients using polymerase chain reaction for the detection of *gag* and *tax* gene proviral DNA.

The CSF has a lymphocytic pleocytosis in 20% of cases, moderate increase in protein in 30%, and often an elevated level of IgG and antibodies to HTLV-1. Thinning of the spinal cord can be seen on MRI, although this is often unavailable in the areas of highest incidence, and is principally useful for excluding other disease processes.

Treatment and prognosis

There is no proven effective therapy, although steroids have been used empirically, usually with only short-term benefits. A pilot study of azothymidine (AZT) as used in AIDS failed to demonstrate a beneficial effect. Commonly, a plateau occurs after the initial deterioration, with phases of more rapid decline interspersed with periods of relative disease inactivity, although never complete remission. Ultimately, 50% require a wheelchair within 10 years, and almost all require some assistance to walk.

Stiff-man syndrome

Definition

Stiff-man syndrome (SMS) is a rare autoimmune CNS disorder characterized by painful muscle spasms and muscular rigidity.

An immunological pathogenesis was suspected after the discovery of increased production of IgG in the CSF in 1980. The demonstration of autoantibodies against glutamic acid decarboxylase (GAD) by Solimena confirmed the autoimmune nature of the disease.

Epidemiology

Men and women appear to be equally affected. The incidence of SMS is not known. HLA-B44, -DR3, and -DR4 antigens are associated with SMS.

Pathogenesis

γ-amino butyric acid (GABA) is an inhibitory neurotransmitter which is synthesized from glutamate by the GAD enzyme. It is believed this transmitter is present in descending spinal pathways responsible for balancing catecholaminergic influences, and hence acts to inhibit muscle tone. The impairment of GABA production by the GAD antibody results in muscular over-activity, manifest clinically in the form of rigidity and spasms.

Pathology

No consistent abnormalities have been found in the CNS of the few affected patients who have come to necropsy; however, histochemical studies have not been performed.

Clinical features

The condition begins in adulthood and follows a variable clinical course, in some cases worsening rapidly for a few weeks before stabilizing, fluctuating, or progressing slowly. Patients complain of an uncomfortable stiffness of their trunk and proximal limb muscles and as a result, their movements can become slow and awkward. Painful spasms of these muscles develops, often provoked by exertion, emotion, or sensory stimuli. Bulbar muscles are only involved in about 25% in contrast to tetanus, which should be considered.

Examination is non-specifc, revealing rigid muscles, but no weakness or reflex changes. Rigidity may lead to joint deformities and contractures, and a hyperlordosis of the lumbar spine is characteristic.

Diagnosis

Like the clinical presentation, results of investigations for diagnostic purposes, are non-specific, the major differential diagnosis being hysteria. EMG findings are indistinguishable from voluntary motor activity, revealing continuous muscle activity which is abolished by sleep, anaesthesia, curare, peripheral nerve blockade, and intravenous diazepam.

Routine CSF findings are unremarkable, although oligoclonal bands can be present, and GAD antibodies are present intrathecally and/or in serum in 60% of cases. Why GAD antibodies are not found in all cases is unclear; however, this may be due to GABAergic autoantigen heterogeneity. These antibodies are also found in a significant proportion of patients with insulin-dependent diabetes mellitus (IDDM). Common associations indude IDDM, present in up two-thirds of patients, pernicious anaemia, vitiligo, autoimmune thyroid disease, and epilepsy.

Treatment and prognosis

The rarity of SMS precludes controlled treatment trials. Drugs that have been tried in the treatment of this condition indude diazepam, clonazepam, baclofen,

clonidine, and valproic acid. Prednisolone and plasma-pheresis have been reported to be beneficial in some cases. Drugs enhancing aminergic activity such as levodopa and methamphetamine typically aggravate the spasms.

Patients have a progressive or fluctuating course. The spasms may be eased by medications; however, the axial rigidity is less responsive, and patients can eventually develop deformities.

Paraneoplastic syndromes

The PNS and CNS may be affected by remote malignancies, the mechanism of which in many cases is autoimmune in nature. It is presumed (and has been demonstrated in some cases such as LES — see p. 272) that the tumour shares antigenic epitopes with neural antigens. The immune system, in mounting a response against the tumour, also produces neurological effects. Often these paraneoplastic syndromes are the initial manifestation of the tumour, and may precede the diagnosis of the cancer by months or years.

Paraneoplastic cerebellar degeneration

Paraneoplastic cerebellar degeneration (PCD) is characterized by the subacute onset of cerebellar symptoms, and has been described with a number of tumours, including Hodgkin's disease, lung, ovarian, and breast cancer. Usually, the neurological disorder precedes the diagnosis of the malignancy. This syndrome was described in 1934, but the association with malignancy was not established until 1951. In 1983, antibodies (subsequently termed anti-Yo after the first two letters of the last name of an index patient) to cerebellar Purkinje cells were reported in association with ovarian cancer in two patients.

Epidemiology

The frequency of paraneoplastic syndromes is dependent upon how actively they are sought. Clinically, relevant manifestations are quite rare, affecting less than 1% of those afflicted with cancer. Conversely, however, as many as half of the patients with subacute cerebellar degeneration have an underlying malignancy. Males and females are equally affected.

Pathogenesis

Anti-Yo antibodies may play a significant part in at least some patients with PCD. At this stage PCD has not been produced in animals by injection of human

IgG, and so it is possible the antibody is simply a marker of the immune response to the underlying malignancy. Alternatively, injected antibody in a healthy animal is unlikely to cross the BBB. Further studies are required to clarify the role of this antibody in PCD. The genetic characteristics are well summarized in Posner's review of CNS paraneoplastic syndromes (see Further reading). Anti-Yo antibodies react with cytoplasmic antigens, and are seen in women with PCD and ovarian, uterine, breast, and adenocarcinomas of unknown origin. They have not, however, been identified in patients with PCD and Hodgkin's disease or lung cancer. They are not present in normal individuals, and with the possible exception of two patients reported by Brashear, anti-Yo antibodies are not seen in patients with cancer without PCD. The levels of antibody are higher in the CSF than serum, suggesting intrathecal synthesis, presumably by B lymphocytes which have invaded the CNS.

Pathology

Characteristically, there is a severe loss of cerebellar Purkinje cells without associated inflammatory cell infiltrates. The deep nuclei are usually well preserved, although there is a diminution of myelinated fibres secondary to the loss of Purkinje cells. Anti-Yo antibodies have been demonstrated at post mortem.

Clinical features

The onset of PCD usually precedes the diagnosis of the underlying tumour. The onset of symptoms is subacute (over weeks); however, patients with anti-Yo antibodies tend to have a more abrupt onset and quicker progression to pancerebellar dysfunction. Gait ataxia is usually the initial manifestation, eventually associated with appendicular ataxia, dysarthria, and nystagmus (especially downbeat).

Diagnosis

In those patients with appropriate tumours, the presence of anti-Yo antibodies (found in serum or CSF) confirms the clinical suspicion. As this antibody is so closely linked to breast or gynaecological malignancies, if discovered, the clinician should undertake an aggressive examination. Examination of the CSF may yield a pleocytosis, elevated protein concentration, and increased IgG levels.

Treatment and prognosis

There appears to be some difference in response to treatment between anti-Yo positive and negative groups. Following treatment of the underlying Hodgkin's disease or small-cell lung cancer (SCLC), anti-Yo negative patients may develop partial or rarely, complete remission, whereas there is no improvement after antineoplastic therapy for patients with anti-Yo antibodies.

Immunosuppressive therapy is generally ineffective. Plasmapheresis, although lowering the serum antibody levels, does not alter the CSF levels, and does not appear to produce any clinical benefits.

The patients overall prognosis is dependent on the underlying tumour. The neurological dysfunction often runs a course independent of the tumour, often stabilizing, although by this stage the disability produced by the PCD is usually severe and often renders the patient confined to a wheelchair.

Paraneoplastic encephalomyelitis

Definition

Paraneoplastic encephalomyelitis (PEM) encompasses a range of diverse neurological syndromes associated with malignancy, including sensory neuronopathy, autonomic neuropathy, myelopathy, cerebellar degeneration, brainstem abnormalities (brainstem encephalitis), and dementia (limbic encephalitis). This syndrome is almost always associated with SCLC, and is associated in some cases with the presence of the anti-Hu antibody.

Introduction

It has long been recognized that neurological problems may develop in patients with malignancies, unexplained by metastases or treatment side-effects. The term PEM was first coined in 1965, although is not accepted as an entity by all neurologists. Anti-Hu antibody was discovered in the 1980s.

About 60% of the patients are women. Most have SCLC, although other neoplasms such as Hodgkin's disease have been associated. Multifocal involvement is evident clinically in about 70%. Sensory neuronopathy is the commonest finding, being seen in over 50% of patients with PEM, while the other manifestations are evident in approximately 25% either solely or as part of a multifocal syndrome.

Pathogenesis

The anti-Hu antibody is a polyclonal complement-fixing IgG present in serum and CSF, which reacts with the nuclei of peripheral and CNS neurons, sparing the nucleoli, and having a lesser cytoplasmic reaction. It is frequently identified in patients with SCLC and PEM, reacting with nuclei of neurons throughout the CNS, dorsal root ganglia, and autonomic ganglia. This antibody has also been identified in patients with PEM and prostate cancer, adenocarcinoma of the lung, neuroblastoma, and chondromyxosarcoma. The antigen to which the antibody reacts is present within all the tumours associated with PEM. As in PCD, the syndrome has not been reproduced in animals experimentally.

Pathology

Pathologically, there is neuronal cell loss with gliosis and inflammatory cell infiltrates (unlike PCD) in various areas of the nervous system. Involvement of the hippocampus produces 'limbic encephalitis', while brainstem involvement most frequently involves the medulla. Motor, sensory, and autonomic neuropathies are produced by involvement of the spinal cord, dorsal root, and autonomic ganglia. Most patients have pathological evidence of involvement in a number of these areas, although clinically there may be only one level obviously affected. Severe autonomic failure is often the cause of death.

Immunohistochemical studies have confirmed the presence of intraneuronal deposits of IgG. In some of these areas there were no or few pathological changes, suggesting that internalization of IgG is required to produce damage to the cell.

Clinical features

The commonest clinical syndrome is a painful sensory neuropathy, characterized by early and often asymmetric involvement of the upper limbs and face involving all modalities. Reflexes are typically absent. Weakness may be present, but is usually not a prominent manifestation, although some patients may present with a syndrome initially indistinguishable from MND. The rapid evolution and development of other neurological manifestations of PEM establishes the diagnosis. It is important to consider the possible coexistence of LES where weakness is present. Autonomic neuropathy may manifest as severe postural hypertension and associated dizziness, impotence, urinary retention, pupillary abnormalities, and constipation.

The cerebellar syndrome is indistinguishable from that of PCD seen with other malignancies, unless other features of PEM are evident. Brainstem abnormalities are highly variable, but can include disabling vertigo, dysarthria, dysphagia, ocular gaze palsies, nystagmus, opsoclonus, and even respiratory failure due to central hypoventilation.

Limbic encephalitis manifests clinically with the subacute onset of a dementia associated with periods of confusion and inappropriate behaviour, and occasionally complex partial or generalized seizures.

Diagnosis

It is sometimes difficult to distinguish the neuropathy seen in PEM (when it occurs in isolation) with a chemotherapy-related complication. Cis-platinum-induced neuropathy differs by producing a neuropathy predominantly involving large fibre functions (vibration and joint position sensation), as distinct from the paraneoplastic sensory neuronopathy which affects all modalities. Nerve conduction studies reveal absent sensory action potentials, often with normal motor conduction velocities.

The EEG may reveal non-specific slowing over the temporal lobes in cases of limbic encephalitis. MRI may show increased signal intensity of the hippocampus early in the course of this condition, although later it is characterized by atrophy.

Treatment and prognosis

There is no specific treatment for PEM. The neurological symptoms do not improve after treatment of the underlying malignancy, and immunosuppressive therapy has not produced any consistent benefits.

As with PCD, the onset is usually subacute, and the condition eventually stabilizes, although by this stage the patient is severely disabled. The patient usually succumbs quite rapidly from the underlying malignancy.

Approximately 10% of patients have identifiable titres of anti-Hu antibody with SCLC, but no evidence of a paraneoplastic syndrome. These patients usually are women and tend to have a better prognosis, as they have limited rather than extensive disease.

Paraneoplastic opsoclonus–myoclonus

Definition

Continuous chaotic saccadic movement of the eyes in both horizontal and vertical planes is termed opsoclonus. This can be a paraneoplastic phenomenon, although it is seen with a variety of conditions including viral infections, intracranial malignancies, hydrocephalus, thalamic haemorrhage, and toxic encephalopathies. The anti-Ri antibody which is associated with this syndrome was described in eight patients by Luque in 1991.

The numbers with this condition reported in the literature is quite small. In adults, opsoclonus–myoclonus is associated with a malignancy in approximately 20% of cases, most commonly with SCLC and breast cancer. Other malignancies reported in association with this syndrome are uterine, ovarian, bladder, and thyroid cancer.

Pathogenesis

In patients with breast cancer and opsoclonus, the anti-Ri autoantibody has been detected. This antibody reacts with a set of 55 and 80 kDa antigens present in the nucleus of neurons, as well as breast cancer cells, and presumably plays an important part in the genesis of the syndrome. Although histochemically appearing to be identical with the anti-Hu antibody seen in PEM, the latter reacts with different proteins (35–40 kDa). The site of the abnormality has not been identified, and the illness has not been reproduced experimentally in animals.

Pathology

Despite the florid neurological symptoms, there is a paucity of abnormalities at autopsy, with only sparse mononuclear perivascular infiltrates being reported.

Clinical features

In patients with SCLC the opsoclonus usually antedates the diagnosis of the tumour. The onset is quite rapid, with nausea and vomiting accompanying the development of the chaotic multidirectional eye movements typical of opsoclonus, which are often exacerbated by fixation. Truncal ataxia generally develops, and myoclonus involving the limbs, head, palate, pharynx, and even diaphragm may be seen in varying combinations. Some patients experience mental state changes.

Opsoclonus precedes the diagnosis of the neuroblastoma in about half the cases, and so can be an important clue to the diagnosis. When associated with opsoclonus, there is a greater than normal incidence of intrathoracic tumours and benign growths.

The anti-Ri antibody, when present, is found in serum and CSF.

Treatment and prognosis

Treatment of the tumour, or trials of prednisolone, thiamine, triazolam or clonazepam may produce remissions in patients with SCLC and opsoclonus–myoclonus. Unlike other paraneoplastic syndromes, the course of paraneoplastic opsoclonus can be relapsing and remitting, suggesting a functional rather than permanent damage to neurons. The course tends to be independent of the underlying malignancy.

Further reading

Keane, R. W and Hickey, W. F. (1996). *Immunology of the Nervous System*. Oxford University Press New York.

Theofilopoulos, A. N. (1995). The basis of autoimmunity: Part I. Mechanisms of aberrant self-recognition. *Immunology Today*, **16** 90–8.

Guillain–Barré syndrome

Asbury, A. K. and Cornblath, D. R. (1990). Assessment of current diagnostic criteria for Guillain–Barré syndrome. *Annals of Neurology*, **27**, 21–4.

Van der Meche, F. G. A. (1994). The Guillain–Barré syndrome. *Baillierés Clinical Neurology*, **3**, 73–94.

Ropper, A. H. (1992). The Guillain–Barré syndrome. *New England Journal of Medicine*, **326**, 1130–6.

Chronic inflammatory demyelinating polyradiculoneuropathy

American Academy of Neurology. (1991). Criteria for diagnosis of chronic inflammatory demyelinating polyradiculoneuropathy. *Neurology*, **41**, 617–18.

Dyck, P. J., Prineas, J. W., and Pollard, J. D. (1993). Chronic inflammatory demyelinating polyradiculoneuropathy. In *Peripheral Neuropathy*, 3rd edn. (ed.) P. J. Dyck, P. K. Thomas, J. Griffin, P. A. Low and J. Poduslo pp. 1498–517. W. B. Saunders, Philadelphia.

Pollard, J. D. (1994). Chronic inflammatory demyelinating polyneuropathy. *Baillierés Clinical Neurology*. **3**, 107–28.

Mendell, J. R. (1993). Chronic inflammatory demyelinating polyradiculoneuropathy. *Annual Review of Medicine*, **44**, 211–19.

Multifocal motor neuropathy

Parry, G. J. and Sumner, A. J. (1992). Multifocal motor neuropathy. *Neurologic Clinics*, **10**, 671–84.

Plexopathies

Russell, J. W. and Windebank, A. J. (1994). Brachial and lumbar neuropathies. *Baillierés Clinical Neurology*, **3**, 173–92.

Paraproteinaemic neuropathy

Kyle, R. A. (1992). Monoclonal proteins in neuropathy. *Neurologic Clinics*, **10**, 713–34.

Yeung, K. B., Thomas, P. K., King, R. H. M., Yeung, K. B., Waddy, H., and Will, R. G. (1991). The clinical spectrum of peripheral neuropathies associated with benign monoclonal IgM, IgG and IgA paraproteinaemia. Comparative clinical, immunological and nerve biopsy findings. *Journal of Neurology*, **238**, 383–91.

Multiple sclerosis

Beck, R. W., Cleary, P. A., Trobe, J. D., Kaufman, D. I., Kupersmith, M. J., Paty, D. W., and Brown, C. H. (1993).

The effect of corticosteroids for acute optic neuritis on the subsequent development of multiple sclerosis. *New England Journal of Medicine*, **329**, 1764–1769.

Compston, A. and Sadovnick, A. (1992). Epidemiology and genetics of multiple sderosis. *Current Opinion Neurol. Neurosurgery*, **5**, 175–81.

Ebers, G. C. (1994). Treatment of multiple sclerosis. *Lancet*, **343**, 275–9.

McDonald, W. I., Miller, D. H., and Thompson, A. J. (1994). Are magnetic resonance findings predictive of clinical outcome in therapeutic trials in multiple sclerosis? The dilemma of interferon-beta. *Annals of Neurology*, **36**, 14–18.

Poser, C. M., Paty, D. W., Scheinberg, L., McDonald, W. I., Davis, F. A., Ebers, G. C., *et al.* (1983). New diagnostic criteria for multiple sclerosis: guidelines for research protocols. *Annals of Neurology*, **13**, 227–31.

Silberberg, D. H. (1994). Multiple sclerosis: approaches to management. *Annals of Neurology*, **36** (Suppl.), S1–162.

Acute disseminated encephalomyelitis and subacute sclerosing panencephalitis

Johnson, R. T., Griffin, D. E., Hirsch, R. L., Wolinsky, J. S., Roedenbeck, S., Lindo de Soriano, I. and Vaisberg, A. (1984). Measles encephalomyelitis–clinical and immunologic studies. *New England Journal of Medicine*, **310**, 137–41.

Johnson, R. T. (1994). The virology of demyelinating diseases. *Annals of Neurology*, **36** (Suppl.), S54–60.

ter Meulen, V. (1991). Virus–cell interactions in the nervous system. *Seminars in Neuroscience*, **3**, 000–000.

Myasthenia gravis

Drachman, D. B. (1994). Myasthenia gravis. *New England Journal of Medicine*, **330**, 1797–810.

Sanders, D. B. (1994). Myasthenia gravis and myasthenic syndromes. *Neurologic Clinics*, **12**.

Tropical spastic paraparesis

Cruickshank, J. K., Rudge, P., Dalgleish, A. G., Newton, M., McLean, B. N., Barnard, R. O., *et al.* (1989). Tropical spastic paraparesis and human T cell lymphotropic virus type I in the United Kingdom. *Brain*, **112**, 1057–90.

Cruickshank, J. K., Corbin, D. O., Bucher, B., and Vernant, J. C. (1992). HTLV-I and neurological disease. *Baillierés Clinical Neurology*, **1**, 61–81.

Paraneoplastic syndromes

Graus, F. and Rene, R. (1992). Clinical and pathological advances on central nervous system paraneoplastic syndromes. *Revue Neurologique*, **148**, 496–501.

Posner, J. B. (1991). Paraneoplastic syndromes. *Neurologic Clinics*, **9**, 919–36.

Luque, F. A., Furneaux, H. M., Ferziger, R., Rosenblum, M. K., Wray, S. H., Schold, S. C. Jr., *et al.* (1991). Anti-Ri: an antibody associated with paraneoplastic opsoclonus and breast cancer. *Annals of Neurology*, **29**, 241–51.

22 Kidney

D. A. Power, A. J. F. d'Apice and A. E. Seymour

Introduction

Much of renal disease is immunologically mediated. This section will focus on the major form of autoimmune renal disease, namely glomerulonephritis. The approach will be, first, to describe the clinical syndromes with which glomerulonephritis can present to the clinician, followed by a discussion of each of the major histological appearances seen on renal biopsy. The diseases (so far as they can be classified as such) associated with each of the histological patterns will be described. Finally, other renal autoimmune diseases such as acute intersitial nephritis and systemic autoimmune diseases will be described, as well as diseases associated with abnormal immunoglobulins.

Renal anatomy

The kidney comprises approximately 1×10^6 nephrons whose anatomy is shown in Fig. 22.1. For discussion of autoimmune renal disease, understanding the structure of the glomerulus is most important. The filtering unit of the nephron is the glomerulus. The glomerular filtration barrier comprises a specialized, fenestrated endothelium, basement membrane, and visceral epithelial cells (podocytes). Holding the capillary loops together is the glomerular mesangium, made up of smooth muscle-like mesangial cells and their extracellular matrix. The glomerulus is surrounded by Bowman's capsule, a basement membrane structure covered in parietal epithelial cells. The glomerular filtrate passes down the tubules through the varying levels of the nephron where it is modified before being passed as urine.

Glomerulonephritis

Classification of glomerulonephritis (Table 22.1)

Classification of glomerulonephritis is unsatisfactory, based largely upon a number of characteristic morphological appearances rather than aetiology or pathogenesis. Diagnosis of a patient with glomerulonephritis can be made potentially at three levels:

(1) mode of clinical presentation;

(2) histological pattern of the renal biopsy;

(3) aetiological diagnosis (e.g. streptococcal infection).

The difficulty in classifying glomerulonephritis is that a similar histological appearance can be produced by different aetiological agents and, probably, pathogenetic processes. In most instances, morphology and mode of clinical presentation are the only information available. This limitation has lead to the creation of 'diseases', such as mesangial proliferative glomerulonephritis, mesangiocapillary glomerulonephritis, and others which may, in fact, be the end product of many different aetiological agents and pathogenetic events. These are not 'diseases' but manifestations of a particular body reaction to a variety of injurious stimuli. In the same way, the body may react in various ways to a specific infectious agent, depending upon dose and immune status.

In occasional individuals, a particular histological appearance may be associated with an aetiological agent, a good recent example being the association of hepatitis C infection with mesangiocapillary glomerulonephritis. Most patients, however, will be left with a diagnosis confined to the histology of their renal biopsy or even, at times, simply their clinical presentation. Despite this, the combination of clinical presentation and morphology correlates reasonably well with prognosis and response to treatment. For

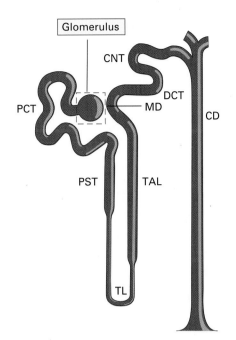

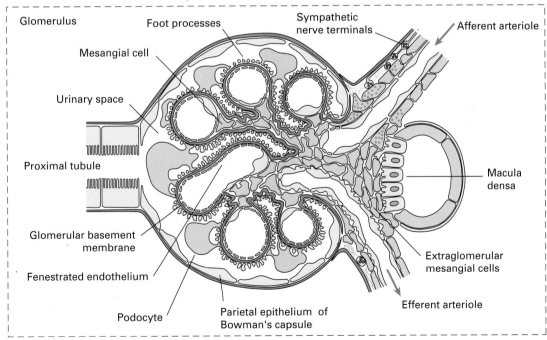

❚ **Fig. 22.1** Structure of the nephron (upper) showing the glomerulus (magnified in the inset diagram) and tubular elements. PCT, proximal convoluted tubule; PST, proximal straight segment of the loop of Henle; TL, thin limb of the loop of Henle; TAL, thick ascending limb of loop of Henle; MD, macula densa; DCT, distal convoluted tubule; CNT, connecting tubule; CD, collecting duct. The blood supply of the nephron is not shown.

▮ **Table 22.1**   Underlying disease in patients with nephrotic syndrome at three ages (expressed as % of all cases at that age)[a]

Age (years)	5	15	60
Minimal change disease	85–90	30	20
Focal and segmental glomerular sclerosis and hyalinosis (FGS)	5	20	5
Membranous glomerulonephritis	—	5	35
Membranoproliferative glomerulonephritis	5	15	5
Proliferative glomerulonephritis[b]	—	20	15
Diabetes	—	—	5
Amyloidosis	—	—	10
Systemic lupus erythemnatosus	—	10	—
Miscellaneous	—	—	5

[a]Table adapted from a number of sources. Percentages are only a rough approximation and have been rounded for simplicity.
[b]Mainly IgA nephropathy.

the purposes of this discussion, histological types of glomerulonephritis which have no known aetiology (i.e. are idiopathic) will be treated as individual diseases.

It is customary to call renal disease secondary when it is a manifestation of a known multisystem disease such as system lupus erythematosus (SLE) or diabetes, whereas glomerular disease occurring on its own is primary.

Clinical syndromes in glomerulonephritis

In common with most forms of disease involving a particular organ, there is a limited spectrum of clinical phenomena which can occur whatever the underlying lesion. In glomerulonephritis, there are six common forms of presentation which are described below. It is important to remember that individuals living in Third World countries or in similar circumstances may have a different range of pathologies underlying the same presenting features. In general, the descriptions given below relate to disease in developed countries. A short description of glomerulonephritis in the Third World is given at the end of this section.

Acute nephritic syndrome

This presentation is typified by children with acute post-streptococcal glomerulonephritis, but is also seen in a number of other conditions including SLE, microscopic polyarteritis, and antiglomerular basement membrane antibody disease. The usual features are a combination of macroscopic or heavy microscopic

haematuria, oedema, hypertension, oliguria, renal impairment, and minor proteinuria. Hypertension is commonly seen in glomerulonephritis, almost always in the setting of one of the other syndromes noted below.

Nephrotic syndrome

The accepted criterion is proteinuria in excess of 3.5 g/day in the adult, or >50 mg/kg per day (or 40 mg/h per m[2]) in a child. This degree of proteinuria leads to hypoalbuminaemia and, usually, to gross oedema. Hypercholesterolaemia also occurs but is not generally regarded as part of the syndrome. The disease causing nephrotic syndrome varies greatly with age (Table 22.1).

Nephritic–nephrotic syndrome

This is an infrequently used term describing patients who have some of the features of the acute nephritic syndrome together with nephrotic-range proteinuria.

Acute renal failure

Glomerulonephritis is a rare cause of acute renal failure but can usually be recognized before renal biopsy because of: (i) the presence of an active urinary sediment; (ii) clinical features that are sometimes associated with the conditions which cause glomerulonephritis; and (iii) the absence of pre-renal acute renal failure, a clear precipitant for acute tubular necrosis, or evidence of obstruction. The syndrome *'rapidly progressive glomerulonephritis'*, actually a combination of clinical and pathological diagnoses, has been used to describe this situation. Despite its problems, this term has been widely adopted and most clinicians would use it in preference to the less specific term acute renal failure when there was clinical evidence to suggest glomerulonephritis. These patients have crescentic glomerulonephritis on renal biopsy.

Chronic renal failure

This is the unfortunate end-point of many forms of glomerulonephritis. Chronic renal failure due to glomerulonephritis may be indistinguishable from that due to other conditions. Usually, the kidneys are small and smooth on renal ultrasound examination.

Asymptomatic urinary abnormalities

The commonest presentation of glomerulonephritis is an asymptomatic abnormality of the urinary sediment, generally detected by dipstick. These can be sub-classified as microscopic haematuria without proteinuria, haematuria with non-nephrotic proteinuria, and isolated non-nephrotic proteinuria. Provided it can be established that haematuria is of glomerular origin, then isolated microscopic haematuria is most commonly due to immunoglobulin (Ig) A nephropathy or thin basement membrane disease in Western communities. Haematuria and proteinuria is most commonly due to IgA nephropathy, whereas a variety of lesions cause isolated proteinuria. Macroscopic haematuria usually occurs without other evidence of the acute nephritic syndrome. It may present 3–4 days after an upper respiratory tract infection (URTI) when it is termed synpharyngitic. Macroscopic haematuria, which comes from the glomerulus, is often due to IgA nephropathy.

The distal form of renal tubular acidosis, so-called type 1 RTA, is a rare feature of glomerulonephritis due, usually, to SLE or Sjögren's syndrome.

Pathogenesis of glomerulonephritis

Mechanisms known to be involved in the pathogenesis of individual forms of glomerulonephritis vary, but some general comments can be made. First, it is convenient to divide them into factors responsible for initiation of disease and those contributing to tissue damage. Secondly, a series of mechanisms for progression have been identified, often unrelated to those causing the original injury.

Initiating factors were, for many years, the major focus of research. It has been stated, based upon this early work, that 95% of cases of glomerulonephritis were due to deposition of preformed circulating immune complexes and 5% to antibodies against the glomerular basement membrane (GBM). More recently, the importance of immune complex deposition from the circulation has been questioned and the interpretation of some of the early data from animal models reviewed. In some forms of glomerulonephritis it now seems that binding of circulating antibodies to endogenous antigens within the kidney or to exogenous antigens that have become trapped in the kidney, so-called *planted antigens*, may be the major initiating mechanism. This has been called *in situ* immune complex formation and the evidence supporting it is best for animal models of membranous glomerulonephritis. It has also been recognized recently that planted antigens may be able to activate the alternative pathway of the complement system directly without antibody binding and immune complex formation.

It seems obvious that identification of the antigens which are the targets for antibody formation would be important. There has, however, been little progress in antigen definition. Even in the case of post-streptococcal glomerulonephritis where the initiating organism is known, the streptococcal proteins responsible for disease remain incompletely defined. In some diseases, immune complexes appear to play no part despite clinical evidence that a circulating factor is involved in the pathogenesis. In particular, minimal change disease and focal and segmental glomerular sclerosis and hyalinosis appear to be due to a non-immunoglobulin circulating factor which may prove to be a lymphokine.

Mechanisms which contribute to the progression of a glomerular lesion once it has been initiated have recently become the subject of increased interest. The local presence and action of cytokines, chemokines, reactive oxygen species, eicosanoids, leukotrienes, and other mediators have all been studied. A general finding has been the unexpected ability of resident cells within the glomerulus, particularly glomerular mesangial cells, to synthesize cytokines, eicosanoids, and chemokines. There is also growing evidence that, in concert with factors produced by infiltrating cells, cytokines play an important part in promoting cellular proliferation and scarring. Another related area has been identification of the mechanisms used by circulating leucocytes to enter the kidney. So far, the mechanisms used by macrophages and lymphocytes to exit the circulation appear similar to those used by cells elsewhere.

Considerable mystery surrounds the origin of cellular infiltrates within the interstitium of the kidney. Generally, these contain mainly T cells with some macrophages, whereas in the glomerulus macrophages predominate and T cells are rare. Why cells infiltrate the interstitium when the primary lesion is within the glomerulus remains unknown. The extent of the interstitial infiltrate is an important predictor of outcome in many forms of glomerulonephritis, often more so than the apparent severity of glomerular lesion, so increasing attention will focus on the mechanisms leading to its accumulation.

The factors contributing to disease progression have excited considerable interest recently as damage may continue after the mechanisms producing the original injury have ceased. These factors include secondary immune phenomena, such as the formation of antibodies to altered glomerular antigens, and both glomerular and systemic hypertension. Any disorder causing reduction in the numbers of glomeruli causes hyperperfusion in the remainder with consequent hypertrophy and either global or segmental sclerosis, the accumulating glomerular damage leading to a vicious cycle. Therefore, treatment of glomerulonephritis includes both measures aimed at minimizing the initial injury and subsequent strategies to control both systemic hypertension and glomerular hyperperfusion.

Animal models have been extremely useful in understanding the pathogenesis of glomerulonephritis. Specific models will be mentioned throughout the text and the most important of these are summarized in Table 22.2.

Histological forms

Renal biopsy appearances are the cornerstone of the day-to-day classification of glomerulonephritis. There are six basic appearances which are described below. A summary of the major diseases encountered clinically appears in Table 22.3.

Acute, diffuse endocapillary glomerulonephritis

Histologically, all glomeruli are very cellular due to increased numbers of endothelial cells, mesangial cells, and infiltrating granulocytes and macrophages. Immunofluorescence shows coarsely granular deposition of C3, sometimes with IgG, along capillary loops; early complement components (C1q and C4) do not occur and their presence indicates another diagnosis such as lupus or evolving mesangiocapillary glomerulonephritis (Fig. 22.2). Electron microscopy shows characteristic subepithelial deposits (humps) with lesser numbers in subendothelial, centrimembranous, and mesangial densities (Fig. 22.3).

The usual cause of this pattern is post-infectious glomerulonephritis. Although a number of infectious diseases can cause glomerulonephritis (Table 22.4), most produce other patterns of damage. The best known and most prevalent cause of acute diffuse

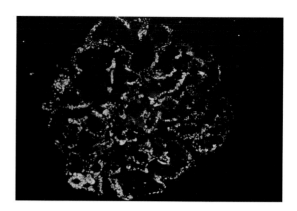

■ **Fig. 22.2** Acute post-infectious glomerulonephritis — coarsely granular ('lumpy-bumpy') staining of capillary walls for C3.

glomerulonephritis worldwide is streptococcal infection. The discussion will centre on acute post-streptococcal glomerulonephritis (APSGN), but it is important to remember that only one-third of glomerulonephritis following infection in Western communities now follows streptococcal infection. The decline is probably due to the combination of improved living standards and antibiotics.

Acute post-streptococcal glomerulonephritis

The classic example of an immune complex nephritis is APSGN. In this disease, an immune response occurs to antigenic components of group A β-haemolytic streptococci which leads to formation of immune complexes of IgG and C3 in mesangial, subendothelial and, particularly, subepithelial locations. A diffuse, proliferative glomerulonephritis ensues which is due to proliferation of local endothelial and mesangial cells and infiltration by neutrophils and macrophages.

Pathogenesis

1. Animal models. The concept of circulating immune complex (CIC) desposition as a cause of glomerular damage arose through study of acute ('one-shot') serum sickness in rabbits (Fig. 22.4). In this model, administration of bovine serum albumin (BSA) on one occasion produced a systemic vasculitis and proliferative glomerulonephritis at about day 10, when circulating antigen-antibody–complexes were being cleared from the circulation. Demonstration of BSA and rabbit IgG in the glomerulus suggested that the disease was due to the trapping of immune complexes in the glomerulus. However, it is equally plausible that BSA becomes 'planted' in the kidney and complexes are subsequently formed

Table 22.2 Principal immunopathological features of experimental autoimmune nephritis

Disease	Stimulus	Species	Strain	Serology	Immunohistology	Human correlate
'One-shot' serum sickness	Bovine serum albumin	Rabbit	—	CIC	Granular IgG + C3 along capillary wall	APSGN
Thy 1.1 model	Anti-Thy 1.1 Ab	Rat	All strains	—	—	Mesangial proliferative glomerulonephritis
Anti-GBM nephritis (Steblay)	GBM + CFA	Sheep	—	Anti-GBM Ab	Linear IgG + C3 on GBM	Anti-GBM disease
		Rat	BN WKY	Anti-GBM Ab	Linear IgG on GBM	Anti-GBM disease
Anti-GBM nephritis (NSN/Masugi)	Anti-GBM Ab	Rat, rabbit	—	Anti-GBM Ab	Linear IgG + C3 on GBM	Anti-GBM disease
Membranous nephritis (active Heymann)	Fx1A + CFA	Rat	LEW, PVG	Anti-gp330 Ab	Granular IgG + C3 along capillary wall	Membranous glomerulonephritis
Membranous nephritis (passive Heymann)	Anti-Fx1A Ab	Rat	All strains	Anti-gp330 Ab	Granular IgG + C3 along capillary wall	Membranous glomerulonephritis
'Lupus' nephritis	Spontaneous	Mouse	NZB/W, BXSB, MRL/lpr	Anti-DNA Ab Polyclonal activation	Granular Ig + C3 along capillary wall	Systemic lupus erythematosus

GBM = glomerular basement membrane; Ab = antibody; MC = mononuclear cell; id = idiotype; TBM = tubular basement membrane; NSN = nephrotoxic serum nephritis

286

Table 22.3 Principal immunopathological features of human glomerulonephritis

Disease	MHC association	Serology	Immunohistology	Pathogenesis	Treatment
Poststreptococcal GN	DR4 (DR1 in Japan)	Anti-strep Ab Variable raised Ig + IC	Subepithelial course granular IgG = C3 (± other Ig)	?Planted Ag	—
IgA nephropathy	DR4, DQw7	Variable raised IgA± IgA–IC ?Anti-mesangial cell Ab	Mesangial IgA + C3 (± IgG)	?IC disease ?Auto-Ab to mesangial cells	?Pred in nephrotic syndrome
Anti-GBM disease	DR2, DR4	Anti-GBM Ab	Linear IgG ± C3 on GBM	Auto-Ab to GBM	PE + Pred + Cyclo
Idiopathic crescentic (Wegener's, Micro. polyart.)	?DR2, DQw7	ANCA Variable raised Ig + IC	Negative or variable scattered IgG ± C3	?Autoimmune	Pred + Cyclo (induction) Pred + Aza (maintenance) PE or pulse MP
Membranous nephropathy	DR3 (DR2 in Japan)	Variable IC	Subepithelial fine granular IgG ± C3	?Auto-Ab to epithelial cells ?Planted Ag	Pred + chlorambucil
Minimal change disease	DR7, DQw2 (DR8 in Japan)	Sometimes raised IgM	Negative or sparse mesangial IgM	Not known ?Role of T cell factors	Pred Cyclo or CsA (relapse)
FGS	—	—	Mesangial IgM	?Stem cell factor	Pred
MPGN 1	—	Variable IC, low C3	Subendothelial granular IgG + C3 (± IgM)	?IC disease	Cyclo or CsA
MPGN II	?DR7	C3NeF, low C3	Linear C3 on GBM	?Auto-Ab to C3bBb	—
SLE	DR3	Anti-DNA Ab Anti-Sm Ab Polyclonal increase Ig ± IC Low C4 ± C3	Subepithelial, subendothelial, and mesangial IgG + IgM + IgA + C3	?Autoimmune ?Planted Ag ?IC disease	Pred ± Cyclo or Aza ?PE or pulse MP (severe)
EMC II	—	Cryoglobulins Paraprotein (IgM) IC + RF Low C4	Subendothelial granular IgM +IgG + C3	IC disease	PE ± Pred ± Cyclo (severe)

GBM = glomerular basement membrane; MPGN = membranoproliferative glomerulonephritis; GN = glomerulonephritis; Ab = antibody; Ag = antigen; IC = immune complex; Cyclo = cyclophosphamide; Aza = azathioprine; CsA = cyclosporin A; FGS = focal and segmental glomerular sclerosis and hyalinosis; Pred = prednisolone; PE = plasma exchange; MP = methylprednisolone; EMC II = essential mixed cryoglobulinemia type II

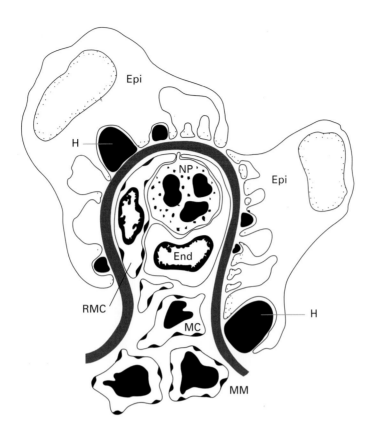

∎ **Fig. 22.3**   Acute endocapillary gomerulonephritis. This is the typical histological lesion of acute post infectious glomerulonephritis. There is accumulation of neutrophils (NP) in the capillary loops and both mesangial (RMC) and endothelial cells (End) proliferate. Immune complex deposits on the subepithelial side of the glomerular basement membrane are typical. MM, mesangial matrix; MC, mesangial cells; Epi, podocytes; H, humps (sub-epithelial deposits).

locally, or '*in situ*'. Not all animals in any experiment develop glomerulonephritis, the disease occurring only in animals with appropriate amounts of antibody production.

2. *Human disease*. The aetiological agent is a nephritogenic strain of group A β-haemolytic streptococcus. The following serotypes have been associated with APSGN: types 1, 2, 4, 6, 12, 18, 25, 31, 47, 49, 51, 52, 55, 57, 59, 60, and 61. Although the disease is most common following URTI in Western communities, some serotypes have been associated with glomerulonephritis following impetigo, notably 47, 49, 55, and 57, and these are commonly responsible for the disease in tropical populations, such as Australian Aborigines. Typing of streptococci is based upon serological differences in cell surface proteins called M-proteins. However, M-proteins are not considered to

be nephritogenic because: (i) evidence that they bind to the glomerulus is weak, and (ii) the correlation between M-type and immunogenicity is poor. Several other antigens appear to be produced relatively specifically by nephritogenic streptococci and are targets for antibody responses in patients with APSGN. Three are currently under study as initiating antigens. *Pre-absorbing antigen* (PA-Ag) is a purified moiety from a crude preparation known as endostreptosin. It activates complement directly by the alternative pathway so it may be the factor which leads to initial complement activation. PA-Ag is anionic, however, so it is difficult to understand how it might localize to the anionic GBM. *Nephritis plasmin binding protein* (NPBP) is an extracellular protein which may protect plasmin from local degradation within the glomerulus, so contributing to glomerular injury. A *cationic proteinase* which might localize rel-

∎ **Table 22.4** Infectious agents associated with endocapillary glomerulonephritis

---

Bacterial infections
  β-haemolytic group A streptococci (skin and throat)
  Staphylococcus aureus and *epidermidis* (visceral abscess, osteomyelitis, meningitis, infective endocarditis)
  Meningococcus pneumoniae (meningitis)
  Streptococcus pneumoniae (pneumonia)
  Streptococcus viridans (infective endocarditis)
  Mycoplasma pneumoniae
  Salmonella typhi
  Mycobacterium leprae
  Yersinia
  Brucella
  Leptospirosis

Viral infections
  Hepatitis B
  Epstein–Barr virus
  Cytomegalovirus
  Measles
  Mumps
  Varicella
  Coxsackie

Parasitic infestation
  Malaria (*falciparum, malariae*)
  Schistiosomiasis (*S. haematobium, S. mansoni*)
  Toxoplasmosis
  Filariasis

Others
  Coxiella
  Candida albicans
  Coccidiodes immitis

---

atively easily to the subepithelial space because of its charge has been identified and sequenced.

Activation of complement is important in this disease because C3 is predominant within the glomerular deposits, reduced C3 levels in serum are characteristic of the disease, and terminal complement components (i.e. C5b–9) are found in the circulation of affected children. Moreover, C3 deposition within the glomerulus may precede detectable IgG deposition, suggesting direct activation by planted antigen. Development of rheumatoid factor activity is common, perhaps related to alteration of the antigenicity of deposited IgG by bacterial neuraminidase, and this may contribute to the immune deposits. Neutrophil exudation into the glomerulus is also a feature; the pathogenetic mechanisms which attract them to the site and those they use to exit the circulation have not been studied.

Only 5–25% of individuals infected in epidemics develop APSGN and clinical disease is commoner in the relatives of those affected. Therefore a human leucocyte antigen (HLA) association has been suspected but while a link between APSGN and HLA-DR4 occurs in unrelated individuals (HLA-DR1 in Japan) it is not strong. Careful studies have shown abnormal urinalyses in many more individuals than those manifesting clinical disease.

Clinical features

APSGN occurs sporadically and as epidemics. Although adults may be affected, it is predominantly a disease of children between the ages of 3 and 8 years; it is extremely rare in children under 2 years and is more common in males (M/F 2:1). The incidence of the disease has declined significantly in Western communities but it remains a common disease in the developing world. Approximately 10 days following an URTI with a group A streptococcus, or about 20 days following a skin infection, usually impetigo due to infected insect bites or scabies, clinical disease occurs. Patients present with anything from microscopic haematuria to florid acute nephritic syndrome with renal failure and, sometimes, the nephrotic syndrome. Typically, they notice passage of small quantities of 'smokey' or dark brown urine and periorbital oedema. Hypertension is common and is usually volume-dependent, emphasizing the profound sodium retention which occurs in this disease. Proteinuria is almost universal, usually <2 g/day, but nephrotic-range proteinuria is reported. Complications such as hypertensive encephalopathy and pulmonary oedema may occur but can usually be prevented once the patient is under medical supervision.

Diagnosis is based upon culture of the organism and serological tests for recent streptococcal infection. The most reliable assay is antibodies to streptococcal DNase B which is positive in 75% of patients in the first week and in even more if it is checked repeatedly. Elevated antistreptolysin O titres (ASOT) are only present in 30% in the first week and are usually negative when impetigo is the initiating infection. Children do not require renal biopsy if the diagnosis is clear. In adults, diagnosis may be more difficult because of the greater range of possible underlying lesions and renal biopsy is often necessary where there may be confusion with other, treatable causes of the acute nephritic syndrome such as microscopic polyarteritis.

Haematuria may continue for 6 months or more and proteinuria for longer but this does not seem to impair long-term renal survival. Reduced serum levels of C3 return to normal within 6–8 weeks. Failure to do so

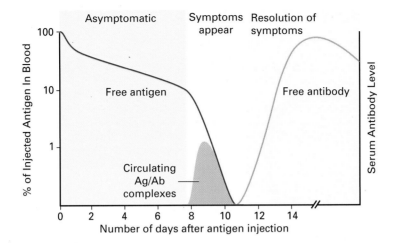

▍**Fig. 22.4** Kinetics of acute serum sickness produced by injection of bovine serum albumin. Appearance of antigen-antibody (Ag/Ab) complexes with the onset of symptoms.

should raise the clinical suspicion of other glomerular diseases associated with low C3 levels such as mesangiocapillary glomerulonephritis, especially in children and adolescents; SLE; and infective endocarditis or shunt nephritis.

Prognosis

There has been prolonged controversy concerning the outcome of this disease. It almost never recurs, in contrast to rheumatic fever, so the initial injury determines the prognosis. In general, adults fare worse than children and the disease appears milder in epidemics. It has been estimated by Cameron that approximately 1% of children die in the acute phase of the disease, 75% will be free of proteinuria in 2–3 years and 95% by 5 years. Only 1–2% develop uraemia in the long term, probably because of severe initial damage. In adults, up to 5% have persisting proteinuria and these have been thought to have a substantial risk of progression to chronic renal failure. However, recent studies indicate that most patients thought to have progressive APSGN actually have IgA nephropathy.

Treatment

In general, supportive therapy is all that is required. Control of hypertension, fluid balance, and potassium intake is critical until a diuresis occurs, generally within 7 days of presentation. Dialysis is not usually required for renal failure. Immunosuppressive drugs have no proven place, even in the presence of crescentic glomerulonephritis.

Mesangial proliferative (mesangiopathic) glomerulonephritis

Light microscopy shows that the mesangial areas are prominent due to deposits, an excess of cells or extracellular matrix, or a combination of all three. Because cellular proliferation is absent in many cases, some authorities prefer to refer to this pattern of glomerulonephritis as mesangiopathic rather than mesangial proliferative. Cellular prominence is due to proliferation of intrinsic mesangial cells and infiltration by macrophages. A number of different conditions give rise to mesangial proliferative glomerulonephritis:

(1) IgA nephropathy;

(2) post-infectious glomerulonephritis in the healing phase;

(3) part of the spectrum of minimal change disease — focal and segmental glomerular sclerosis and hyalinosis;

(4) an early manifestation of Alport's syndrome in children;

(5) IgM nephropathy;

(6) C3 and other so-called complement nephropathies;

(7) SLE.

In these conditions, the immunofluorescence and electron microscopic appearances will differ. However, by far the commonest cause of this appearance is IgA nephropathy.

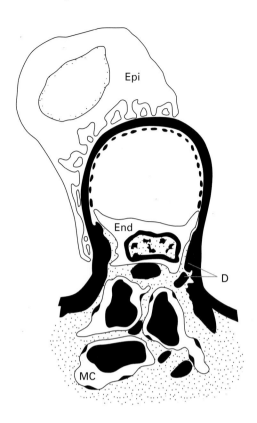

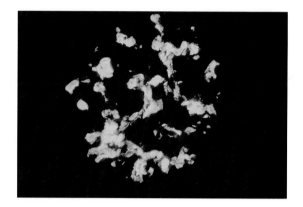

▮ **Fig. 22.6** IgA nephropathy — staining for IgA is restricted to the mesangium and resembles the outline of a deciduous tree in winter.

the main constituent of the enlarged mesangium and focal proliferation or sclerosis is very common. Immunofluorescence shows mesangial IgA with C3, IgG, IgM, and other immunoreactants in lesser numbers of biopsies (Fig. 22.6). IgA forms dense deposits seen within the mesangial matrix by electron microscopy. Occasionally, crescents with foci of necrosis and neutrophil infiltrates can be seen and these are usually associated with episodes of macroscopic haematuria or acute renal failure. Impressive interstitial and periglomerular mononuclear infiltrates are present in some biopsies and, with segmental glomerular lesions and obsolescent glomeruli, are predictive of progressive disease.

Pathogenesis

Three clinical observations underlie most of the current ideas concerning the aetiology and pathogenesis of this disease. First, the disease is due, at least in part, to deposition of a circulating factor. IgA nephropathy recurs regularly in renal transplants (about 50%) and disappears from grafts with IgA nephropathy which have been inadvertently transplanted into patients with a different renal disease. Secondly, genetic factors are probably important because the disease is commoner in families and some racial groups, such as Asians. Finally, the phenomenon of synpharyngitic haematuria suggests that mucosal immunity may be the source of the IgA deposited in IgA nephropathy.

IgA deposits in the mesangium have several unique characteristics. They are always IgA_1 and do not possess a secretory piece. They stain with reagents for J chain and are always, at least in part, polymeric. These findings have been compared with the properties of mucosal and serum IgA. Most (90–95%) circu-

▮ **Fig. 22.5** Glomerular capillary loop showing mesangial proliferative glomerulonephritis. There is proliferation of mesangial cells (MC), extracellular matrix accumulation and formation of immune deposits (D), which typically contain IgA (IgA nephropathy). There is no change in the appearance of the endothelium (End) or podocytes (Epi).

IgA nephropathy

This is the commonest primary glomerulonephritis in the Western world. It was first described in 1968 when anti-IgA reagents became available. The diagnosis rests upon the demonstration of mesangial deposits of IgA with varying degrees of mesangial cell proliferation and extracellular matrix accumulation.

Pathology

Light microscopy shows mesangial expansion of varying degrees due to a combination of mesangial cellular proliferation, slight macrophage infiltration, and increased mesangial matrix (Fig. 22.5). Generally, either cellular proliferation or extracellular matrix accumulation predominates but hyaline deposit may be

lating IgA is monomeric, originating in the spleen, bone marrow, and lymph nodes whereas mucosal IgA is mainly polymeric. Circulating IgA is 84% IgA1, 16% IgA2 whereas mucosal IgA is 40% IgA2. The phenomenon of synpharyngitic haematuria has suggested that increases in mucosal IgA may lead to IgA deposition within the mesangium and that this may be the usual route leading to its accumulation. The problem is how to explain the lack of IgA2 in the deposits if the IgA originates from a mucosal surface. At present there is no solution.

IgA nephropathy has been associated with an increased incidence of HLA-B35, -DR4, and -DQw7. No autoantigen has been well characterized. A fascinating piece of work suggests that the initiating factor may be antimesangial cell autoantibodies of IgG class. Description of the autoantigen in these reports has so far been very preliminary. There is also a problem when one attempts to include these observations in the pathogenesis of IgA nephropathy: How does IgA fit in? Although mesangial proliferative glomerulonephritis with other immune reactants is well known, and these reactants may change in sequential biopsies, IgA deposition is predominant in Western communities so that it is very likely that IgA is involved in the pathogenesis in some way.

Various abnormalities of IgA synthesis have been reported in these patients;

(1) overproduction of IgA by B cells *in vitro*;

(2) increased T-cell help for the heavy chain switch to IgA;

(3) differences in glycosylation of the heavy chain of IgA;

(4) polymorphisms in the immunoglobulin heavy chain switch region (this has not been confirmed).

There is also good evidence that local complement activation is important in the pathogenesis of IgA nephropathy. Approximately 75% of patients have serological evidence of alternative pathway activation at some time during their course, consistent with IgA deposition, and a smaller number have activation of the classical pathway. The membrane attack complex (MAC) of complement (C5b-9) is found consistently within the mesangium by immunohistochemical staining using monoclonal antibodies. There is some evidence for an increased frequency of genetic abnormalities in complement genes, such as homozygous null C4 alleles and particular variants of the C3 gene but the significance of these observations is uncertain.

Study of the factors leading to mesangial cell proliferation, macrophage infiltration and extracellular matrix accumulation has increased greatly in recent years, perhaps because of the possibility that therapeutic intervention in these 'down-stream' events may prove successful. Certainly, years of research into the mechanisms surrounding the initial insult in IgA nephropathy have, as in so may other areas of glomerulonephritis research, yielded no new therapeutic approaches.

1. Animal models. There is no really satisfactory model of IgA nephropathy. In general, those models where IgA can be found within the mesangium produce relatively unimpressive histological changes in the mesangium.

Models producing IgA deposition. It is possible to produce a lesion similar to IgA nephropathy in mice by administration of IgA immune complexes or by stimulating *in vivo* formation of such complexes by immunization with dextrans, which incite a strong IgA response. Although the histological changes are not marked, these data demonstrate that IgA can localize as an immune complex within the mesangium to produce histological changes. In keeping with the postulated mucosal origin of IgA, oral immunization can also give rise to mesangial IgA deposition. However, the changes seen in the mesangium are relatively minor.

The *Thy 1.1 model* is the most widely studied model of IgA nephropathy despite fundamental differences between the two diseases (Table 22.2). The roughly sequential evolution of cellular infiltration, mesangial cellular proliferation, and extracellular matrix accumulation over a short period has provided a convenient tool for researchers who wish to study these processes. However, the model is in no way dependent on IgA deposition. It depends upon mesangial cell surface expression of the cell surface protein Thy 1.1. Intravenous administration of heterologous goat or rabbit antibodies against rat Thy 1.1 produces a lesion which evolves through initial lysis of mesangial cells (day 1) followed by cellular proliferation (days 3–5) and subsequent accumulation of mesangial matrix (day 10). The disease is self-limiting and returns to normal within 2–3 months.

This model has been widely used to identify cytokines important in the proliferative and sclerotic phases of mesangial proliferative glomerulonephritis (MPN). Platelet-derived growth factor (PDGF), especially the BB isoform, appears particularly important in the proliferative phase of this model and in human disease whereas transforming growth factor β (TGFβ) has been implicated in mesangial matrix expansion. Transfection of glomeruli *in vivo* with cDNA encoding PDGF leads to profound mesangial cellular proliferation and TGFβ causes significant scarring. The ability to produce mesangial cell 'disease' *in vivo* by gene transfer has generated great interest in the therapeutic possibilities of this technique. Evidence that antibodies against PDGF or TGFβ can modify the Thy 1.1 model suggests that gene therapy which inhibits the action of cytokines such as PDGF and TGFβ may prove beneficial.

Mesangial cells also synthesize a variety of other cytokines which may be involved in the pathogenesis of MPN such as basic fibroblast growth factor, inter-leukin (IL) 1 and IL-6. Chemokines such as Hermes, IL-8, and macrophage chemotactic protein-1 are pro-duced by mesangial cells and appear likely to con-tribute to the cellular infiltrate seen in MPGN. Platelets and macrophages also contribute to the pathogenesis of this model by release of soluble mediators, includ-ing cytokines.

2. *Human disease: cytokines involved.* In human renal disease, PDGF and IL-6 have been most strongly implicated. Both have been localized to mesangial cells in some biopsies by immunohistochemistry. They may be involved in the proliferative phase of the disease because both are potent mitogens for mesan-gial cells *in vitro*. IL-6 can also be detected in urine of patients with IgA nephropathy and the level has been correlated with the histological severity of the renal lesion. However, infection in the renal tract also pro-duces elevated levels so that the diagnostic utility of the assay may be limited in clinical practice.

Clinical

The usual presentation is asymptomatic microscopic haematuria with varying degrees of non-nephrotic pro-teinuria. Less common presentations include episodes of macroscopic haematuria which may be recurrent, chronic renal failure, hypertension, nephrotic syn-drome, and acute renal failure. Episodes of macro-scopic haematuria may be precipitated by infection, especially URTI, and heavy exercise. Macroscopic haematuria following an URTI occurs about 2–3 days after the commencement of the infection (synpharyn-gitic), in contrast to about 10 days with post-streptococcal glomerulonephritis, and may be accom-panied by loin pain and fever. These episodes usually settle in a day or so without treatment.

IgA nephropathy may occur in a number of condi-tions characterized by high serum levels of IgA: hepatic cirrhosis and gluten enteropathy but mesangial IgA deposition occurs in a minority and clinical mani-festations are unusual. IgA nephropathy is also associ-ated with dermatitis herpetiformis and ankylosing spondylitis.

Serum IgA is elevated in about 50% of patients and IgA rheumatoid factors have been described in a similar percentage but these are of no diagnostic or prognostic value.

Prognosis and treatment

Progression to renal failure occurs in about 20% of patients within 10 years. There is a further increase at 20 years but the small numbers of patients followed so far make more exact estimation of risk difficult. Approximately 15% of patients on dialysis pro-grammes have IgA nephropathy. Attempts to identify those individuals likely to progress using clinical or laboratory data have not been very successful. A poor prognosis may be indicated by: older age, proteinuria (especially >1 g/day), raised serum creatinine, hyper-tension, absence of episodes of macroscopic haema-turia and persistently high (>100 × 10⁶ RBC/l) urinary erythrocyte excretion. Some of these are simply conse-quences of progression rather than predictors. Histologically, presence of glomerular sclerosis and interstitial scarring, extracapillary proliferation (cres-cents) and, perhaps, extension of IgA deposits on to the peripheral capillary loops have all been associated with a poorer outcome.

There is no definitive therapy for IgA nephropathy. Despite the association of synpharyngitic haematuria with URTI, there is no evidence that tonsillectomy or prophylactic antibiotics have any influence on the disease. Immunosuppressive agents are not routinely used. Recurrence occurs (~50%) in renal transplants but is usually mild and an infrequent cause of graft failure.

Mesangial proliferative glomerulonephri-tis without IgA deposition

This is an uncommon and very heterogeneous group. Several 'diseases' which were named on the basis of absent IgA and mesangial deposition of another immunoreactant, namely IgM nephropathy, C1q and C3 nephropathy, are probably not real entities. The clinical features and prognosis of mesangial prolifera-tive glomerulonephritis without IgA remain ill-defined.

Crescentic glomerulonephritis

Crescents are groups of cells which line Bowman's capsule and are made up of macrophages and prolifer-ating parietal epithelial cells; they may occur in any form in any form of glomerular damage associated with rupture of capillary loops and have no diagnostic specificity. The histological appearance of crescents has long been recognized as a poor prognostic feature regardless of the aetiology of the glomerulonephritis.

There are three major groups of diseases associated with this finding which have been subclassified according to immunofluorescent findings within the glomerular loops:

1. Linear IgG along the GBM. This is anti-GBM antibody disease and includes the so-called

Goodpasture's syndrome of haemoptysis, renal failure, and anaemia.

2. No immune reactants found within the glomerulus ('pauci-immune'). Microscopic polyarteritis and Wegener's granulomatosus are the major diseases.

3. Prominent granular fluorescence. The commonest diseases in this group are Henoch–Schönlein purpura, SLE, MPGN, post-streptococcal glomerulonephritis, and IgA nephropathy.

Pathological and pathogenetic considerations

Initially considered due to proliferation of parietal epithelial cells of Bowman's capsule, it is now known that crescents are very heterogeneous even in the same renal biopsy with macrophages predominating in some and parietal epithelial cells in others. It also appears that macrophages and some T lymphocytes predominate in crescents where Bowman's capsule has been breached. Various pathological considerations such as the presence of circumferential or localized crescents and, particularly, the percentage of 'viable' glomeruli affected by crescents influence the prognosis. The underlying disease is also important with anti-GBM disease having a worse prognosis than idiopathic crescentic glomerulonephritis of comparable histological severity.

Crescent formation appears to require breaks in the continuity of the glomerular filtration barrier and the presence of circulating fibrinogen. Fibrin in the urinary space may be the stimulus to crescent formation, although the way in which it does so remains unknown. Evidence from the nephrotoxic serum nephritis model of anti-GBM disease suggests that interactions between ICAM-1 (CD54) and ICAM-2 (CD102) and the monocyte ligands LFA-1 (CD18/CD11a) and, especially, CR3 (CD18/CD11b) are important in monocytes leaving the circulation to surround Bowman's capsule. There is no information concerning the importance of other ligands such as the selectins and of PECAM-1. The mechanisms leading to activation of ICAM-1 and the possible importance of chemokines are not yet known.

Antiglomerular basement membrane antibody glomerulonephritis

In humans, anti-GBM disease is due to circulating IgG antibodies against the non-collagenous N-terminal domain of the $\alpha 3$ chain of collagen IV. This leads to a crescentic glomerulonephritis in the kidney. The lung may also be involved, because of shared antigens between glomerular and alveolar basement membranes, giving rise to Goodpasture's syndrome.

Pathogenesis

1. *Animal models.* Arguably the best studied models of anti-GBM disease are: (i) passive anti-GBM antibody disease, nephrotoxic serum nephritis (NSN) or Masugi nephritis, and (ii) active anti-GBM antibody disease or Steblay nephritis (Table 22.2).

NSN may be induced in rats or rabbits with heterologous antibody against GBM which then localizes to the GBM and acts as a planted antigen. Two days later a heterologous phase occurs characterized by neutrophil accumulation and proteinuria. Within 2 weeks the autologous response to the foreign immunoglobulin leads to a proliferative, crescentic nephritis which is the model for anti-GBM disease. In addition to the response against the heterologous antibody, there is a response to poorly defined autoantigens. This phase is similar to human disease and is dependent for full expression on complement, neutrophils, and macrophages (Fig. 22.7)

Depletion studies have shown that local fibrin deposition is required for crescent formation. This seems to be produced by local cleavage of fibrinogen. In the glomeruli, there is an increase in procoagulant activity mediated in part through expression of tissue factor by infiltrating macrophages. This leads to activation of the extrinsic pathway of complement through fixation of factor VII and culminates in fibrin formation. How fibrin deposition then leads to crescent formation is unknown.

Anti-GBM antibody disease can also be produced by active immunization with heterologous or even homologous extracts of GBM. Steblay first produced a model of anti-GBM disease in sheep by immunizing with homologous or heterologous GBM extracts and Freund's adjuvant. Similar models have been studied in inbred rats where there is strain dependence of the disease. The genes involved have not been identified but may include the major histocompatibility complex (MHC).

2. *Human disease.* In humans, anti-GBM disease is associated with circulating anti-GBM antibodies of restricted IgG subclass distribution. They are directed against the non-collagenous (NC1) domain of the $\alpha 3$ chain of collagen IV. Six α chains have been described for collagen IV. While $\alpha 1$ and $\alpha 2$ are the major constituents of basement membrane collagen IV, localized predominantly in the subendothelial region, the $\alpha 3$ and $\alpha 5$ chains have a restricted distribution. Although it is not known whether these two chains may be associated, it is of interest that sera from patients with anti-GBM disease do not react with the GBM of patients with Alport's syndrome. The $\alpha 5$ chain is the abnormal collagen in the X-linked form of Alport's syndrome, suggesting that these two minor chains may be physically associated in the GBM. Finally, details of the

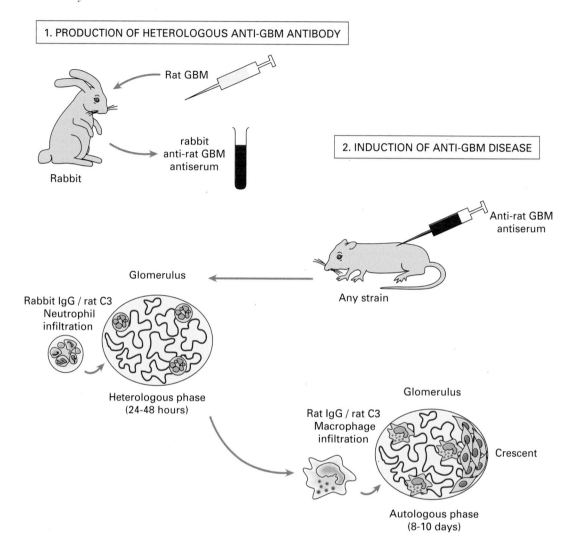

▮ Fig. 22.7 Nephrotoxic serum nephritis. The two steps are (1) production of a rabbit antibody to rat glomerular basement membrane (GBM), and (2) injection of rabbit antibody into rats. This leads to the development of acute changes, due to the direct action of the injected antibody (heterologous phase) and later changes due to the formation of anti-rabbit immunoglobulin antibodies (autologous phase). The autologous phase is usually used as a model of anti-GBM disease.

manner in which the anti-GBM autoantibody is formed are obscure, at present, but the large majority of patients with this disease possess HLA-DR2.

Pathology

Varying numbers of crescents are seen histologically, with focal necrotizing glomerulonephritis seen in the glomerular tufts. The latter is a characteristic appearance comprising areas of necrosis and neutrophil degeneration within the glomerulus. The hallmark, however, is linear deposition of IgG and complement along the GBM (Fig. 22.8). This can be confused, with the linear accentuation of capillary walls for IgG seen in diabetic glomerulosclerosis, although the intensity of staining is much less in diabetes. It is also possible to detect circulating IgG antibodies against extracts from the GBM by ELISA (enzyme-linked immunosorbent assay) or radioimmunoassay; the latter is available as a commercial kit. This is a less sensitive assay than direct immunofluorescence of a renal biopsy specimen and its major usefulness is determining when it is safe to perform a renal transplant in a patient who

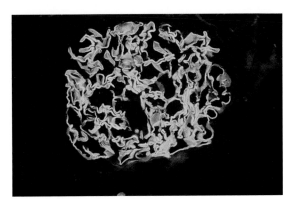

▌ Fig. 22.8 Antibasement membrane disease — uniform and smooth, linear staining of the capillary wall for IgG.

has had anti-GBM disease. About 5% of patients have a positive p-anti-neutrophil cytoplasmic antibody (ANCA) which is often IgM. These patients may have an associated small vessel vasculitis on renal biopsy.

Clinical features

There are two peaks of incidence, one in young adults and the other in the elderly. Males predominate (MF: 1.4:1). About two-thirds have pulmonary involvement and anaemia is common. Typically, patients present with acute nephritic syndrome and haemoptysis and life-threatening pulmonary haemorrhage occasionally occurs. Pulmonary haemorrhage is more common in patients who smoke or have intercurrent pulmonary infections and a minority of patients have only lung haemorrhage, although renal biopsies show linear IgG, without other changes. The balance between renal and lung damage may alter during the course of the disease and the factors determining localization of tissue damage are not understood. Most patients have no evidence of an associated immunological disease, although Goodpasture's disease is recognized as a rare complication of idiopathic membranous glomerulonephritis. About 5% of patients have histological evidence of a small vessel vasculitis. Recurrence of the disease is rare. Anti-GBM antibodies can persist with no evidence of ongoing disease.

Treatment

Immunosuppression with cyclophosphamide and steroids together with plasma exchange continues to be the standard treatment. Controversy still surrounds the part of plasma exchange but most groups would advocate its use, especially in patients with life-threatening pulmonary haemorrhage where it may be dramatically effective. Prognosis for retention of some renal function is best if the serum creatinine is <600 mmol/l at the time of presentation. Most patients who present with a serum creatinine >600 mmol/l will rapidly develop irreversible end-stage renal failure. However, treatment is still worthwhile in this group as occasional patients respond. The presence of oliguria (urine output <400 ml/day) or, especially, anuria (<50 ml/day) is a more ominous sign and these patients virtually never recover useful renal function. Whether the latter should be subjected to aggressive immunosuppressive therapy in the absence of pulmonary disease is doubtful. In those who have some preservation of renal function, plasma exchange is generally continued for 2 weeks and immunosuppressive drugs maintained at high doses for this period before being tailed off and stopped at 3 months. Recurrences are rare but can be managed in the same way. Transplantation is not contraindicated once serum anti-GBM antibody levels are no longer detectable.

Idiopathic, 'pauci-immune', crescentic glomerulonephritis

It has been increasingly recognized over recent years that virtually all of these patients have a systemic vasculitis. Renal biopsies show necrotizing glomerulonephritis with a variable number of crescents. There are, however, no immune deposits within the glomerulus (therefore, 'pauci-immune'). Clinical features characteristic of microscopic polyarteritis or Wegener's granulomatosus may also be seen. It is often impossible, however, to distinguish these two disorders by clinical criteria or renal biopsy. Practically, treatment is the same although prognosis and course of the disease may differ. To some extent, distinctions between Wegener's granulomatosus and microscopic polyarteritis are now made on the basis of the pattern of ANCA.

Wegener's granulomatosus and microscopic polyarteritis

Renal disease is common in Wegener's granulomatosus but is not the usual presenting feature. Patients presenting with ENT or pulmonary disease, however, frequently have an active urinary sediment with glomerular red blood cells, non-nephrotic proteinuria, granular and red cell casts. Development of acute renal failure due to crescentic nephritis is a feared complication and an occasional presenting feature.

1. *Pathology.* Histologically, there is focal necrotizing glomerulonephritis and a variable number of crescents. Granulomas adjacent to glomeruli or in the interstitium, often in the wall of small arterioles, are very uncommon but useful diagnostically when they occur. Patients with acute renal failure (so-called rapidly progressive glomerulonephritis) may have

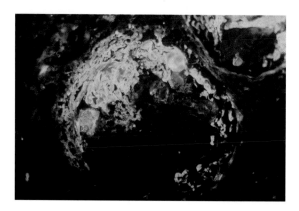

▌ Fig. 22.9 Crescentic glomerulonephritis — intense staining for fibrin among the cells of a crescent that surrounds the glomerulus.

crescents in >80% of glomeruli. Immunofluorescence in cellular glomeruli is negative aside from staining of fibrin in the crescents (Fig. 22.9) and irregular staining of sclerosed glomeruli or necrotic tissue. Virtually all patients are positive for c-ANCA and have antibodies against proteinase-3.

Diagnosis of Wegener's granulomatosus is often difficult unless there is obvious disease in the upper respiratory tract or lungs; the major problem is in distinguishing the condition from microscopic polyarteritis. Although treatment of the two conditions is identical so that there is not really a therapeutic issue, renal disease in Wegener's granulomatosus probably has a slightly better prognosis. Renal biopsy can be helpful but the availability of ANCA has assisted diagnosis because c-ANCA is almost always present in Wegener's whereas p-ANCA is the more common pattern in microscopic polyarteritis. Microscopic polyarteritis often presents with non-specific symptoms such as lethargy and muscle aches and an active urinary sediment is then found on examination. Alternatively, acute renal failure or the acute nephritic syndrome are common presentations. Renal biopsy shows identical features to those in Wegener's granulomatosus, aside from the presence of granulomata in Wegener's granulomatosus.

2. Treatment. Treatment is identical for the two conditions. The cornerstone of treatment is cyclophosphamide combined with high-dose steroids. This also applies to patients with acute renal failure due to crescentic glomerulonephritis. In this dramatic clinical situation, however, two additional therapies have been used. First, plasma exchange has its advocates but the clinical trial supporting its use suggests that it is beneficial only in dialysis-dependent patients. Other studies have suggested there is no benefit. Pulse doses of methylprednisolone are effective but whether there is any advantage over oral therapy is debated.

Most patients will improve on immunosuppressive treatment. Improvement in renal function often occurs in patients with a minority of viable glomeruli on renal biopsy and after several months of dialysis; in stark contrast to the experience in anti-GBM disease. Particular care is required when using cyclophosphamide in renal failure and, especially, in the elderly who are very susceptible to intercurrent and opportunistic infection while receiving this therapy.

Rarely, patients do not respond adequately to cyclophosphamide and steroids. In these cases, plasma exchange or even intravenous immunoglobulin are short-term options of unproven effectiveness. Cyclosporin has been used in occasional patients with apparent success whereas cotrimoxazole has yet to achieve an established place in the treatment of Wegener's but may be considered as an adjunct to other therapy.

Although the outlook for Wegener's or microscopic polyarteritis treated with cyclophosphamide and steroids is good, relapses are common. They are best detected by a change in the urinary sediment in the presence of a positive ANCA. The frequency of relapses makes it difficult to stop therapy but the long-term complications of cyclophosphamide, in particular, may necessitate it. Options are to stop cyclophosphamide after at least 12 months of inactive disease and substitute azathioprine or to use pulse intravenous cyclophosphamide from the outset. The latter is of unproven efficacy in this condition and some evidence suggests that it may be inferior to daily oral cyclophosphamide.

Churg–Strauss syndrome

Renal disease is uncommon in Churg–Strauss syndrome. When it does occur, the pattern is often of focal necrotizing glomerulonephritis so that histological differentiation from other forms of vasculitis may be difficult. The presence of eosinophilic granulomas is classical but unusual, and it is more common to see large numbers of eosinophils. Features suggestive of Churg–Strauss in a patient with renal vasculitis include asthma, eosinophilia >1.5 × 10^9/l and, to a lesser extent, mononeuritis multiplex. Vasculitic disease may affect other organ systems (e.g. heart, bowel, skin, etc.), although Churg–Strauss is often less severe than other forms of systemic necrotizing vasculitis. ANCAs occur in up to 70% and are mainly of the p-ANCA type, although c-ANCA has also been reported. Treatment with steroids alone may be adequate but the presence of significant renal disease is an indication for additional cytotoxic therapy, especially cyclophosphamide.

Classic polyarteritis nodosa

Most patients thought to have classic polyarteritis prove to have a combination of classic polyarteritis nodosa (affecting medium-sized arteries) and microvascular polyarteritis. Occasionally, only the classic pattern occurs. The urinary sediment in classic polyarteritis is normal and renal biopsy shows normal glomeruli and segmental vasculitis of arcuate and interlobar arteries. The diagnosis is best made by demonstration of aneurysms by means other than renal biopsy such as visceral angiogram because risks of bleeding after biopsy are said to be increased and the diagnostic yield is low.

Membranous glomerulonephritis

One of the more common causes of nephrotic syndrome in the adult is membranous glomerulonephritis (MN), a disease where subepithelial immune complexes of IgG and C3 are formed together with a gradual accumulation of new basement membrane-like material between the complexes, termed subepithelial spikes. The GBM is thickened but there is no increase in cellularity within the glomerulus. Immunofluorescence shows granular staining for IgG (Fig. 22.10), sometimes with C3, along the basement membrane and electron microscopy demonstrates electron dense deposits along the epithelial side of the basement membrane. The electron dense deposits come to be surrounded by new basement membrane-like material, giving the appearance of subepithelial 'spikes' on light microscopic silver stains, and are then encased within

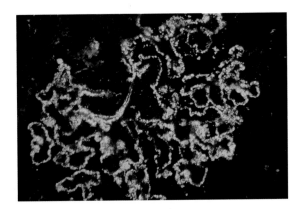

▌ **Fig. 22.10** Membranous glomerulonephritis — granular staining of capillary walls for IgG; the granules are finer and more numerous than in post-infectious glomerulonephritis.

it, producing a 'train-track' pattern in silver stains. Occasionally, in stage I disease (see below) the deposits may be so small and closely spaced that an initial impression on immunofluorescence microscopy may be of linear staining.

Four stages in the evolution of the lesion are recognized: (Fig. 22.11).

1. Subepithelial deposits (stage I).
2. Argyrophilic spikes between deposits (stage II).
3. Deposits encased in basement membrane-like material (stage III).
4. Resorption of the deposits within the thickened basement membrane (stage IV).

Some groups recognize stage V, when resolution of the lesion leaves a distorted membrane containing residual lucencies in place of the resorbed deposits. There is gradual refashioning of the membrane to a normal pattern.

Pathogenesis

1. Animal models. Experimentally, a histological lesion which is, for practical purposes, identical in appearance to MN can be produced in two ways: (i) administration of heterologous antibodies against a proximal tubular extract, and (ii) administration of a cationic antigen which becomes planted on the epithelial side of the basement membrane (Fig. 22.12).

Heymann nephritis (HN) (Fig. 22.13). The most important antigen in Fx1A preparations is a complex of a 330 kDa protein termed gp330 and receptor-associated protein (RAP), a 44 kDa protein related to human α2-macroglobulin receptor-associated protein. Gp330 is an anionic glycoprotein present both in the proximal tubular epithelium and in the clathrin-coated pits of glomerular epithelial cells. It is a member of the low-density lipoprotein (LDL)-receptor gene family and does not appear to be involved in the pathogenesis of human MN. Binding of anti-Fx1A antibodies to the gp330/RAP antigenic complex leads to insertion of the membrane attack complex of complement (C5b-9) into the glomerular epithelial cell surface. This is followed by endocytosis, transcellular passage and urinary excretion of C5b-9. Insertion of C5b-9 activates the visceral epithelial cell, leading to proteinuria. The anti-Fx1A/gp330/RAP/C5b-9 complex is also shed from the cell on to the basement membrane, leading to subepithelial immune complexes.

In situ *immune complex formation.* Administration of a cationic foreign antigen such as cationized heterologous IgG leads to deposition of the IgG on the epithelial side of the GBM. This is followed by an autologous anti-IgG response, *in situ* immune complex

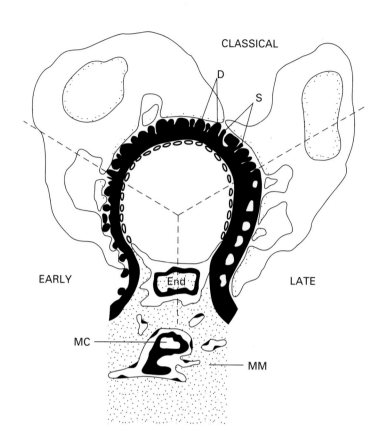

▍**Fig. 22.11** Capillary loops showing membranous glomerulonephritis. It is divided into early (stage I), classical (stages II and III), and late (stage IV) stages. In the early stage (subepithelial deposits — stage I), IgG-containing immune complexes are seen on the epithelial side of the glomerular basement membrane, but there is no reaction of the basement membrane. In the classical stage, osmophilic spikes of basement membrane are seen between the immune deposits (spike formation — stage II), and subsequently the immune deposits (D) become surrounded by new basement membrane (incorporation of immune deposits — stage III). In the later stage the immune deposits within the basement membrane begin to disappear leaving a very thickened vacuolated basement membrane (deposit resorption — stage IV). There are no changes in the endothelium (End), mesangial cells (MC) or mesangial matrix (MM) but foot process fusion is common.

formation and proteinuria. The lesion resembles MN, morphologically, but there is no passage of C5b-9 into the urine. As in HN, proteinuria is dependent on local C5b-9 formation.

2. *Human disease*. Evidence that some cases of human MN are similar in pathogenesis to HN comes from the histological similarities between the two con-

ditions and the presence of C5b-9 in urine in both conditions. The latter is specific, in humans, for MN but occurs in less than 50%. Whether the remainder have a pathogenesis similar to that of experimental immune complex MN or represent quiescent disease is unknown. In HN only certain strains develop the active form of the disease and, in humans, there is an increased risk of MN in patients who possess the hap-

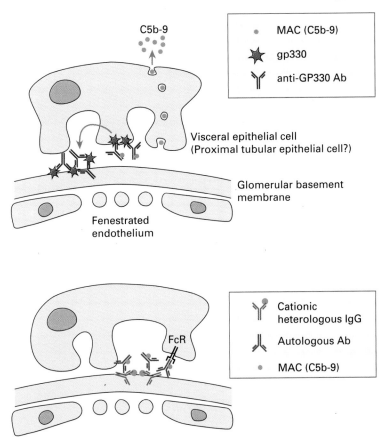

▮ Fig. 22.12 Two models of membranous glomerulonephritis. The upper panel shows the events which occur in Heymann nephritis. Antibodies against GP 330 and other antigens cross the glomerular basement membrane, bind GP330 and fix complement. The membrane attack complex (MAC or C5b-9) damages the cell and is also excreted from the urinary side of the visceral epithelial cell, so appearing in the urine and serving to distinguish this form of injury from others. The complex of GP300/anti-AP330 is extruded from the cell membrane onto the glomerular basement membranes so forming immune complexes. The lower panel shows a model of injury where cationic heterologous IgG crosses the glomerular basement membrane to act as a planted antigen on the epithelial side. Autologous antibody also crosses the basement membrane, fixes complement and causes local damage. This form of injury is not associated with the appearance of C5b-9 in the urine.

lotype HLA-A1-B8-DR3 or one or more of its constituent genes, especially DR3. In the Japanese, the association is with HLA-DR2. The association of MN and malignancy is well known, as is the occurrence of MN after administration of certain drugs (Table 22.5). Moreover, MN is the commonest form of *de novo* transplant glomerulonephritis; i.e. glomerulonephritis occurring in the transplanted kidney of a patient whose original renal disease was different.

Clinical features

Most patients present with proteinuria, frequently of nephrotic range. The disease is commonest in middle-aged or elderly males and rare in children or adolescents unless they are infected with hepatitis B. The outlook for a patient with MN is unpredictable, but is now recognized to be much better than previously thought. In adults, about 40% will be in remission within 10 years and only 10% will have developed renal failure. Relapses are also well described in those who remit. Prognosis is most strongly influenced by the presence of nephrotic syndrome and impaired renal function.

Although MN is associated with malignancy, especially of the lung and colon, these are usually clinically apparent at the time the renal disease presents; there-

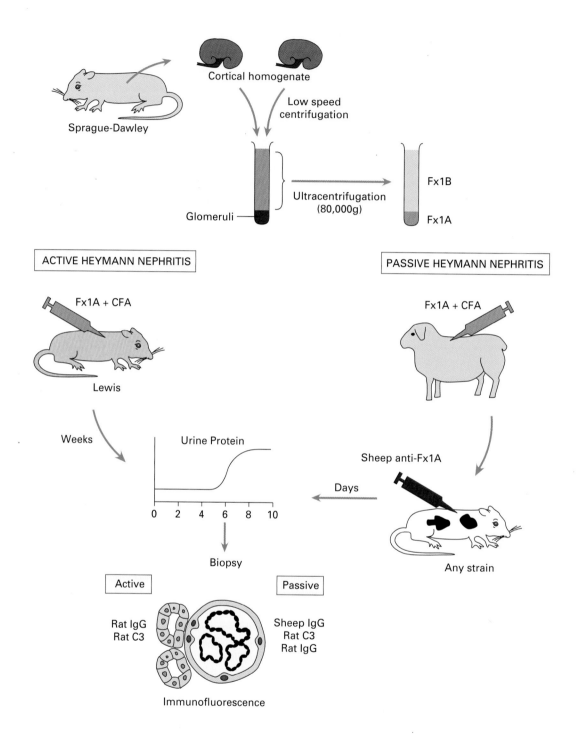

▮ Fig. 22.13 The Heymann model of membranous glomerulonephritis. First, rat kidneys are used to produce a tubular extract, called Fx1A. This can then be used to immunize rats directly to produce the active model (which is strain specific), or to immunize sheep to produce anti-Fx1A antibody. The latter can be used to induce passive Heymann nephritis in any strain of rat.

▌ **Table 22.5** Diseases associated with membranous glomerulonephritis

---

Common
 Cancer: lung, colon (usually apparent)
 Systemic lupus erythematosus
 Drugs: gold, penicillamine
 Hepatitis B
 Renal transplantation

Uncommon
 Congenital and secondary syphilis
 Chronic transplant rejection
 Sarcoidosis
 Schistosomiasis

---

fore, a prolonged or complicated search for malignancy is not warranted.

Treatment

The unpredictability of the course of MN leads to substantial difficulties in the interpretation of clinical trials and, even more so, when planning therapy for the individual patient. Steroids in daily or alternate day doses have not shown evidence of sustained benefit in most trials and have been abandoned as monotherapy. Addition of one of the alkylating agents, chlorambucil or cyclophosphamide, has shown benefit in some of the relatively small trials conducted so far. In patients whose prognosis is expected to be poor, treatment for a period with cyclophosphamide or chlorambucil and steroids may be used empirically. The difficulty is in identifying such patients but those with nephrotic syndrome, hypertension, and early impairment of renal function might be treated, particularly if they are male. There is no guidance concerning the optimal dose or duration of therapy but good results have been reported with alternating pulses of chlorambucil and methylprednisolone.

 Transplantation of those who progress to end-stage renal failure is not contraindicated; although MN occurs *de novo* in about 1% of transplants, recurrent disease occurs in only 10% of patients whose original disease was MN.

Idiopathic nephrotic syndrome

Three conditions are sometimes collected under this heading, namely minimal change disease (MCD), minimal change with some mesangial cellular proliferation, and focal and segmental glomerular sclerosis, and hyalinosis (FGS). Despite the dissimilarity in histological appearances and the differences in outcome, there are compelling reasons to consider the three disorders, part of a spectrum when they present with nephrotic syndrome. These include: (i) development of FGS in patients whose initial biopsy (apparently adequate) did not show this lesion; (ii) loss of mesangial proliferation in biopsies which initially showed this lesion; (iii) steroid responsiveness may occur in all three variants, although it is commonest in typical MCD; and (iv) FGS may recur in and MCD has been demonstrated *de novo* in renal transplants. However, the usual clinical courses of MCD and FGS are so different that accurate differentiation is important, whatever the conceptual similarities between the conditions.

Minimal change disease

As its name implies, the appearances of renal biopsy specimens are normal by light microscopy and immunofluorescence is negative. Electron microscopy, however, shows effacement of the normal podocyte foot processes so that the body of the podocyte comes to lie directly on the GBM (Fig. 22.14). This is the typical picture of MCD but some patients show mesangial cellular proliferation with minor deposits of immunoglobulin, especially IgM. A suggestion that mesangial IgM deposits indicate a poor prognosis has not been confirmed by most observers. The widespread belief that foot process effacement is a non-specific phenomenon occurring in all forms of the nephrotic syndrome is incorrect. The presence of diffuse foot process loss is an important diagnostic sign of MCD if FGS can be excluded, most importantly by a response to corticosteroid therapy.

Incidence

The annual incidence in children in Western communities has been estimated at about 2 per 100 000 compared with about 3 per 1 000 000 in adults. In children, MCD accounts for 60–90% of cases of nephrotic syndrome with a slight male predominance (2:1); whereas there is no sex bias in adolescents and adults and it accounts for only about 25% of nephrotic syndrome. Some racial groups are more susceptible, especially Asians, Indians, and Japanese.

Pathogenesis

The barrier to loss of protein in the glomerular filtrate conceptually comprises a set of pores of approximate molecular radius 55 Å and a strong anionic charge on the glycoproteins of the GBM and visceral epithelial cells. Proteinuria in MCD has been considered due to loss of the anionic charge on the GBM so that smaller molecules such as albumin (radius 40 Å), which are excluded from the urine by their charge alone are able

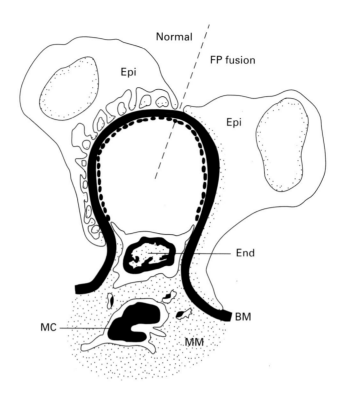

▊**Fig. 22.14** Foot process (FP) fusion or effacement, as seen in minimal change disease, and focal and segmental glomerular sclerosis and hyalinosis. This appearance can also be superimposed on other forms of glomerulonephritis where it is associated with heavy proteinuria. MM, mesangial matrix; MC, mesangial cells; End, endothelium; EPI, podocytes.

to cross. Larger molecules will still be excluded by their size. Several studies have shown a reduction in the anionic charge of the GBM in this condition, although all have been criticized. Moreover, there is evidence that the reduction in anionic charge may be generalized, affecting other cell membranes and even circulating albumin.

In 1974, Shalhoub proposed that a circulating lymphokine produced through T-cell dysfunction was the aetiological agent in MCD. Current evidence for this view includes: (i) the therapeutic response to steroids and alkylating agents; (ii) cases of remission occurring in measles (an immunosuppressive disease); (iii) the association of MCD with activity in Hodgkin's disease; (iv) occurrence of MCD in apparent response to allergic stimuli such as pollens, bee stings, and food; and (v) the association of MCD with HLA tissue type; the evidence seems to be strongest for DR7 and DQw2. More recently, it has been suggested that a cationic factor produced by the immune system may

lead to neutralization of charge on the GBM. This suggestion has fuelled much subsequent research but the factor remains ill-defined. For example, a T-cell hybridoma produced from the peripheral blood of a patient with MCD has been reported to secrete a 'glomerular permeability factor' which induces proteinuria in rats. This factor has not yet been purified or identified

Clinical features

Almost all cases of MCD are idiopathic, especially in children. There are, however, well described associations of MCD with administration of non-steroidal anti-inflammatory drugs (NSAIDs) (in the elderly), when it usually coexists with interstitial nephritis; malignancy; and IgA nephropathy. The association with lymphoproliferative disorders, especially Hodgkin's lymphoma has reinforced the view that MCD is due to a circulating lymphokine. From a practical standpoint, it is generally not worth investigating these patients for occult malignancy as any tumour is usually obvious when the nephrotic syndrome occurs.

Although the peak age for MCD is about 5 years, this disease is responsible for about 25% of all cases of nephrotic syndrome at any age. Patients present with the nephrotic syndrome which may be severe. Typical findings are pitting oedema, sometimes in non-dependent areas, frothy urine which contains large amounts of protein and, usually, little or no micro-scopic haematuria. Ascites and pleural effusions are uncommon but may give rise to dyspnoea and so cause confusion with heart failure. Rarely, patients develop oliguria due to the very rapid development of nephrotic syndrome. The usual explanation is loss of intravascular volume due to reduced oncotic pressure but the evidence for this is very poor. It is more likely that the ability of water and its solutes to cross the glomerular filtration barrier (known technically as the glomerular ultrafiltration coefficient or Kf) is acutely reduced by the pathological changes. Patients are usually normotensive and, apart from the unusual cir-cumstance noted above, have normal renal function. A peculiar form of MCD occurs in elderly patients taking NSAIDs where it is combined with interstitial nephri-tis. These patients often have abnormal renal function. MCD in children may be associated with IgA deposits, probably because of the coincidental occurrence of the two common disorders. The response to steroids is the same.

Proteinuria in children is often selective (i.e. the passage of smaller molecules such as albumin as a pro-portion of serum concentration is much greater than that of larger molecules such as IgG), but this is not usual in adults. Serum IgG may also be reduced and, perhaps, accounts for the marked susceptibility of chil-dren with MCD to pneumococcal infection.

Treatment

The natural history of untreated patients is that most will lose their proteinuria if followed for 3–4 years. Chronic renal failure almost never occurs whatever treatment is given. The nephrotic syndrome, however, is unpleasant and dangerous so that all patients should be given treatment with steroids. In children, the usual dose of prednisolone is 60 mg/m^2 per day for 6–8 weeks or until a week following remission followed by a period of alternate day dosage or a reducing daily course. From the International Study of Kidney Disease in Children (ISKDC) data, 93% will go into remission within 6–8 weeks on this regimen, 36% will never experience a relapse, 18% will relapse infre-quently, and 30% will become either frequent relapsers or steroid dependent (i.e. steroids cannot be withdrawn without immediate recurrence of symptoms). In the latter two groups, a course of cyclophosphamide 3 mg/kg per day for 8 weeks is very effective and may allow complete cessation of steroids. However, the risk of gonadal toxicity, in particular, is a problem which has made this therapy less attractive in recent years particularly when the long-term outcome of the condition for most patients is good.

In adults, a dose of 1 mg/kg per day of oral pred-nisolone for a similar period has been recommended. Doses used in Australia and the UK tend to be slightly lower than this. Adults respond more slowly and less completely to steroids but, once a remission has been achieved, they relapse far less often.

Occasional patients do not respond to steroids, especially adults. When this occurs the most likely reason is that the diagnosis is incorrect and the patient has FGS. A remission can sometimes be induced with cyclophosphamide in the odd patient who does not respond to steroids. Cyclosporin can also be used to produce remission but, unfortunately, most will relapse once the drug is stopped.

Focal and segmental glomerular sclerosis and hyalinosis

The light microscopical lesion of FGS is not specific. Most commonly, this pattern is seen as a manifestation of glomerular hyperperfusion, occurring in a wide variety of renal disorders usually as a consequence of glomerular destruction but occasionally in glomerular enlargement (glomerulomegaly) of unknown cause. However, there is a small, important and specific group in which FGS is an apparently primary lesion presenting as idiopathic and corticosteroid-resistant nephrotic syndrome and progressing more or less rapidly into chronic renal failure. This group, described below, is distinguished from the other, non-specific forms by diffuse effacement of epithelial foot processes.

Pathology

FGS affects the juxtamedullary glomeruli first so that a superficial renal biopsy will miss the lesion and detect only foot process effacement. Such biopsies may be misdiagnosed as MCD. By light microscopy, FGS appears as obliteration of portion of the glomerulus by collapse, adhesion to Bowman's capsule and the accu-mulation of hyaline debris, often with aggregates of foam cells. There is often moderate, although irregular, mesangial proliferation. The visceral epithelial cells around the lesions are enlarged and vacuolated, corre-sponding to areas of separation of the cells from the GBM by electron microscopy; elsewhere there is total effacement of podocyte foot processes. Immunofluorescence microscopy of unaffected

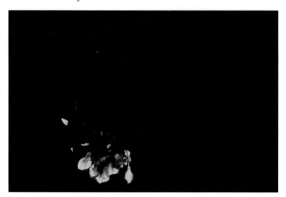

▮ **Fig. 22.15** Focal glomerulosclerosis — segmental 'blobby' staining for IgM corresponding to hyaline in the sclerotic lesion. Similar, non-specific staining may be seen in segmental glomerular scarring from any cause and in the insudative lesions of diabetic glomerulosclerosis.

glomeruli is negative but the areas of sclerosis may show non-specific, segmental staining for IgM and C3 (Fig. 22.15). Unfortunately, even this pattern is not absolutely specific. Prolonged proteinuria from any cause may lead to areas of capillary collapse, usually adjacent to the proximal tubule (the 'glomerular tip lesion'). Therefore, rarely patients with MCD and other glomerular disorders may develop FGS-like lesions and can be distinguished from true FGS only by response to corticosteroids.

Pathogenesis

FGS is probably due to the action of a circulating factor. It recurs in at least 20% of renal transplants in these individuals, sometimes as soon as the blood flow to the graft is restored. The risk of recurrence is much higher, however, in those patients <20 years who had a rapid course into renal failure. Several studies have described factors present in serum from some individuals with FGS which induce proteinuria in experimental animals. None has yet proceeded to complete identification. A recent study reported that a murine model of FGS was due to a circulating factor produced by cells originating from bone marrow stem cells. In common with minimal change disease, FGS is postulated to be due to a circulating lymphokine or cytokine.

Clinical features

These patients present with nephrotic syndrome. Distinguishing FGS from MCD is a common problem to which there is no clear solution. Patients with FGS may have microscopic haematuria and renal impairment but these are also seen, albeit less commonly, in

MCD. Generally, this disease is suspected when a child with nephrotic syndrome does not respond to steroids or an adult with apparent MCD either does not respond or has deteriorating renal function. Some adults, of course, are detected by the initial renal biopsy. A particular problem with FGS is maintenance of severe proteinuria despite severe renal failure. In most glomerular diseases (excepting amyloid, on occasion), proteinuria declines as the kidneys fail. It may be necessary to infarct or remove the kidneys if proteinuria leads to malnutrition.

Associated diseases

FGS in patients who are nephrotic is mainly idiopathic. However, it may be seen in association with malignancy, especially Hodgkin's disease and non-Hodgkin's lymphoma where the course of the nephropathy parallels that of the malignancy. A particularly aggressive form of FGS in patients who are infected with human immunodeficiency virus (HIV) has been reported increasingly in recent years. Termed collapsing FGS, the entire glomerular tuft is affected by the disease and these patients progress rapidly into renal failure. It has supplanted other forms of drug-associated nephropathies in groups at risk and has also been identified in patients with no demonstrable precipitating factors.

Treatment

A small number of patients with apparent FGS respond to steroids. Therefore, all patients with FGS should have a 6–8 week trial of steroids. If they respond then the prognosis is probably better than for the cohort that does not. Relapses are more likely than in steroid-responsive children with MCD. If steroids are ineffective there is little that can be offered. Cyclophosphamide has been the subject of conflicting reports but does not appear to be of major benefit in adults or children. Cyclosporin may have temporary effects in some patients and these can be long-lived in a very few. Individuals who respond to cyclosporin generally do so within the first month so that it is worth a trial.

Transplantation may prove disastrous in these individuals because the disease often recurs and may do so immediately, leading to massive proteinuria. As this is an unpredictable event, these patients may be grafted once using an organ from a cadaveric donor to determine what the outcome will be. Recurrent disease in one graft indicates a very high probability of recurrence in further grafts.

Prognosis

The major determinant of outcome in childhood nephrotic syndrome is response to steroid therapy. In those who do not respond, so-called primary non-responders, FGS is a common finding on renal biopsy (approximately 40%). About 50% of nephrotic patients with FGS will develop end-stage renal failure within 10 years.

Membranoproliferative (mesangiocapillary) glomerulonephritis

The histological appearance of MPGN is due to a combination of mesangial cellular proliferation or leucocyte infiltration together with thickening of the GBM. By an accident of publication, two completely unrelated diseases are frequently combined under this diagnosis. An early and influential paper on MPGN found two patterns of disease distinguished by electron microscopy — one characterized by subendothelial deposits, so-called type 1; and the other typified by dense transformation of the GBM, so-called type 2. Further studies have shown that the 'type 2' form, better called dense deposit disease, more often shows focal and segmental proliferation or simple glomerular enlargement than the MPGN pattern. However, the original division, unfortunately, has become established in the literature. To complicate the issue further, yet another pattern of MPGN has been identified in which electron microscopy shows massive deposits disrupting the GBM and this form has been termed 'type 3' MPGN. Probably, this 'type 3' lesion is merely another pattern of the so-called 'type 1' lesion, both representing chronic immune complex glomerulonephritis. The nature of the dense material in dense deposit disease, so called 'type 2', is unknown and there is no evidence that it represents immune complex deposit.

In summary, the three lesions are often grouped under the rubric MPGN:

1. *Type 1* — a chronic immune complex glomerulonephritis characterized by an MPGN pattern. This pattern is diffuse glomerular enlargement produced by mesangial proliferation with thickening of capillary walls. Electron microscopy shows that the capillary wall thickening is produced by extravasation of material from the mesangium around the capillary wall, between the basement membrane and the endothelium (hence the alternative term mesangiocapillary glomerulonephritis). Silver stains by light microscopy show the membrane and new mesangial material as two layers — double contours. Immunofluorescence microscopy usually shows granular mesangial and capillary wall staining for IgG, C1q, and C3 but may reveal a lobular pattern with staining only for C3 (Figs. 22.16, 22.17 and 22.18).

2. *Dense deposit disease* (so-called type 2) — a distinct lesion characterized by electron microscopy showing dense, agranular transformation of the glomerular and tubular basement membranes, Bowman's capsule and other structures by material of unknown composition. Light microscopy may show MPGN but more commonly reveals irregular glomerular enlargement with variable segmental proliferation or sclerosis. Immunofluorescence shows intense, ring-like mesangial deposits (doughnuts) of C3 with weak linear C3 staining of glomerular and tubular basement membranes (Fig. 22.19).

3. *Type 3* — a variant of type 1 with similar light and immunofluorescence findings but massive dense deposits by electron microscopy causing disruption of the GBM.

Pathogenesis

The aetiologies of the two major forms of MPGN appear to be distinct. Type 1 is often associated with a chronic response to infection, while dense deposit disease is probably due to a circulating factor because it recurs in >90% of transplants performed in these individuals, often rapidly.

1. *Complement abnormalities.* MPGN is commonly associated with low levels of serum complement. In approximately 50–60% of patients with MPGN, CH_{50} levels in serum are depressed. In MPGN, low C3 is often associated with the presence of an unusual autoantibody directed against the alternative pathway C3 convertase, C3bBb. Called C3 nephritic factor (C3NeF), this autoantibody can be detected in about 60% of patients with *dense deposit disease* and in 20% of those with type 1. It stabilizes the alternative pathway convertase, preventing its normal degradation by factor H, factor I, and CR1, so increasing the rate of C3 breakdown. Assays for the detection of C3NeF measure the ability of serum from patients with C3NeF to cause C3 breakdown in serum from normals. It is not a routine assay and there are no accepted clinical indications for its measurement. There is no correlation between complement or C3NeF levels and progression of the renal lesion in patients with MPGN.

C3NeF is also associated with partial lipodystrophy, an acquired loss of subcutaneous fat predominantly over the arms and upper body. The correspondence between partial lipodystrophy, MPGN, and C3NeF is not complete so that most patients with partial lipodystrophy and C3NeF have no renal disease.

The explanation for the relationship between complement deficiency and MPGN is obscure. Major

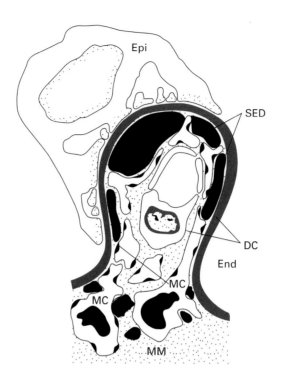

▌ **Fig. 22.16** Membranoproliferative (mesangiocapillary) glomerulonephritis type I. This is a commoner form of this lesion, and comprises mesangial hypercellularity and thickened glomerular basement membranes. Mesangial hypercellularity is due to a combination of mesangial cell proliferation (MC) and macrophage infiltration, while subendothelial immune deposits (SED) and the interposition of mesangial cell cytoplasm (MC) between the glomerular basement membrane and the endothelium (End) lead to the appearance of a thickened glomerular basement membrane with a double contour (DC).

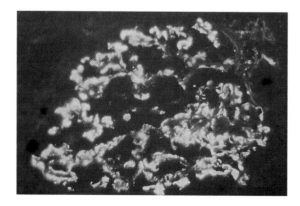

▌ **Fig. 22.17** Membranoproliferative glomerulonephritis (type 1) — granular staining of mesangia and capillary walls for IgG; similar staining was also present for C1q and C3.

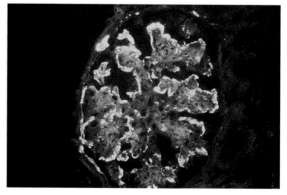

▌ **Fig. 22.18** Membranoproliferative glomerulonephritis (type 1) — an alternative pattern in this condition is granular, lobular staining of capillary walls for C3 only.

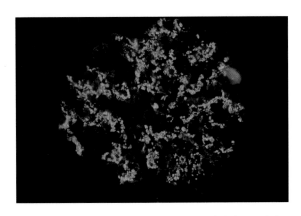

∎ **Fig. 22.19** Dense deposit disease — bright, nodular staining of mesangia for C3; careful examination of these nodules at a higher power would reveal non-staining centres (doughnuts). There is usually also linear C3 staining of glomerular and tubular basement membranes, not seen well in this photograph.

theories are: (i) complement deficiency leads to inefficient clearance of CICs (ii) complement activation itself is pathogenetic and causes the injury; and (iii) the primary abnormality in the glomerulus leads to secondary complement activation and formation of an autoantibody as a by-product of the continuous presence of C3bBb.

None is satisfactory as an explanation for all of the observed phenomena. In particular: (i) dense deposit disease does not resemble an immune complex disease; (ii) it has not been possible to reproduce the injury by continuous complement activation in animals; and (iii) bilateral nephrectomy does not reduce complement activation in patients with MPGN. The third hypothesis seems particularly doubtful because dense deposit disease recurs rapidly and frequently in renal transplants using kidneys from normal, unrelated individuals.

2. *Associated diseases.* The decline in incidence of the idiopathic form of MPGN has led to an increasing number of cases of type 1 MPGN occurring secondary to an underlying disease. The commonest of these are SLE, infection with hepatitis B and C, infective endocarditis, infected ventriculo-atrial shunts and essential mixed cryoglobulinaemia. The association with hepatitis C infection has been reported only recently; these patients have type 1 MPGN with mixed cryoglobulinaemia. The renal disease may respond to treatment with α-interferon.

Clinical features

MPGN is predominantly a disease of children and young adults, with the mean age of presentation for type 1 about 25 years and for dense deposit disease about 15. Dense deposit disease is almost as common as type 1 in children whereas, in adults, type 1 is far commoner. Interestingly, however, the incidence of type 1 MPGN has declined in most Western countries over the past 20 years while the incidence of dense deposit disease has remained constant. It has been suggested that the parallel reduction in incidence of post-streptococcal glomerulonephritis has contributed to this decline, although MPGN is rarely seen in the former condition. In Third World countries and populations living in poor conditions, type 1 MPGN is sometimes the commonest single form of glomerulonephritis suggesting an association with infection.

In children, the commonest presentation is with nephrotic syndrome and about 12–15% of childhood nephrotic syndrome is due to MPGN. In adults, presentation with asymptomatic haematuria and non-nephrotic proteinuria is the commonest single presentation but other presenting syndromes seen include nephrotic syndrome, chronic renal failure and, occasionally, rapidly progressive glomerulonephritis with crescents on renal biopsy. Episodes of macroscopic haematuria occur in a minority but hypertension is found in 80–90% at presentation. Unexplained anaemia may occur, perhaps due to the effects of continuing complement activation.

Prognosis

Although a small percentage (perhaps 5%) will undergo spontaneous remission, the outlook for preservation of renal function is bleak with 50% dead or in end-stage renal failure at 10 years and 90% at 20 years.

Treatment

If there is an association with the presence of infection, then attempts should be made to eradicate it. This is not usually the case even in populations with a high incidence, so several lines of therapy have been devised based on the presumed pathogenesis of the disease. Steroids may slow disease progression, probably via their anti-inflammatory effects but at the cost of steroid-induced side-effects. The anticoagulant and anti-platelet drugs warfarin, aspirin, and dipyridamole have also been used in clinical trials, sometimes with other agents. The rationale is to reduce glomerular deposition of fibrin. Analysis of these trials, however, suggests that there is no statistical difference in kidney survival between treated and untreated patients. There is also a substantial risk in the use of some of these agents, especially warfarin. Immunosuppressive agents such as cyclophosphamide have also been used, generally in combination with other agents. Controlled trials of therapy with cyclophosphamide, dipyridamole, and aspirin have not shown any statistically significant benefit. Plasma exchange may benefit some patients but the experience is small.

Overall, there is no convincing evidence that any therapy is of benefit in patients with MPGN and, in general, they should probably be offered no treatment. However, where the evidence is so mixed and the disease probably heterogeneous, it has been argued that some patients should be given a therapeutic trial of anticoagulants and antiplatelet agents or even steroids. This is not a generally accepted view. More aggressive treatment has been advocated for the small number of patients who have crescentic disease. Therapy similar to that outlined for anti-GBM disease has been used but the long-term outcome has been poor in the anecdotal studies reported.

Transplantation of patients with MPGN is not contraindicated. Although dense deposit disease recurs in 90% it is usually mild and of little consequence to the graft. Type 1 MPGN probably recurs less commonly — although careful studies have not been performed — but is more prone to cause progressive graft damage.

Hereditary glomerulonephritis

There are three patterns of hereditary glomerulonephritis. The most common, thin GBM disease is very common in Western communities and typically presents as microscopic haematuria. The mode of inheritance is unclear but diagnosis is more common in women; the nature of the membrane defect is unknown. The Alport lesion is usually inherited in a sex-linked recessive pattern and affected males present initially with microscopic haematuria, later developing proteinuria and progression into chronic renal failure. Diagnosis is by electron microscopy, the GBM showing variation in width and texture, especially a lamellated pattern. The defect is absence of the $\alpha5$ (occasionally the $\alpha6$) chain of type IV collagen in the GBM. A minority of patients (about 15%) develop antibasement membrane glomerulonephritis following transplantation, after exposure to the antigen missing from their own kidneys. A rare pattern of hereditary glomerulonephritis, characterized by the presence of fibrillary collagen in the GBM, occurs in association with orthopaedic abnormalities in the nail-patella syndrome; the nature of the defect is unknown.

Glomerular disease in the third world

The characteristics of glomerular disease in the Third World are very different from those in developed countries. Although the incidence of glomerulonephritis is increased through much of the developing world and the occurrence of certain diseases very different from that in Western countries, there is a great deal of variation between individual Third World countries such that it is not possible to discuss them together. A few general comments can be made. First, the incidence of nephrotic syndrome is often very high and both APSGN and type 1 MNGN are far more common causes. Chronic renal failure also appears to be much more common in these communities than in the West, although the precise reason is unknown. There are several characteristic disease such as MNGN due to infection with *Schistosoma mansoni* and amyloidosis with leprosy. Quartan malaria, too, is alleged to produce a characteristic histological appearance, generally in children and young adults presenting with nephrotic syndrome. Different characteristics are found in displaced indigenous populations in Western countries, such as American Indians and Australian Aborigines (so-called 'Fourth World', populations). In addition to an excess of infection-related glomerulonephritis, these peoples are devastated by complications of diabetes and appear to show glomerular enlargement of unknown cause with progressive damage caused by focal glomerulosclerosis,

Acute interstitial nephritis

A number of conditions give rise to acute interstitial nephritis (Table 22.6). However, most cases that come to clinical attention now are due to drugs, particularly penicillins, sulphonamides, rifampicin, and NSAIDs. Although the majority of these patients present with acute renal failure, interstitial nephritis is a relatively rare cause of this syndrome, accounting for approximately 1% of cases.

Penicillins

Methicillin is the major culprit but cases associated with many other β-lactam antibiotics have been reported. Patients can be of any age and the illness generally occurs about 2 weeks following initiation of antibiotic therapy. Typically, affected individuals have one or more of fever, rash, arthralgias, and eosinophilia. The presence of eosinophilia suggests that this disease may involve type 1 hypersensitivity. Eosinophiluria is also well described but is relatively non-specific. Renal biopsy shows expansion of the interstitium by oedema containing aggregates of activated mononuclear cells admixed with eosinophils. Renal failure may be non-oliguric. The disease is self-

∎ **Table 22.6**   Causes of acute interstitial nephritis

Drugs
   penicillins (especially methicillin)
   cephalosporins
   rifampicin
   sulphonamides

Non-steroidal anti-inflammatory drugs
   propionic acid derivatives (fenoprofen, naproxen)
   others

Infections
   septicaemia
   leptospirosis
   others

Malignant infiltration
   myeloma
   lymphoma
   leukaemia

Systemic autoimmune disease
   systemic lupus erythematosus
   Sjögren's syndrome
   sarcoid

Idiopathic

---

limiting provided the antibiotic has been stopped but steroids have been reported, anecdotally, to reduce the duration of renal failure. A short course of oral prednisolone, sometimes with initial bolus doses of methylprednisolone is frequently administered but the evidence supporting its efficacy remains inconclusive.

Non-steroidal anti-inflammatory drugs

This form of the disease has been increasingly recognized in elderly patients. It can probably occur with any NSAID but is commonest with the propionic acid derivatives, especially fenoprofen. Duration of therapy preceding diagnosis is long at 5–6 months and the fever, rash, and eosinophilia characteristics of other types of drug-induced interstitial nephritis are usually absent. A striking association with nephrotic syndrome due to MCD has been noted. Renal biopsy shows an interstitial nephritis with, usually, few eosinophils and the glomeruli reveal only diffuse obliteration of epithelial foot process. NSAID-induced interstitial nephritis appears to be mediated, at least partly, by CD8+ T cells which infiltrate the kidney. There is little evidence to implicate type I hypersensitivity. The simulta-

neous occurrence of MCD may be due to inhibition of the cycloxygenase pathway in the infiltrating T cells, leading to shunting of arachidonic acid through the leukotriene pathway. Treatment of this disease with steroids is probably unnecessary and cessation of the NSAID is all that is required. The syndrome may recur with further NSAID usage and these drugs should be avoided in such patients.

Systemic disease affecting the kidney

Diabetes mellitus

Diabetes is one of the most common systemic diseases leading to glomerular disease. There is, however, nothing to suggest that immunological mechanisms contribute to the lesions within the kidney. Rather, they appear to be the consequence of abnormal glucose metabolism.

Incidence

Only 25% of insulin-dependent diabetics will ever develop overt nephropathy; the greatest risk occurs in the second decade following diagnosis. The frequency is lower in non-insulin-dependent diabetics, but may be as high as 50% after 20 years in some racial groups.

Pathology

The histological findings are those of a diffuse increase in thickness of the GBM and increased volume of the mesangium due, largely, to additional matrix. This is known as diffuse diabetic glomerulosclerosis; because the GBM normally contains small amounts of IgG, the increase of basement membrane is usually accompanied by linear IgG accentuation (not to be confused with true linear staining) but this has no immunopathological significance. Formation of large acellular nodules in the mesangium follows organization of microaneurysms and leads to the Kimmelsteil–Wilson lesion of nodular diabetic glomerulosclerosis. In addition, accumulations of hyaline material (insudative lesions) beneath Bowman's capsule (a 'capsular drop') or over a capillary loop (a 'fibrin cap') may be seen but are not specific. Accumulation of hyaline material in both afferent and efferent arterioles is said to be specific for diabetic nephropathy.

Clinical features

Proteinuria, hypertension, and renal failure are the hallmarks of diabetic nephropathy. Almost all patients with juvenile-onset diabetes who have nephropathy will have retinopathy but the reverse does not hold.

Also, the relationship is much less strong for maturity-onset diabetes. Patients with diabetic nephropathy often have a number of other diabetic complications, especially vascular disease, autonomic neuropathy, and neuropathic ulcers.

Treatment

The first clinical finding is microalbuminuria in the range 20–200 μg/min. Patients who have microalbuminuria are at risk of progression to overt nephropathy, defined as proteinuria >0.5 g/day. Control of glycemia at this stage can correct microalbuminuria. Once overt nephropathy develops, good control has little impact on progression of the lesion but control of hypertension and moderate protein restriction can greatly slow progression to end-stage renal failure. There is evidence that angiotensin-converting enzyme (ACE) inhibitors, by reducing intraglomerular filtration pressure, reduce progression of renal disease both in those with microalbuminuria and established nephropathy. This effect is independent of their antihypertensive action.

Systemic lupus erythematosus

Renal disease occurs in up to 75% of patients with SLE, if they are followed for long enough. Together with cerebral vasculitis, it is the major determinant of survival. Many patients, however, will not require specific therapy for their renal lesion.

Pathology

Several typical histological findings may occur in the kidney in SLE. These include: (i) prominent glomerular cell proliferation and infiltration by leukocytes; (ii) immune deposits in the mesangial, subepithelial, and subendothelial areas, the latter giving rise to the characteristic wire-loop lesion; and (iii) presence of IgG, IgA, and IgM with C3, C4, and C1q in a single biopsy, the so-called 'full house' characteristic of SLE. The immunofluoroscence findings correspond to the general patterns described below but are always granular and may be accompanied by granular staining of tubular basement membranes, usually for IgG, C1q, and C3.

It is now usual practice to grade lupus nephritis according to the WHO classification, although the pattern at any stage of the disease represents only a 'snapshot' of the immune status of the patient and may change from time to time. The five grades are:

1. *Normal* (grade I).
2. *Mesangial glomerulonephritis* (grade II). This grade is subdivided into IIA where the mesangium contains immune deposits and IIB where there is

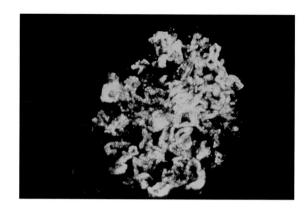

▌ **Fig. 22.20** Severe lupus glomerulonephritis (type 4) — granular staining of mesangia and capillary walls for IgG with confluent aggregates along capillary walls corresponding to large subdneothelial deposits (wire loops). There was similar staining for IgM, IgA, C1q, and C3 — a 'full house' pattern.

also mesangial cellular proliferation. Only IIB is usually associated with an abnormal urinary sediment.

3. *Focal proliferative glomerulonephritis* (grade III). This is defined as a lesion affecting <50% of glomeruli. Findings are those of immune deposits, cellular proliferation, and infiltration affecting glomeruli in a segmental manner and diffuse deposition of IgG, C3, and other immune reactants (Fig. 22.20). Areas of fibrinoid necrosis and crescent formation may occur. These patients generally have microscopic haematuria and proteinuria, sometimes of nephrotic range, but normal renal function.

4. *Diffuse proliferative glomerulonephritis* (grade IV). Findings are similar to those noted above but affect >50% of glomeruli and are usually more severe. This is the most common form of lupus nephritis and also the most serious. These patients often have renal impairment together with heavy proteinuria, haematuria, and hypertension. Serological findings are usually significant with high levels of anti-dsDNA antibodies and low complement levels.

5. *Membranous glomerulonephritis* (grade V). This is very similar to the idiopathic form except that the immune deposits may contain a 'full house' of reactants and there are often immune deposits in other sites apart from the subepithelium. These patients usually have proteinuria, often of nephrotic range. The prognosis for renal function is good, although occasional patients deteriorate.

Pathogenesis

The mechanisms leading to renal injury in lupus are probably similar to those involved in producing disease in other organ systems. High-affinity anti-dsDNA antibodies can be eluted from kidneys affected by SLE. To some extent the physicochemical properties of the antibodies and immune complexes may influence the lesion produced, with large anionic complexes becoming trapped in the mesangium and subendothelium and leading to cellular infiltration whereas smaller cationic complexes may cross the GBM and produce subepithelial deposits without cellular infiltration. The importance of antibodies which cross-react with antigenic determinants on the surface of renal cells or on basement membranes and the role of cellular mechanisms within the glomerulus remain ill-defined. Certainly, leucocyte infiltration within the interstitium of the kidney is likely to be a primary determinant of outcome but the mechanisms leading to its accumulation have not been well studied.

Several murine models of SLE have been described (Table 22.2) and have given some insight into the pathogenesis of the disease.

Clinical features

The presentation is extremely variable. Renal disease is often the first manifestation of SLE. Acute nephritic syndrome and the nephrotic syndrome are common, as is the finding of an abnormal urinary sediment in a patient known to have SLE.

Immunological tests

Autoantibody and complement assays have two major uses in the assessment of renal lupus — first, as a predictor of renal involvement and, secondly, in monitoring known renal lupus so as to guide immunosuppressive therapy. The major predictors of renal lupus are high titre anti-dsDNA antibodies and low complement levels. Antibodies to extractable nuclear antigens (ENAs) may help predict the risk of renal involvement. Antibodies against Sm are associated with severe renal disease, especially in Asians, while antibodies against Ro predict a lack of renal involvement.

Assessing the response of patients who have just commenced immunosuppressive treatment or predicting relapse in patients with controlled lupus on low-dose medication are the principal situations in which serological tests are used to help guide therapy. As a general rule, it is easier to suppress the autoantibody response than to modify the renal lesion. A fall in autoantibody levels must, therefore, not be accepted as conclusive evidence that the disease is under control. Regular checks of renal function and the urinary sediment are essential; occasionally, a repeat of the renal biopsy will provide useful information.

Relapse is common in patients with renal SLE who have either stopped immunosuppressive therapy or, more commonly, have reduced treatment to low maintenance doses. The clinical problem is to detect relapse before it has become so advanced that it is clinically obvious. While relapse can occur without increased antinuclear antibodies, an elevation in anti-dsDNA antibodies, particularly when coupled with low complement levels is highly predictive. However, the sensitivity of these tests in prediction of relapse varies in individual patients. It is very important to continue to monitor renal function, proteinuria, and the activity of the urinary sediment as well as autoantibody and complement levels in patients with renal lupus. One particular concern is the patient with inactive serology who has continuing renal disease. These patients almost invariably have an active urinary sediment but it can be difficult to distinguish an abnormal sediment due to past disease which has produced scarring and current disease activity. Renal biopsy is very helpful in this situation and can be performed every few years, if necessary.

Treatment

There is now little doubt that immunosuppressive therapy reduces the risk of renal failure in patients with severe lupus nephritis, although a placebo-controlled trial has never been performed. The question for the individual patient is what the risk of renal failure is and whether therapy will modify the outcome. These are difficult questions. In recent years, treatment has been guided by the combination of clinical and laboratory findings with renal biopsy appearances. Patients whose biopsy shows WHO grade IV disease require aggressive treatment, even more so if they have adverse clinical features such as nephrotic syndrome, hypertension, and renal failure. The usual regimen now is intravenous pulse cyclophosphamide therapy with high-dose steroids tapering to a maintenance dose. At the end of 6–12 months of this treatment, options are to continue pulse cyclophosphamide at longer intervals or to change to a steroid-sparing agent such as azathioprine. Treatment must be continued in the long-term with regular monitoring for relapses. Indications for therapy are less clear in WHO grade III, but many of these patients will receive treatment with steroids and another agent, especially if the number of glomeruli affected approaches 50% or they have adverse clinical features. Generally, patients in grades II and V are not treated for their renal lesion alone unless there are particular indications.

Prognosis

The outlook for WHO grade IV lesions is now very good, with over 80% maintaining renal function over 10 or more years. Properly managed patients with SLE should rarely progress to end-stage renal failure.

Transplantation

In those patients with SLE who come to dialysis, transplantation is not contraindicated. Lupus rarely recurs in transplanted kidneys for reasons which are obscure. One particular problem, however, is that the use of prolonged immunosuppressive therapy prior to development of end-stage renal failure makes it difficult to use marrow suppressants such as azathioprine after transplantation, probably due to reduced marrow reserve.

Henoch–Schönlein purpura (HSP)

This is often viewed as a systemic form of IgA nephropathy. It occurs in adults and children but is commonest in children under 6 years. The renal lesion is indistinguishable from that of IgA nephropathy. The major clinical difference is that the nephropathy of HSP has a greater tendency to relapse and remit whereas IgA nephropathy is often a chronic, 'smouldering' disease. This distinction is not, however, absolute. Episodes of rapidly progressive glomerulonephritis which may culminate in end-stage renal failure are commoner in HSP than in IgA nephropathy. Treatment of these episodes is controversial, but the usual range of therapies used for rapidly progressive glomerulonephritis have been advocated with, as yet, no consensus.

Haemolytic uraemic syndrome (HUS) and thrombotic thrombocytopenic purpura (TTP)

These related diseases comprise microangiopathic haemolytic anemia, thrombocytopenia, purpura, and varying degrees of renal failure. In TTP, fever and neurological manifestations also occur. Although many cases are idiopathic, HUS in children has been associated with bloody diarrhoea due to an *Escherichia coli* producing verocytotoxin. Cases in adults may be associated with malignancy (especially in those undergoing chemotherapy), lupus anticoagulant, pregnancy and the oral contraceptive, and the immunosuppressive drugs cyclosporin and FK-506.

Pathology

Arterioles and glomerular capillaries are principally affected. Intraluminal platelet thrombi are characteristic of TTP whereas additional subintimal fibrin deposition and intimal proliferation (thrombotic angiopathy) are typical of HUS, although there is probably considerable overlap between the conditions.

Pathogenesis

There are three major theories concerning the origin of these disorders.

1. Increased levels of a platelet aggregator. Candidate molecules include von Willebrand factor (vWF) which occurs in this disease as multimers of large size, and a cysteine protease, calpain, which may activate vWF enzymatically.

2. Reduced levels of a platelet aggregation inhibitor.

3. Endothelial cell injury and activation.

Treatment

The rationale of current therapy is to attempt to remove platelet aggregators and to replace them with inhibitors of platelet aggregation. In adults, it is now usual to advocate plasma exchange with a replacement solution of fresh frozen plasma. Although there has been no placebo-controlled trial, it does appear that this has produced a substantial increase in survival when results are compared with historical controls. In children, the outcome of HUS is often good with supportive treatment alone, so that the indications for this treatment are not so strong. Some patients who have more chronic disease may respond to oral steroids instead of plasma exchange.

Scleroderma

The renal lesion of scleroderma renal crisis is similar to that seen in malignant hypertension, comprising intimal proliferation and fibrinoid necrosis of arteries and arterioles. Scleroderma, however, affects arcuate and interlobar blood vessels as well as smaller arteries and arterioles whereas only the latter are affected in malignant hypertension. The treatment of scleroderma renal crisis is well known, comprising increasing doses of ACE inhibitor to counteract the high levels of renin seen in this condition. A minority of patients with diffuse scleroderma will develop clinically significant renal scleroderma, usually within the first 5 years after diagnosis. Patients who have anticentromere antibodies are usually spared.

Diseases due to a circulating paraprotein

Essential mixed cryoglobulinaemia (EMC)

EMC produces a very distinctive renal lesion. These patients have circulating IgMκ rheumatoid factor autoantibodies which precipitate with polyclonal IgG in the cold. Renal disease is a relatively late manifestation, occurring about 5 years after the onset, and comprises three histological lesions within the glomerulus: (i) profound microphage infiltration; (ii) intraluminal thrombi, of cryoprecipitate; and (iii) a double contour of the GBM due to macrophage interposition beneath the endothelium. The overall appearance is that of a cellular MPGN and often is associated with vasculitis characterized by massive immune deposit. By electron microscopy, some deposits, especially in those patients with monoclonal paraproteins, have a microtubular substructure. Patients present in a variety of ways, including acute nephritic syndrome, nephrotic syndrome, and chronic renal failure. Optimal treatment is not well defined but steroids and cyclophosphamide are often used to control renal disease.

Diseases associated with myeloma

A number of renal lesions can be produced by myeloma. These include: myeloma kidney; hypercalcaemia; plasma cell infiltration of the kidney; radiocontrast-induced renal injury; cryoglobulinaemia; renal tubular dysfunction; disease associated with disproportionate production of light chains or, rarely, heavy chain amyloidosis.

Myeloma kidney

The typical appearance is of fractured proteinaceous casts in the tubules. There is often an interstitial infiltrate which may comprise some giant cells and granulomas in relation to areas of tubular disruption. These patients usually present with renal failure, often acutely following dehydration or administration of radiocontrast media. The outlook is very poor and the value of dialysis is often difficult to determine in the individual patient.

Disease due to free light or heavy chain

Three renal conditions result from unbalanced light or heavy chain production by a myeloma that may be clinically occult. They usually present with a combination of nephrotic syndrome and renal failure. The particular pattern of disease (i.e. amyloidosis or light chain disease) depends on the properties of the monoclonal light chain involved.

Amyloidosis is due to deposition of mainly λ light chains within the glomerulus. This produces irregular obliteration of capillary walls and lumina by amorphous, eosinophilic material that is congophilic and has an apple green appearance under polarized light. Electron microscopy shows non-branching amyloid fibrils that cannot be distinguished from AA amyloid. The deposits usually stain with anti-light chain antibodies but, if not, can be identified by their lack of staining for AA proteins.

Light chain disease is generally due to κ light chains which possess sufficient constant region to react well with these reagents. The deposits accumulate in basement membranes and are granular rather than fibrillar on electron microscopy. There is thickening of tubular and GBMs with a pattern resembling diabetic glomerulosclerosis in some patients and, sometimes, the deposition of amyloid-like material in vessels and elsewhere.

Patients with both patterns of light chain deposition often present with nephrotic syndrome and renal failure. Interestingly, patients who have one of these diseases do not usually develop myeloma kidney.

Heavy chain disease is very rare. Heavy chain antisera usually stain the deposits which can form fibrils or granular deposits depending on their physicochemical characteristics.

Treatment of all of these disorders is similar. Courses of melphalan and prednisolone identical to those used in treatment of myeloma (with the dose of melphalan adjusted according to renal function) can often preserve or improve renal function. Therapy should be designed to reduce levels of the paraprotein in serum to undetectable levels.

Fibrillary and microtubular glomerulonephritis

These disorders are characterized by the accumulation of fibrils of varying size within the glomeruli. The light microscopic features are variable and diagnosis is restricted to electron microscopic examination. Fibrils may be encountered in the glomeruli in several conditions including amyloidosis, cryoglobulinaemia, and some examples of lupus glomerulonephritis. In these two recently recognized conditions the fibrils are of different size and significance. Fibrillary glomerulonephritis is characterized by fibrils approximating 20 nm diameter and appearing to consist predominantly of IgG4. In contrast the fibrils in mictrotubular (immunotactoid) nephropathy are about 40 nm in diameter. Little is yet known about these conditions but evidence to date suggests that microtubular (immunotactoid) nephropathy has an underlying lymphoproliferative disorder in most cases, with a circulating paraprotein in some cases. Both conditions appear to have the capacity to cause progressive renal damage but information about prognosis and possible therapeutic strategies is so far fragmentory.

Further reading

A Report of the International Study of Kidney Disease in Children (1981). The primary nephrotic syndrome in children: identification of patients with minimal change nephrotic syndrome from initial response to prednisone. *Journal of Paediatrics*, **98**, 561–64.

Austin, H. A., III, Boumpas, D. T., Vaughan, E. M., and Balow, J. E. (1994). Predicting renal outcomes in severe lupus nephritis: contributions of clinical and histologic data. *Kidney International*, **45**, 544–50.

Boumpas, D. T., Austin, H. A., III, Vaughan, E. M., *et al.* (1992). Controlled trial of pulse methylprednisolone versus two regimens of pulse cyclophosphamide in severe lupus nephritis. *Lancet*, **340**, 741–45.

Cameron, J. S., Turner, D. R., Heaton, J., *et al.* (1983). Idiopathic mesangiocapillary glomerulonephritis. Comparison of types I and II in children and adults and long-term prognosis. *American Journal of Medicine*, **74**, 175–92.

Cameron, J. S. (1993). The long-term outcome of glomerular disease. In *Diseases of the kidney*, 5th edn, (edn, R. W. Schrier and C. W. Gottschalk), pp. 1895–958. Little, Brown and Co., Boston.

Couser, W. G. (1988). Rapidly progressive glomerulonephritis: classification, pathogenetic mechanisms, and therapy. *American Journal of Kidney Diseases*, **11**, 449–64.

Couser, W. G. (1993). Pathogenesis of glomerulonephritis. *Kidney International*, **44**, S19–26.

D'Amico, G. (1987). The commonest glomerulonephritis in the world: IgA nephropathy. *Quarterly Journal of Medicine*, **64**, 709–27.

D'Amico, G., Colasanti, G., Ferrario, F., and Sinico, R. A. (1989). Renal involvement in essential mixed cryoglobulinemia. *Kidney International*, **35**, 1004–14.

Floege, J., Eng, E., Young, B. A., *et al.* (1993). Infusion of platelet-derived growth factor or basic fibroblast growth factor induces selective mesangial cell proliferation and matrix accumulation in rats. *Journal of Clinical Investigation*, **92**, 2952–62.

Fogo, A., Qureshi, N., and Horn, R. G. (1993). Morphologic and clinical features of fibrillary glomerulonephritis versus immunotactoid glomerulopathy. *American Journal of Kidney Diseases*, **22**, 367–77.

Glotz, D. and Druet, P. (1992). Immune mechanisms of glomerular damage that affect the kidney. In *Oxford textbook of nephrology*, (ed. S. Cameron, A. M. Davison, J-P.

Grünfeld, D. Kerr, and E. Ritz), pp. 240–62. Oxford University Press.

Guasch, A., Deen, W. M., and Myers, B. D. (1993). Charge selectivity of the glomerular filtration barrier in healthy and nephrotic humans. *Journal of Clinical Investigation*, **92**, 2274–82.

Jennette, J. C. and Falk, R. J. (1994). The pathology of vasculitis involving the kidney. *American Journal of Kidney Diseases*, **24**, 130–41.

Johnson, R. J., Gretch, D. R., Yamabe, H., *et al.* (1993). Membranoproliferative glomerulonephritis associated with hepatitis C virus infection. *New England Journal of Medicine*, **328**, 465–70.

Kallenberg, C. G. M., Brouwer, E., Weening J. J., and Cohen Tervaert, J. W. (1994). Anti-neutrophil cytoplasmic antibodies: current diagnostic and pathophysiological potential. *Kidney International*, **46**, 1–15.

Kashgarian, M. (1994). Lupus nephritis: lessons from the path lab. *Kidney International*, **45**, 928–38.

Korbet, S. M., Schwartz, M. M., and Lewis, E. J. (1994). Primary focal segmental glomerulosclerosis: clinical course and response to therapy. *American Journal of Kidney Diseases*, **23**, 773–83.

Lewis, E. J., Hunsicker, L. G., Bain, R. P., and Rohde, R. D. (1993). The effect of angiotensin-converting enzyme inhibitor on diabetic nephropathy. *New England Journal of Medicine*, **329**, 1456–62.

Neilson, E. G. (1989). Pathogenesis and therapy of interstitial nephritis. *Kidney International*, **35**, 1257–70.

Nolasco, F., Cameron, J. S., Heywood, E. F., Hicks, J., Ogg, C., and Williams, G. D. (1986). Adult-onset minimal change nephrotic syndrome: a long-term follow-up. *Kidney International*, **29**, 1215–23.

Orlando, R. A., Kerjaschki, D., Kurihara, H., Biemesderfer, D., and Farquhar, M. G. (1992). gp330 associates with a 44-kDa protein in the rat kidney to form the Heymann nephritis antigenic complex. *Proceedings of the National Academy of Sciences, USA*, **89**, 6698–702.

Ruggenenti, P., Galbusera, M., Cornejo, R. P., Bellavita, P., and Remuzzi, G. (1993). Thrombotic thrombocytopenic purpura: evidence that infusion rather than removal of plasma induces remission of the disease. *American Journal of Kidney Diseases*, **21**, 314–18.

Sharma, K. and Ziyadeh, F. N. (1994). The emerging role of transforming growth factor-β in kidney diseases. *American Journal of Physiology*, **266**, F829–42.

Sissons, J. G. R., West, R. J., Fallows, J. *et al.* (1976). The complement abnormalities of lipodystrophy. *New England Journal of Medicine*, **294**, 461–5.

Turner, N., Mason, P. J., Brown, R., Fox, M., Povey, S., Rees, A., and Pusey, C. D. (1992). Molecular cloning of the Goodpasture antigen demonstrates it to be the alpha 3 chain of type IV collagen. *Journal of Clinical Investigation*, **89**, 592–601.

van Es, L. A. (1992). Pathogenesis of IgA nephropathy. *Kidney International*, **41**, 1720–29.

Wilson, C. B. (1991). The renal response to immunologic injury. In *The kidney*, 4th edn, (ed B. M. Brenner and F. C. Rector, Jr), pp. 1062–181. W. B. Saunders, Philadelphia,

23 Cardiovascular system

S. L. Wesselingh, M. LeMire and J. Finlay-Jones

Introduction

A common theme which emerges in the study of infectious agents in cardiovascular disease is that the antimicrobial immune response may not only lead to microbial clearance but also, if excessive or if induced in a way which breaks tolerance to self antigens, may lead to tissue destruction (acute or chronic), perhaps including autoimmunity. A second common theme is that of genetic diversity, both with respect to the infectious agents (not all strains leading to significant host tissue damage on infection) and to the host [the major histocompatibility complex (MHC) phenotype of the host being a determinant in the breaking of tolerance].

Rheumatic fever

Definition

A non-suppurative sequel to upper respiratory tract infection by group A streptococci (*Streptococcus pyogenes*), involving primarily the heart, joints, subcutaneous tissue, and central nervous system.

Introduction

Rheumatic fever has been of major interest for many years for it demonstrates very clearly the role of the immune system not only in clearance of a pathogen but also in the development of tissue damage. It did, however, take some time for the association between streptococcal infection and rheumatic fever to be identified. Chorea was first described by Sydenham in 1666, and the association between rheumatism and carditis recognized by Charles Wells in 1812. Specific myocardial lesions in the myocardium were noted in 1904 by Aschoff and in the 1930s it became accepted that rheumatic fever arose as a consequence of streptococcal upper respiratory tract infections. In the 1960s there was a rapid decline in the incidence of acute rheumatic fever (ARF) but in the 1980s there have been sporadic epidemics and a possible resurgence of the disease.

Epidemiology and environmental factors

The epidemiology of ARF is fascinating and still has not been completely clarified. A complete understanding will require not only an understanding of the aetiological agent but also of differential host susceptibility. It has been noted repeatedly that even in epidemics of group A streptococcus infection, rheumatic fever affects only a small proportion of infected persons. The attack rate varies from 0.9 to 3%. Familial aggregation of rheumatic fever has also been noted. These epidemiological studies have not only demonstrated the absolute need for prior infection with group A streptococcus, but have also demonstrated that only certain strains of group A streptococcus are capable of causing disease. They have also provided suggestions that host/genetic characteristics may be equally important with microbial factors in the pathogenesis of the disease. Recent molecular epidemiology studies have reinforced this possibility, with evidence for increased susceptibility in patients with certain human leucocyte antigen (HLA) types.

Crowding seems to be by far the most significant environmental risk factor with epidemics occurring in both crowded ghettos and army barracks.

The incidence is highest among children in the 6–15-year-old group, with no clear-cut sex association, although there is a female preponderance in cases of mitral stenosis and Sydenham's chorea, which are associated with ARF.

Although there has been a dramatic decline in the second half of the twentieth century in the number of cases of rheumatic fever seen in the developed world, it is important to recognize the global impact of this disease. Rheumatic fever and its consequences are still the major causes of cardiac-related morbidity and mortality in the developing world. Recent events suggest the possibility of resurgence of ARF in the USA. Beginning in early 1985, an epidemic of the disease occurred in Salt Lake City, Utah, and the surrounding area, and there were several other recent small epidemics of ARF in the USA. Interestingly, these have occurred in patients of middle class origin rather than in the poor crowded ghettos. Over this period of time there has also been an increase in other serious toxin-related streptoccocal infections.

Pathogenesis

It was previously thought that ARF occurs only after respiratory and not cutaneous group A streptococcal infection but it appears from recent studies among Australian Aborigines that cutaneous infections may be able to initiate ARF. It is, however, essential that infection occurs with rheumatogenic strains of specific M protein types. The interaction between group A streptococcus and the immune system is therefore of fundamental importance and it is thus critical to understand the important components of the bacteria.

The major components of the bacteria which are relevant to the pathogenesis of the disease are presented in Table 23.1.

Figure 23.1 summarizes the sequence of events which leads to the development of ARF starting with pharyngeal (or perhaps cutaneous) infection, development of an appropriate or inappropriate immune response and subsequent tissue damage. The reason for the development of an inappropriate response is not completely understood. The most widely accepted hypothesis concerning the pathogenesis of infection is that the disease results from an autoimmune response induced by the similarity of certain streptococcal antigens (such as the M protein, group A carbohydrate, and membrane of the streptococcal cell wall) to human tissue antigens. This is strain specific. The cell wall also contains muramyl peptide (peptidoglycans), which can be potent immunological adjuvants capable of amplifying the host antibody response. Figure 23.2 is a simplified diagram of the surface of the group A streptococcus, which highlights some possible initiators of an inappropriate immune response.

Heart-reactive antibodies that cross-react with streptococcal antigens have been documented as has deposition on heart tissue of immunoglobulin and complement component C3. However, the passive transfer of antiheart antibodies has no pathogenic effect, suggesting that T-cell-mediated immune responses may also be required. CD4+ T lymphocytes are found in affected cardiac tissue, (and catalase production may play a potent part in the production of damage) and they almost certainly play a critical role in the dysregulation of the host immune response and the generation of both antibody and cell-mediated tissue damage

Clinical features

There is usually a latent period of about 2–3 weeks between the onset of the streptococcal sore throat and the onset of ARF. There is no difference between the latency period for recurrent attacks compared with initial episodes.

Initially, ARF can present with *polyarthritis, carditis, subcutaneous nodules,* or *erythema marginatum,* or very rarely *chorea.* Approximately 75% of ARF

▮ **Table 23.1**   Components of *Streptococcus pyogenes* and the pathogenesis of acute rheumatic fever

Bacterial component	Role in pathogenesis
1. Cell wall	Contains epitopes which cross-react with components of cardiac myosin
2. Muramyl peptide (peptidoglycan)	Contains potent immunological adjuvants which may amplify host responses
3. Group A carbohydrate (basis for Lancefield classification)	Cross-reactivity with structural glycoprotein of heart valves
4. M protein (multiple different types)	May determine rheumatigenicity
5. Hyaluronate capsule	May induce autoantibody production
6. Extracellular products: haemolysins erythrogenic toxins deoxyribonucleases streptokinases	Responsible for haemolysis, erythema, breakdown of nucleoproteins, and conversion of plasminogen to plasmin
7. Lipoteichoic acid	Mediates adherence to epithelial cells

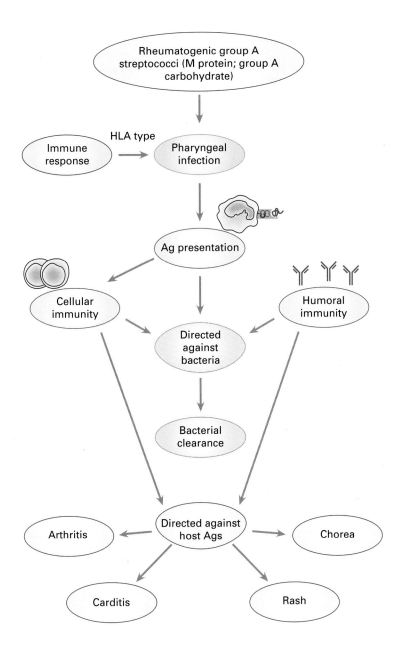

▌ **Fig. 23.1** Acute rheumatic fever (ARF): immunological and clinical events after streptococcal infection. This figure summarizes the sequence of events which leads to the development of ARF, starting with infection, the development of an appropriate or inappropriate immune response, and subsequent tissue damage. HLA, human leucocyte antigen; Ag, antigen.

patients present with polyarthritis. Carditis is the next most common presentation affecting 35–45% of patients. Eventually, chorea may develop in 15%, and subcutaneous nodules and erythema marginatum in fewer than 10%. Younger children are most likely to present with carditis and older children with arthritis.

1. *Carditis*. Cardiac involvement can present with symptoms of acute pericarditis or congestive heart

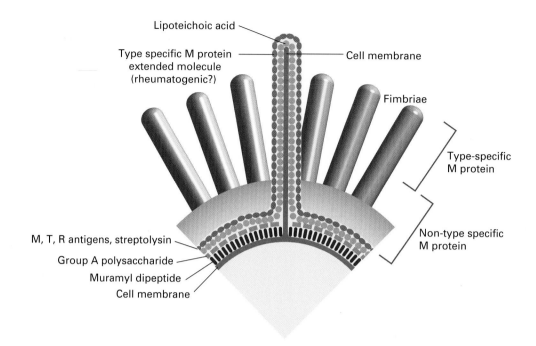

Lipoteichoic acid

Type specific M protein
extended molecule
(rheumatogenic?)

Cell membrane

Fimbriae

Type-specific
M protein

Non-type specific
M protein

M, T, R antigens, streptolysin

Group A polysaccharide

Muramyl dipeptide

Cell membrane

■ **Fig. 23.2** Cell wall associated structures of group A streptococci. Adapted from figure 204.1 of *Streptococcus pyogenes* by G. H. Stollerman. Ch. 204; In *Infectious Diseases* (ed. S. L. Gorbach, J. G. Bratlett, and N. R. Blacklow). Philadelphia. W. B. Saunders.

failure, or can be asymptomatic. The clinical signs of carditis include the development of new heart murmur(s), cardiac enlargement, congestive heart failure or pericardial friction rubs. The development of fatal heart failure during ARF is quite rare. In contrast, long-term changes involving the myocardium and endocardium are relatively common and may lead to chronic valvular disease and a significant risk of cardiac failure or bacterial endocarditis. Importantly, the carditis can be relatively asymptomatic and yet still give rise to valvular damage and other long-term consequences.

2. *Polyarthritis.* Patients can present with a range of symptoms from arthralgia to severe arthritis with warmth, swelling, redness, and tenderness. The arthritis is often migratory in nature, and in most cases subsides within 4 weeks of onset leaving no residual articular damage.

3. *Nodules.* Subcutaneous nodules are painless and are often very small. They are usually associated with carditis and present later in the illness, 2–3 weeks

after the first symptoms, and last about a week. Nodules can be found over bony surfaces and tendons such as those adjacent to elbows, knees, wrists or ankles, and over Achilles tendons.

4. *Sydenham's chorea.* Patients with Sydenham's chorea demonstrate emotional lability, and rapid, involuntary purposeless movements. The choreiform movements disappear during sleep. The period between the onset of chorea and the streptococcal pharyngitis can be up to 2–3 months, making diagnosis difficult. Also of interest is the fact that while it is seen in both male and female children, in adults it is seen in females only, and is worsened by pregnancy.

5. *Erythema marginatum.* This is an erythematous eruption that moves rapidly from place to place, and is characterized by an erythematous edge and clear centre.

6. *Minor manifestations.* These occur commonly in association with ARF, but are not diagnostic or specific for ARF. Most common are arthralgia and fever.

▍ **Table 23.2**   Features of acute rheumatic fever

Major	Carditis
	Polyarthritis
	Chorea
	Subcutaneous nodules
	Erythema marginatum
Minor	Fever
	Arthralgia
	Erythrocyte sedimentation rate elevated
	Previous rheumatic fever

Diagnosis

The diagnosis requires evidence of streptococcal infection and can be achieved by serology for antibodies to extracellular products of group A streptococcus (e.g. streptolysin O, DNase B, and hyaluronidase) *plus* the presence of either two of the major manifestations of disease (see Table 23.2), or one major and two minor manifestations.

Treatment and management

The primary aim of all therapy for ARF is only to treat the symptoms, as there is currently no treatment which affects the underlying process. The treatment is therefore aimed at pain control, fever reduction, and treatment of cardiac failure. Salicylates, non-steroidal anti-inflammatory drugs (NSAIDs), and if necessary corticosteroids are given for pain control and fever reduction. Carditis may require corticosteroids, bed rest, oxygen, and diuretics. Sedation and a quiet environment may be used for those with chorea. Reactivation of symptoms, or 'rebound', may occur especially after the cessation of corticosteroid therapy.

Outcome and prognosis

Patients who have had one attack of ARF are at increased risk of further attacks of the disease following subsequent streptococcal infections. The risk is highest within the first few years after the initial attack and then declines but continues into adult life. Increased risk of recurrence is associated with higher levels of the antistreptococcal antibody response and more advanced pathology at first occurrence. However, the most significant morbidity and mortality is not associated with recurrence of ARF but with the long-term sequelae of damaged heart valves and consequent development of cardiac failure and/or bacterial endocarditis. The majority of these patients ultimately require prosthetic valve insertion.

▍ **Table 23.3**   Secondary prophylaxis of ARF

Determinant	Duration of prophylaxis
If carditis present	10 years post-ARF or until age 25
If no carditis	5 years post-ARF or until 18 years

ARF, acute rheumatic fever.

Prevention

The most widely used regimen for the prevention of recurrence is a single monthly injection of 1.2 million units of penicillin G benzathine. This regimen has been extremely effective, but compliance may be limited due to the discomfort of the injection.

Oral regimens include penicillin V 250 mg twice daily or sulphadiazine 1 g daily, or if penicillin allergy exists, erythromycin 250 mg twice daily.

The duration of secondary prophylaxis is debated and some physicians think it should be life-long. Recent recommendations are presented in Table 23.3. In addition to the prevention of recurrences of ARF, patients with residual rheumatic valvular disease must be protected from bacterial endocarditis. This is discussed in the section on bacterial endocarditis (below).

Myocarditis

Definition

Inflammation of the heart muscle due to infectious or non-infectious causes.

Introduction

The major interest in myocarditis stems from the hypothesis that idiopathic-dilated cardiomyopathy most often results from an acute viral myocarditis. This may be either due to persistent cardiac viral infection or secondary to an autoimmune response to a recent viral infection. The current management of myocarditis and idiopathic dilated cardiomyopathy is presently empirical at best. It is therefore likely that an increased understanding of the basic immunopathogenesis of myocarditis and idiopathic dilated cardiomyopathy will have a major impact on treatment of virus or immune-mediated heart disease.

Environmental factors

Clinical, serological, histological, and molecular data all suggest that viruses are the most important agents in the development of myocarditis. Myocarditis can occur following measles, mumps, and influenza. However, most investigators have concentrated on the group B coxsackievirus. These are the most common viruses associated with myocarditis and have been demonstrated in inflamed cardiac tissue by *in situ* hybridization and by reverse transcriptase–polymerase chain reaction (RT–PCR) of mRNA extracted from homogenized tissue.

Utilizing PCR techniques and employing a combination of primers and probes that identify a wide range of enteroviruses, viral sequences have been demonstrated not only in acute myocarditis and end-stage idiopathic dilated cardiomyopathy, but also in other cardiac conditions, as well as in normal heart. This suggests the possibility that both normal and abnormal heart may represent a site of latent or low-grade infection, but that the development of significant myocardi-

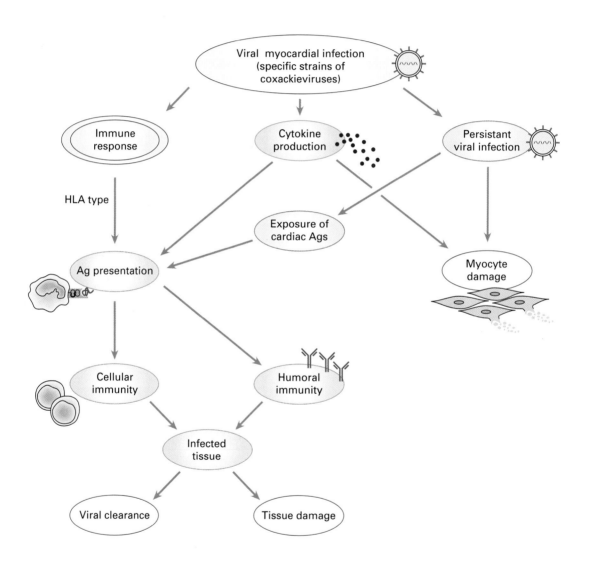

▮ **Fig. 23.3** Myocarditis: immunological and clinical events after viral infection. This indicates the likely scenario in the development of myocarditis; highlighted are the important roles of viral strain and cytokine production in the development of immune mediated tissue damage, and the possible role of viral persistence. HLA, human leucocyte antigen; Ag, antigen.

tis requires both the presence of the virus and certain host characteristics. It is also possible that the pathogenesis of infection has similarities to ARF, as described above, in that specific viral subtypes are required to elicit an immune response typical of myocarditis.

Immunopathogenesis

Most information regarding the immunopathogenesis of myocarditis has come from models utilizing coxsackievirus B3 (CVB3) or encephalomyocarditis virus infection of mice.

The following are the major findings of these studies:

1. Susceptibility to myocarditis is dependent on the age, sex, and genetic background of the host, and the myocarditic nature of the virus strain. In addition ethanol, forced exercise, and increased left ventricular pressure and drug therapies such as corticosteroids that are likely to increase viral replication have all been shown to increase the severity of myocarditis.

2. Increased expression of MHC antigens during acute viral infection may play a part in the initiation of clones of cytolytic T cells that recognize and lyse both infected and uninfected myocytes.

3. Again reminiscent of the immunopathogenesis of ARF, results from studies in mouse models have suggested that there may be development of autoreactive antibodies during the acute viral infection which then play a part in the development of chronic myocarditis.

4. The role of cytokines in the development of myocarditis is of great interest. Recent studies showed that mouse strains genetically resistant to CVB3 myocarditis will develop the disease when given either tumour necrosis factor (TNF) or interleukin-1 during the acute infection. In some models, anti-TNF antibody treatment significantly reduced the severity of the inflammation. Interestingly, early treatment with nitric oxide inhibitors significantly increased the morbidity and mortality.

Clinical presentation and diagnosis

Patients presenting with a history of fever, malaise, arthralgia, and upper respiratory tract infections in association with evidence of any cardiac disease such as arrhythmias (supraventricular tachycardia and ventricular extrasystoles), chest pain, or cardiac failure, should be carefully evaluated for further evidence of myocarditis. If definitive evidence of myocarditis is present then evidence of viral infection should be sought using:

(1) serology;

(2) culture of throat and faecal specimens; and, if clinically indicated

(3) endomyocardial biopsy for (i) histology, (ii) viral culture, (iii) *in situ* hybridization or PCR for detection of viral nucleic acid.

Treatment and management

The mainstay of therapy is the appropriate treatment of the cardiac failure and bed rest. Corticosteroids given early in the course of the disease have been associated with poor outcome in both humans and mice, presumably because of increased viral replication. Corticosteroids are therefore contraindicated and especially so if there is any evidence of an antecedent viral infection. Most immunosuppressant trials have been uncontrolled and have had varied results. However, a recent large controlled trial demonstrated no benefit from immunosuppressants suggesting that specific therapy will rely on the development of appropriate antivirals.

Outcome and prognosis

The outcome of acute viral myocarditis is quite variable, with most resolving spontaneously, but a small proportion progress to severe cardiomyopathy and cardiac failure. If, however, as is suggested by some authors, most idiopathic cardiomyopathy is the end-stage of viral myocarditis, the frequency and prognosis may be quite different than was previously thought.

Pericarditis

Definition

Inflammation of the pericardium due to infectious or non-infectious causes.

Introduction

Pericarditis is a relatively common reason for presentation to hospital. It often mimics myocardial ischaemia and can be associated with a number of common viral conditions. In addition, it can be due to pyogenic, tuberculous, or mycotic infections or be the manifestation of systemic diseases.

∎ **Table 23.4**   Common causes of pericarditis

Infectious	Viral	Coxsackievirus
		Influenza virus
		Echovirus type 8
		Mumps virus
	Pyogenic bacterial	*Staphylococcus aureus*
		Streptococcus pneumoniae
		Haemophilus influenzae
	Mycobacterial	*Mycobacterium tuberculosis*
	Fungal	*Candida albicans*
		Aspergillus
		Cryptococcus neoformans
Non-infectious	Associated with non-immune systemic illness	Myocardial infarction
		Uraemia
		Trauma
		Radiation
		Malignancy
	Associated with immune-mediated disease	Rheumatic fever
		Collagen vascular disease
		Rheumatoid arthritis
		Systemic lupus erythematosus
		Scleroderma
		Drug induced
		Post-cardiac injury syndrome
		Dresslers syndrome
		Postpericardiotomy
		Post trauma

Pathogenesis

The pathogenesis of the infectious causes of pericarditis essentially involves the introduction of a virulent pathogen into the pericardial space. Viruses spread to the pericardium haematogenously, and pericardial inflammation ensues. Myocarditis may also develop. A number of patients develop recurrent 'viral pericarditis'. This is thought not to be due to persistent viral infection but to autoimmune phenomena as described below for post-cardiac injury syndrome.

Pyogenic pericarditis can be secondary to:

(1) local spread from a pulmonary infection;

(2) endocarditis;

(3) a postsurgical focus;

(4) bacteraemia.

Similarly, tuberculous pericarditis can develop from a local spread or by lymphatic or haematogenous spread.

The pathogenesis of post-cardiac injury syndrome, drug-induced pericarditis and pericarditis associated with immune-mediated illness probably involves similar mechanisms to those involved in the pathogenesis of ARF, with the generation of autoimmunity directed against cardiac antigens exposed by the trauma, surgery, or infarction of tissue. The local production of cytokines both by intrinsic cardiac cells and by systemic cellular infiltrating cells may also be involved in the upregulation of MHC antigens and the generation of an environment in which autoantigens can be successfully presented, and cellular and humoral immunity directed against cardiac antigens can be generated. Some authors have suggested an alternative hypothesis involving latent viruses rather than immune responses in the production of long-term damage.

The pathogenesis of pericarditis involves the development of inflammation within a confined space, often with development of an effusion. If this occurs rapidly or if the effusion is very large, it may precipitate obstruction to the inflow of blood to the ventricles resulting in cardiac tamponade which may be fatal if not quickly treated.

Clinical features

Manifestations of pericarditis comprise:

(1) retrosternal chest pain; which is increased by deep inspiration(s) and lying down and which radiates to both arms and shoulders;

(2) prodromal flu-like illness;

(3) fever;

(4) shortness of breath.

On examination the following signs:

(1) friction rub high-pitched scratching and grating, transitory;

(2) tamponade: pulsus paradoxus greater than 10 mmHg, with a prominent x descent with loss of y descent

Diagnosis/Laboratory investigations

(1) based on a history of typical symptoms;

(2) ECG; ST segment elevation and later T wave inversion which may be persistent;

(3) chest X-ray, computerized tomography, magnetic resonance imaging;

(4) echocardiography;

(5) viral isolation from throat and stool specimens;

(6) pericardiocentesis for viral culture, PCR, etc.

Treatment and management

Treatment of pyogenic, fungal, and mycobacterial pericarditis requires urgent therapy with appropriate antimicrobials and pericardial drainage via pericardiostomy. These conditions, however, often require surgical intervention, with decortication and resection. The treatment of viral pericarditis is (at this point in time) currently symptomatic. However, as with myocarditis, steroids are contraindicated in the acute phase. Patients are also advised to avoid alcohol and excessive exercise.

Pericarditis-associated non-infectious systemic disease requires optimal treatment of the systemic illness.

Outcome and prognosis

The outcome of viral pericarditis is generally good, but is commonly associated with recurrence. A small number of patients are left with permanent cardiac defects. Pyogenic, fungal, and mycobacterial pericarditis each have significant morbidity and mortality and therefore require prompt and appropriate therapy.

Infective endocarditis

Definition

Infective endocarditis is an infection involving the endocardial lining of the heart, usually the valvular endocardium, with a range of associated microorganisms. The term is preferable to bacterial endocarditis because fungi, rickettsiae, and chlamydiae are also implicated. The terms acute and subacute are also used to describe, respectively, the fulminant course of staphylococcal endocarditis with death in less than 6 weeks or the more prolonged course, often of several months, in streptococcal endocarditis.

Introduction

Until the advent of modern antimicrobial therapy in the mid-twentieth century endocarditis was almost always fatal. With current treatment mortality has fallen to approximately 10–20%.

Epidemiology

The incidence of infective endocarditis is estimated at two to four per 100 000 person years or about 1 per 1000 hospital admissions in the USA. Considerable change in patient characteristics has occurred over the last 30 years. Patients are older, as rheumatic fever has become less frequent. As rheumatic valvular disease has diminished other cardiac risk factors including prosthetic valves, congenital heart disease and mitral valve prolapse have assumed greater importance. Noncardiac risk factors such as intravenous drug abuse and intravascular catheters have also become more common.

Causative organisms

Changes have occurred over the last few decades in the organisms recognized as causes of infective endocarditis (see Table 23.5). Viridans streptococci, normal flora of the pharynx, remain the commonest causative organism accounting for half to two-thirds of cases. However, *Staphylococcus aureus* now causes approximately one-quarter of cases and is particularly common in intravenous drug users. Coagulase-nega-

❚ **Table 23.5**   Aetiology of infective endocarditis*

Organism	Approximate incidence
Viridans streptococci	50–70%
Enterococci	5–10%
Staphylococcus aureus	25%
S. epidermidis	2–5% but only seen in prosthetic valves (25% of prosthetic valves endocarditis are positive for *S. epidermis*)
HACEK† organisms; other Gram negative bacilli; miscellaneous, e.g. fungi rare pathogens	5–10%
Culture negative	5–10%

*Figures refer to patients without a history of intravenous drug use.
†HACEK = *Haemophilus* spp., *Actinobacillus actinomycetemcomitans*, *Cardiobacterium hominis*, *Eikenella* spp., and *Kingella kingae*.

tive staphylococci, such as *Staphylococcus epidermidis*, are the most common causes of early prosthetic valve endocarditis. About 5–10% of cases are attributable to enterococci, and a similar number to uncommon pathogens such as Gram-negative bacilli, *Legionella*, Chlamydiae, Rickettsiae, and fungi. Some uncommon pathogens do not grow in blood culture media and present as 'culture negative' endocarditis.

Pathogenesis

In the majority of cases there is a predisposing cardiac lesion or prosthesis. It is thought that valvular heart disease may initially lead to non-bacterial thrombotic endocarditis. Turbulent flow distal to a valve orifice may cause denudation of the valvular (and/or mural) endocardium. Adherence of platelets and fibrin deposition may result and a non-infected vegetation is formed.

Subsequent bacteraemia can lead to colonization of the vegetation in which organisms are protected from normal phagocytic defences by overlying fibrin and platelets.

Bacteraemia has a varied aetiology. Poor dental hygiene with gingival disease is associated with relatively frequent and usually transient episodes of bacteraemia. It is probably peridontal disease rather than dental procedures which causes bacteraemia and endocarditis. Other aetiologies of bacteraemia include intravenous drug use, hospital use of intravascular devices and some procedures involving the urinary or gastrointestinal tracts.

Infective endocarditis manifests via a variety of pathogenic mechanisms in the heart and other organs. Cardiac involvement with virulent organisms such as *S. aureus* may lead to rapid valve destruction and myocardial abscess formation. Pyogenic infection is found in distant sites as a consequence of septic emboli. In contrast, less virulent organisms such as viridans streptococci are slower to produce valve damage and systemic manifestations of infection. Streptococcal endocarditis may manifest with immune-complex-mediated disease. The presence of very large quantities of antigen in the intravascular space elicits a vigorous antibody response. Immune complexes deposit in skin, joints, glomeruli, and are phagocytosed in the spleen. A vasculitis sometimes occurs as a result and renal changes range from mild proteinuria or haematuria to rapidly progressive (crescentic) glomerulonephritis.

Clinical features and diagnosis

The clinical presentation of infective endocarditis is extremely varied. Examples include fever of unknown origin, septicaemia, and major embolic events. Constitutional symptoms include fever, sweats, anorexia, malaise, and weight loss. These may have a gradual onset (e.g. streptococcal endocarditis) or present acutely (*S. aureus* endocarditis). However, these changes are non-specific and the diagnosis is supported by cardiac or other organ manifestations.

1. *Heart.* Most cases will present with a murmur on auscultation. However, some congenital lesions and right-sided endocarditis are exceptions. The finding of a new regurgitant murmur is of particular value in the diagnosis of endocarditis. The mitral valve alone is most frequently involved, followed by the aortic valve alone. Next most frequent is the involvement of both mitral and aortic valves, then tricuspid valve (and then congenital lesions). Infection of prosthetic valves is encountered with increasing frequency. Congestive cardiac failure is the most important cardiac complication and usually results from valve destruction. Less commonly arrhythmia, conduction disturbance, and myocardial abscess may occur.

2. *Skin.* Peripheral stigmata of endocarditis are seen in the skin, nails, and eyes. Petechiae may be seen in the extremities and conjunctivae and are associated with emboli or vasculitis. Splinter haemorrhages are found in the nail beds but are also associated with trauma. Clubbing is found in patients presenting relatively late. *Janeway lesions* are painless haemorrhagic lesions of the palms and soles and result from septic emboli. *Osler's nodes* are caused by immune complexes and are painful nodules found in the finger or toe pads.

3. *Eyes.* Signs in the eyes include conjunctival petechiae and *Roth spots*, which are pale-centred haemorrhagic areas seen on fundoscopy.

4. *Kidney.* There is frequently involvement of the kidneys with glomerulonephritis being the most common lesion. Other renal lesions include embolism, abscess, and acute tubular necrosis due to severe sepsis.

5. *Other.* Virtually any vascular organ may be involved in endocarditis. Splenomegaly is common in subacute presentations. Arthritis may be associated with immune complex deposition. Cerebral infarction, abscess or haemorrhage from mycotic aneurysm rupture are not common but dreaded consequences of endocarditis. Infarction and abscess also occur in the spleen, kidneys, and lungs (in cases of right-sided endocarditis).

Laboratory findings

Non-specific laboratory findings in endocarditis include normocytic anaemia, leucocytosis, and elevated erythrocyte sedimentation rate and C-reactive protein. Immunological markers include a positive rheumatoid factor; elevated immunoglobulins; hypocomplementaemia, and the presence of immune complexes. Protein, blood, and red cell casts may be present in the urine.

The blood culture is the most important laboratory test in the diagnosis of infective endocarditis. (Persistently positive blood cultures, usually all being positive, are typically seen). A series of blood cultures is taken over a 24 h period and these are usually positive in typical cases. Culture-negative endocarditis may be due to a fastidious or non-bacterial organism or partially treated endocarditis. In cases where endocarditis is suspected, a minimum of three sets of blood cultures in the first 24 h is recommended. Serology is recommended for unusual causes such as chlamydia, *Legionella*, and *Coxiella burnetii* if cultures are negative but suspicion is strong.

Echocardiography has become a valuable tool in the diagnosis of endocarditis and assessment of cardiac complications. The sensitivity of transoesophageal

∎ **Table 23.6** Duke University Criteria (abridged)

Outcome	Criteria	Findings
Definite infective endocarditis	Pathological criteria Clinical criteria	Culture and/or histologically proven from surgical or autopsy specimens. Two of the following major criteria: (1) bacteraemia with a 'typical'[a] organism or persistent bacteraemia with an organism consistent with endocarditis,[b] (2) echocardiographically demonstrated vegetation, abscess, or new partial dehiscence of a prosthetic valve; (3) auscultatory finding of a new regurgitant murmur; Or One major and three of the following minor criteria: (1) predisposition: predisposing heart condition or intravenous drug use; (2) fever: 38.0°C (100.4°F); (3) vascular phenomena: major arterial emboli, septic pulmonary infarcts, mycotic aneurysm, intracranial haemorrhage, conjunctival hemorrhages, Janeway lesions; (4) immunological phenomena: glomerulonephritis, Osler's nodes, Roth spots, rheumatoid factor (5) microbiological evidence: positive blood culture but not meeting major criterion as noted previously *or* serological evidence of active infection with organism consistent with infective endocarditis (6) echocardiogram: consistent with infective endocarditis but not meeting major criterion as noted previously. Or Five minor criteria
Possible infective endocarditis		Findings are consistent with endocarditis but fall short of 'definite'.
Rejected		Firm alternative diagnosis established; *or* Resolution of manifestations of endocarditis within 4 days of commencing antibiotic therapy; *or* No pathological evidence of endocarditis at surgery or autopsy after >4 days of antibiotic therapy.

[a] Two separate blood cultures positive with either viridans streptococci, *Streptococcus bovis*, HACEK organisms (HACEK = *Haemophilus* spp., *Actinobacillus actinomycetemcomitans*, *Cardiobacterium hominis*, *Eikenella* spp., and *Kingella kingae*), community-acquired *Staphylococcus aureus* or enterococcus without another definable primary focus.
[b] Three of three or three of four separate blood cultures positive with an organism consistent with infective endocarditis, or positive cultures taken more than 12 h apart.

echocardiography is 85–90%, and is superior to transthoracic echocardiography (50–60%) for vegetations. In addition, abscess and prosthetic valve dehiscence are better seen. However, the advantage is less clear with imaging of the right-sided valves.

Diagnostic criteria

Despite the fact that infective endocarditis is an uncommon problem, it is a frequently considered diagnosis particularly in cases of fever of unknown origin. The difficulty in confirming the diagnosis has led to the development of clinical criteria such as those of the Duke University Medical Center (see Table 23.6).

Treatment and outcome

High doses of a bactericidal antibiotic given intravenously usually for 4 weeks are recommended because of the difficulty in penetrating to the site of infection and also because of the altered metabolic state of bacteria within vegetations. A β-lactam antibiotic (penicillin for streptococci and flucloxacillin for most staphylococci) is usually employed with addition of an aminoglycoside for 5–14 days because of some synergistic activity and earlier clearance of bacteraemia. Longer courses (6 weeks) may be required for more resistant organisms such as enterococci and shorter course therapy (2 weeks) is adequate for uncomplicated highly sensitive streptococci and *S. aureus* right-sided endocarditis. Recent trials of domicilary once-daily ceftriaxone in streptococcal endocarditis suggest this is a reasonable alternative in uncomplicated cases of streptococcal endocarditis, although extensive experience is lacking.

Surgery is required for cases in which antimicrobial therapy is inadequate, e.g. fungal endocarditis, when valvular dysfunction leads to congestive cardiac failure or impaired valve opening, when abscess or prosthetic valve dehiscence occurs and in the event of multiple embolic episodes. Infection of a prosthetic valve usually requires surgical replacement of the valve and mortality is about 50%.

Prognosis is best for highly sensitive (viridans) streptococcal endocarditis with mortality approximately 10%. Relapse is more common with more resistant organisms such as enterococci. *Staphylococcus aureus* in intravenous drug abusers has a relatively good outcome, 90% cure, but in left-sided endocarditis a mortality rate of approximately one-third is seen.

Further reading

Bayer, A. S. (1993). Infective endocarditis (review article). *Clinical Infectious Diseases*, **17**, 313–22.

Bayer, A. S., *et al.* (1994). Evaluation of new clinical criteria for the diagnosis of infective endocarditis. *American Journal of Medicine*, **96**, 211–19.

Durack, D. T., Bright, D. K., and Lukes, A. S. (1994). Duke Endocarditis Service. New criteria for diagnosis of infective endocarditis: utilisation of specific echocardiographic findings. *American Journal of Medicine*, **96**, 200–9.

Fowler, V. G. and Durack, D. T. (1994). Infective endocarditis. *Current Opinion in Cardiology*, **9**, 389–400.

Korzeniowski, O. M. and Kaye, D. (1992). Endocarditis. In *Infectious diseases*, (ed. S. L. Gorbach, J. G. Bartlett, and N. R. Blacklow), pp. 548–57. W. B. Saunders, Philadelphia.

Scheld, W. M. and Sande, M. A. (1990). Endocarditis and intravascular Infections. In *Principles and practice of infectious disease*, 3rd edn (ed. G. L., Mandell, R. G. Douglas, and J. E. Bennett), pp. 670–706. Churchill Livingstone, New York.

Mason, J. W. (1995). A clinical trial of immunosuppressive therapy for myocarditis. *New England Journal of Medicine*, **333**, 269–75.

Section IV

Systemic immunological disease

24 Systemic lupus erythematosus

N. Manolios and L. Schrieber

Definition

Systemic lupus erythematosus (SLE) or lupus is a clinical syndrome characterized by breakdown in tolerance, production of autoantibodies and inflammation in multiple organs leading to a wide range of clinical manifestations. The cause remains unknown, although both genetic and environmental factors appear to play an important part in the induction and perpetuation of the disease.

Introduction

The incidence and prevalence of SLE varies according to ethnic background, being more prevalent in black Americans and Chinese compared with Caucasians. The commonest age of disease onset is between 20 and 40 years, with females affected more frequently than males (9:1). Age-specific prevalence rates in the USA are one in 250 for black females and one in 1000 for white females aged 15–64 years.

The clinical manifestations are protean ranging from mild skin rashes and arthralgia to life-threatening renal failure. Lupus is a heterogeneous disorder resulting in a variety of clinical syndromes. These include idiopathic SLE, drug-related lupus, phospholipid antibody syndrome, subacute cutaneous lupus erythematosus, discoid lupus, and neonatal lupus erythematosus (NLE). The range of therapies used to treat patients with SLE is diverse and includes non-steroidal anti-inflammatory drugs (NSAIDs), antimalarials, corticosteroids, and immunosuppressive drugs. Treatment depends on the severity and extent of organ system involvement. The prognosis of SLE has improved dramatically over the past two decades. It is now considered a chronic rather than an acute fatal disease.

Genetics

It has been proposed that for any disorder to be considered genetic in origin there should be supporting data from twin studies, evidence of familial aggregation, studies of ethnicity, and tissue typing as well as experimental models of the disease. In SLE, supporting data for each of these parameters make the case for genetic predisposition compelling.

1. *Twin studies*. The concordance rate for SLE in monozygotic twins is 24–69%. The concordance rate for dizygotic twins ranges from 5 to 15%, similar to that for other first-degree relatives. This marked discordance for autoimmunity has been attributed to differences in environmental exposure, although X-chromosome inactivation and genetic imprinting are also potential biological sources of variation between monozygotic twins.

2. *Familial aggregation*. In American blacks with disease onset less than 30 years of age, familial aggregation is particularly marked. In these studies, 10% of probands have an affected relative. The commonest matches are sister–sister and mother–daughter — not surprising in a disorder with a striking female predominance.

3. *Ethnicity*. Although SLE occurs in all populations the prevalence rate varies in different ethnic groups. There is an over-representation of American blacks compared with whites, even after adjustment for socio-economic class. African blacks do not have the same high prevalence of SLE observed in American blacks, suggesting an environmental factor superimposed on their genetic background. Chinese have been reported to have a higher prevalence of SLE and to exhibit disease of greater severity than Caucasians.

4. *Tissue typing*. In Caucasians, SLE is associated with human leucocyte B8 DR3/DR2 antigens (HLA) and with the C4AQO allele. The strong

linkage disequilibrium among different genes in the major histocompatibility complex (MHC) makes it difficult to assess which genes are primarily responsible for susceptibility to SLE. Some groups have proposed that the C4AQO alleles are the critical determinants, while others have argued that DR/DQ MHC class II molecules are the most important. In Japanese, the C4AQO gene is not associated with lupus and the HLA-DR2 haplotype is most frequently identified as the primary risk factor. This suggests that immune complex clearance by C4AQO may play only a modest part in disease pathogenesis and is not the decisive factor increasing SLE susceptibility. Recently, both the haplotypes B7/DR2 and B8/DR3 have been shown to be MHC-linked susceptibility genes for Caucasians with SLE. The DQB1AZH (now called DQB1*0502) allele confers risk for the development of nephritis, whereas HLA-DR4 is negatively associated with nephritis. Inherent complement deficiencies (C2, C4) also predispose to SLE.

Class II MHC (-DR, -DQ) gene associations with SLE may be better explained by association with autoantibody subsets. For example, anti-SS-A/Ro antibodies are found in association with HLA-DR2 and HLA-DR3, and more closely with DQ genes (DQw2.1).

Possible gene candidates outside of the HLA locus involved in disease susceptibility include those on the X-chromosome, the T-cell antigen receptor, and immunoglobulin genes. The strongest evidence implicating X-linked loci is the high female to male ratio. In addition, genes known to affect immune regulation/inflammation mapped to the X-chromosome include the properdin gene, a tyrosine kinase involved in B-cell differentiation, the ligand for CD40 which plays a central part in T–B-cell interaction, and the gene for tissue inhibitor of metalloproteinases.

Experimental models

There are a number of inbred strains of mice that spontaneously develop an SLE-like syndrome. They share many characteristics with their human counterpart and exhibit strong genetic predisposition. While most strains have female predominant disease (NZB/NZW, MRL-lpr/lpr), the BXSB strain is unusual in that it is the male members of the strain that bear the brunt of clinical disease expression.

Transgenic mouse models have provided invaluable insights into the mechanisms of tolerance, immunopathogenesis and treatment of autoimmune disease. Transgenic mice expressing viral (SV40 T antigen, lymphocytic choriomeningitis virus, influenza virus haemagglutinin), cytokines [interferon (IFN) γ, tumour necrosis factor, interleukin (IL) 2], immunoglobulin, T-cell receptor, proto-oncogenes, and MHC transgenes have been established. They have provided invaluable information on the pathogenetic mechanisms of autoimmunity. The nature, amount, timing of antigen presentation and state of maturation of the immune system may influence tolerance in a multistep manner.

Environmental factors

Genetic factors in combination with environmental agent(s) have been implicated in the induction and perpetuation of SLE. Agents known to affect disease include ultraviolet radiation which may exacerbate a lupus flare, and a number of drugs which may induce drug-related lupus. Other possible factors include infectious agents (retroviruses, superantigens) and foods containing psoralens (celery, parsley) that could potentially increase photosensitivity. L-canavanine which is structurally related to hydrazine (which is implicated in drug-related lupus), is found in alfalfa seeds, sprouts, and legumes. Severe emotional and physical stress can also induce disease flares. Other less well studied factors include hair dyes, exposure to vinyl chloride and implantation of silicone polymers.

Microbes

While a microbial aetiology for autoimmune diseases remains a popular theory supportive evidence in SLE is limited. Earlier studies described electron dense, presumed viral, particles within renal biopsies of SLE patients. This has not been confirmed. Patients with SLE frequently have high titres of antibodies to a variety of microbes. This is now thought to occur as a result of an anamnestic response to exogenous as well as endogenous antigens, rather than selective antigenic drive. In inbred SLE mice vertical transmission of type C viruses has been described. Nevertheless, in cross-breeding studies type C viral expression can be dissociated from disease casting doubt on their pathogenic role. Recent reports of autoimmune features in patients with human immunodeficiency virus (HIV) infection have increased interest in a pathogenic role for retroviruses in autoimmunity. Although a few HIV-infected adults have developed lupus, the association may be coincidental. Paradoxically, patients with established SLE who have contracted HIV infection experience a decrease in lupus disease activity, perhaps reflecting a decrease in T-helper cell activity. An endogenous retroviral RNA transcript, 8.4 kb, has recently been detected at high levels in the thymus of lupus but not normal mice. Studies seeking evidence of retroviral infection in patients with SLE are in progress.

Sex hormones

There is persuasive evidence that sex hormones play a part in disease pathogenesis. The disorder has a striking female predominance and is most common during the reproductive age groups. Inbred SLE mice with early oophorectomy are protected against disease expression. Exogenous oestrogens given to male mice exacerbate disease, while testosterone has an ameliorating effect. Oestrogen metabolism may be abnormal in patients with SLE and the disorder is commoner in Klinefelter's syndrome. Oestrogen-containing preparations in patients with SLE have not been demonstrated to exacerbate disease, but predispose to thrombosis. The mechanism by which sex hormones exert an effect is uncertain, but binding to oestrogen receptors expressed by T cells may lead to modification of immune responses.

Immunopathogenesis

There is compelling evidence that the immune system plays a pathogenic part in disease. SLE is the prototype autoimmune disorder with immune dysregulation involving stem cells, T and B cells, natural killer (NK) cells and the reticuloendothelial (or mononuclear phagocytic) system, as well as cytokine abnormalities. Immune function abnormalities in patients with SLE are shown in Fig. 24.1.

Tolerance

Breakdown in immunological tolerance, either central or peripheral is a fundamental process in autoimmune disease. Central tolerance involves thymic deletion of self reactive cells (negative selection) and positive selection of T cells with low affinity for self MHC. In contrast, there are four, non-mutually exclusive hypotheses that have been proposed to explain peripheral T-cell tolerance, which are involved in the prevention of tissue specific autoimmune disease. These include: anergy (loss of co-stimulatory signals, down-regulation of receptors critical for T-cell activation); deletion of reactive T cells; ignorance of the antigen by the immune system; and suppression of autoreactive T cells. Tolerance once induced does not necessarily persist. A breakdown in any of these mechanisms may lead to autoimmune disease.

Failure to become tolerant to self antigens (central or peripheral tolerance), cross-reactivity and molecular mimicry (such as after viral infections), development of anti-idiotypic antibodies that cross-react with self antigens, the development of altered self antigens (drugs, infections), and polyclonal stimulation of naturally occurring autoantibody producing cells may underly the initiation and perpertuation of autoantibody secretion.

Cellular defects

Stem cells

A number of stem cell abnormalities have been noted in mice. Lethally irradiated normal recipients receiving bone marrow stem cells from lupus-prone mice develop autoimmunity. This suggests that either the stem cells are phenotypically abnormal or have the genetic ability to induce autoimmunity. Other abnormalities include a greater propensity for bone marrow stem cells to give rise to an increased number of B-cell colonies and for each B cell to produce more antibody. Stem cell abnormalities in humans remain to be determined.

T cells

The major abnormality in T-cell function thought to contribute to disease pathogenesis is the failure to suppress B-cell antibody production or provide excess help to autoantibody-producing B cells. T-cell abnormalities noted in SLE patients are shown in Table 24.1.

B cells

In SLE patients, there is an increase in the number and/or activity of B cells at all stages of lymphocyte maturation (Table 24.1). Autoreactive B cells do not differ from conventional B cells, CD5+ B cells are specifically skewed towards autoantibody formation. Low-affinity immunoglobulin (Ig) M autoantibodies produced by the CD5+ B cells do not appear to be pathogenic compared with the high-affinity IgG autoantibodies, which are usually produced by CD5+ B cells.

Natural killer cells

In SLE patients, NK cells are reduced both in number and functional capability. This impairment may be due to cytokine abnormalities (e.g. insensitivity to IFNγ) or high levels of circulating immune complexes (CIC) binding to their Fc receptors and altering their function. The consequences of dysregulated function of NK cells may be to allow an uncontrolled expansion of autoantibody producing lymphocyte clones, thereby amplifying inflammation.

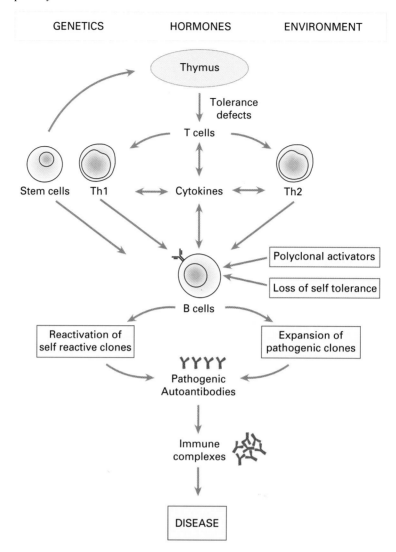

▮ **Fig. 24.1** An illustrative summary showing the multifactorial nature and disordered immune sites found in systemic lupus erythematosus (SLE). A primary stem cell defect has been shown to exist in animal models of SLE. Thymic defects include defective thymic processing, loss of tolerance and decreased thymic factors. Decreased suppressor–inducer subset of T cells in conjunction with increased production of factors (IL-5, IL-6, BCGF, IL-4) by Th2 cells may play a part in the induction and maintenance of B-cell hyperactivity. The defective suppressor T cell function may also fail to regulate B cells. Abnormalities in IL-2 responsiveness may cause further imbalances. Abnormalities in B-cell number and function exist. B cell may be stimulated by polyclonal activators or the result of tolerance defects. the secretion of autoantibodies may further impair T-cell function (anti-lymphocyte antibodies) as well as causing tissue damage. Failure to clear immune complexes by the reticuloendothelial system has been noted.

Reticuloendothelial system (RES)

The inability to efficiently clear CIC by the RES may lead to their increased tissue deposition and the maintenance of inflammation. The clearance of CIC by the RES occurs primarily in the liver (mediated by C3b receptors) and spleen (Fc-receptors, Fig. 24.2). In patients with SLE there is defective splenic Fc receptor-mediated and hepatic C3b receptor-mediated clearance of immune complexes from the circulation.

▌ **Table 24.1**   T- and B-cell abnormalities in lupus patients

T cells

Abnormalities in T-cell number and phenotype
  Lymphopenia. May be due to antilymphocyte antibodies
  Decreased supressor-inducer subset (CD4+CD45R+, 2H4+)
  Decreased 'naive' cells (CD4/8CD45RA+). Correlates with active renal disease
  Decreased 'memory' cells (CD4/8CD29). Negative correlation with anti-DNA antibody production
  Decreased suppressor cell activity
  Increased activated cells (CD4+, DR+)

Abnormal signalling and proliferative responses
  Abnormal calcium response to phytohaemagglutinin (PHA)
  Defective anti-CD2 proliferation
  Circulating anti-CD45 antibodies

B cells

Abnormalities in B-cell function
  Polyclonal B-cell activation
  Intrinsic B-cell abnormalities
  Increased responsiveness to stimulatory cytokines

Whether these defects are secondary to saturation of the RES by immune complexes or due to primary RES defects is uncertain.

Cytokines

Cytokines are molecules released from activated cells that have the ability to influence a variety of immune effector mechanisms. A number of cytokine abnormalities has been noted in SLE. These include, decreased quantities of IL-1 produced from monocytes and lower production and responses by T cells to IL-2. There is also an elevation of cytokines [IL-6, IL-4, B-cell growth factor, IL-5] controlling B-cell differentiation and antibody formation during active disease. Serum-soluble IL-2 receptors are elevated and are a sensitive predictor of disease activity.

Role of antibodies in SLE

Antibodies mediate tissue inflammation and injury in SLE either by a direct pathogenic effect (e.g. anti-SS-A/Ro activity against skin), and/or due to their association with antigens to form immune complexes [e.g. anti-double-stranded (ds) DNA/dsDNA] either in the circulation or *in situ* (e.g. glomeruli).

Direct pathogenic role

Anti SS-A/Ro antibodies may contribute to the cutaneous and cardiac lesions in the NLE syndrome as well as to the skin lesions in patients with subacute cutaneous lupus erythematosus (discussed below).

Immune complexes

Elevated levels of CIC are consistently found in patients with active SLE and contribute to tissue inflammation following their deposition. Under physiological conditions antibodies are produced in response to microbial infection, and form CIC (Fig. 24.2). Those that bind serum complement are transported in the circulation associated with erythrocytes bound to C3b receptors. In the liver and spleen they are removed from the blood following binding to C3b and IgG Fc receptors, respectively. In SLE a wide range of abnormalities contribute to the persistence of high levels of CIC as outlined in Fig. 24.2. The net result is prolonged high levels of CIC which become available for deposition at non-lymphoid sites, e.g. glomeruli. Their deposition in tissues may result in complement activation, polymorphonuclear leucocyte chemotaxis and the release of tissue mediators of inflammation leading to vascular injury. Why CIC deposit in the kidneys (Fig. 24.3) in some patients, in the skin, choroid plexus and/or synovium in others is uncertain.

In situ immune complex formation

The mechanisms of glomerular immune complex deposition are depicted in Fig. 24.4. In the glomeruli

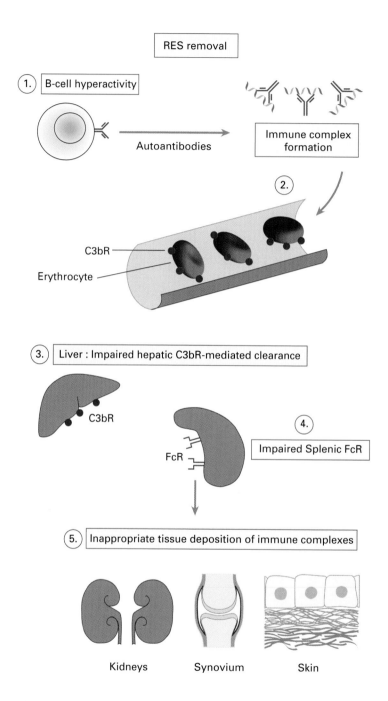

∎ Fig. 24.2 Schematic model of role of circulating immune complexes (CIC) in pathogenesis of systemic lupus erythematosus. Abnormalities have been described at a number of levels including: (1) exaggerated immune complex formations due to B cell hyperactivity; (2) an acquired defect in erythrocyte C3b receptor expression (C3bR); (3) impaired hepatic C3bR-mediated clearance of CIC; (4) impaired splenic Fc receptor (FcR) mediated clearance of CIC; leading to (5) inappropriate tissue deposition of non-lymphoid sites such as kidneys, synovium, or skin. RES, reticuloendothelial system.

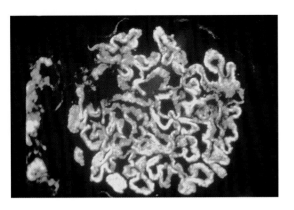

∎ **Fig. 24.3** Deposition of immune complexes on glomerular basement membrane assessed by direct immunofluorescence techniques using flurores-ceinated antibodies against human immunoglobulins.

of SLE patients immune complexes may form *in situ*. The glomerular basement membrane (GBM) is nega-tively charged due to its high content of heparan sul-phate and other glycosoaminoglycans. Histone, a basic protein which is a component of the nucleosome, when infused experimentally into animals, deposits on the negatively charged GBM. Free dsDNA which is subse-quently infused binds to the deposited histone. Circulating antibodies to dsDNA bind to the deposited DNA resulting in *in situ* immune complex formation. It is likely that both CIC and *in situ* immune complex deposition contribute to glomerular nephritis in SLE.

Anti-idiotypic antibodies

The designated acronym 16/6 idiotype has been given to a series of human IgM monoclonal anti-DNA anti-bodies. These antibodies when transfused in rodent experimental models induce the disease, while anti-DNA antibodies lacking the 16/6 idiotype do not. The 16/6 anti-idiotype to anti-ds DNA may be associated with the development of lupus nephritis in patients, by forming 16/6 anti-idiotype containing immune com-plexes, which deposit in glomeruli.

Clinical features

The clinical expression of SLE is protean and encom-passes a wide range of clinical features, Table 24.2. The American Rheumatism Association have pub-lished a set of 11 criteria for the classification of SLE, commonly used in diagnosis, research, and clinical studies. These include clinical and laboratory abnor-malities which are characteristic of SLE and have a high sensitivity (96%) and specificity (96%). The pres-ence of four or more features is diagnostic of SLE. The presence of three criteria makes the diagnosis prob-able, whereas two, places the diagnosis as possible.

Constitutional manifestations such as fatigue, fever, weight loss, and malaise are common when the disease is active. Musculoskeletal symptoms occur in 90% of patients, manifesting as polyarthralgia or arthritis. Joints commonly affected include interphalangeal and

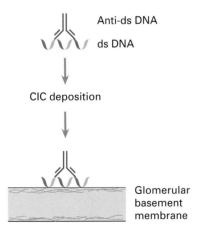

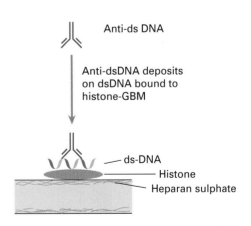

∎ **Fig. 24.4** Mechanisms of immune complex deposition in glomeruli: (a) circulating immune complex (CIC) depo-sition; (b) *in situ* immune complex formation. GBM, glomerular basement membrane; ds, double stranded.

∎ **Table 24.2** Common clinical manifestations of systemic lupus erythematosus

Organ	Symptom
Musculoskeletal	Arthralgia/arthritis, myalgia, tenosynovitis
Dermatological	Rashes, photosensitivity, alopecia, mouth ulcers, livedo reticularis
Renal	Nephritis, proteinuria
Haematological	Haemolytic anaemia, thrombocytopenia, lymphopenia
Pulmonary	Pleurisy, pleural effusions
Central nervous system	Psychosis, seizures
Heart	Pericarditis, endocarditis
Vascular disease	Recurrent abortions, thrombosis, vasculitis

metacarpophalangeal joints and wrists. The arthritis/arthralgia may be evanescent, recurrent, and at times rheumatoid-like. Synovial fluid analysis shows less inflammatory cells and a reduced level of complement compared with synovial fluid in rheumatoid arthritis. Other manifestations include ischaemic necrosis of the bone, e.g. femoral or humeral head, and rarely Jaccoud's arthritis, a deforming but non-erosive form of arthritis which affects the hands.

Skin manifestations are myriad and involve both cutaneous and mucous membranes. The classical, butterfly rash occurs over the malar bones and the nose, in up to 40% of SLE patients (Fig. 24.5). The skin rash may be erythematous and diffuse — macular or maculopapular; vasculitic ulcerations, nodules, infarcts, or livedo reticularis; or discoid. The demonstration of immune deposits at the dermo-epidermal junction of skin by direct immunofluorescence in clinically involved or uninvolved sites, although not specific, is supportive of the diagnosis of SLE.

Serositis with involvement of the pleura and pericardium is present in 25% of cases. Pleurisy with or without an effusion is the commonest pulmonary presentation. Pleural fluid is exudative, with modest leucocytosis, decreased complement, increased immune complexes, increased protein levels, normal glucose, and pH >7.3. This contrasts with rheumatoid pleural fluid which has a low glucose level and an acidic pH. Other clinical manifestations include pneumonitis; pulmonary haemorrhage, especially in patients with lupus glomerulonephritis; interstitial infiltrates and occasionally dyspnoea associated with dysfunctional diaphrams and diminished lung volumes.

Central nervous system (CNS) involvement represents one of the last clinical frontiers of SLE. Current knowledge about pathogenesis and diagnostic criteria is incomplete. Clinical features include organic brain syndrome with impaired intellect, memory lapses, and cognitive dysfunction, seizures, focal neurological

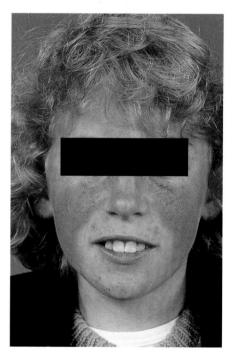

∎ **Fig. 24.5** Butterfly rash, typical of systemic lupus erythematosus.

lesions (chorea, cerebral vascular accidents, transverse myelitis, infarcts, peripheral neuropathies), and psychosis or severe behavioural disturbances in the absence of secondary causes such as drugs, infection, hypertension, and/or other organ dysfunction. *Grand mal* seizures are the most common form of epilepsy, although *petit mal*, temporal lobe and Jacksonian seizures have been reported. Immune complex-induced vasculitis, thromboembolic events, hypercoagulability, antiphospholipid antibodies and antineuronal antibodies, may all contribute to the pathogenesis of CNS involvement. Magnetic resonance imaging scanning is

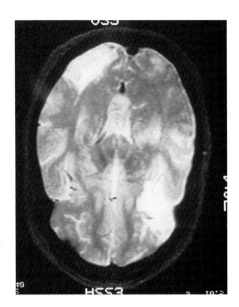

∎ **Fig. 24.6** MRI brain scan showing multiple focal abnormalities.

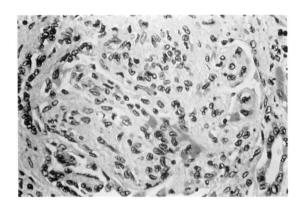

∎ **Fig. 24.7** Light microscopy of renal glomerulus showing diffuse proliferative glomerulonephritis.

currently the best means for imaging focal lesions (Fig. 24.6). Antineuronal antibodies have been associated with diffuse cerebritis and cognitive defects, and antiribosomal P antibodies with psychosis. There are no agreed criteria for the diagnosis of CNS involvement in SLE.

The major threat to long-term survival is renal involvement. While 60% of patients have proteinuria, only 30% have serious renal disease. The early features of renal involvement include a positive urinary sediment with proteinuria and red cell casts. Elevated serum urea and creatinine are a late feature. Histologically, the renal changes may include mesan-

gial abnormalities, focal or diffuse proliferative glomerulonephritis, membranous glomerulonephritis tubulo-interstitial inflammation, or any combination of these. Renal biopsies with diffuse proliferative changes have the worst prognosis. (Fig. 24.7).

Cardiac involvement may contribute to the morbidity and mortality of SLE and is more common than previously recognized. Features include pericarditis, in which clinically detected effusions are uncommon and it is mostly noted on echocardiography; myocarditis, presenting as unexplained resting tachycardia, electrocardiogram (ECG) changes, unexplained congestive cardiac failure; and endocarditis manifest as valvular verrucae, emboli, secondary infection, especially affecting the mitral valve.

Variants of SLE

Subacute cutaneous lupus erythematosus

This defines a subgroup of SLE patients who are often antinuclear antibody (ANA) negative, have antibodies to SS-A/Ro and are HLA-DR3 positive. Clinically, patients are characterized by photosensitivity, nonscarring dermatitis, mild systemic features, and a low prevalence of nephritis (Fig. 24.8). The anti-SS-A/Ro antibodies are thought to play a pathogenic part in the production of the cutaneous lesions. The disorder is usually responsive to antimalarial drugs and has a good prognosis.

Neonatal lupus erythematosus

This uncommon syndrome occurs in the offspring of some mothers with SLE, as well as patients with

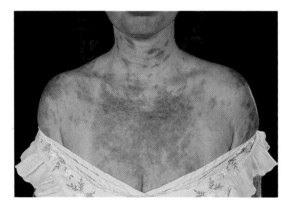

∎ **Fig. 24.8** Photosensitive skin rash in subacute cutaneous lupus erythematosus.

Sjögren's syndrome. Its clinical manifestations include transient cutaneous and haematological abnormalities and a permanent cardiac lesion, isolated congenital heart block (CHB). The transient clinical features include a photosensitive skin eruption (Fig. 24.8), discoid lesions, thrombocytopenia, Coomb's positive haemolytic anaemia, and leucopenia, which develop at or shortly after birth and resolve without sequelae within 3 months. CHB may develop *in utero* during the second half of pregnancy, or become apparent after birth.

This syndrome represents an example in which the physiological process of transplacental transfer of IgG antibodies from the maternal to fetal circulation leads to disease. Infants with this syndrome tested during the first 3 months of life nearly always have serum antibodies to SSA/Ro or SS-B/La, as does their mother's blood. However, in babies tested after 6 months of age these autoantibodies are undetectable. In women with SLE (and those with Sjögren's syndrome) who have IgG antibodies to SSA/Ro or SS-B/La, these may cross the placenta and target the fetal skin and/or heart where they deposit and produce an inflammatory reaction. Experimental studies have demonstrated that anti-SSA/Ro antibodies are able to target to human, but not murine skin *in vivo*. The maternally derived IgG SSA/Ro antibodies are catabolized by the infants and disappear from the circulation by 3 months of age. This parallels the resolution of the skin eruption.

In CHB, anti-SS-A/Ro antibodies target to the myocardial tissue, and induce inflammation leading to fibrosis of the conducting tissue. The infant suffers from brachycardia due to complete atrioventricular block, which may result in sudden death or the need for a cardiac pacemaker. Mothers of these infants may be asymptomatic at the time they deliver an affected infant, but may subsequently develop SLE or Sjögren's syndrome. They are at significant risk (approximately 25%) of a subsequent pregnancy being complicated by NLE.

Phospholipid antibody syndrome

Patients with SLE may have a biological false positive test for syphilis (BFP-VDRL) anticardiolipin antibodies and/or *in vitro* evidence of abnormal coagulation tests which fail to correct with the addition of normal plasma, i.e in the presence of the lupus anticoagulant. These three test abnormalities are due to antibodies directed against phospholipids. The lupus anticoagulant is detected in a functional assay, in which antibodies bind to the phospholipid used in the partial thromboplastin time assay, resulting in prolongation of coagulation times. The BFP-VDRL is due to antibodies that bind to the cardiolipin antigen — the substrate used in this test. Anticardiolipin antibodies are detected using an ELISA (enzyme-linked immunosorbent assay). Paradoxically, *in vivo* these autoantibodies are associated with a thrombotic rather than a bleeding tendency.

Phospholipid antibodies are not restricted to patients with SLE and are found in a variety of autoimmune, inflammatory, and infectious disorders, e.g. HIV infection. The term phospholipid antibody syndrome refers to patients with venous and/or arterial thrombosis, recurrent spontaneous abortion, and thrombocytopenia occurring in association with antiphospholipid antibodies.

The phospholipid antibodies detected in these three assays probably recognize slightly different antigenic determinants (Fig. 24.9). In some patients all three assays are positive while in others only one. Antibodies of the IgG class are most strongly associated with thrombosis. The mechanisms by which they produce a thrombotic tendency are complex. Phospholipid antibodies stimulate platelet aggregation, inhibit endothelial prostaglandin I_2 production, and interfere with protein S and C activity, proteins that are important in fibrinolysis. Any combination of the above effects may contribute to the thrombotic tendency. Krilis and coworkers (1991) have identified α_2-glycoprotein (α_2-GPI), also known as apolipoprotein H, as an important target for pathogenic anticardiolipin antibodies. In patients with SLE, anticardiolipin antibodies are directed at cardiolipin co-associated with α_2-GPI. By contrast, in HIV infection the antibodies are associated only with cardiolipin. The α_2-GPI antigen plays a part in the regulation of coagulation/fibrinolysis and antibodies which interfere with this protein and its function may contribute to thrombosis.

Drug-related lupus (DRL)

This entity occurs on exposure to certain drugs and is comprised of a photosensitive skin eruption, polyarthralgia or polyarthritis and pleuropericarditis in association with a homogeneous immunofluorescence pattern of ANAs and antihistone antibodies. CNS and renal involvement is unusual. Of the 60 drugs implicated in the development of drug-related lupus only a few have been definitely associated. These include procainamide, hydralazine, α-methyldopa and chlorpromazine. Typically, patients are older than those with idiopathic SLE — no doubt related to the patient group who receive antihypertensive and antiarrhythmic medications. The ANA show specificity only to histones, unlike patients with idiopathic SLE

LUPUS
ANTICOAGULANT

ANTICARDIOLIPIN
ANTIBODIES

BFP-VDRL

▮ **Fig. 24.9** Schematic model showing overlap of phospholipid antibodies using Venn diagram. BFP-VROL (test for syphilis).

who also usually have antibodies to dsDNA. The symptoms rapidly resolve with the cessation of the inducing drug, although the autoantibody levels diminish slowly. It may take months to years before they disappear. Routine assays for antihistone antibodies and its subclasses are not generally available. With the introduction of new anti-arrhythmic and antihypertensive drugs the syndrome has become rare.

Laboratory findings

Laboratory investigations can reveal a number of haemotological, serological, and biochemical abnormalities that may be the direct consequence of disease, complications of disease, or secondary to treatment. Many of the tests performed (immunoglobulin levels, complement levels, autoantibodies) are not diagnostic or predictive of disease activity in their own right and should be interpreted within the context of the individual clinical situation.

Antinuclear antibodies

ANA are autoantibodies reactive with nuclear antigens and are found in over 95% of patients with SLE. They are best detected by indirect immunofluorescence using a variety of substrates (rat liver, HEp 2 cells, *Crithidia lucilia*). The ANA titres, which provide a semiquantitative measure of the level of antibody in serum are usually lower if an animal organ (mouse liver, rat kidney) is used as a substrate compared with cell culture lines (HEp 2). Another feature of ANAs is the type of immunofluoresence pattern noted (Fig. 24.10). There are three basic patterns (homogeneous, rim or ring, speckled), which may be helpful in defining clinical subsets of SLE. More than one pattern can be noted in an individual. Although it is a very sensitive test it has a low specificity and is useful as a screening test. The clinical significance of several commonly encountered autoantibodies are listed in Table 24.3 and discussed below.

Antibodies to DNA

These frequently occur in SLE patients and include antibodies to ss-DNA and ds-DNA. The currently used

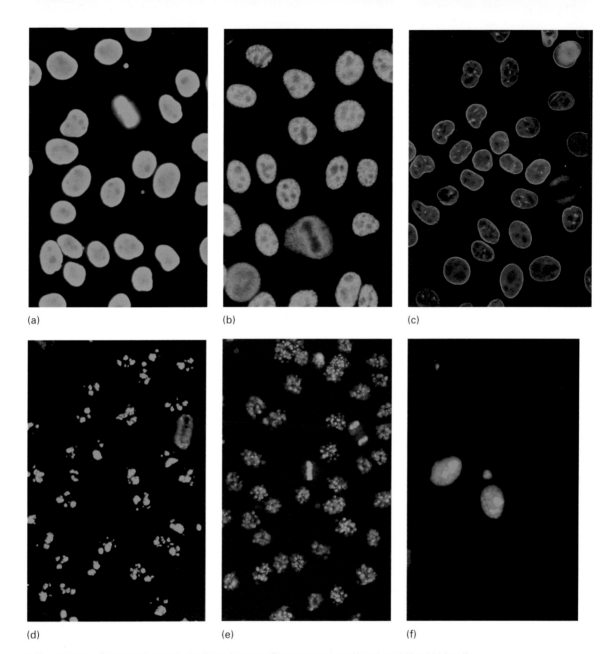

(a)   (b)   (c)

(d)   (e)   (f)

❚ Fig. 24.10   Pattern of ANA by indirect immunofluorescence on Hep-2 and Hep2000 cells.
(a) Homogeneous. The nuclei stain uniformally. The autoantibody specificities associeted with this pattern are to native (ds) DNA, histones and deoxyribonucleoprotein
(b) Speckled staining. The pattern on Hep-2 cells shows a speckling through the nucleus. The nucleoli appear as unstained areas within the speckled nucleus. The pattern is due to antibodies directed to extractable nuclear antigens—SM, U1RNP, Scl 70 (DNA topoisomerase I), SS-A/Ro, SS-B/La or other unspecified antigens.
(c) Nuclear lamin. Found in a few patients with SLE. More common in those with hepatitis, cytopenias with a circulating anticoagulant or cardiolipin antibodies, leucocytoclastic vascultis, or cerebral vasculitis.
(d) Nucleolar. An intense homogeneous staining of nucleoli which is often associated with less intense staining of the rest of the nucleus. Seen most commonly in systemic sclerosis and associated with autoantibodies to DNA topoisomerase, RNA polymerase and fibrillin.
(e) Centromere. Scattered throughout the nucleus are medium sized fluorescent points. In mitosis these points are related to the chromosome configuration and during metaphase and anaphase localization is to chromosomes. Found in the limited form of scleroderma, CREST; also in primary biliary cirrhosis. Rarely found in same sera as Scl-70 (topoisomerase I).
(f) Appearance with anti Ro seen with Ro transfected Hep-2 cells (Hep-2000).
(Slides by courtesy of Immunoconcepts).

▌ **Table 24.3**   Autoantibodies noted in SLE and their clinical relevance

Site	Antigen	Clinical features
Nucleus	ds-DNA	Characteristic of SLE/nephritis
	ss-DNA	Non-specific
	U1-RNP	Present in a variety of connective tissue disease including SLE, mixed connective tissue disease and overlap syndromes (myositis, sclerodactyly, Raynaud's)
	Sm	Characteristic of SLE
	Histones	Present in drug-related lupus
	SSB/La	Presence associated with decreased nephritis
	SSA/Ro	Present in a number disorders, including SLE, Sjögrens syndrome, congenital heart block, neonatal lupus
	PCNA	Presence characteristic of SLE
Cytoplasm	Ribosomal P-protein	Psychosis, depression
Cell membranes	Red cells	Coomb's positive haemolytic anemia
	White cells	Lymphopenia
	Platelets	Thrombocytopenia
	Phospholipid	Associated with thrombosis, recurrent abortions

SLE, systemic lupus erythematosus.

methods for detecting and quantitating anti-ss DNA and anti-ds DNA are radioimmunoassays, ELISA, and immunofluorescence. Immunofluoresence with *Crithidia luciliae* is used for detecting anti-dsDNA antibodies only. Antibodies to ss-DNA are found frequently in a variety of inflammatory and autoimmune diseases and have little diagnostic specificity. Elevated levels of antibodies to dsDNA are highly specific for SLE (98%) and may fluctuate with disease activity. However, they are present in only 60% of patients with SLE. Antibodies to ds-DNA have a pathogenic role, and are associated with nephritis. They are useful in monitoring disease activity and response to therapy.

Antibodies to non-histones

Antibodies to Smith (Sm) and ribonucleoprotein antigens

The term extractable nuclear antigens (ENA) includes antibodies to Sm and nuclear ribonucleoprotein (nRNP) antigens — two non-histone antigens. These antigens are comprised of five distinct uridylate-rich RNPs that associate with proteins. They form a functional unit termed a spliceosome, that functions to post-translationally modify mRNA (Fig. 24.11a). These particles are recognized by specific autoantibodies in some SLE patients. Autoantibodies to the U1-RNP particle are termed anti-U1RNP antibodies whereas antibodies to the U1-U5-RNP complex are termed anti-Sm antibodies.

This heterogeneous group of antibodies can be detected by immunodiffusion methods (Ouchterlony double-diffusion gels) using the appropriate antigen extracts and reference serum (Fig. 24.12), counter-immunofluorescence or by immunoprecipitation. Antibodies to U1RNP and Sm are found in 40–50% and 10–30% of SLE patients, respectively. The latter are highly specific for SLE and do not characterize any clinical subgroup. Antibodies to U1RNP are found in patients with SLE, particularly those with Raynaud's disease and myositis, or in SLE patients with overlapping features of scleroderma, and polymyositis. Typically, patients with anti-U1RNP antibodies do not have anti-dsDNA antibodies and have mild disease with infrequent renal involvement.

SSA/Ro and SSB/La autoantibodies

Another pair of small nRNPs (SSA/Ro, SSB/La) cooperate with RNA polymerase III during transcription of mRNA. SSA/Ro, a 60 or 52 kDa protein associated with one of five cytoplasmic RNAs (referred to as hY1-hY5), and SSB/La (48 kDa) antigen were initially defined as cytoplasmic in origin in patients with SLE and Sjögrens syndrome (Fig. 24.11b). These antigens vary in expression at different stages of the cell cycle and can be localized either in the cytoplasm or nucleus. Ro and La antigens are identical to SSA and SSB antigens, respectively. Production of autoantibodies to these antigens is linked to HLA-DQ loci.

(a)

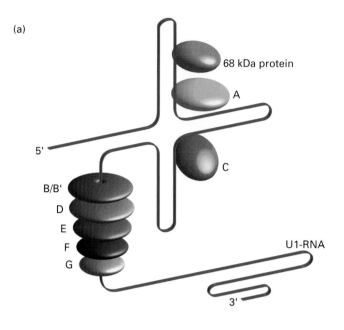

(b)

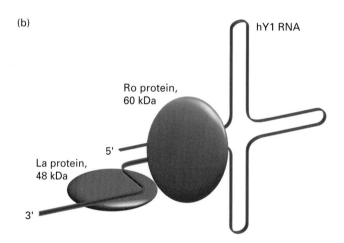

∎ **Fig. 24.11** (a) Schematic representation of all the constituents of a spliceosome apparatus. The function of this unit is to excise introns from heteronuclear RNA and join the exons to form mRNA. It is composed of a group of uridine rich RNAs (U1, U2, U4-6, and U-6) with a subset of proteins (70 kDa, A, B/B1, D, E, F, G) attached to them. Anti-Sm antibodies are directed against U1, U2, U4-6, and U5 particles. Anti-U1RNP antibodies are specific for U1 particles only. This results in partial identity between anti-Sm and anti-U1 RNP. (b) The SS-A/Ro, SS-B/La RNA protein complex. One of five RNAs (hY1-5) bind at least two proteins (SS-A/Ro and SS-B/La).

Anti-SS-A/Ro and anti-SSB/La are found in 25–40% and 10% of SLE patients, respectively. Antibodies to SS-A/Ro occur without antibodies to SS-B/La, but not vice versa. Patients with both anti-SS-A/Ro and anti-SS-B/La antibodies have less fre-quent and less severe renal disease, than those with anti-SS-A/Ro alone. The increased renal involvement in patients with anti-SS-A/Ro alone may be a reflection of the presence of anti-DNA antibodies associated with this autoantibody profile. Anti-SS-A/Ro-

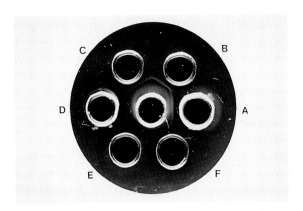

▌ **Fig. 24.12** Double immunodiffusion in agar (Ouchterlony analysis). The interaction of antigen with antibody in agar forms stable immune complexes which can be analysed visually. Reaction patterns are those of identity, non-identity or partial identity. Shown are complete identity between wells (B) and (C) and partial identity between wells (B) and (A) (anti-Sm and anti-U1RNP). Middle well contains the substrate (rabbit thymus extract). Agar plate courtesy of Ms C. Stoudt, Sutton Laboratory, RNSH.

positive SLE patients often have photosensitivity, prominent sicca symptoms, rheumatoid factor, and hypergammaglobulinaemia Anti-SS-A/Ro antibodies are also found in patients with Sjögren's syndrome alone and have a similar clinical profile to that noted above. Anti-SS-A/Ro antibodies are occasionally found in normal individuals (3%), relatives of patients with autoimmune diseases and patients with SLE features but who are ANA-negative.

Haematological autoantibodies

A number of autoantibodies have a direct effect on the haematological system. Antibodies to any of the cellular components of blood can be found in lupus patients. The commonest manifestations are antibodies to lymphocytes due to anti-T-cell antibodies, red cells (Coombs' positive haemolytic anaemia), and platelets (idiopathic thrombocytopenia). Leucopenia ($<4000/mm^3$) occurs frequently and may involve granulocytes as well as lymphocytes.

Antibodies to ribosomal P-protein

Autoantibodies that react with the P-protein of ribosomes, or a portion of the RNA that combines with the P-protein to form GTPase activity, are largely limited to patients with lupus (5–10%). The previously noted clinical association of these antibodies with severe depression or lupus psychosis is now being questioned.

Proliferating cell nuclear antigen (PCNA)

This autoantibody is specific for SLE and not found in other connective tissue disorders. It is, however, present only in a minority of SLE patients (5%). Patients with this autoantibody may have a higher incidence of diffuse proliferative glomerulonephritis.

Treatment

Owing to the wide spectrum of clinical manifestations and disease severity it is not possible to offer a standard treatment to all SLE patients. Treatment needs to be tailored to the severity and extent of disease in the individual patient. General measures include a nutritious low saturated fat diet, cessation of smoking, and a regular exercise programme to maintain ideal body weight. Photoprotection is important and includes avoidance of sunlight during the middle of the day, the use of high-grade blockout (SPF 15+) and the wearing of long sleeves and broad-rimmed hats. Exposure to ultraviolet-B sunlight can activate skin disease and a systemic flare.

Medication

For skin disease topical corticosteroids are helpful. Polyarthralgia and polyarthritis is treated initially with NSAIDs. If these measures fail to adequately control skin or joint symptoms then an antimalarial drug, usually hydroxychloroquine (Plaquenil), should be introduced. This drug is not only effective in skin and joint disease but may protect against the development of systemic disease. The usual starting dose is 400 mg/day, subsequently reducing to 200 mg/day. Ophthalmological assessment at baseline and on a 4–6 monthly basis is mandatory to detect the uncommon but potentially serious complication of retinal toxicity.

Corticosteroids

Low-dose corticosteroids (e.g. prednisolone 5–10 mg/day) may be used to control difficult skin and joint manifestations. High-dose corticosteroids and immunosuppressive drugs are reserved for those with major organ or life-threatening disease, such as diffuse proliferative glomerulonephritis. Treatment is usually commenced with oral prednisone 50–100 mg/day or with intermittent intravenous pulses of methyl pred-

▮ **Table 24.4** Treatment of systemic lupus erythematosus

Antimalarials
    Hydroxychloroquine
    Chloroquine
    Quinacrine

Corticosteroids
    Prednisone or prednisolone (oral)
    Methylprednisolone (i.v.)

Immunosuppressives
    Azathioprine
    Methotrexate
    Cyclophosphamide (oral or i.v.)
    Chlorambucil
    Cyclosporin A (experimental)

Androgens
    19-nortestosterone
    Danazol

Physical modalities
    Plasmaphoresis
    Total nodal irradiation

Dietary
    Arachidonic acid analogues, e.g. eicasopentanoeic
    acid

Immunotherapy
    Immunoadsorption of anti-DNA antibodies
    Intravenous gammaglobulin
    Monoclonal antibodies against CD4 or CD5

---

nisolone (500–1000 mg). These must be continued for several weeks until disease activity is suppressed, and then tapered slowly.

Immunosuppressive agents

Cyclophosphamide has been shown to decrease the likelihood of end-stage renal failure in patients with severe lupus nephritis, but not prolong overall life expectancy. Intravenous pulses of cyclophosphamide (every 4–6 weeks for at least six courses) is more effective and less toxic than continuous daily oral cyclophosphamide. There is an increased risk of infection (especially herpes zoster), infertility (especially in women over 35 years of age) and malignancy, particularly after long-term oral usage. Intravenous pulses of cyclophosphamide produces less bladder toxicity (haemorrhagic cystitis) and malignancy than oral cyclophosphamide. There is less clinical experience

with chlorambucil and methotrexate. Azathioprine is less toxic than cyclophosphamide but is less effective in severe renal disease. Its major role is as a steroid-sparing agent in patients whose prednisone dose cannot be reduced below 12–15 mg/day without flares in disease. There is limited experience with cyclosporin A and concerns about its nephrotoxicity.

Physical modalities

Plasma exchange has been used in patients with SLE without clear evidence of benefit, but at great expense. It may have a role in crises, e.g. evolving renal failure as part of a severe lupus flare. Total nodal irradiation has been used in some patients with severe SLE, but is toxic. It cannot be recommended for routine use.

Immunotherapy

There are a number of experimental approaches that are being evaluated including intravenous γ-globulin (especially in thrombocytopenia, monoclonal antibodies directed against T- and B-lymphocyte subsets, and immunoabsorption techniques to remove anti-DNA antibodies from the circulation.

Dietary therapy

In SLE mice a diet enriched in polyunsaturated fatty acids, e.g. eicosopentanoeic acid prevents and ameliorates lupus nephritis. In humans with SLE a significant benefit of this approach has not been demonstrated. Androgen therapy has been evaluated anecdotally and may have anti-inflammatory effects in females with SLE. However, its viralizing effect makes this treatment unacceptable to most patients. In males with SLE androgens may exacerbate disease.

Monitoring

The monitoring of patients with SLE involves assessing the clinical features and laboratory indices of organ involvement. Renal involvement is monitored by 24 h urinary protein, creatinine clearance tests and examination of urine for the presence of red cell casts, and monitoring of blood pressure. For skin or joint disease, the occurrence of a rash and polyarthralgia/polyarthritis are monitored. There are a number of disease activity indices that have been developed including the Systemic Lupus Erythematosus Disease Activity Index (SLEDAI) which uses clinical and laboratory parameters. However, these are not practical for routine clinical use and are largely confined to research studies.

Serum immunological markers that are useful for monitoring disease activity include antibody titres to dsDNA, and C3 and C4 complement levels. In some patients an increase in titre of antibodies to dsDNA and a decrease in C3 and C4 levels antedates a disease flare. In general, treatment is based on clinical features occurring in conjunction with abnormalities in laboratory tests rather than on the basis of laboratory tests *per se*. Full blood count and platelet counts need to be monitored closely in patients on immunosuppressive drugs. Ophthalmological review is essential for those on hydroxychloroquine.

Prognosis

The outlook for patients with SLE has improved dramatically over the past two decades. The disorder can no longer be considered an acute fatal disorder but rather as a chronic one. Studies in the 1980s and early 1990s have revealed that 80–90% of patients are alive at 10 years. Less certain is what happens in the second decade and beyond. Data are now emerging that the majority do not succumb from active disease. The long-term concerns are similar to those experienced by long-term survivors of renal transplants — the development of premature atheroma and infections. Premature myocardial infarction and cerebrovascular accidents are a significant complication. Infections are an ever-present risk in those on immunosuppressive therapy.

A number of treatment strategies will need to be addressed to prevent the development of atheroma. They include cessation of smoking, monitoring of serum lipids, close monitoring and control of blood pressure, and maintenance of ideal body weight. Corticosteroids and circulating immune complexes may themselves be risk factors for atheroma.

Further reading

Deapen, D., Escalante, A., Weinrib, L., *et al.* (1992). A revised estimate of twin concordance in systemic lupus erythematosus. *Arthritis and Rheumatism*, **35**, 311–18.

Donadio, J. V. and Glassock, R. J. (1993). Immunosuppressive drug therapy in lupus nephritis. *American Journal of Kidney Diseases*, **21**, 239–50.

Elkon, K. B. (1994). Autoantibodies in SLE. In *Rheumatology* (ed. J. H. Klippel, and P. A. Dieppe), pp. 4.5–4.10. Mosby Year Book Europe Limited.

Fessel, W. J. (1988). Epidemiology of systemic lupus erythematosus. *Rheumatic Disease Clinics of North America*, **14**, 1–4.

Gladman, D. D. (1991). Prognosis of systemic lupus erythematosus and the factors that affect it. *Current Opinion in Rheumatology*, **3**, 789–96.

Handwerger, B. S. (1991). T cell and B cell function in lupus. *Current Opinion in Rheumatology*, **3**, 157–79.

Harley, J. B. and Schofield, R. H. (1991) Systemic lupus erythematosus: RNA protein autoantigens, models of disease heterogeneity and theories of aetiology. *Journal of Clinical Immunology*, **11**, 297–316.

Hauptman, H. W. (1991). Variants/subsets of SLE. *Maryland Medical Journal*, **40**, 909–16.

McNeil, H. P., Chesterman, C. N., and Krilis, S. A. (1991). Immunology and clinical importance of antiphospholipid antibodies. *Advances in Immunology*, **49**, 193–280.

Miller, J. F. A. P. and Morahan, G. (1992). Peripheral T cell tolerance. *Annual Review of Immunology*, **10**, 51–69.

Pisetsky, D. (1992). Antinuclear antibodies. *Rheumatic Disease Clinics of North America*, **18** (2), 283–505.

Reveille, J. D. (1991). The molecular genetics of systemic lupus erythematosus and Sjögren's syndrome. *Current Opinion in Rheumatology*, **3**, 722–30.

Steinberg, A. D. *et al.* (1991). Systemic lupus erythematosus. *Annals of Internal Medicine*, **115**, 548–51.

Stevens, M. B. (1991). The clinical spectrum of SLE. *Maryland Medical Journal*, **40**, 875–85.

Tan, E. M., Cohen, A. S., Fries, J., Masi, A. T. *et al.* (1982). The 1982 revised criteria for the clarification of systemic lupus erythematosus. *Arthritis and Rheumatism*, **25**, 1271–7.

Teh, L. S. and Isenberg, D. A. (1994). Review: antiribosomal P protein antibodies in systemic lupus erythematosus: A reappraisal. *Arthritis and Rheumatism*, **37**, 307–15.

Yung, R. L. and Richardson, B. C. (1994). Drug-induced lupus. *Rheumatic Disease Clinics of North America*, **20**, 61–86.

This disorder was first recognized in Naples in the mid-eighteenth century by Dr Carlo Curzio and originally considered a bland fibrotic disorder of unknown aetiology. In more recent times, it has been recognized as an inflammatory, vascular, and fibrotic disorder in which immunological factors probably play an important part. While many of the pathogenetic mechanisms are being elucidated, its aetiology is largely unknown.

Introduction

Incidence and mortality

Population-based studies suggest that the annual incidence of scleroderma is between 1 and 20 per million people, with a peak between 40 and 50 years of age, with about three times more women than males. Onset in childhood and familial occurrence are rare. Hospital clinic-based studies of scleroderma are biased in that they contain a high percentage of patients with diffuse disease. None the less, they suggest a mortality of about 50% at 5 years, with most patients dying of either respiratory or cardiac disease.

Occupational and environmental factors

It is very difficult to identify with certainty environmental triggers implicated in the genesis of scleroderma. Environmental factors suggested as being of possible significance have largely been reported as isolated cases or small series. These include vinyl chloride, silica, organic solvents (e.g. toluene, trichloroethylene, hexachloroethane), epoxy resins, silicone in breast implants, and drugs (e.g. bleomycin, pentazocin).

Genetic factors

There are no clear-cut genetic associations of scleroderma, although there may be weak associations with human leucocyte antigen (HLA) B8 DR3. The HLA haplotype DR3/DRW52a represents a significant genetic risk factor for the development of pulmonary fibrosis in scleroderma (discussed below).

Pathogenesis

Scleroderma is a disorder in which abnormalities occur in three major areas: the fibroblast with overproduction of collagen and other matrix proteins, the vascular endothelium, and the immune system. Any hypothesis seeking to explain the pathogenesis of scleroderma must take into account and interrelate these three areas (Fig. 25.1).

Although, the triggering or perpetuating antigen is not known, scleroderma is thought to be an autoimmune disease. The reasons for this include its association with other autoimmune diseases, the presence of antinuclear antibodies, the mononuclear cell infiltrate that characterizes the early scleroderma lesion, and the occurrence of a very similar disorder in chronic graft-versus-host disease following bone marrow transplantation. The immunoregulatory abnormalities thought to play a key part in the aetiology of autoimmunity are discussed elsewhere in this book. The lymphocyte also regulates macrophage activation through its capacity to secrete cytokines such as interferon (IFN) γ. As in most chronic inflammatory processes, the macrophage is an important determinant of the nature of the pathological process. This is due to the enormous range of bioactive macrophage mediators many of which act on adjacent mesenchymal cells such as fibroblast and endothelial cells.

Fibrosis is the hallmark of scleroderma and represents the end result of a balance between interacting

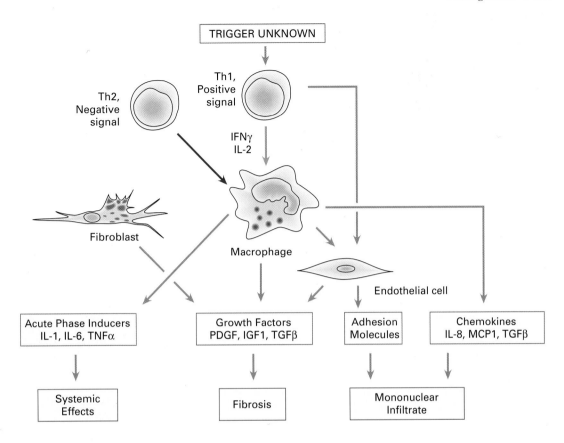

▌Fig. 25.1 Major pathogenic mechanisms in scleroderma.

factors (Figs 25.2 and 25.3), predominantly cytokines, which both stimulate fibroblast proliferation and enhance the synthesis of collagen and other matrix proteins such as proteoglycans and fibronectin. In the skin the sources of these cytokines include macrophages, endothelial cells, keratinocytes, Langerhans cells, and dermal fibroblasts. The fibroblast itself has largely been considered as a collagen producing cell. However, as with most mesenchymal cells it is capable of producing a wide range of cytokines including fibrogenic cytokines such as platelet-derived growth factor-A (PDGF-A), transforming growth factor (TGF) β and insulin-like growth factor (IGF) 1. While there is little direct evidence for this role in scleroderma, it is known that fibroblasts, when stimulated by a wide range of different growth factors including PDGF and IGF-1, can also respond by synthesizing IGF-1 and PDGF-A.

Scleroderma fibroblasts differ from normal skin fibroblasts in that they replicate faster and produce more collagen. Cytokines such as TGFβ and/or PDGF

are believed to induce the overgrowth within the skin of a fibroblast subpopulation with these characteristics. Further stimulation by cytokine especially TGFβ results in matrix protein synthesis from this amplified cell subpopulation. The chronic inflammatory response that triggers the fibrosis in scleroderma may well be a relatively short-lived reaction in the skin, which once it passes, leaves an irreparably damaged organ.

It has been assumed that the endothelial damage that plays a part in the pathogenesis of scleroderma must involve immunologically mediated cytotoxic mechanisms. It is also likely that the endothelium is involved in the genesis of the fibrotic response. Initial lesions are perivascular and include fibrosis and infiltration of lymphocytes and macrophages. PDGF has also been detected in this location and PDGF-B receptors, not expressed in normal skin, have been found in perivascular fibroblasts. Additionally, collagen mRNA and histochemical studies both suggest that the major site for synthesis of collagen is in fibroblasts adjacent to blood vessels in the deep dermis.

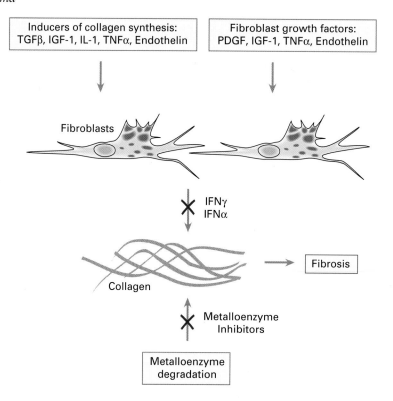

| Inducers of collagen synthesis: TGFβ, IGF-1, IL-1, TNFα, Endothelin | Fibroblast growth factors: PDGF, IGF-1, TNFα, Endothelin |

Fibroblasts

IFNγ
IFNα

Collagen → Fibrosis

Metalloenzyme Inhibitors

Metalloenzyme degradation

■ **Fig. 25.2** Regulation of fibroblast collagen production

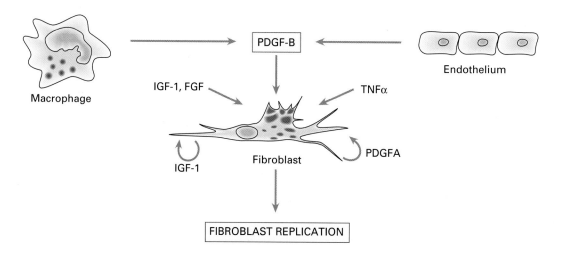

Macrophage → PDGF-B ← Endothelium

IGF-1, FGF   TNFα

IGF-1   Fibroblast   PDGFA

FIBROBLAST REPLICATION

■ **Fig. 25.3** Regulation of fibroblast replication. FGF, fibroblast growth factor; TNF, tumour necrosis factor PDGF, platelet-derived growth factor.

The endothelium plays a pivotal part in directing leucocyte traffic and is also capable of producing a range of important cytokines. The endothelial cells in scleroderma skin express adhesion molecules which may help to localize the extravasation of inflammatory cells. These endothelial changes, perhaps triggered in part by cytokines released from surrounding mononuclear cells, may be directly linked to fibrosis through the capacity of the endothelium to release cytokines. Two potential endothelial cell mediators of fibrosis are PDGF and endothelin. PDGF is a powerful growth factor for fibroblast whose synthesis can be induced by cytokines and injury and which has been histopathologically localized to the scleroderma lesion. Endothelin is released from activated and injured endothelium and plasma levels are elevated in scleroderma subjects. As well as induction of a vasospastic response, this molecule is known to induce both increased fibroblast replication and collagen synthesis.

Clinical features

In most instances the diagnosis of scleroderma is not difficult, but there are a number of other disorders to it which it bears some similarities. These include mixed connective tissue disease, chronic graft-versus-host disease, the toxic oil syndrome, eosinophilic myalgia, and eosinophilic fasciitis. Discussion in this chapter will be limited to scleroderma, of which there are two major forms, limited and diffuse scleroderma, which are separated by the extent of skin involvement. Localized forms of scleroderma (e.g. morphea, linear scleroderma) also occur in which the process is confined to patchy areas of skin without spread to systemic involvement. Recognition of the different forms of scleroderma is important as they are associated with varying complications and carry different prognostic implications.

Both limited and diffuse scleroderma are multisystem diseases and their manifestations are summarized in Table 25.1. To some degree, skin involvement, Raynaud's phenomenon, and oesophageal disease is present in virtually all subjects. Also very common are lower gastrointestinal tract disease and mild pulmonary disease. Severe pulmonary disease, cardiac disease, myositis, and renal disease are all uncommon.

Skin disease

The skin disease is the hallmark of scleroderma and is its most important diagnostic criterion. The changes in the skin consist of thickening with loss of subcutaneous tissue and adnexal structures such as hair and sweat glands. In the early stages, this thickening is more easily felt than seen. With time the skin takes on a shiny wrinkle-free and often pigmented or depigmented appearance and may become very hard to the touch. Skin involvement usually commences in the fingers and progresses proximally up the arms. The skin of the face (especially peri-orally) is frequently also involved early in the disease. In limited scleroderma skin involvement is confined to the fingers, hands, and face but sometimes progresses up the arms. If skin involvement (excluding the face) progresses further than the elbows, the scleroderma is defined as having become diffuse in type. Diffuse scleroderma is often associated with truncal involvement and is generally a more aggressive and rapidly progressive disorder.

Tight skin over flexural surfaces predisposes to ulcers which may be very difficult to heal. Severe skin involvement may sometimes lead to contractures with limitation of movement especially of fingers and jaw. The contractures associated with this condition can be very debilitating and difficult to treat.

Subcutaneous calcification or calcinosis is frequently observed in scleroderma. It may be widespread but occurs most frequently in the fingers. Calcific lesions tend to ulcerate and discharge mineral crystals. These may become superinfected and may not heal without surgical removal of the calcified material.

The histopathological appearance of the skin is essentially that of a chronic inflammatory fibrotic lesion and there are no specific diagnostic features. The early advancing lesions demonstrate dermal infiltration with mononuclear cells with prominent perivascular localization. There is oedema, dermal thickening, and later an increase in collagen occurring as tightly packed bundles. In time the chronic inflammatory process disappears leaving a fibrotic dermis, lacking adnexal structures.

Treatment

Penicillamine is the only drug of proven benefit for scleroderma skin involvement.

Vascular disease
Large vessel disease

Raynaud's phenomenon is a major feature of this disorder. It is usually the earliest symptom of scleroderma and may be present some years before any other disease features are obvious. Without Raynaud's phenomenon, the diagnosis of scleroderma should only be made with care as its absence is rare. Typically, in contrast to the idiopathic Raynaud's phenomenon, it first begins in adulthood rather than childhood, may be asymmetrical and associated with digital ulceration (Fig. 25.4). It is

▮ **Table 25.1** Manifestations of scleroderma

	Diffuse form	Limited form
Vascular		
Raynaud's phenomenon	+++	++++
Digital ulceration and gangrene	++	+++
Pulmonary hypertension	+	++
Coronary artery constriction	+	++
Pulmonary		
Pleural effusion	+	+
Interstitial lung disease	+++	++
Bronchiolitis	++	++
Pulmonary hypertension	+	++
Cardiac disease		
Pericardial effusion	+	+
Arrhythmias	++	++
Cardiomyopathy	++	+
Coronary artery constriction	+	++
Renal disease		
Malignant hypertension	+	+/−
Gastrointestinal disease		
Sicca symptoms	+++	+++
Reflux oesophagitis	++++	++++
Malabsorption	++	++
Constipation or diarrhoea	+++	+++
Anal incompetence	+	+
Musculoskeletal		
Myositis	++	+
Calcinosis	++	++
Inflammatory or mechanical arthritis	+	+
Bone resorption	++	+++
Skin		
Skin thickening (below elbow)	++++	++++
Skin thickening (above elbow and trunk)	++++	−
Telangiectasia	+++	+++
Pigmentation/depigmentation	++	++
Loss of adnexal structures	+++	+++
Ulceration	++	+++

probably a manifestation of both narrowing of digital blood vessels and vascular hyperreactivity.

While involvement of digital blood vessels of the arms is clinically the most obvious, vascular involvement of the arteries of the legs and the pulmonary vasculature also occurs. In the latter instance this leads to pulmonary hypertension (discussed below). Involvement of peripheral vessels often leads to digital ulceration. This problem is invariably worse during the colder weather, but with more severe disease can also occur in warm seasons. In some patients, severe ulceration can lead to gangrene and digital loss. Ulceration is often complicated by infection which can sometimes involve bone and joint as well as soft tissue. Ulcers often heal slowly, presumably because of the poor blood supply. Severe vasospastic phenomena are particularly associated with the presence of a centromere pattern antinuclear antibody.

Arterial involvement is characterized by intimal proliferation in which myointimal cells are arranged

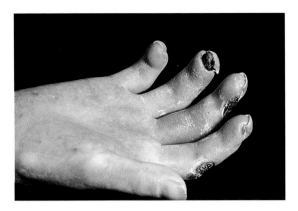

▌ **Fig. 25.4** Hand of a patient with sclero-derma showing digital ulceration, skin thickening and telangiectasia.

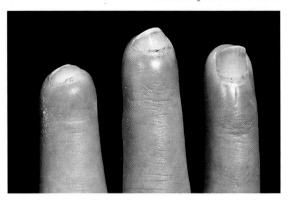

▌ **Fig. 25.6** These fingers of a patient with scleroderma demonstrate small nail bed infarcts.

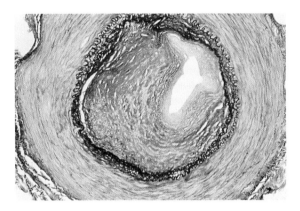

▌ **Fig. 25.5** Scleroderma digital artery demonstrating marked intimal proliferation.

concentrically in a mucoid and fibrilar matrix (Fig. 25.5). Adventitial fibrosis is frequent and marked narrowing becomes associated with thrombosis and luminal occlusion.

Capillary abnormalities

Microcirculatory abnormalities involving both skin and major organs represents the dominant vascular pathology in scleroderma. The damage to, and decrease in number of capillaries contributes to poor tissue nutrition and predisposes to digital ulceration and poor wound healing. Abnormal capillaries (Fig. 25.6) can be consistently visualized at the nail bed by either a magnifying glass or capillary microscopy. Viewed this way the vessels appear decreased in number and display increased tortuosity. Superficial capillary malformations visible as small telangiectasia also occur (Fig. 25.6). These are sometimes widespread, especially on the face, but may also involve

mucosal surfaces and the gastrointestinal tract. These capillary abnormalities, if present in large numbers on mucosal surfaces are prone to bleeding and may cause epistaxis or occult gastrointestinal blood loss.

Perivascular mononuclear cell infiltration and evidence of endothelial injury are prominent in early disease, often preceding fibrosis. This injury is manifest by endothelial cell swelling and vacuolization, gaps between endothelial cells, and reduplication of the basal lamina. Endothelial destruction and increased cell turnover is also present.

Treatment of digital ulceration

Prevention is the mainstay of treatment of digital ulceration. General measures include, effective home heating, dressing very warmly whenever venturing outside, and even moving to a warm climate if possible. Warm covering must extend to the whole body as just warm gloves to Raynaud's affected extremities are insufficient. Vasodilators such as the calcium channel blockers and nitroglycerine patches can also provide some relief during the cold weather. The onset of digital ulceration requires careful management which includes, the most effective vasodilatation possible, treatment of infections, appropriate local wound care, assessment of viability of the affected area, and sometimes the use of powerful parenterally administered vasodilators such as prostaglandin E_2 and prostacyclin. Procedures such as sympathectomy provide only transient relief and in most instances are not advisable.

Gastrointestinal disease

The whole gastrointestinal tract is affected in most patients with scleroderma. The essential element in this process seems to be an abnormality in the motor control of the gastrointestinal tract causing a generalized decrease in motility. Recent evidence suggests this is associated with high serum levels of gastrointestinal regulatory peptides but the pathogenesis is poorly understood.

Oesophageal disease

Oesophageal involvement of some degree is almost universal in diffuse and limited scleroderma. This is due to an oesophageal motility disorder that can best be visualized with motility studies. These demonstrate decreased and sometimes absent peristalsis in the lower half of the oesophagus and an incompetent lower oesophageal sphincter.

The symptoms exhibited are typically those of oesophageal reflux accompanied by a variable element of dysphagia. The latter may be due to decreased oesophageal motility, scarring around the gastro-oesophageal sphincter or severe sicca symptoms from associated Sjögren's syndrome. Occasionally, the tone of the gastro-oesophageal sphincter is markedly decreased resulting in reflux of such a degree that bending causes free regurgitation of stomach contents.

Histopathologically, this is characterized by atrophy of distal oesophageal musculature and replacement by fibrous tissue. The lamina propria and submucosa also display increased collagen and the changes of oesophagitis may also be present. The ganglia of the Auerbach's plexus, which are important in motor control appear histologically normal.

Treatment

Until the advent of powerful inhibitors of acid secretion, oesophagitis was a major cause of morbidity. Because of damage to the gastro-oesophageal sphincter feeding gastrotomies were even sometimes required. These types of major complications have largely disappeared with the regular use of agents such as cimetidine, ranitidine, and more recently omeprazole.

Fundoplication is a useful surgical procedure if disabling free reflux of gastric contents is present.

Small bowel disease

Clinically, significant small bowel hypomotility is substantially less common than oesophageal disease. The development of chronic diarrhoea and weight loss provides the clinical clue to its presence. Stasis may cause small bowel overgrowth of bacteria with resultant diarrhoea and malabsorption. This can be detected with the ^{14}C breath test. Occasionally, small bowel disease may present as unexplained weight loss with apparently normal bowel motions. However, in these instances it will usually be due to the normalization of bowel habit in a previously constipated patient.

The most prominent histopathological finding is an increase in submucosal and serosal collagen with atrophy of the muscularis externa. The villus architecture is normal but there may be a mild inflammatory infiltrate. As in the oesophagus, the myenteric neurons appear normal.

Treatment

This complication can usually be treated quite readily by nutritional supplementation and long-term administration of antibiotics to decrease bowel flora.

Large bowel disease

Constipation is a common symptom in scleroderma and is due to large bowel hypomotility. In most instances it is not severe and can be readily managed. Of much greater concern is dysfunction of the anal sphincter which can lead to faecal incontinence. This is not common and in women may be exacerbated by local trauma during childbirth.

Histopathologically, like the small bowel, the large bowel is characterized by mucosal and submucosal collagen deposition and variable atrophy of the muscularis externa. This leads to the development of the characteristic asymptomatic wide mouth diverticuli on the antimesenteric border.

Treatment of the generalized hypomotility

There are several drugs including metaclopramide, cisapride, and octreotide that are known to increase oesophageal, gastric, and small bowel motility. In some situations they may partially reverse the motility abnormalitiies of scleroderma.

Lung disease

Respiratory symptoms are common in scleroderma and include a non-productive cough and shortness of breath which may worsen with time. Various studies estimate the frequency of lung involvement between 25 and 75%. Aside from occasional pleurisy, involvement of the lung occurs at three major levels: the pulmonary interstitium, the pulmonary artery, and the bronchiole. From an aetiological point of view it is important to bear in mind that more than half of the patients with scleroderma have sicca symptoms. Sjögren's syndrome is also associated with pulmonary complications including lymphoid interstitial pneumonitis, obliterative bronchiolitis, and bronchitis. The differentiation between scleroderma and Sjögren's syndrome as the cause of pulmonary disease is of some practical importance as lymphoid interstitial pneumonitis seems to be relatively sensitive to treatment.

Investigations play a key part in the management of lung involvement in scleroderma. Their aim is to categorize the type of lung disease, determine its severity and ascertain the presence of an ongoing inflammatory response. This is not a simple process because of the invasive nature of open lung biopsy methods, and the limitations of other pulmonary investigations. Transbronchial biopsies have no real place in the investigation of these processes and there are inherent difficulties in many other respiratory investigations. These include lack of sensitivity (e.g. chest X-ray: CXR), incapacity to differentiate fibrosis from inflammation (e.g. CXR, respiratory function tests), and lack of standardization and technical difficulty (bronchoalveolar lavage). A variety of investigations are therefore performed, the most useful, of which include respiratory function studies, high resolution computerized tomography (CT), and gallium lung scanning. The bronchoalveolar lavage is particularly useful, but only where there is experience both in its performance and sample analysis. If pulmonary hypertension is suspected, echocardiography is helpful. If mild tricuspid incompetence is present it is possible to estimate pulmonary artery pressure non-invasively.

Interstitial lung disease

This is the commonest cause of severe morbidity and mortality in scleroderma. It is characterized by decrease in lung volumes and gas diffusion (D_{LCO}), increased gallium lung uptake, an alveolar pattern of change on high resolution CT scan, and abnormal bronchoalveolar lavage. CXR will often be normal except late in the disease.

Bronchoalveolar lavage has been particularly useful in providing an analysis of the types of abnormalities present in the lung in scleroderma. It shows increased cellularity and an increased percentage of either neutrophils (increased from 0–1% to 5–10%) or lymphocytes (increased from 20–30% to 40–60%). These two patterns tend to be mutually exclusive. The lymphoid interstitial pneumonitis pattern, at least in some instances may represent lung disease secondary to Sjögren's syndrome and not scleroderma. It is generally felt to carry a somewhat better prognosis and there is less impairment of the D_{LCO}. The neutrophilic alveolitis is probably directly attributable to scleroderma and is associated with greater depression of D_{LCO}.

Both the anti-Scl-70 antibody and the HLA haplotype DR3/DRW52a represent a significant genetic risk factor for the development of pulmonary fibrosis in scleroderma. The presence of both carries a relative risk of 16.7 for the development of pulmonary fibrosis.

Pulmonary histopathological changes are indistinguishable from those of cryptogenic fibrosing alveolitis. They consist of an increased number of intra-alveolar macrophages with occasional neutrophils and lymphocytes and an interstitial infiltrate with lymphocytes and plasma cells. A variable amount of fibrosis is also present and any pulmonary vascular changes are confined to parts of the lung affected by the interstitial process. The unaffected regions or lobes, when examined by electron microscopy are often ultrastructurally abnormal.

Treatment

In rare selected cases lung transplantation may be feasible for end-stage disease.

Pulmonary hypertension

Pulmonary hypertension occurs as a consequence of severe interstitial lung disease or as a 'primary' phenomenon. This section deals specifically with the latter group. Estimates suggest it occurs in up to 10% of scleroderma subjects, particularly in those who have a centromere antibody and the limited form of the disease. Early pulmonary hypertension is suggested by a markedly depressed D_{LCO} (often less than 50% of predicted), which is out of proportion to changes of an interstitial pulmonary process such as decrease in lung volumes. In some instances echocardiography may provide further evidence of pulmonary vascular disease, but direct measurement of pulmonary artery pressure by cardiac catheterization is required for unequivocal confirmation.

While the aetiology of pulmonary hypertension is not well understood, the identification of a family of potent endothelial-derived vasospastic and smooth muscle proliferative compounds, the endothelins, has suggested a part for them in this disorder. The endothelins probably also play a part in the more generalized vascular disease of scleroderma. Raised endothelin levels are seen in scleroderma generally but are more elevated in those with pulmonary vascular disease. Additionally, there is evidence for its local production within the lung in this condition. This suggests that endothelin release from the pulmonary vasculature may cause pulmonary vasoconstriction and eventual proliferation of arterial smooth muscle cells leading to pulmonary hypertension.

Treatment

While vasodilators, including prostaglandins are often tried, there is currently no satisfactory treatment for pulmonary hypertension and most patients die within 2 years of diagnosis. In rare individual cases heart/lung transplantation may also be a feasible option.

Bronchiolitis

This probably occurs in 13–25% of scleroderma patients and is frequently asymptomatic. The usual indication of the presence of small airways disease is a decrease in the maximal mid-expiratory flow rate (MMEFR). While smoking is a common confounding cause of a depressed MMEFR, this test is not markedly affected by interstitial pulmonary disease.

There is some evidence for an association of a depressed MMEFR with a bronchoalveolar lavage lymphocytosis, perhaps because of washout of these cells from the terminal airways. The dominant association of bronchiolitis may well be with Sjögren's syndrome rather than scleroderma itself.

Histopathological confirmation of small airways disease can sometimes be undertaken successfully by transbronchial biopsy. Microscopic changes include chronic submucosal inflammatory infiltrate affecting mainly the terminal and respiratory bronchioles with variable bronchiolar metaplasia, fibrous scarring, and luminal constriction.

Treatment

If treatment is necessary, there is some evidence that the bronchiolitis may be responsive to corticosteroids.

Cardiac disease

Cardiac involvement is another important determinant of mortality in scleroderma. It is most commonly asymptomatic and occurs in about 50–80% of subjects. It is commonly manifest by conduction abnormalities, less frequently ventricular dysfunction, and uncommonly pericardial effusions. The conduction abnormalities of scleroderma are most likely due to primary disease of the conduction pathways, rather than a consequence of cardiomyopathy. Clinically significant cardiomyopathies are uncommon.

Like other arterial beds, the coronary vasculature in scleroderma patients also displays an increased sensitivity to cold. This may manifest as angina, or simply abnormalities of cardiac perfusion or function. It has been suggested that recurrent insults of this type may lead to the cardiac fibrosis observed histologically.

Histopathologically, the cardiac lesion is characterized by patchy fibrosis and occasionally inflammatory infiltrates. It is not known whether similar to scleroderma elsewhere, the fibrosis is usually preceded by inflammatory changes.

Treatment

Arrhythmias are treated on their own merits. At least on a short-term basis, cold-induced changes in coronary vasculature may be corrected by nifedipine.

Inflammatory cardiomyopathies may be treated as discussed in, or rarely by cardiac transplantation.

Renal disease

This complication manifests usually as malignant hypertension which can cause headaches, visual symptoms, cardiac failure, seizures, and ultimately renal failure and death. The onset is usually sudden and often accompanied by a rapid deterioration in renal function. This is an uncommon complication that seems to have decreased in prevalence in recent years. It has been suggested that advances in the treatment of hypertension over the last 20 years, especially the use of angiotensin-converting enzyme inhibitors, may have favourably influenced the development of malignant hypertension in this disorder.

The histopathological abnormality is essentially that of scleroderma vascular disease (described previously) involving the small arteries and arterioles.

Treatment

The advent of powerful antihypertensive agents, especially the angiotensin-converting enzyme inhibitors, have made a dramatic difference to the outlook of patients with this complication. Organ transplantation has been successfully undertaken if renal failure results.

Musculoskeletal disease

Bone resorption

Osteolysis is a frequent feature of severe acral disease and usually affects the fingers causing resorption (Fig. 25.7). It can rarely affect other bones and is presumed to occur on the basis of impairment of blood supply.

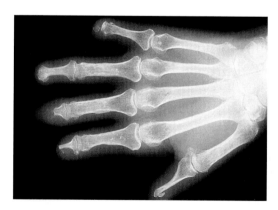

▌ **Fig. 25.7** Hand X-ray of a patient with scleroderma showing erosion of distal phalanges.

Myositis

Myositis is an uncommon occurrence and is usually of mild degree. Pain and stiffness is commoner than major limitation of proximal muscle function. In contrast to polymyositis, it is usually responsive to corticosteroids, often in low doses.

Arthritis

Deformity and limitation of movement, especially in the hands, occurs with some frequency due largely to contractures. True inflammatory arthritis is less common and usually responds to non-steroidal anti-inflammatory drugs or low doses of corticosteroids

Immunological abnormalities

Using the standard immunofluorescence assay significant titres of antinuclear antibodies detected are negative in many patients with scleroderma. More sophisticated assessment of antibodies to nuclear protein components suggests that antinuclear antibodies of various types are probably present in most if not all scleroderma patients (Fig. 25.8). The two most widely detected antibodies are those directed at topoisomerase I (Scl-70) and the centromere which identify mutually exclusive groups of patients. The Scl-70 antibody is associated with the diffuse variant of scleroderma and carries a worse prognosis. The centromere antibody is found in those with limited scleroderma and is associated with vasospastic phenomena including pulmonary hypertension.

More recently, other antinuclear antibodies have also been detected that are not yet widely used in clinical practice. These include anti-Th ribonuclear protein antibody associated with limited scleroderma and anti-PM-Scl associated with a scleroderma–polymyositis overlap syndrome. Of most significance are antibodies to RNA polymerase I, II, and III, which all co-associate. Antibody to RNA polymerase III is highly specific for scleroderma being found in about 50% of those with diffuse disease and rarely in those with limited disease. It does not co-associate with the Scl-70 antibody or any of the other scleroderma specific antibodies, suggesting that it identifies a separate disease subset. It tends to be associated with a lesser frequency of major organ involvement than the Scl-70 antibody, which is found in 30% of patients with diffuse scleroderma.

Markers of inflammation, the acute phase proteins, are often either normal or mildly elevated. Sometimes, however, there is clear evidence of a marked

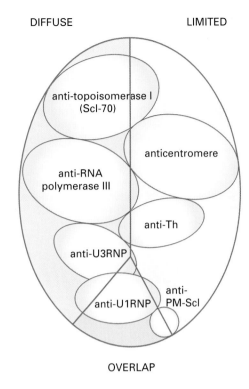

▌ **Fig. 25.8** Distribution of autoantibodies in scleroderma.

inflammatory response and at least one study of early disease suggests that this identifies a poor prognosis group.

Treatment

Controlled therapeutic studies of scleroderma are difficult to perform because of the low prevalence of this condition, the presence of disease subsets, the scarcity of objective and readily quantifiable markers of disease activity or good surrogate markers, and the difficulty of obtaining patients early in the course of their illness. Late-stage, largely fibrotic, disease may be unresponsive to therapy, whereas early inflammatory disease may quite sensitive to anti-inflammatory drugs. Thus far, penicillamine is the only drug widely used in the therapy of the pathogenic processes of scleroderma. It has been shown to improve the degree and extent of skin thickening and the D_{LCO}. However, it is not effective in all subjects and its action is slow. By and large it is not sufficiently powerful for aggressive and rapidly progressive manifestations of severe scleroderma. Because of its frequency and life-threatening nature interstitial lung disease is the complication of most concern in this regard. There is a small double-blind study of immunosuppression with chlorambucil suggesting no efficacy and there are anecdotal reports and small studies suggesting the efficacy of immuno-suppression with drugs such as prednisone and cyclophosphamide, methotrexate, or cyclosporin. Other modalities under trial and of possible benefit include IFNγ and -α, and photophoresis. In the absence of clear guidelines, and when faced with a patient with aggressive scleroderma, many clinicians experienced in the treatment of this disorder would recommend immunosuppression.

While at this stage successful, strategies for the modification of the inflammatory/fibrotic process of scleroderma are limited, in many instances symptomatic therapy can greatly improve quality of life. These approaches include vasodilator therapy, treatment of oesophageal reflux, and improvement of bowel motility; and these are discussed in the appropriate chapters of this section.

Further reading

Lotti T., and Cerinic, M. M. (ed.) (1994). Elsevier *Clinics in dermatology*, New York.

Current Opinion in Rheumatology (1992) Vol. 4, No. 6.

Current Opinion in Rheumatology (1993) Vol. 5, No. 6.

Current Opinion in Rheumatology (1991) Vol. 3, No. 6.

Gay, S., Trabandt, A., Moreland, L. W., and Gay, R. E. (1992). Growth factors, extracellular matrix, and oncogenes in scleroderma. *Arthritis and Rheumatism*, **35**, 304–10.

Mauch, C., Eckes, B., Hunzelmann, N., Oono, T., Kozlowska, E., and Krieg, T. (1993). Control of fibrosis in systemic scleroderma. *Journal of Investigative Dermatology*, **100**, 92–6S.

Silman, A. J. (1992). Pregnancy and scleroderma. *American Journal of Reproductive Immunology*, **28**, 238–40.

26 Sjögren's syndrome

T. P. Gordon and M. Reichlin

Definition

Sjögren's syndrome (SS) is a common inflammatory autoimmune disorder characterized by lymphocytic infiltration and destruction of exocrine glands, notably the lacrimal and salivary glands giving rise to dry eyes (keratoconjunctivitis sicca: KCS) and dry mouth (xerostomia). SS may exist on its own (primary SS) or in association with other autoimmune diseases when it is called secondary SS. The secondary form is usually associated with rheumatoid arthritis but can also occur with systemic lupus erythematosus (SLE), progressive systemic sclerosis, inflammatory myopathies, overlap syndromes, and primary biliary cirrhosis.

Introduction

Other features of SS include systemic or extraglandular involvement (particularly in the primary type) and generalized lymphoproliferation which may terminate as a malignant lymphoma. Primary SS affects women more often than men in a ratio of 9:1 and can develop at any age from 15 to 65 years. It is associated with human leucocyte antigen (HLA) DR3 and the linked gene HLA B8. In secondary SS the age and sex distribution and immunogenetics follow that of the associated disease.

Pathogenesis

The cause of SS and the mechanisms of lymphocytic infiltration and glandular destruction are unknown. Several viruses have been implicated including Epstein–Barr virus, vesicular stomatitis virus, hepatitis C virus, human immunodeficiency virus (HIV) 1 and human T-cell lymphotrophic virus, but rigorous proof is lacking. There appears to be little self-tolerance to sequestered autoantigens such as Ro and La in the B- or T-cell compartments. Whatever the initiating agent (viral, chemical, or other), it is hypothesized that epithelial cell injury is an early event leading to up-regulation of major histocompatibility complex (MHC) class II molecules and presentation of self (e.g. La) or foreign (e.g. viral) antigens to CD4+ T cells. Release and uptake of sequestered La/Ro RNPs by antigen-presenting cells (APC) and B cells would also allow presentation of La and Ro peptides to CD4+ T cells, production of cytokines [interleukin (IL) 2 and γ interferon] and generation of anti-Ro/La autoantibodies (Fig. 26.1). Release of cytokines such as IL-1 and tumour necrosis factor from epithelial cells and APC would contribute to the lymphocytic infiltration and tissue damage. Circulating immune complexes (e.g. Ro/anti-Ro) may be involved in tissue damage in both glandular and extraglandular sites.

Clinical features and diagnosis

Ocular symptoms include a gritty sensation, soreness, and photosensitivity as well as dry eyes. Schirmer's test can be used to estimate tear secretion (less than 5 mm wetting of filter strip in 5 min is considered abnormal). The diagnosis of KCS is confirmed by detecting corneal epithelial erosions on Rose Bengal and slit-lamp examination. Most patients complain of a dry mouth and may also note lip-cracking, oral soreness, and difficulty in swallowing dry food. Dryness of the upper airways may result in persistent cough or hoarseness. Several methods are available to assess salivary gland involvement but the simplest is to weigh a sponge before and after it has been placed in the mouth for 2 min (the Saxon test).

Intermittent swelling of the parotid glands occurs in about one-third of patients whereas persistent

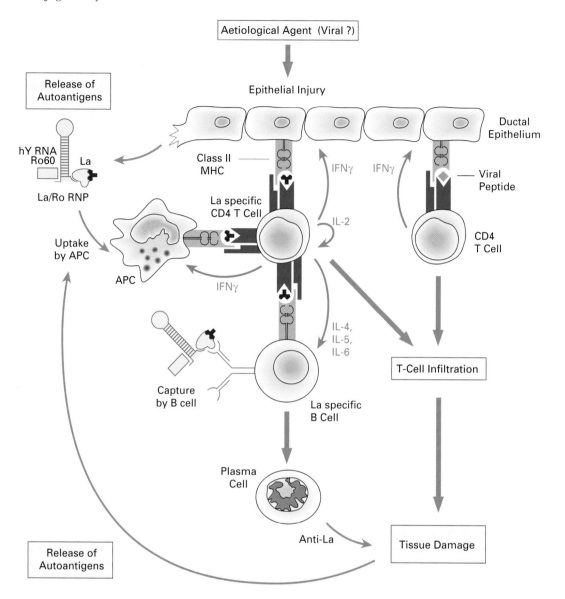

∎ **Fig. 26.1** Schematic representation of the pathogenesis of Sjögren's syndrome. Epithelial cell injury leads to upregulation of major histocompatibility complex (MHC) class II molecules and presentation of self (La) or foreign (viral) peptides to CD4+ T cells. Released La/Ro RNPs are internalized and processed by antigen-presenting cells (APC) and antigen-specific B cells with additional presentation of La peptide–MHC class II complexes. Spreading of the response to Ro following initiation of immunity to La may occur via capture of La/Ro RNPs by Ro-specific B cells and presentation of La determinants to primed La-specific T cells (or vice versa).

enlargement should raise the possibility of malignancy (Fig. 26.2). Other causes of salivary gland enlargement include acute and chronic infections, sarcoidosis, and tumours. Histological evidence of salivary gland involvement in SS is best obtained by minor salivary gland (labial) biopsy. Parotid gland biopsy is indicated if malignancy is expected. There is a lymphocytic infiltrate by mature lymphocytes and occasional plasma cells into the salivary gland lobules with occasional germinal centre formation and variable acinar

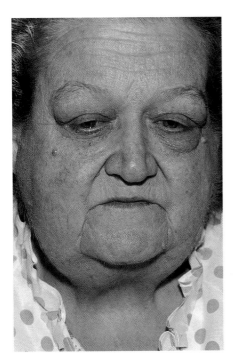

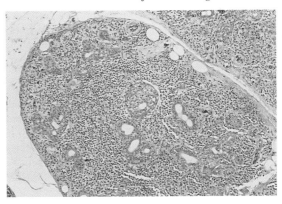

▌ **Fig. 26.3** Labial salivary gland biopsy showing lymphocytic infiltration and epimyoepithelial islands of ectasia in the ducts. The lobular architecture is preserved.

▌ **Fig. 26.2** Sjögren's syndrome. Facial appearance due to enlarged salivary glands especially involving the parotid glands. Subsequent biopsy revealed non-Hodgkins lymphoma.

obliteration. Proliferative and metastatic changes occur in the ductal cells with the formation of epimyoepithelial islands which when seen are pathognomic of the disease. The lobular architecture is generally preserved helping in differentiation from lymphoma (Fig. 26.3).

A number of other organ systems can be involved in SS and are responsible for many of its clinical manifestations (Table 26.1). Hypokalaemia and metabolic acidosis are occasionally seen with overt renal tubular acidosis. Interstitial cystitis has recently been recognized as a feature of the disease. Pulmonary abnormalities are common but may be of little clinical significance. The exact prevalence of central nervous system involvement is unknown, but both focal and diffuse presentations have been reported. Raynaud's phenomenon, non-erosive arthritis, purpuric vasculitis, and cryoglobulinaemia may be observed in primary SS. A past history of adverse drug reactions particularly to antibiotics is frequently obtained. Myositis in SS may be distinctive with a normal or slightly elevated creatine phosphokinase and a biopsy which shows either vasculitis or perivascular infiltrates.

In clinical practice the diagnosis of primary SS is strongly suggested by the characteristic signs and symptoms of KCS and xerostomia together with laboratory evidence of autoantibodies (anti-Ro; anti-La;

▌ **Table 26.1** Extraglandular features of Sjögren's syndrome

	Symptoms
Respiratory	Nasal crusting; tracheobronchitis; peribronchial lymphatic infiltration; lymphocytic interstitial pneumonitis; interstitial fibrosis
Renal	Renal tubular acidosis; interstitial nephritis; glomerulonephritis; interstitial cystitis
Neurological	Organic brain syndromes; focal events such as hemiparesis, visual loss; ataxia and transverse myelitis; aseptic meningitis; sensory and motor peripheral neuropathy; myositis
Gastrointestinal tract	Dysphagia; primary biliary cirrhosis; chronic active hepatitis; recurrent pancreatitis; atrophic gastritis
Articular	Arthralgia; non-erosive arthritis
Other	Thyroiditis; Raynaud's phenomenon; normocytic anaemia; purpuric vasculitis; monoclonal gammopathies; cryoglobulinaemia; lymphoproliferative disorders

rheumatoid factor); and by the exclusion of other causes of glandular enlargement and ocular and oral dryness. In some patients it may be necessary to confirm the diagnosis by demonstrating extensive lymphocytic infiltration on minor salivary gland biopsy.

A diagnosis of secondary SS is made when there are sufficient clinical features to diagnose another autoimmune rheumatic disease such as rheumatoid arthritis, SLE, or systemic sclerosis. Patients with SLE and SS share many of the clinical features of primary SS and have similar serological and immunogenetic characteristics. For this reason the term SS/SLE overlap is often used.

SS should be considered an autoimmune disorder and distinguished from age-related atrophy of salivary glands occurring in elderly subjects. In contrast to SS, these older patients with sicca symptoms do not have an inflammatory infiltrate on salivary gland biopsy or serological abnormalities, such as anti-Ro or anti-La autoantibodies.

Immunological findings

Common serological findings include polyclonal hyperglobulinaemia, presence of rheumatoid factors and a raised erythrocyte sedimentation rate (ESR). The C-reactive protein is generally normal but is elevated in patients with vasculitis. Mixed cryoglobulinaemia with monoclonal rheumatoid factors correlates with the presence of extraglandular disease, low serum C4 levels, and anti-Ro (SS-A) antibodies.

A number of organ-specific autoantibodies are found including antisalivary duct, antithyroid, and antigastric parietal cell antibodies.

Antibodies to the extractable nuclear antigens Ro (SS-A) and La (SS-B) are a feature of primary SS and SS/SLE. The two responses are strongly linked, reflecting the structural association of the Ro and La proteins in ribonucleoprotein complexes (RNP). The reported prevalence of these two autoantibodies varies among different centres, but anti-La appear to be relatively specific for primary SS while anti-Ro antibodies may occur in patients with other systemic rheumatic diseases. Anti-Ro antibodies with or without anti-La are associated with vasculitis, photosensitivity, hyperglobulinaemia, rheumatoid factor, HLA-DQ1/DQ2 heterozygosity, and congenital heart block. These autoantibodies are often detected in SS/SLE overlap syndrome but are uncommon in RA with secondary SS. There are two Ro molecules of Mr 60 and 52 kDa; the majority of anti-Ro sera from SS patients react with both forms. Anti-Ro sera which have accompanying precipitins to the U1 RNP particle react almost exclusively with the 60 kDa Ro molecule. Virtually all patients with this profile have SLE.

The majority of the salivary gland lymphocytes are CD4+ T cells with a smaller number of CD8+ T cells and B cells. MHC class II antigens are present on the CD4+ T cells and epithelial cells. Clonally expanded B cells may be detected as immunoglobulin gene rearrangements on Southern blotting. In the sicca syndrome observed rarely with HIV-1 infection there is an infiltration of the salivary glands with a predominance of CD8+ T cells.

Treatment and prognosis

Many patients with SS have sicca symptoms alone which can be managed with tear substitutes, lubricating eye ointments, skin lotions, and oral fluoride. Stomatitis, dental caries, and oral candidiasis (without obvious white fungal plaques) are common complications of xerostomia. No treatments have been shown to alter the natural history of primary SS but the prognosis is generally better than rheumatoid arthritis or SLE. Patients with systemic vasculitis and cryoglobulinaemia may require corticosteroids and immunosuppressives, but the role of these agents in cutaneous vasculitis and lung and neurological complications is unclear. Patients with mild systemic features (fatigue, joint symptoms, and an elevated ESR or C-reactive protein) may benefit from a non-steroidal anti-inflammatory drug or antimalarial therapy. In secondary SS the underlying disease should be treated accordingly. Patients with SS may develop extensive lymphocytic infiltration with CD4+ T cells and present with lymphadenopathy, splenomegaly, and organ involvement. The term pseudolymphoma has been used to describe those lesions which disrupt normal architecture but do not meet histological criteria for malignancy. The risk for developing non-Hodgkin's lymphoma is increased by a factor of 44. They are usually of B-lymphocyte origin, can occur in glandular or extraglandular sites, and may be heralded by falling levels of serum immunoglobulins and autoantibodies.

Further reading

Aziz, K. E., Montanaro, A., McCluskey, P. J., and Wakefield, D. (1992). Sjögren's syndrome: review with recent insights into pathogenesis. *Australian and New Zealand Journal of Medicine*, **22**, 671–8.

Fox, R. I., and Kang, H-I. (1992). Pathogenesis of Sjögren's syndrome. *Rheumatic Disease Clinics of North America*, **18**, 517–40.

Fox, R. I., Howell, F. V., Bone, R. C., and Michelson, P. (1984). Primary Sjögren's syndrome: clinical and immunopathologic features. *Seminars in Arthritis and Rheumatism*, **14**, 77–105.

Gordon, T., Topfer, F., Keech, C., Reynolds, P., Chen, W., Rischmueller, M., and McCluskey, J. (1994). How does autoimmunity to La and Ro initiate and spread? *Autoimmunity*, **18**, 87–92.

Smith, D. L. and Lucas, L. M. (1987). Sjögren's syndrome. *Postgraduate Medicine*, **82**, 123–31.

Talal, N. (1989). Sjögren's syndrome. *Clinical Aspects of Autoimmunity*, **1**, 7–18.

27 Rheumatoid arthritis

P. J. Roberts-Thomson and R. N. Maini

Definition

Rheumatoid arthritis (RA) is a chronic systemic autoimmune disorder of unknown aetiology whose main clinical manifestation is a symmetrical polyarthritis. The disease preferentially affects females and the peak age of onset is in the fourth and fifth decade. X-rays of involved joints characteristically show soft tissue swelling, marginal bony erosions, and loss of articular cartilage. Immunoglobulin (Ig) M rheumatoid factor (RF), an autoantibody reactive against the Fc fragment of IgG, is observed in 80% of patients. There is no known cure for RA, but effective suppression of the inflammatory synovitis or extra-articular manifestations is possible. The term 'rheumatoid disease', in contrast with 'rheumatoid arthritis' emphasizes the multisystem nature of this autoimmune disorder.

Introduction

Historical

RA appears to be a disease of modern times with the first complete description being ascribed to the Parisian A. Landre-Beauvais (1772–1840) in 1800. A. Garrod coined the term rheumatoid arthritis in 1858 to distinguish it from the well characterized gouty arthritis and other forms of rheumatism including rheumatic fever and osteoarthritis. Another name for RA common at that time was arthritis deformans, the name emphasizing the destructive changes seen in the joints. Before the eighteenth century little evidence can be found to suggest the prior recognition of RA either in contemporary medical or popular literature or in works of art. Furthermore, extensive archaeological examination of skeletal remains from earlier times has also not supported the existence of RA in medieval

Europe. However, there is some palaeopathological evidence that in ancient times, a symmetrical, erosive, and deforming arthritis may have occurred in North American native populations and this has led to the speculation that RA may be an infectious disorder transmitted to the Old World by the returning Spanish conquistadors.

Prevalence

RA has a worldwide distribution but the prevalence varies depending on the population studied. In studies involving Caucasians the prevalence varies from 1 to 3% (generally closer to 1%) but lower figures are reported for Chinese and Asians. In rural eastern South Africa the prevalence for black Africans is very low and when the disease occurs it appears mild in nature. Higher frequencies are found for urban black populations in these regions. There is some evidence that the prevalence figures for RA in Europe may be declining in females, while for each subsequent generation the mean age of onset may be increasing. The incidence of RA is approximately 1/10 of the prevalence rate and females are more likely to be affected than males with the ratio being 3:1. Felty's syndrome, while relatively common in Caucasians with RA, is very rare in black populations.

Pathogenesis

Current dogma views RA as a systemic autoimmune disorder in which unknown trigger factor(s) initiate, in genetically susceptible individuals, an immune hypersensitivity response which occurs predominantly in synovial linings (Fig. 27.1). This immune response involves a variety of immune and inflammatory effector mechanisms which lead to gross joint inflammation with subsequent bone and cartilage destruction, which are the pathological hallmarks of RA.

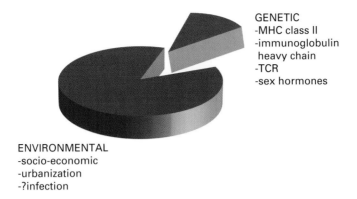

GENETIC
-MHC class II
-immunoglobulin
 heavy chain
-TCR
-sex hormones

ENVIRONMENTAL
-socio-economic
-urbanization
-?infection

∎ **Fig. 27.1** Identified genetic and environmental factors in rheumatoid arthritis. MHC, major histocompatibility complex; TCR, T-cell receptor.

A full understanding of the pathogenesis of RA requires a detailed knowledge of the cellular, humoral, and molecular mechanisms involved in inflammation and in immunological hypersensitivity.

Genetic factors

Population, family, and twin studies have demonstrated the involvement of genetic factors in the predisposition to RA with possibly 30% of the expression of RA being explicable by the operation of these genetic factors (Table 27.1). Genetic factors are also involved in the phenotype (or severity) of the disease. Most emphasis has been on the major histocompatibility

∎ **Table 27.1** Comparison of concordance rates (CR) for classical and definite rheumatoid arthritis related to the presence of risk factors

Risk factor	Value (%)
Male population prevalence	0.7
Female population prevalence	1.6
Male sibship CR	3.0
Sibling CR	4.9
Dizygotic twin CR	5.0
Female sibship CR	9.3
HLA identical sibship of the same sex CR	15.5
Seropositive HLA identical sibship of the same sex CR	20.5
Seropositive monozygotic twin CR	30.0

HLA, human leucocyte antigen.

complex (MHC) found on the short arm of chromosome 6; however, other genetic loci linked with RA are known including those coding for the immunoglobulin heavy chain, T-cell receptor and genes involved in the production of sex hormones.

Human leucocyte antigen (HLA) class II loci in the MHC appears to be particularly important and may account for 37% of the genetic factors involved. Early studies demonstrated an association of RA with HLA-DR4 (British, Asian, Japanese, Maoris, North Indians, Latin American, Mexican, and American blacks) and DR1 (Israeli Jews and Indians), although both these associations seemed to be absent in Greek rheumatoid patients.

Furthermore, the more severe cases of RA, especially those with systemic complications such as vasculitis and Felty's syndrome, were even more likely to be DR4 than patients with less aggressive disease confined to joints.

Mixed leucocyte culture typing and DNA analysis has now defined several HLA-DR4 subtypes. It is of considerable interest that while the subtypes HLA-Dw4 and -Dw14 are associated with RA in several studies, Dw15 is only associated with RA in the Japanese, while Dw10 and Dw13 are not associated with RA in any ethnic group. A recent study has also shown that in DR4 homozygotes Dw4/Dw14 individuals develop more severe RA than Dw4/Dw4.

At the phenotypic level, the importance of HLA class II molecules lies in their participation in a trimolecular reaction involving the HLA antigen-binding cleft formed by the α and β chains of an antigen-presenting cell (APC) binding to a processed linear

∎ **Table 27.2**   HLA-DR associations with RA defined by DR β_1 sequence positions 70–74

DR type	Sequence					Association with RA
	70	**71**	**72**	**73**	**74**	
DR4						
W4	Q	K	R	A	A	positive
W14	Q	R	R	A	A	positive
W15	Q	R	R	A	A	positive
DR1	Q	R	R	A	A	positive
DR4						
W10	D	E	R	A	A	negative
W13	Q	R	R	A	E	negative

Q, glutamine; K, lysine; R, arginine; A, alanine; D, aspartic acid; E, glutamic acid; HLA, human leucocyte antigen; RA, rheumatoid arthritis.

peptide antigen usually between nine and fifteen amino acids, and the HLA–antigen complex in turn binding to the variable portion of the T-cell receptor.

Nucleotide sequencing of HLA-DR $\beta1$ exons coding amino acid residues 70–74 has revealed that HLA-DR4 subtypes -Dw4, -Dw14 and -Dw15 share similarities with each other (with a conservative substitution of glutamine with lysine at position 71 in Dw4) and with HLA-DR1 (Table 27.2). The sequence predicts susceptibility to RA and, for example, is associated with RA in 83% of Caucasians in Britain. In contrast, negative associations are observed in individuals who are DR4-w10, in whom the positively charged basic amino acids glutamine and arginine in positions 70 and 71 are replaced by the negatively charged acidic amino acids aspartic and glutamic acid. In Dw13 individuals, in whom a negative association is also observed, arginine is substituted for glutamic acid in position 74. Molecular modelling studies suggest that amino acid residues 70–74 are located in the α-helix forming the wall of the peptide binding groove, and thus likely to be involved in antigen binding. Acidic substitutions could profoundly alter protein structure and thereby alter affinity for peptide antigens.

These findings have lent support to the shared epitope hypothesis, i.e. the susceptibility to RA is related to a shared epitope (common structural configuration) on the class II molecule. This hypothesis is supported by the co-segregation of susceptible HLA class II phenotypes detected by monoclonal antibodies. However, whether the susceptibility to RA is due to permissive binding of specific peptides such as those on autoantigens or on environmental antigens, whether superantigens may initiate disease by binding specifically to the HLA molecules, or whether selection or tolerance of the T-cell repertoire are also involved, remains to be elucidated.

Environmental factors

Little is known concerning the presumed environmental factors in the aetiopathogenesis of RA. RA is more common in urbanized tribal South African blacks compared with their rural cousins and, as is found in a number of chronic rheumatic disorders and is more common in people in lower socio-economic classes. Many infectious agents have been implicated in the aetiopathogenesis of RA. These include Epstein–Barr virus (EBV), *Mycobacterium* tuberculosis, mycoplasma, *Proteus mirabilis*, rubella virus, parvo virus, and retroviruses. However, time and space clustering of cases has not been clearly demonstrated arguing against an infectious agent.

Other studies have sought to implicate infectious microbes by seeking evidence of immune hyperreactivity to these microbiological antigens. EBV is of special interest in that RA patients seem to demonstrate impaired cellular immunity with enhanced antibody levels and an induced RA nuclear antigen (RANA) to this DNA virus but these associations do not explain the occurrence of RA in patients who have never been infected with EBV or why only a small proportion of patients infected with this ubiquitous virus go on to develop RA.

Autoimmunity

Evidence in favour of RA being a systemic autoimmune disorder includes the preferential occurrence in females during their child-bearing years, a family history of other systemic autoimmune disease, RA showing MHC restriction, the presence of a variety of circulating antibodies including RF, antinuclear antibody, antiperinuclear antibody, antikeratin antibody, and antibodies against native type II collagen, the presence of immune pathology in affected tissues (e.g. infiltration of synovium with T cells showing evidence of cellular activation), the response to immunosuppresive or immunomodulating drugs (e.g. cyclosporin) or techniques which deplete the body of T cells and the amelioration of symptoms in RA patients infected with the T-cell cytotrophic human immunodeficiency virus. All these clinical and pathological features strongly support an autoimmune basis for the occurrence and progression of RA. However, the explanation for the loss of immune tolerance and the disordered immunoregulation in these patients is still not understood.

Pathology

Synovitis, pannus formation, cartilage loss, and *bony erosions* are the major pathological hallmarks of RA while a variety of extra-articular manifestations can also be observed.

Synovitis

RA is a disorder in which inflammation of synovial membranes is a prominent feature. These membranes line synovial joints and tendons and in RA symmetrical involvement is common. The earliest changes include hyperplasia of the synovial lining layer which is normally two cells in depth and contains type A, macrophage-like, cells and type B cells, fibroblast-like, cells secreting hyaluronic acid. New vessel formation in the sublining layer is also an early feature. With time increasing cellularity of the sublining layer occurs with infiltration of lymphocytes, CD4 T cells being predominant and occurring in a perivascular distribution, numerous macrophage-like cells, infrequent B cells but abundant plasma cells.

In some inflamed synovium formation of typical germinal follicles occurs. The advanced inflammatory synovium is a highly vascularized immune tissue with prominent villi projecting into the joint space. The majority of the infiltrating cells and the lining layer demonstrate evidence of activation, their cell surface membranes being rich in HLA class II proteins, adhesion proteins, and receptors for cytokines. Indeed, a common feature of activated cells in general is their augmented production of soluble cytokines and expression of cytokine receptors.

Pannus

The junction between synovial tissue, cartilage, and bone is the site of early erosive damage in RA. This

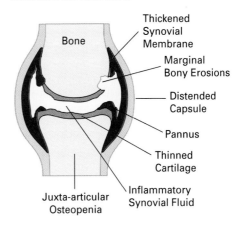

▌ Fig. 27.2   Pathological hallmarks of rheumatoid arthritis.

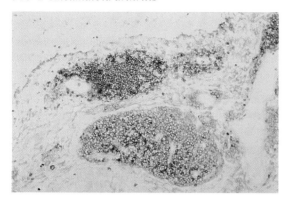

▌ Fig. 27.3 Double label immunohistochemistry of rheumatoid synovium demonstrating infiltrating T cells (blue) and upregulation of major histocompatibility complex class II DR antigen (brown) on some of the T cells and on the synovial macrophage-like cells (courtesy of Dr M. D. Smith).

site becomes filled and overlaid by a blanket vascular tissue termed pannus. The lining layer of pannus is in continuity with the lining layer of hypercellular synovium lining the capsule of joints and has been regarded as being derived from it, although islands of pannus may be seen at sites distant from the margin. The cellular pannus forms a distinct junction with underlying cartilage which shows many characteristics of degradation, including loss of matrix, water content, and chondrocyte depletion. The conventional view is that pannus has an invasive degradative effect on underlying cartilage mediated by the secretions of enzymes such as metalloproteinases. This is associated with further loss of cartilage as a result of enzymatic destruction of matrix by chondrocytes themselves, coupled with a lack of synthesis of newly formed matrix. Pannus also appears to erode adjacent bone by a similar process involving degradation of bone matrix, but in addition involving active bone resorption by osteclasts.

A second type of pannus may also be observed, especially in the marginal area of cartilage in weight-bearing joints. This consists of vascular pannus overlying cartilage with an indistinct intervening multi-layered zone of cells with a 'fibroblastic' morphology. In contrast, the underlying cartilage of this pannus does not show degradative changes with loss of matrix. This type of pannus has been regarded as representing a fibrotic healing phase, but has alternatively been termed a 'transitional' fibroblastic zone because of cytoplasm of these cells contains cartilage components such as keratan sulphate, chondroitin sulphate, and collagen type II. It has been considered that these cells are either derived from chondrocytes as a result of metaplastic changes or are undifferentiated mesenchymal cells. The finding of proinflammatory cytokines capable of cartilage degradation such as interleukin -1 (IL-1) 1 and tumour necrosis factor (TNF) in pannus cells contiguous with cartilage in the invasive type of erosion contrasts with absence of these cytokines in transitional fibroblastic zones. Instead, the latter type of pannus shows the presence of only transforming growth factor (TGF) β, which (as TGFβ stimulates collagen and matrix production) is compatible with the proposal that the tissue is in an anabolic state of healing or differentiation.

Synovial fluid

In active RA the nature and volume of the joint fluid change concomitantly with the inflammation in the synovium. The volume of the fluid increases considerably adding to the clinical swelling of the joint and the fluid is characterized by the presence of inflammatory cells with loss of its normal viscous properties. The predominant cell is the polymorph which paradoxically is only rarely found in the synovial membrane. The polymorph may contribute up to 90% of the total cell count, the remaining cells comprising T cells (CD8+ >CD4+), macrophages, B cells, and dendritic cells. The synovial fluid can be considered a plasma filtrate enriched with locally synthesized proteins and contains most of the plasma proteins, the larger proteins, e.g. IgM, α_2-macroglobulin being proportionally much reduced because of their large size. In synovial inflammation there is some loss of the integrity of this blood–synovial fluid permeability barrier. Locally produced are rheumatoid factor containing immune complexes, complement products, and cytokines and their solubilized receptors particularly those cytokines derived from macrophage or macrophage-like cells (e.g. TNFα, IL-1, IL-6, IL-8, and TGFβ).

Extra-articular manifestations

Local

These are more common in long-standing and severe seropositive cases. Rheumatoid nodules are the commonest, and are found in areas susceptible to trauma, such as elbows and fingers. They consist of a palisade of macrophages surrounding a central area of necrotic debris.

Systemic manifestations

In response to cytokines produced by the inflamed synovium a number of systemic changes occur. These include an acute phase response of the liver induced by IL-6 and IL-1 and characterized by elevation of C-reactive protein (CRP), serum amyloid A and fibrinogen, mild normochromic anaemia and thrombocytosis. Weight loss may occur.

In more severe cases there may be:

(1) vasculitis of venules or small or medium arteries;

(2) fibrosis of lungs which may progress to significant fibrotic impairment of lung function;

(3) granuloma formation characterized by nodule formation;

(4) serositis as characterized by pericarditis and pleurisy, commonly asymptomatic;

(5) Felty's syndrome: enlargement of the spleen with lymphadenopathy, fever, leg ulcers, and susceptibility to bacterial infections due to neutropenia;

(6) lymphadenopathy, particularly of those nodes draining inflamed joints.

Immunopathogenesis

Current concepts concerning the immunopathogenesis of RA are illustrated schematically in Fig. 27.4. It is likely that this scheme will be considerably modified as new knowledge accumulates in coming years.

The earliest changes observed in the rheumatoid synovium include proliferation of the lining synovial cells, formation of new vessels in the sublining layer, and the recruitment to and retention in this layer of a variety of cells of lymphohaematopoietic origin to this layer. Increased expression of a variety of cellular adhesion proteins (e.g. ICAM-1, E-selectin, VCAM-1) is observed on the synvoial endothelium and lining layer and is likely induced by the cytokines TNFα, IL-1, etc. High endothelial venules (HEV) are also found which specifically facilitate the exit of circulating T cells into the synovium. A number of chemokines and chemotactic factors have been identified which provide the molecular signals for this egress from the circulation into the synovium. These include IL-8, a chemokine for polymorphs and T cells, RANTES, a chemokine for memory CD4+ T cells, and monocytes, LTB4, C3a, and C5a chemotactic for polymorphs.

Within the lining synovium it is postulated that APC process antigen and present it in the grove of the MHC class II molecular complex to T cells which bear a receptor (TCR) specific for that antigenic peptide. A number of cell types may act as APCs and these include the plentiful macrophages, the less abundant dendritic cells and B cells, and possibly chondrocytes. The nature of the stimulating antigenic peptide is not known; it could be exogenous from a processed

microbe or endogenous and need not necessarily be constant or uniform during the ongoing immune response. Indeed to date there is little evidence for the presence in the synovium of a specific T-cell idiotype common to all patients and if one were to be detected it would presumably be necessary to investigate patients very early in the disease as a large number of T cells of various specificities are recruited into the synovium during the ongoing immune response.

T cells comprise up to 50% of the cells extracted from inflamed synovial membranes with CD4+ T cells outnumbering CD8+ T cells. The CD4+ cells tend to accumulate as perivascular nodules while CD8 cells are more diffusely scattered. The majority of the CD4 cells are of the primed or memory phenotype (CD2a+ CD45RO+) and bear activation membrane markers, e.g. HLA class II and IL-2 receptor (IL-2R). Most of the T cells contain $\alpha\beta$ TCRs with a small number (but increased relative to blood) of the $\gamma\delta$ receptor. The nature and function of these latter T cells is unclear. The cytokine profile of the CD4+ cells, as determined by polymerase chain reaction (PCR) and analysis of T-cell clones derived from synovium suggests they have some of the characteristics of the Th1 subtype despite a paucity of IL-2, interferon, and TNFβ at protein level. The reason for this discrepancy is not yet known but TGFβ which inhibits cytokine production at a post-translational level, may be responsible. Proinflammatory cytokines (e.g. IL-1, TNFα, IL-8, and IL-10) are abundant in the rheumatoid joint and are predominantly derived from macrophages. The spectrum of cytokines present in joints have pleiotropic effects, displaying a wide variety of actions on many cell types and also demonstrate much redundancy in their biological properties. Important target cells could be monocytes/ macrophages, which are abundant in the deeper layers of the synovial membrane and pannus, but also the lining layer type A and type B cells. These effector cells, on activation, release a wide variety of proinflammatory mediators including prostanoids, proteolytic enzymes, oxygen-derived free radicals, and a wide array of cytokines.

Both proinflammatory, e.g. IL-1, TNFα, and IL-6 and anti-inflammatory, e.g. IL-10 and TGFβ cytokines are found in rheumatoid synovium and synovial fluid (Table 27.3). In addition, an extensive range of cytokine inhibitors are being recognized including soluble TNF receptors and the IL-1 antagonist protein. These cytokines have a local effect influencing cells in the immediate microenvironment but can also circulate and have a systemic effect (e.g. TNFα, IL-6). TNFα appears to be a pivotal inflammatory cytokine and may induce and synergize with other cytokines and has potent effects on endothelium, chondrocytes, osteo-

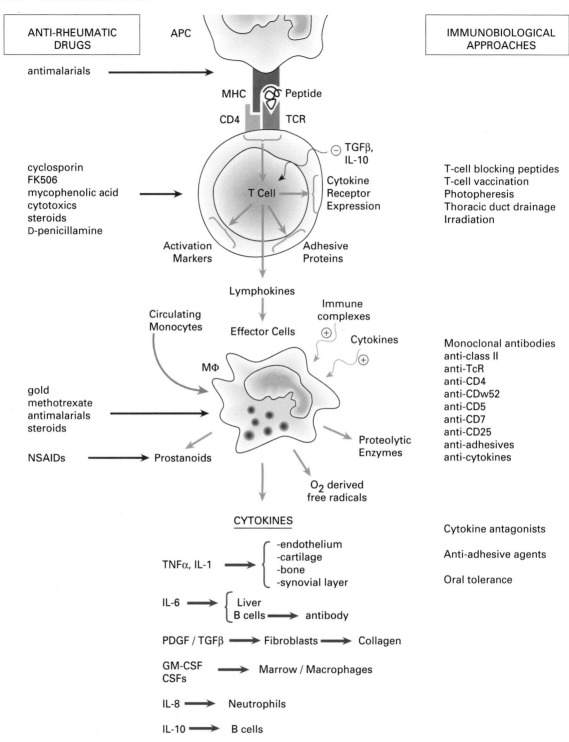

ANTI-RHEUMATIC
DRUGS

APC

IMMUNOBIOLOGICAL
APPROACHES

antimalarials

MHC   Peptide

CD4   TCR

⊖ TGFβ,
IL-10

cyclosporin
FK506
mycophenolic acid
cytotoxics
steroids
D-penicillamine

T Cell

Cytokine
Receptor
Expression

T-cell blocking peptides
T-cell vaccination
Photopheresis
Thoracic duct drainage
Irradiation

Activation
Markers

Adhesive
Proteins

Lymphokines

Circulating
Monocytes

Immune
complexes

Effector Cells   ⊕

⊕ Cytokines

MΦ

gold
methotrexate
antimalarials
steroids

Monoclonal antibodies
anti-class II
anti-TcR
anti-CD4
anti-CDw52
anti-CD5
anti-CD7
anti-CD25
anti-adhesives
anti-cytokines

Proteolytic
Enzymes

NSAIDs   Prostanoids

O₂ derived
free radicals

CYTOKINES

Cytokine antagonists

Anti-adhesive agents

Oral tolerance

TNFα, IL-1   { -endothelium
-cartilage
-bone
-synovial layer

IL-6   { Liver
B cells   antibody

PDGF / TGFβ   Fibroblasts   Collagen

GM-CSF
CSFs   Marrow / Macrophages

IL-8   Neutrophils

IL-10   B cells

∎ **Fig. 27.4**   Immunopathogenesis of rheumatoid arthritis and postulated sites for therapeutic intervention.

▌ **Table 27.3** Factors present at initial evaluation which have been found to influence outcome in patients with rheumatoid arthritis

---

Sociodemographic
  Older age at onset
  Female sex
  Lower level of formal education
  Employment requiring moderate-heavy labour

Clinical
  Insidious onset
  Longer duration of disease at initial visit
  Greater number of joints affected
  Presence of extra-articular features, especially subcutaneous nodules
  Greater degree of physical disability or worse health status or functional class

Laboratory
  Positive test for rheumatoid factor, especially in high titre
  Presence of erosions on joint radiographs
  Elevated erythrocyte sedimentation rate
  Presence of HLA-DR4, especially homozygosity

HLA, human leucocyte antigen.

clasts, and other phagocytic cells. Neutralizing chimeric anti-TNF antibodies have been shown to rapidly suppress synovial inflammation and the systemic manifestations in RA emphasizing the central role of this cytokine in pathogenic networks. The cytokines IL-6 and IL-10 are potent co-stimulatory cytokines for the activation and differentiation of B cells into plasma cells and may facilitate the synthesis of high quantities of RF in the synovium. IL-1 and IL-10 may also activate the CD5 subset of B cells giving rise to the natural antibodies including a range of autoantibodies. Circulating IL-6 is also an important cytokine in inducing an acute phase response in the liver.

With this complex network of cytokines in RA, each having a myriad of biological effects it is important that we have an understanding of the regulation of this network both at the transcriptional level and in the secreted form. Soluble cytokine receptors to most of the cytokines have been described while IL-1 has a specific IL-1 receptor antagonist protein (IL-1 ra). However, the role of all these inhibitors is still uncertain in RA. Furthermore, certain aspects of T-cell function leading to the gross impairment of systemic delayed-type hypersensitivity is noted in active RA. Hence, the regulation of cytokine synthesis and secretion and the nature of natural inhibitors requires further characterization and offer therapeutic potential.

Within the fertile immune environment of the inflamed synovium it is not surprising to find an abundance of plasma cells secreting a variety of antibodies. These include the autoantibodies RF, antiperinuclear factor, and anticollagen II which are closely associated with the rheumatoid disease process together with other antibodies reflecting the recently augmented B-cell repertoire of the host, e.g. tetanus toxoid antibodies following toxoid immunization. Presumably these latter B cells are recruited into the synovium in a non-specific fashion. RF is found in 80% of patients with RA and can be found in all the immunoglobulin classes, namely, IgM, IgG, and IgA. However, routine diagnostic assays usually detect IgM RF because of its potent agglutinating and precipitating activity. In general, there is a good correlation between the presence of IgM RF and IgG RF. RF is not specific for RA as it is found in low or moderate levels in a wide variety of chronic infective and autoimmune disorders. Most healthy subjects will secrete for short periods small quantities of RF (either *in vivo*, or *in vitro* using blood mononuclear cells) following immune stimulation, e.g. immunization. The presence of persisting RF, however, may pre-date the onset of RA and high levels at onset has adverse prognostic significance. Antiperinuclear factor, antikeratin, and anti-RA33 antibodies occur less frequently in RA than RF but are found infrequently in other diseases, i.e. these antibodies show high specificity for the presence of RA. The pathogenic significance of these autoantibodies is uncertain but their importance lies in appearing early in the disease and in a proportion of patients being present in the absence of RF and therefore of diagnostic value.

Finally, high levels of RF containing immune complexes are observed together with polymorphs in the rheumatoid synovial fluid. The immune complexes can activate the complement cascade and the resultant complement breakdown components can act as chemotactic factors facilitating polymorph influx into the synovial fluid. These immune complexes can also activate these phagocytic cells via their Fc and C3b receptors with subsequent release of proteolytic enzymes, prostanoid's and oxygen-free radicals with potential to damage the cartilage. It is known that the half-life of these polymorphs in the joint fluid is only 1–2 days suggesting that the inflamed joint can be considered as a giant graveyard for these inflammatory cells. It is also likely that the immune complexes formed in the joint can escape into the circulation and be responsible for some of the systemic vasculitic manifestations.

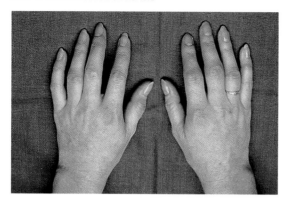

▌ **Fig. 27.5** Early rheumatoid arthritis of hands showing mild swelling of metacarpophalangeal and proximal interphalangeal joints in a symmetrical distribution.

In summary, the pathogenesis of RA involves a complex interplay between the vascular endothelium, the lining synovial layer, the multiple cell types of the immune system and the secretory products of all these cell types. We still do not understand what initiates this disorded immune response and only have a preliminary insight into the regulatory mechanisms of this interplay.

Clinical features

Initial presentation

The initial clinical manifestations of RA are quite variable. A common onset is the insidious development of a symmetrical synovitis involving the metacarpophalangeal (MCP), proximal interphalangeal (PIP), and wrist joints and metatarsophalangeal joint (MTP) of the foot.

Symptoms include pain, stiffness, and swelling. However, redness of the skin overlying involved joints is distinctly unusual in RA and if present should suggest an alternative arthritic disorder, e.g. gout. Prolonged early morning stiffness of variable duration is characteristic of RA and if synovitis involves the small joints of the hand there is difficulty in making a fully closed fist in the period immediately after awakening from sleep. Disease onset involving a wider distribution of small and large joints may also occur, although early involvement of the hip joints is unusual. Involvement of the synovial zygo-apophyseal joints of the upper cervical spine is common but RA rarely involves synovial joints of the lower spine.

Together with joint symptoms, the patients may also complain of general fatigue. With synovitis involving the hand, weakness of hand grip is often noted but this weakness is due to pain and discomfort causing inability to make a strong functional grip, rather than reflecting muscular weakness. Onset in the older patient may be associated with shoulder girdle pain and stiffness and difficulty in turning over in bed at night and in performing the usual daily activities involved in hygiene and grooming. This is called a polymyalgic onset reflecting the similar symptoms found in polymyalgia rheumatica. Occasionally, elderly patients are seen who have an explosive onset of widespread synovitis, evidence of pleuritis, pericarditis, debility, weight loss, and mild fever. This is called a systemic onset. The palindromic onset is also uncommon and consists of acute swelling, pain, and effusion in one or more joints which rapidly settles over several days. These episodes, not necessarily involving the same joint, may re-occur over several years before chronic synovitis develops. Patients with rheumatoid robusta may be seen occasionally, who complain of relatively few symptoms, but have extensive erosive disease.

Initial investigations

Useful investigations in the early phases of patients with suspected RA include a complete blood picture, ESR, antinuclear antibody, RF, CRP, and X-rays of involved joints together with a standard request for X-rays of the hands, wrists, and feet. A complete blood picture may reveal a mild normochromic normocytic anaemia with normal white cell count and a slight to moderate thrombocytosis. The severity of these haematological findings generally reflects the severity of the arthritis. The erythrocyte sedimentation rate is generally elevated and correlates with an elevated CRP, both indices reflecting an acute phase response. The CRP (corrected for the surface area of the involved joints) correlates best with the joint index. RF may be elevated in the early phases of the disease in approximately 75% of patients while the antinuclear antibody is frequently positive and of a homogeneous pattern. X-rays in the early stages may show only soft tissue swelling around involved joints but should be closely examined for small marginal bony erosions or ghosting of the bone margins and for joint cartilage thinning. The earliest erosions are often seen in the feet and examination of the MTP (particularly fifth) may show erosions, even when there is an absence of symptomatic foot discomfort. If a large joint is swollen it may be possible to aspirate synovial fluid for analysis. An increased white cell count (predominantly polymorphonuclear) will confirm the inflammatory nature of the fluid and in RA the synovial fluid white cell count is generally between 5000 and 50 000/mm³. Crystals will be absent and on occasion RF in the joint fluid will be at a higher level than in the corresponding serum suggesting local synthesis of RF in the synovium.

Early differential diagnosis

Differential diagnosis in the early phase of RA is extensive involving many disorders which present with chronic mono-, oligo-, or polyarthritis or with systemic manifestations. With acute monoarthritis it is important to examine the synovial fluid of the involved joints for evidence of crystals and/or infection. In oligoarthritis, a search for clues to psoriasis should be intense, e.g. skin plaques, particularly in the scalp, behind the ear, hair line, natal cleft or umbilicus, nail pits, etc. With an acute or chronic polyarthritis a long list of diagnostic possibilities should be entertained. These include viral infections (e.g. parvo virus, Ross River virus); bacterial infections (e.g. endocarditis or Lyme disease); mycoplasma infections (e.g. Reiter's disease); crystal-induced disease (e.g. chondrocalcinosis); other inflammatory states (e.g. polymyalgia rheumatica, B27-associated arthropathies or reactive arthropathies, various forms of vasculitis, etc.); other connective tissue disorders (e.g. systemic lupus erythematosus); lymphoproliferative disorders (e.g. multiple myeloma and amyloidosis). The finding of an elevated RF in the appropriate clinical situation is a useful confirmatory test for the suspected clinical diagnosis of RA, while the finding of early marginal erosions is characteristic of any inflammatory arthritis including RA (but can occur in other inflammatory arthritides, e.g. psoriatic arthritis).

Natural history and prognostic indicators

The natural history of RA is very variable. In a group of 50 patients with RA (mean aged 33 years, mean duration of symptoms 5 months) who were followed for 5.7 years and who had only minimal or no treatment with disease modifying drugs, three patterns of disease progress were observed (Fig. 27.6). The monocyclic pattern (approximately 10% of patients) seen in patients who have had a single episode of synovitis followed by remission. In contrast, the progressive pattern (approximately 10% of patients) consists of patients who have persistent synovitis with increasing numbers of involved joints over time. The majority (80% of patients) had a polycyclic pattern which could be subdivided into two types, an intermittent type (30%) defined as two or more cycles of synovitis separated by complete remission for at least 6 months and a continuous type (50%) defined as continuing synovitis without complete remission and without increasing involvement of other joints.

Other studies have investigated possible prognostic features at onset. Results of these studies vary according to the group of patients studied (Table 27.4). One of the largest of these outcome studies involves 681 consecutive RA patients studied for a mean period of 11.9 years. The results suggested that in general, older

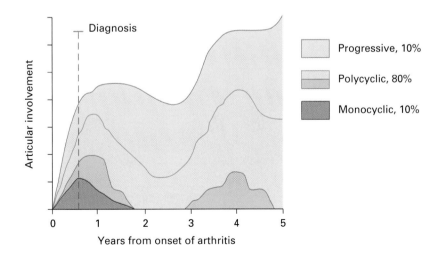

▌**Fig. 27.6**   Patterns of disease progress.

▮ **Table 27.4** Summary of cytokines produced by rheumatoid arthritis synovial cells

Cytokine	mRNA	Protein
IL-1α	+	+
IL-1β	+	+
TNF-α	+	+
LT	+	−
IL-2	+	−
IL-3	−	−
IL-4	?	−
INF-γ	+	−
GM-CSF	+	+
IL-8	+	+
G-CSF	+	?
M-CSF	−	?
TGF-β	+	+
EGF	+	+
PDGF-A	+	+
PDGF-B	+	+

female patients with impaired function, together with high levels of RF or presence of rheumatoid nodules and radiological evidence of extensive erosions have poorer functional outcomes. Age was found to be one of the most powerful predictors of disability. Alternatively, other studies have suggested that an insidious onset with early progression to systemic disease may also signify a worse long-term outcome. Disability and radiological progression appears to develop most rapidly during the first 5 years after disease onset and then assumes a slow linear rate of increase after 10 years (Fig. 27.7). This information has important implications with regard to early intervention with disease modifying drugs. Radiological erosions occur early in the disease (28% of patients show changes by 1 year, 71% by 5 years) and occurs more commonly and at an earlier stage in the feet compared with the hands. Men may have a greater risk of developing rheumatoid nodules, evidence of vasculitis and other extra-articular manifestations and elderly men may also be more prone to an acute severe onset

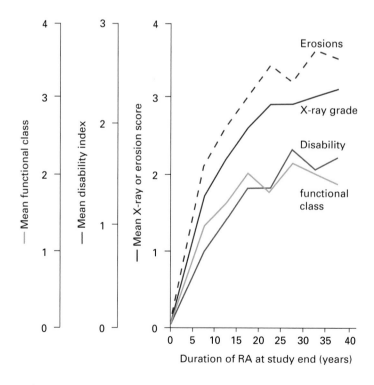

▮ **Fig. 27.7** Rate of disability and radiological progress. RA, rheumatoid arthritis.

which subsequently settles. Patients with RA have a substantially reduced life expectancy (with females dying on average 10 years earlier) and increased morbidity and mortality is associated with arthritis causing severe disability and with arthritis of long duration. These patients have a greater risk of dying from an infective cause. Patients with RA also have increased morbidity and perhaps mortality due to the adverse effects of their drug therapy or surgical intervention.

Clinical outcome

The natural history of RA in many patients involves slow but progressive articular and tendon destruction and development of systemic or extra-articular manifestations. Articular involvement is generally of a symmetrical fashion and involves both large and small synovial joints. The initial joint swelling progresses to gross destruction of the joint with large marginal bony erosions and articular cartilage loss, subluxation, and deformities. This leads to the classical rheumatoid deformity seen in the hands which include the well known features of swan neck or Boutonniere deformity of the digits due to the impairment of the intrinsic muscles of the hand, palmar subluxation at the MCP joint (Fig. 27.8), ulna deviation of the digits and the wrist, wasting of the small muscles of the hand, carpal collapse, presence of features of medial nerve compression at the wrist and flexor tenosynovitis. All these changes characteristically occur in a symmetrical fashion. The disease may also involve larger joints including the cervical spine, wrist, knee, and ankle

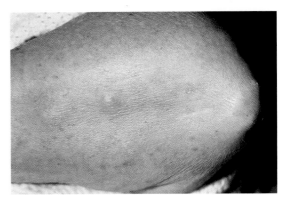

∎ **Fig. 27.9** Development of early rheumatoid nodules over the olecranon.

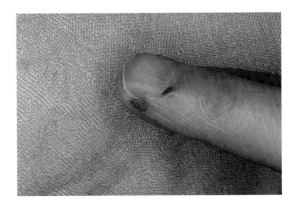

∎ **Fig. 27.10** Nail bed infarcts seen in rheumatoid vasculitits.

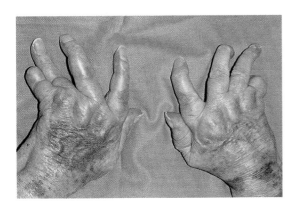

∎ **Fig. 27.8** More advanced rheumatoid arthritis of hands showing subluxation and ulnar deviation at the metacarpophalangeal joints and destructive involvement of the proximal interphalangeal joints.

joints but further description of these changes is beyond the scope of this chapter. However, involvement of the lower spinal synovial facet joints, and sacro-iliac joints is uncommon or rare in RA.

Extra-articular manifestations are numerous and include rheumatoid nodules, particularly on surfaces exposed to friction and trauma, e.g. olecranon, fingers, sacrum (Fig. 27.9); vasculitis manifesting as palpable purpura, nailfold infarcts (Fig. 27.10), skin ulceration and mononeuritis multiplex; pleuritis, pericarditis, mild peripheral neuropathy, and low-grade fever and weight loss. Eye involvement may manifest as a simple keratitis sicca or as a more severe scleritis which may progress to the feared scleromalacia perforans. Rheumatoid respiratory manifestation include rheumatoid nodules in lung parenchyma, pleuritis, fibrosing alveolitis, and bronchiolitis obliterans. Clinically significant renal or hepatic involvement in

RA is uncommon. Lymph node enlargement, particularly involving nodes draining inflamed joints is common and the nodes may reach a size of 2–3 cm. Lymphoedema may occur over the dorsum of the hands and wrists. Felty's syndrome is seen infrequently after many years of progressive synovitis and is defined as the constellation of splenomegaly, neutropenia, and lower limb skin ulcers occurring in a patient with RA. Felty's patients have very high levels of RF and circulating immune complexes and because of their neutropenia they are at risk of severe bacterial infections (particularly if the absolute white cell count is less than 100/mm^3).

Management

The management of patients with RA involves a team approach generally co-ordinated by the general practitioner/specialist rheumatologist working together with physiotherapists, occupational therapists, podiatrists, rehabilitation consultants, orthopaedic and plastic surgeons, nurse educators, and personnel from the domiciliary services. Each of these contributes to the overall care of patients with RA. There are four general groups of drugs useful in the management of RA:

(1) simple analgesics, e.g. paracetamol;

(2) non-steroidal anti-inflammatory drugs (NSAIDs);

(3) slow-acting antirheumatic drugs (SAARDs) also called the disease modifying antirheumatic drugs (DMARDs) or more recently the symptom modifying drugs;

(4) corticosteroids: different preparations and routes of administration.

NSAIDs

These include a large number of preparations which all have anti-inflammatory, antipyretic, and analgesic properties. The precise mechanism for their anti-inflammatory properties are unknown but may in part relate to potent inhibition of cyclooxygenase activity and the suppressive effects on neutrophil migration, activation, and secretion of inflammatory mediators. More recently, the considerable morbidity and mortality associated with NSAIDs have been recognized, particularly in the elderly, but if carefully used can provide long-standing and effective relief of symptoms. NSAIDs do not influence the natural history of arthritis and have no or minimal effect on laboratory indices of inflammation (e.g. ESR, CRP) and on immune indices (e.g. RF).

SAARDs

In contrast to NSAIDs these effectively suppress rheumatoid synovitis and do reduce the laboratory indices. The SAARDs drugs include antimalarials, intramuscular and oral gold, d-penicillamine, salazopyrin, methotrexate, cyclosporin, and cytotoxic drugs. They are scientifically proven in their efficacy in the short term (e.g. over a period of 1–5 years) but it is still to be proven whether they influence the long-term outcome of RA. Each of the SAARDs have their own spectrum of adverse side-effects and require careful monitoring (e.g. antimalarials can cause retinal toxicity; gold causes marrow suppression and membranous nephritis; methotrexate causes hepatic fibrosis). One of the limitations of the SAARDs is the re-emergence of active synovitis after 1–2 years despite an initial good suppressive effect. This loss of control varies from patient to patient and SAARD to SAARD but it is frequently necessary to use, in each patient, an increasing number of these SAARDs either sequentially or in combination. In recent years methotrexate has become popular as an effective SAARD possibly because it is well tolerated with approximately 50% of patients continuing to have benefit after 5 years of treatment (compared with 15% with intramuscular gold).

Corticosteroids

The most potent anti-inflammatory drugs known and are very useful in the management of patients with RA but have to be used carefully and selectively. Injections of steroids into the involved synovial compartment are of particular value in controlling synovitis over the short term, e.g. 3–6 weeks and can be repeated into the same joint three to four times a year. However, the long-term local effects of more frequent administration of steroids into joints is still uncertain. Both large and small joints can be injected, the smaller joints requiring a smaller total dose of steroids. Generally, the steroid is mixed directly with a local anaesthetic, and provided a no-touch technique is used the steroid can be administered safely in the consulting room.

Single pulses of steroids intravenously, intramuscularly, or orally can also be useful in gaining rapid control of inflammation in patients with widespread polyarthritis or in patients with systemic manifestations but in this situation should be used in conjunction with the initiation of a SAARD. Low-dose steroids, e.g. prednisolone 5–10 mg/day gives useful symptomatic benefit to patients who are difficult to control with SAARDs or in the elderly patients who are intolerant of other therapies. However, the adverse effects of long-term steroids should be carefully noted and where appropriate measures should be taken to minimize these (e.g. assessment of bone densitometry and possible use of calcitriol as a prophylaxis, measurement of blood pressure and the use of antihypertensive drugs, etc). Moderate- to high-dose corticosteroids are not indicated in RA because of their hazardous side-effects except when life-threatening complications, e.g. vasculitis and pericarditis, occur.

Monitoring of disease

Patients with RA require regular supervision to assess the activity of their arthritis, to note the development of any complications and to monitor the efficacy and possible toxicity of their medication. Following the initial assessment and/or commencement of specific medication each patient is reviewed at regular intervals, e.g. 3 monthly until the disease becomes well controlled and 6 monthly thereafter. At each visit the visual analogue score for pain and stiffness, a count of the number of painful/swollen joints, and a global assessment of current clinical status are recorded. Every 2 years a health assessment questionnaire is recommended, the score providing a simple assessment of functional capacity. For patients on SAARDs, blood tests may be required for appropriate monitoring of side-effects of drugs at more frequent intervals, but in addition, a blood picture, ESR or CRP and RF titre taken every 3 months when plotted on a graph compared with a clinical status gives a global view of progress over time. (Fig. 27.11).

In general, patients who respond to a disease suppressant will show evidence of a progressive decline in their CRP and RF. The patient's clinical status, blood tests, and if indicated urine tests are also monitored at regular intervals for any evidence of side-effects due to the SAARD and this is frequently delegated to the general practitioner. At each visit consideration is given to any local, systemic, or general medical problems which require further assessment and possible referral to appropriate experts (e.g. podiatrist, orthopaedic surgeon, cardiologist, etc.).

RA should be viewed as an ongoing long-term disorder and accurate medical records are vital if maximum benefit for each patients is to be achieved.

Future developments

Several pivotal questions remain to be answered concerning the aetiopathogenesis and management of RA. What are the environmental triggers that initiate and perpetuate RA? What factors are important in the exacerbation and amelioration of the disease activity? How does pregnancy cause suppression of synovitis? What prognostic factors are important in determining long-term outcome and likely response to treatment? Does treatment with SAARDs influence the long-term disability and joint deformity or are they only of symptomatic benefit useful in the short term?

New therapeutic approaches appear likely in the future. These include monoclonal antibody reagents which will selectively deplete the CD4+ T-cell subset or interfere with the expression or upregulation of cellular adhesion proteins in the inflamed synovium. It is also possible that TCRs, specific for the postulated trigger agent for RA may be identified which will allow direct attack by monoclonal antibodies to its idiotype or alternatively lead to peptide blockade (given intramuscularly or even by the oral route). Furthermore the clonotypic T cells might be able to be selectively anergized or depleted by molecular techniques in predisposed individuals. Neutralizing chimeric antibodies to TNFα appear to be particularly effective in suppressing inflammation and clinical trials are currently underway. Cytokine inhibitors, e.g. soluble receptor for TNFα or IL-1 or the use of the natural IL-1 antagonist, or use of anti-inflammatory cytokines, e.g. IL-4 and IL-10 may also be shown to have a part in the therapy of this autoimmune inflammatory condition. A number of new drugs are in development. These include both new NSAIDs and SAARDs, e.g. T-cell selective antifungal preparations and new alkaloid SAARDs. Different combinations of SAARDs are also being trialled. A better understanding of the benefits and hazards of current and new corticosteroid preparations is likely to aid in the better management of patients with RA. New joint prostheses, particularly for the knee, ankle, shoulder, and elbow are also likely to improve functional capacity of patients with deformity of these joints.

Further reading

Arnett, F. C., *et al.* (1988). The American Rheumatism Association 1987 revised criteria for the classification of rheumatoid arthritis. *Arthritis and Rheumatism*, **31**, 315–324.

∎ **Fig. 27.11** Mean change in various clinical and laboratory indices following 24 weeks of chrysotherapy. CIC, circulating immune complexes; CRP, C-reative protein; CS, clinical score; HAQ, health assessment questionnaire; RF, rheumatoid factor; ESR, erythrocyte sedimentation rate.

Boers, M. and Ramsden, M. (1991). Long-acting drug combinations in rheumatoid arthritis: A formal overview. *Journal of Rheumatology*, **18**, 316.

Brennan, F M., Field, M., Chu, C. Q., Feldmann, M., and Maini, R. N. (1991). Cytokine expression in rheumatoid arthritis. *British Journal of Rheumatology*, **30**, 76–80.

Brooks, P. M. and Day, R. O. (1991). Nonsteroidal antiinflammatory drugs: Differences and similarities. *New England Journal of Medicine*, **324**, 1716.

Gregersen, P. K., *et al.* (1987). The shared epitope hypothesis. *Arthritis and Rheumatism*, **30**, 1205–13.

Harris, E. D. Jr. (1990). Rheumatoid arthritis: pathophysiology and implications for therapy. *New England Journal of Medicine*, **322**, 1277.

Maini, R. N. and Feldman, M. (1993). Immunopathogenesis of rheumatoid arthritis. In *Oxford textbook of rheumatology*, (ed. P. J. Maddison, D. A. Isenberg, P. Woo, and D. N. Glass), Vol. 2, pp. 621–38. Oxford University Press.

28 Idiopathic inflammatory myopathies

A. M. Heitz, P. N. Hollingsworth, R. L. Dawkins

Definition

The idiopathic inflammatory myopathies (IIM), also referred to as polymyositis, are a heterogeneous group of conditions. They are characterized clinically by proximal muscle weakness and histologically by muscle fibre necrosis, regeneration, and a mononuclear inflammatory infiltrate. Infectious, vasculitic, and granulomatous myosis as well as non-inflammatory myopathies, are not usually included, and will not be discussed here.

Introduction

Classification

The definitions and classification of Bohan and Peter (Tables 28.1 and 28.2) remain in use for clinical and research purposes. Recent morphological studies indicate that a simpler pathological classification can be attempted comprising of three entities:

(1) dermatomyositis (DM);

(2) pure polymyositis (PM);

(3) inclusion body myositis (IBM).

Table 28.1 Abbreviated version of the criteria for polymyositis/dermatomyositis advocated by Bohan and Peter

1. Symmetrical weakness of limb girdle muscles.
2. Muscle fibre necrosis, phagocytosis, and regeneration.
3. Increased muscle enzymes in serum.
4. Electromyographic changes.
5. Dermatomyositis rash.

Table 28.2 Classification of idiopathic inflammatory myopathies according to Bohan and Peter

I   Primary idiopathic polymyositis.

II Primary idiopathic dermatomyositis.

III Dermatomyositis or polymyositis with neoplasia.

IV Childhood dermatomyositis or polymyositis with vasculitis.

V   Polymyositis or dermatomyositis with collagen vascular disease.

On the other hand a larger number of syndromes can now be recognized taking into account the presence or not of systemic lupus erythematosus (SLE), mixed connective tissue disease (MCTD), scleroderma, progressive systemic sclerosis (PSS), and Sjögren's syndrome; associated cancer; other tissue involvement, particularly skin and lung; as well as autoantibodies and human leucocyte antigen (HLA) associations.

The morphological entities PM, and DM, and IBM are not uniquely associated with particular syndromes. Each of these can occur alone, or be associated with another process such as human immunodeficiency virus (HIV) or malignancy. One such process may be linked with more than one of PM, DM, or IBM, although the relative frequencies of these associations are variable (Fig. 28.1).

Although numerous IIM syndromes occur, three main morphological types of muscle damage can be recognized: DM, PM, and IBM. Recent morphological observations imply that myofibre ischaemia secondary to capillary loss is the mechanism of muscle death in DM whereas T-cell mediated cytotoxicity directed to the muscle fibres themselves is the predominant mechanism in PM and in IBM.

Certain autoantibodies occurring specifically in IIM appear to mark particular syndromes, to predict natural

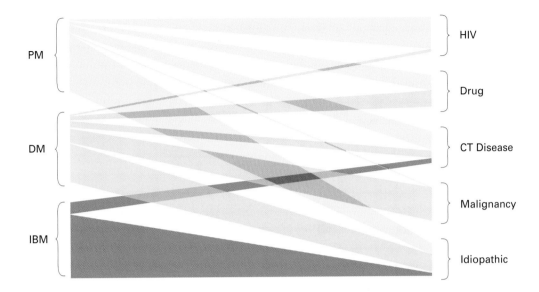

∎ **Fig. 28.1** Relationships between the three histopathological types of idiopathic inflammatory myopathies (left), and potentially causal associations (right). PM, polymyositis; DM, dermatomyositis; IBM, inclusion body myositis; CT, connective tissue.

history and response to treatment, and, in some cases also to correlate with HLA type.

While the cause of these syndromes is not known, these recent developments implicate an autoimmune response directed at intracellular structures involved in transcription and particularly translation of the genetic code into protein. The potential role of viruses in triggering this autoimmunity will be discussed.

Epidemiology

The incidence of IIM is five cases per million per year. DM afflicts children and adults with a female preponderance and PM adults over the age of 20. IBM rarely occurs before age 50, with a male to female ratio of approximately 3:1.

Immunogenetics

Most studies indicate an association between PM and DM and HLA-B8 and -DR3 (the 8.1 haplotype). Mixed connective tissue disease shows entirely different associations; with DR4 and DQ3. In d-penicillamine-associated DM there is an increase in DR4 due to the presence of rheumatoid arthritis for which d-penicillamine is a therapy. While some of these associations may reflect the antigen-presenting

functions of the HLA genes (class I and II), other major histocompatibility complex (MHC) genes including complement genes, tumour necrosis factor (TNF) genes and genes for other ligands and receptors are likely to be involved. The 8.1 haplotype, associated with many autoimmune diseases, has a deleted C4A gene, and a particular TNF α allele. Individuals with 8.1 haplotype have increased responses to various immune stimuli, and homozygotes have a deficient antibody response to hepatitis B vaccine. It is likely that these findings will be explained by combinations of alleles of non-antigen-specific MHC genes.

Viruses and myositis

A viral aetiology has long been postulated for IIM, the main candidates being the picorna viruses and the retroviruses. Picorna viruses are implicated because of their ability to cause a transient myositis and because of demonstrations of binding of coxsackie virus to histidyl t-RNA synthetase (HRS), the antigen for the most common myositis specific autoantibody, anti-Jo-1. As a t-RNA synthetase, HRS joins histidine to native t-RNA, but also to genomic RNA of the picorna virus. The virus–synthetase complex could then be presented to the immune system as foreign. If the resulting immune response was also directed at the

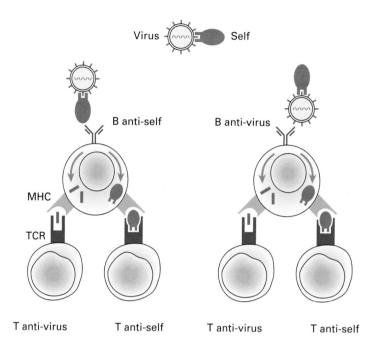

▌**Fig. 28.2** Postulated mechanism of viral induced autoimmune response to an to an intracellular protein, e.g. a tRNA synthetase. A self tRNA synthetase bound to a virus forms a particle that may be bound by an antiviral B cell or by an anti-cell tRNA synthetase B cell. In each case both viral and cell peptides will be presented by the B cell both antiviral and anti-self T-helper cells and B cells may then be engaged, activated and driven to proliferate. TCR, T-cell receptor; MHC, major histocompatibility complex.

native complex, and this response was persistent, autoimmunity would result. (Fig. 28.2).

Extensive investigation including *in situ* hybridization and polymerase chain reaction have failed to demonstrate persistence of viral particles in muscle. The virus may act as a trigger. How the process becomes self-sustaining, or what role autoantibodies have in muscle damage is unknown, but will be discussed below.

The retroviruses human T-lymphotropic virus (HTLV) I, HIV and simian retroviruses show the most convincing association with the inflammatory myositides. HIV-associated PM may occur at any stage of infection, suggesting that the virus itself rather than immune modulation is the causative factor. Clinical, electomyographic (EMG), pathological, and immunocytochemical characteristics are identical with seronegative disease. HIV antigens cannot be localized on muscle fibres but only in surrounding lymphoid cells. This implies that viral replication does not occur in muscle fibre. Rather the same T-cell-mediated and MHC-I restricted cytotoxic process demonstrated in

'idiopathic' PM is triggered in susceptible individuals by the retrovirus.

Similar immunopathological features have been described for HTLV-I. In Jamaica, where HTLV-I is endemic, the rate of PM is nine times higher in HTLV-I infected patients than in matched uninfected individuals. In rhesus monkeys, simian retrovirus-1 and simian immunodeficiency virus produce immunodeficiency and polymyositis.

The positive amyloid staining of vacuolated fibres in IBM may suggest an alternative infective agent. Prions have the same size and amyloidogenic properties as these fibres. The prolonged and indolent course of prion associated neurological disease is not inconsistent with the insidious onset of IBM and the age group in which it occurs.

Pathology

The features required for histological diagnosis of any IIM on muscle biopsy are segmental myofibre necrosis, regeneration occurring *pari passu*, and associated inflammatory infiltrate. The three major subgroups show characteristic variations which distinguish them and suggest separate pathogenetic mechanisms (Fig. 28.3).

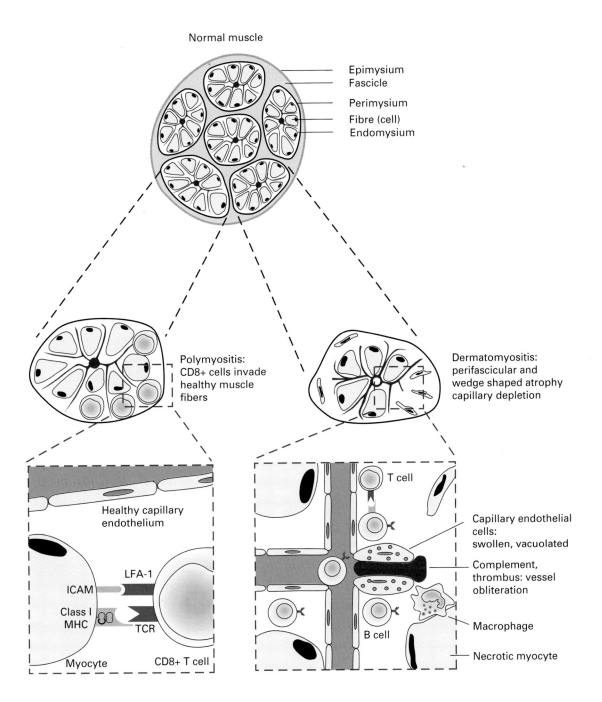

∎ Fig. 28.3 Schematic summary of muscle injuring mechanisms in idiopathic inflammatory myopathies. Vascular (capillary) injury leads to ischaemic necrosis in juvenile dermatomyositis and dermatomyositis, whereas direct cytotoxic T cell injury of muscle cells predominates in inclusion body myositis and pure polymyositis. TCR, T-cell receptor; MHC, major histocompatibility complex; ICAM, intercellular adiesion molecule.

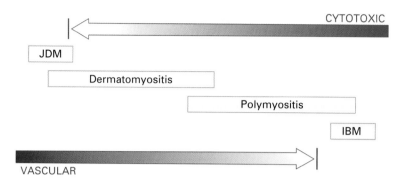

∎ **Fig. 28.4** Relative contributions of vascular injury and direct cellular cytotoxicity to muscle fibre necrosis in idiopathic inflammatory myopathies. IBM, inclusion body myositis; JDM, juvenile dermatomyositis.

The observations of Engle and colleagues imply that the basis of DM is vascular injury. This precedes, and is topographically related to, myofibre necrosis. Endothelial cell swelling and hyperplasia, and platelet and fibrin thrombi are seen in the central supplying vessel or its branches. These vessels may be obliterated or depleted. Atrophy and ischaemic necrosis occurs in the area of hypoperfusion, usually at the edge of the fascicle (perifascicularly) or in a wedge distribution. Inflammatory infiltrates are found, mainly in fibrous septa adjacent to lymphatics. The cells consist mainly of B cells, in close proximity to CD4+ T cells. Macrophages are present but invasion of non-necrotic muscle is rarely observed. Deposition of the membrane attack complex and other complement components and sometimes immunoglobulin is seen in vessel walls. This suggests an antibody- and complement-mediated capillary microangiopathy with ischaemic necrosis and secondary muscle phagocytosis.

In PM and IBM, capillary distribution and architecture are normal. The earliest change is invasion of non-necrotic fibres by lymphocytes. These T lymphocytes are predominantly (80%) CD8+, cytotoxic and bind abnormally upregulated MHC-I and ICAM-1 molecules on the surface of otherwise healthy muscle fibres. T-cell receptor gene rearrangement studies indicate that the receptors, whether α/β or γ/δ, are clonal, although the antigen that they recognize has not been identified.

IBM is histologically similar to PM with three main distinguishing features: rimmed vacuoles, angulated fibres, and, by electron microscopy, tubular filaments. Rimmed vacuoles are slit-like vacuoles surrounded by basophilic granular inclusions. Eosinophilic cytoplasmic inclusions with amyloid staining are also present around vacuoles. Small groups of angulated fibres are found. Rimmed vacuoles are not specific for IBM.

Electron microscopic examination is essential and will demonstrate abnormal intracytoplasmic tubular filaments adjacent to vacuoles in the myofibre nucleus. Intracytoplasmic inclusions may be sparse and can be missed. The proportion of hypertrophied muscle fibres is three to four times that found in PM/DM and an important distinguishing feature.

In some cases of PM or DM a mixed picture may be seen (Fig. 28.4), although one or other process is usually predominant.

Clinical features

Common features

All of these diseases are characterized by muscle weakness, generally symmetrical and proximal. Distal involvement occurs relatively early in IBM and late in PM/DM. The onset may rarely be acute and severe associated with systemic illness with high fever, malaise, high creatine kinase (CK), and myoglobulinuria. This pattern is associated with the anti-signal recognition particle (SRP) antibody. Most cases show progression over weeks or months; more insidious weakness suggests IBM.

Limb muscles are most commonly involved, followed by pharyngeal musculature and neck flexors, with respiratory muscle weakness late in disease. Facial involvement is rare. Ocular muscle involvement is not documented in IIM. If present it implies disease of nerve or neuromuscular junction.

Wasting may occur with disease progression and may be prominent in IBM. Reflexes are preserved except for depression proportional to wasting. Myalgia occurs early and is more prominent with DM. Sensory changes are not present.

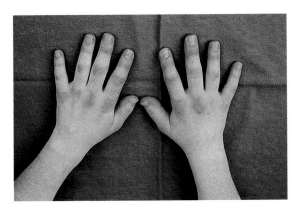

▌**Fig. 28.5** Typical appearance of hands in dermatomyositis.

Features of inclusion body myositis

IBM is characterized by its slow progression, by the frequent occurrence of falls due to distal weakness which may be asymmetrical and by a poor response to steroids. CK may be normal and is never more than modestly elevated. No myositis specific autoantibodies are present and the incidence of associated connective tissue disease is 15%.

Features of dermatomyositis

DM is defined by its typical skin changes, of heliotrope rash, periorbital oedema, Gottron's papules — erythematous raised smooth or scaly patches over the knuckles of the IP or metacarpophalangeal and other extensor joint surfaces; violaceous rash over the V-neck or shawl distribution, and nailed changes with dilated capillary loops. Subcutaneous calcification occurs in juvenile DM, and occasionally in adult DM and is resistant to treatment.

Other features

Involvement of heart, lungs, and gastrointestinal tract may be present. Dyspnoea and cough may be a reflection of interstitial lung disease, or secondary to respiratory muscle involvement, aspiration pneumonia from pharyngeal muscle weakness, methotrexate toxicity, or congestive cardiac failure from cardiomyopathy. Palpitations secondary to abnormalities of arteriovenous conduction and tachy- and bradyarrhythmias as well as dilated cardiomyopathy with a depressed ejection fraction may occur.

Gastrointestinal involvement is present in up to 60% of cases and may be due to myositis of striated muscle in the pharynx and upper third of the oesophagus, manifest by dysphagia, odynophagia, and regurgitation; to scleroderma-like changes in the oesophagus and bowel in overlap syndromes; or to vasculitis, ischaemia, and ulceration in adult or juvenile DM, producing pain, cramping, and altered bowel habit. Gastric ulceration occurs in juvenile DM and as a treatment complication in adults.

Malignancy

An association between DM, polymyositis, and neoplasms has been generally accepted for some 50 years. However, more recent analyses indicate that PM is uncommonly associated with cancer. On the other hand DM is a marker of internal malignancy. Some 25% of patients with DM will have malignancy, and in approximately a third of these the malignancy precedes the diagnosis of DM, in one-third it coincides with, and in one-third it follows the diagnosis. Skin involvement is an important predictor of malignancy. This includes the classical DM rash and the less common fiery red rash which may be superimposed on the classical rash and which is highly associated with malignancy. A poor response of either the myositis or the rash to immunosuppressive treatment also indicates an increased probability of malignancy. These correlates apply to adolescents and young adults as well as to older people.

Diagnosis

Plasma CK is increased in most inflammatory myopathies, due to release of the enzyme from injured muscle cells. In IBM, CK is usually less than 10 times normal, and may be normal. It is usually higher in the other myopathies, but is not a reliable distinguishing feature. Resolution of inflammation results in a fall in the CK, but returning of the CK activity to normal does not guarantee resolution of the myositis. Increased plasma myogenic lactic dehydrogenase and transaminases may occur, but are less specific than CK as markers of muscle injury.

The EMG is 80% sensitive and specific for a myopathic process. It may demonstrate myopathic potentials and/or spontaneous fibrillations or complex repetitive discharges. These are not specific for IIM. The usefulness of EMG is in demonstrating active myopathy, excluding a neuromuscular process, and monitoring activity.

Recent trials have shown ultrasound and magnetic resonance imaging scanning, in experienced hands, to be similar to EMG in detecting histologically proven inflammatory myopathy. Reliable distinction between the types of inflammatory myopathy is not possible, but chronicity, severity, distribution of disease, and selection of muscle for biopsy and response to treatment can be assessed using these modalities.

Muscle biopsy is recommended in all cases to confirm the diagnosis and thereby justify immunosuppressive treatment.

Autoantibodies are clinically useful in confirmatory testing and some are predictors of prognosis, response to treatment and extramuscular pathology. They have no role in screening for, or excluding, PM and DM because of their low diagnostic sensitivity.

Autoantibodies

Clinical consideration

Up to 80% of patients with IIM express an autoantibody, reactive with nuclei or cytoplasm a detectable by immunofluorescence, for example on HEp-2 cells or by immunodiffusion or immunoblotting (Table 28.3). These have usually been given eponymous names such as Jo-1 pending identification of the antigen. Of these, approximately 40% are myositis specific, comprising mostly antisynthetases, with the most important others being anti-SRP and anti-Mi2.

Anti-Jo, the prototype antisynthetase, binds to a conformational epitope of a cytoplasmic antigen, histidyl t-RNA synthetase and is named for the first patient to demonstrate this antibody. The five known

▮ **Table 28.3** Autoantibodies in the idiopathic inflammatory myopathies

	Frequency %	Syndrome	HLA	Associated conditions
A				
Specific to myositis				
(i) Antisynthetase			DR3	} Fever, ILD, Arthritis
				}
Jo	18–20	PM>DM		}
PL7	3	}		}
PL12	3	}		}
OJ	2	}PM>DM		
EJ	2	}		
(ii) Non-synthetase				
				Severe and cardiac
Anti-SRP	4	PM		fever, ILD, arthritis
KJ	<1	PM		
fer	<1	Nodular myositis	DR7	Alcoholic rhabdomyolysis
MAS	1	PM		Florid Rash
Anti-Mi-2	8	DM		
B				
Connective tissue disease associated				
	1	}		SLE
Anti-Ku	12	}	DR4	MCTD
U1RNP	4	}		SSC
U2RNP	10	} Overlap	DR3	Sjögren's syndrome
Ro/SSA	5	}	DR3	SLE
La/SSB	8	}		SSc
PM-Scl				
Common to PM, DM and connective tissue disease	87	PM or DM or Overlap		Any IIM
Anti-56 kDa				

PM, pure polymyositis; DM, dermatomyositis; SLE, systemic lupus erythematosus; IIM idiopathic inflammatory myopathies; ILD, interstitial lung disease; MCTD, mixed connective tissue disease; HLA, human leucocyte antigen.

antisynthetases show no cross-reactivity, and no patient has more than one. Clinically, the antisynthetases are strongly associated with interstitial lung disease, arthritis and Raynaud's phenomenon (the 'synthetase syndrome'), glomerulonephritis (rare), a mediocre response to steroid therapy and with HLA-DR3 or DR-6. Antisynthetase is not a marker for interstitial lung disease (ILD) without myositis, though occasionally the lung disease may clinically precede muscle disease.

Anti-SRP (signal recognition particle) is the most clinically useful of the non-synthetase–myositis-specific antibodies. SRP is involved in the transloca-tion of secretory proteins to the endoplasmic reticulum. Anti-SRP is strongly associated with PM. Ten per cent of patients have clinically significant car-diomyopathy but none have ILD or arthritis. Patients with this antibody often have severe steroid-resistant

myositis and the worst prognosis amongst the antibody defined subgroups.

Anti-Mi2 is an antinuclear antibody and always associated with DM. It is linked with a florid rash, steroid responsiveness, and a good prognosis.

Almost no patients have more than one myositis specific antibody, although non-myositis specific anti-bodies may coexist or be the only antibodies present. Antibodies to Ro/SSA, La/SSB U1RNP, and U2RND are often seen in overlap syndromes. Although they may present with myositis alone, other features usually develop. Anti-Ku is strongly associated with an overlap syndrome and anti-PMScl is found in 8% of myositis patients and 3% of patients with systemic sclerosis.

Relationship to disease pathogenesis

Antisynthetase antibodies demonstrate characteristics (Table 28.4) which suggest they are antigen driven and

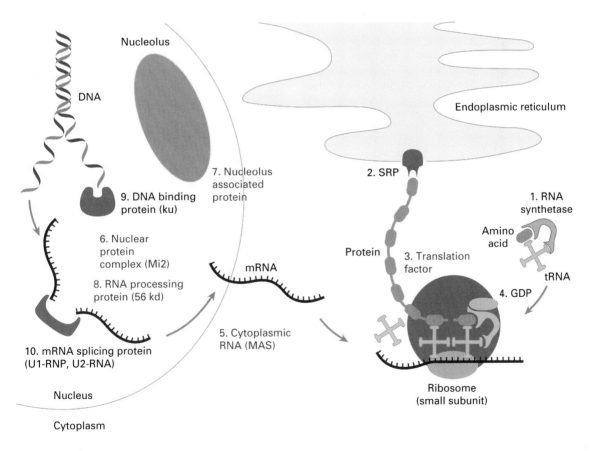

∎ **Fig. 28.6** Autoantibodies in idiopathic inflammatory myopathies bind molecules involved in translation of the genetic code. (1) RNA synthetase (synthetase); (2) signal recognition particle (SRP); (3) translation factor (fer); (4) elongation factor 1-a (KJ); (5) cytoplasmic RNA (MAS); (6) nuclear protein complex (Mi-2); (7) nucleolus associ-ated protein (PM-Scl); (8) RNA processing protein (56 kDa); (9) free end DNA binding protein (ku); (10) mRNA splicing protein (U1-RNP, U2-RNA); (11) SSA/Ro and SSB/La. (Antigens of unknown function are shown in red.)

∎ **Table 28.4**   Features of antisynthetase antibodies

1. Unique to pure polymyositis and dermatomyositis.
2. Antigens vary widely in size and structure.
3. Bind only one type of tRNA synthetase.
4. Only one type of antisynthetase in any patient.
5. Inhibit synthetase quantitatively.
6. Affinity maturation.
7. Predominantly IgG1.
8. Vary independently of total IgG.
9. May precede onset of disease.
10. Vary with disease activity.

reactive with elements of a functional system. Other myositis associated autoantibodies target diverse nuclear and cytoplasmic particles involved in gene transcription and translation (Fig. 28.6). These observations suggest a role for viruses in induction of autoimmunity.

A model for a virus initiated, but autoantigen driven response to a t-RNA synthetase is suggested in Fig. 28.6. The immune system is initially ignorant, or not completely tolerant-hypoergic-, of the intracellular t-RNA synthetase. B cells and T cells specific for t-RNA synthetase exist but in low numbers. They are not activated because the concentration of t-RNA synthetase in the extracellular fluid is too low, and/or because of hypoergy.

If a picorna virus infects the muscle, t-RNA synthetase may bind to it, forming a particle containing both self and non-self proteins. B cells with receptors specific for epitopes of either virus or self t-RNA synthetase would bind, internalize, and digest the particle and present both self t-RNA synthetase and viral peptides.

An antiviral T-helper cell could then provide help to both self reactive and virus reactive B cells. Similarly, both antiviral and anti-self T cells could be activated. In this way, clones of anti-self t-RNA synthetase T and B cells would be expanded and activated. A response could now be driven by low amounts of t-RNA synthetase, and the autoimmunity perpetuated.

The major difficulties in implicating autoantibodies as direct agents of muscle injury are the limited access of the immune system to intracellular antigens, the ubiquity of the antigens, which are not restricted to muscle tissue, and the appearance of the same antibody in two processes with apparently differing mechanisms, namely PM versus DM.

Other investigations

The extent of investigation for other organ involvement should be guided by symptoms. Chest X-ray (CXR) can be supplemented by measures of differing capacity. Single breath diffusing capacity (D_{LCO}) is abnormal in 50% of patients, even with normal CXR. Echocardiogram or isotope imaging of the myocardium may be useful to detect cardiac myositis, and videofluoroscopy for pharyngeal and oesophageal involvement.

Extensive radiological investigation for underlying malignancy is not recommended by most authorities. Yearly history and examination, including rectal and vaginal examination, with urinalyses, full blood count biochemistry, mammogram, and CXR is a reasonable approach. Some features, such as malignant erythema, the 'fiery red rash', vasculitis, a poor response to treatment, the Mi2 autoantibody or a family history of cancer would prompt a more extensive evaluation.

Treatment

No large case-controlled trials of therapy for IIM have yet been performed. All treatment regimens to date have been empiric. The aim of treatment is to restore muscle strength and function while minimizing drug toxicities.

Corticosteroids are used also as first-line therapy or in conjunction with other immunosuppressants. A high dose of 1 mg/kg per day is continued until the CK is normal and muscle strength is returning, followed by a gradual tapering over 3–4 months to a maintenance dose of 5–15 mg/day. If no improvement is seen, a second agent should be added. If initial response is noted, followed by relapse, a second steroid induction is attempted. Steroid myopathy or atrophy of type I muscle fibres may supervene or may coexist with persisting or recurring myositis and the two can be clinically indistinguishable. Associated features such as a deterioration in the CK or autoantibody titres or extramuscular manifestation suggestive of PM/DM or of steroid toxicities may be informative, as well as repeat biopsy.

Other therapies may be added as steroid-sparing agents, as alternative drugs in case of steroid resistance or for patients with rapidly progressive disease. Azathioprine and methotrexate are most commonly used but have not been tested or compared in clinical trials. They have similar rates of toxicity and are roughly equally preferred. Cyclophosphamide may be especially indicated in interstitial lung disease. Plasmapheresis is ineffective. Cyclosporin has been usefully employed in a number of small uncontrolled trials in childhood DM and resistant adult disease. Intravenous γ-globulin therapy shows some promise; a recent double blind cross-over trial of high-dose γ-globulin (2 g/kg per month) in 15 treatment-resistant patients showed a response in 14. Drawbacks were the prohibitive cost and rapid relapse on discontinuation. Trials utilizing lower doses or immunoglobulin Fc particles are awaited.

CXR and electrocardiography (ECG) can be supplemented by D_{LCO}, which is abnormal in 50% of patients, even with normal CXR. ECG, echocardiogram, and myocardial scintography can be used to assess for heart involvement, and video fluoroscopy for pharyngeal and oesophageal involvement.

Prognosis

The expected rate of remission is approximately 50% in children and somewhat lower in adults. Mortality studies for adults demonstrate improvement over the past decade, with a death rate of 20–30% over 5 years. The course may be monocyclic with complete remission, relapsing, chronically stable or chronically progressive. Poor prognosis is predicted by increasing age, cardiac or pulmonary involvement, dysphagia, severity of weakness, autoantibody status, and presence of malignancy.

Further reading

Benbassat, J., Gefel, D., Larholt, K., Sukenik, S., Morgenstern, V., and Zlotnick. A. (1985). Prognostic factors in polymyositis/dermatomyositis: A computer-assisted analysis of ninety-two cases. *Arthritis and Rheumatism*, **28**, 249.

Bertorini, T. E. (1989). Histopathology of the inflammatory myopathies. In *Polymyositis and dermatomyositis* (ed. M. C. Dalakas), p. 157. Butterworth, Boston.

Bohan, A (1988). Clinical presentation and diagnosis of polymyositis and dermatomyositis. In *Polymyositis and dermatomyositis* (ed. M. C. Dalakas), p. 19. Butterworth, Boston.

Bohan, A. and Peter, J. B. (1975). Polymyositis and dermatomyositis. *New England Journal of Medicine*, **292**, 344–7 and 403–7.

Bunch, T. W. (1988). The therapy of polymyositis *Mount Sinai Journal of Medicine*, **55**, 483.

Callen, J. P. (1984). Myositis and malignancy. *Clinics in Rheumatic Diseases*, **10**, 117–30.

Carpenter, S. (1989). Resin histology and electron microscopy in inflammatory myopathies. In *Polymyositis and dermatomyositis*, (ed. M. C. Dalakas), p. 195. Butterworth, Boston.

Engel, A. G. and Arahata, K. (1986). Mononuclear cells in myopathies: Quantitation of functionally distinct subsets, recognition of antigen-specific cell-mediated cytotoxicity in some diseases, and implications for the pathogenesis of the different inflammatory myopathies. *Human Pathology*, **17**, 704.

Hochberg, M. C., Feldman, D., and Stevens, M. B. (1986). Adult onset polymyositis/dermatomyositis: An analysis of clinical and laboratory features and survival in 76 patients with a review of the literature. *Seminars in Arthritis and Rheumatism*, **15**, 168.

Hollingsworth, P. N. and Dawkins, R. L. (1992). Autoimmune diseases of muscle. In *The autoimmune diseases*, II, (ed. R. Thomas), Orlando, FL. Academic Press.

Lachanpal, S., Bunch, T. W., and Melton III, L. J. (1986). Polymyositis-dermatomyositis and malignant lesions: does an association exist? *Mayo Clinic Proceedings*, **61**, 645.

Lotz, B. P., Engel, A. G., Nishino, H., Stevens, J. C., and Litchy, W. J. (1989). Inclusion body myositis: Observations in 40 patients. *Brain*, **112**, 727.

Matthews, M. B. and Bernstein, R. M. (1983). Myositis autoantibody inhibits histidyl–tRNA synthetase: A model for autoimmunity. *Nature*, **304**, 177.

Plotz, P. H., Dalakas, M., Leff, R. L., Love, L. A., Miller, F. W., and Cronin, M. E. (1989). Current concepts in the idiopathic inflammatory myopathies: Polymyositis, dermatomyositis, and related disorders. *Annuals of Internal Medicine*, **11**, 143.

Roifman, C. M., Schaffer, F. M., Wachsmuth, S. E., Murphy, G., and Gelfand, E. W. (1987). Reversal of chronic polymyositis following intravenous immune serum globulin therapy. *Journal of the American Medical Association*, **258**, 513.

Targoff, I. N. (1993). Humoral Immunity in polymyositis/dermatomyositis. *Journal of Investigative Dermatology*, **100** (Suppl.), 116–23S.

29 Juvenile chronic arthritis

D. M. Roberton

Introduction

Inflammatory joint disease in childhood may be due to or associated with a wide variety of conditions. Infection of the joint (septic arthritis) or contiguous bone (osteomyelitis), either as a primary disorder or as part of a systemic infective process, is the most important cause of acute arthritis in children because of its potential to destroy growing bone. Synovitis may also occur in association with infection elsewhere in the body without direct infection of the joint or periarticular tissues, and is usually transient. Other forms of synovitis may also be transient (e.g. transient synovitis or 'irritable hip'), although such a diagnosis can only be made by exclusion. Arthritis may also be the presenting feature of other systemic disorders in childhood, such as leukaemia, inflammatory bowel disease, metabolic disorders, and a number of congenital syndromes.

Definition of juvenile chronic arthritis

Chronic arthritis in childhood is defined as an arthritis that persists for a minimum of 6 consecutive weeks in one or more joints, commencing before the age of 16 years and after active exclusion of other causes.

The clinical criteria necessary for the diagnosis of arthritis are:

> swelling or effusion in a joint or joints;
> or two of the following three criteria:

(1) heat in the joint on palpation;

(2) pain on movement of the joint;

(3) limitation of movement.

Juvenile chronic arthritis may be due to many different causes (Tables 29.1 and 29.2). Some confusion occurs because of minor differences in nomenclature. European literature discusses juvenile chronic arthri-

■ **Table 29.1** Features of juvenile rheumatoid arthritis

Systemic onset
  high remittent fever and one or more of:
    rash, hepatomegaly;
    splenomegaly, serositis;
    lymphadenopathy, myalgia, or arthralgia at onset with arthritis not necessarily present at onset

Pauciarticular onset
  four or fewer joints involved (usually large joints, e.g. knees, ankles, wrists, elbows)
  There are two major patterns of onset:
    young children, with many having positive antinuclear antibody results, and a relatively high risk of chronic iridocyclitis
    older children (usually boys) with a high incidence of HLA-B27.

Polyarticular onset
  five or more joints involved during the onset period. The majority are rheumatoid factor negative, but a subgroup of older girls may be IgM rheumatoid factor positive with progressive disease.

▌ **Table 29.2**   Other forms of juvenile chronic arthritis

Juvenile psoriatic arthritis
  defined as chronic arthritis in childhood in association with skin lesions of psoriasis, or three of:
    nail pitting,
    a family history of psoriasis in a first-degree relative,
    a psoriasis like rash, and
    dactylitis

Juvenile ankylosing spondylitis
  often onset in boys from age 9 years onwards, with involvement of large joints of lower limbs, enthesopathy,
  and initial absence of sacro-iliitis and lumbar spine involvement.

Arthropathy associated with connective tissue disorders
  systemic lupus erythematosus, juvenile dermatomyositis, scleroderma, overlap syndromes, vasculitis
  syndromes

Arthropathy of inflammatory bowel disease
  commonly Crohn's disease, which may present with little in terms of specific bowel sympatomatology, but with
  weight loss, rash, an arthropathy, and enthesopathy

Reactive arthritis
  includes Reiter's syndrome and arthritis of enteric infection

---

tis, including systemic, pauciarticular, and polyarticular onset disease as forms of chronic arthritis in childhood, and tends not to favour the term juvenile rheumatoid arthritis (JRA) except for rheumatoid factor positive disease. North American classification proposals describe JRA (systemic, pauciarticular, and polyarticular types) as subtypes of juvenile chronic arthritis. Diagnostic classification is also made difficult by the evolution of some forms of chronic arthritis in childhood, and tends not to favour the term juvenile rheumatoid arthritis except for rheumatoid factor positive disease. North American classification proposals describe juvenile rheumatoid arthritis (systemic, pauciarticular and polyarticular types) as subtypes of juvenile chronic arthritis. Diagnostic classification is also made difficult by the evolution of some forms of chronic arthritis in childhood, for example, an apparent pauciarticular onset may later prove to be the early manifestation of juvenile psoriatic arthritis, or juvenile ankylosing spondylitis.

The various forms of juvenile rheumatoid arthritis (JRA) are classified according to their features during the first six months after the onset of symptoms. The three major categories of juvenile rheumatoid arthritis and their distribution frequencies are:

systemic onset	approximately 10% of JRA
pauciarticular onset	approximately 50% of JRA
polyarticular onset	approximately 40% of JRA

The major features of these categories are listed in Table 29.1. Other important forms of juvenile chronic arthritis are listed in Table 29.2. New classification criteria have been proposed recently, but have yet to be accepted universally.

Epidemiology of juvenile chronic arthritis

Few satisfactory studies have been performed of the incidence and prevalence of chronic arthritis in childhood. A Finnish community study reported the incidence of chronic arthritis in urban children to be 18.9 per 100 000 children <16 years of age. A recent regional population study in South-western Sweden has suggested an average annual incidence of juvenile chronic arthritis, as defined by EULAR criteria, of 10.9 per 100 000 children <16 years of age. In these studies, the term juvenile chronic arthritis encompasses juvenile rheumatoid arthritis and other persisting inflammatory arthropathies of childhood.

Juvenile rheumatoid arthritis

Juvenile rheumatoid arthritis has a bimodal pattern of age of onset, with a peak incidence in the second year of life and a second peak at around the age of 9–10 years. Females are affected more commonly than males. Particular features of juvenile rheumatoid arthritis compared to adult rheumatoid arthritis are the absence of classical IgM rheumatoid factor, the frequent presence of ANA in serum, the pauciarticular and asymmetrical distribution of joint involvement in the majority, the occurrence of uveitis, the systemic form of onset in some children, and the high probability of disease remission with time in many children. Familial occurrence is very rare but affected siblings have been described in a number of reports, usually with similar patterns of disease.

Aetiology of juvenile rheumatoid arthritis

The aetiology of JRA remains unknown. Although agents such as rubella have been suggested as likely causes, there have been no epidemiological or laboratory studies to date to confirm infection in the pathogenesis. There has been extensive study of human leucocyte antigen (HLA) expression in children with JRA and other connective tissue disorders, with evidence of association of particular HLA alleles with specific disease manifestations. These findings suggest predisposition to disease in some children, either as a result of altered immune responsiveness or susceptibility to environmental risk factors or infectious agents. Study of cell populations in and related to affected joints may offer some clues to aetiology as it is now possible to define the antigenic specificity and T-cell receptor (TCR) usage of synovial T-cell populations. Polymerase chain reaction (PCR) allows exquisitely sensitive detection of infectious antigens in the synovial space, and will enable more precise study of the potential of infectious agents to cause JRA.

Pathology

Examination of synovium from children with JRA does not show any differentiating features between the clinical subtypes nor from the synovial biopsy appearances of adult RA. There is hypertrophy of villi, hyperplasia and hypertrophy of the synovial lining layer, and hypervascularity. Synovial biopsy is not usually a useful procedure in diagnosis except in some children presenting with monoarticular arthritis, where the exclusion of other disease processes is important. Erosions may occur at a later stage in severe progressive disease, usually polyarticular, but are not as common or as early as in adult disease.

In children with pauciarticular or polyarticular onset disease, the erythrocyte sedimentation rate (ESR) and C-reactive protein (CRP) may be within

normal limits for age. A microcytic hypochromic anaemia is common, due to a combination of the effects of the chronic inflammatory process and to poor nutritional intake. Classical immunoglobulin (Ig) M rheumatoid factor (RF) is not persistently present except in the small subgroup of RF-positive polyarticular onset disease. Antinuclear antibodies (ANA) will be present in 60% or more of patients, with the highest prevalence in early-onset pauciarticular arthritis (EOPA-JRA) in girls.

Pathogenesis

The pathogenesis of the inflammatory joint lesions in the various forms of juvenile chronic arthritis remains unknown. Immunological factors are important, with the inflammatory lesions being likely to be a response to exogenous or endogenous antigen. Abnormal immunoregulation of the inflammatory response may be an inportant factor in persistence of arthritis. Some of the more recent findings in studies of JRA are described below.

Synovium

The sequence of synovial changes in JRA is initial synovial congestion; cellular infiltration by polymorphonuclear cells then lymphocytes; synovial lining cell hyperplasia and elongation; and vascular proliferation.

Between 5 and 10% of CD3+ cells in inflamed synovium have been reported as TCR $\gamma\delta$ positive in patients with JRA, a finding similar to RA, and it is possible that $\gamma\delta$ T cells are important in the pathogenesis. In JRA, there are approximately equal proportions of Vδ1 and Vδ2 cells, compared with a Vδ1 predominance in RA. In contrast, in peripheral blood, the TCR $\gamma\delta$ lymphocytes have been shown to be mainly Vδ2, suggesting that there may be preferential homing or expansion of the Vδ1 subset in both RA and JRA synovium. The TCR $\gamma\delta$ lymphocytes are present mainly in lymphoid-like tissues and in perivascular areas: only a few TCR $\gamma\delta$ cells are present in the synovial layer. $\gamma\delta$T cells in the synovium in JRA express the activation antigens CD69 and HLA-DR in greater proportions than in peripheral blood. The Vδ1 cells express the high molecular weight isoform CD45RA; most of the Vδ2 have CD45RO.

Synovial fluid

Synovial fluid in JRA has a predominance of polymorphonuclear cells, but it is likely that lymphocytes present have important effects in the pathogenesis of the arthritis. There are low numbers of B cells (CD19) and increased numbers of T cells in synovial fluid in JRA in comparison with peripheral blood. Many of the synovial fluid T cells are activated (DR+). CD4+ cells have been shown to be present in synovial fluid in decreased numbers: those present are CD2hi, CD29+ and have the CD45R0 phenotype — this phenotype is associated with binding to extracellular matrix and is also associated with 'primed' T cells. There is minimal increase in CD25 in synovial fluid. Synovial fluid T cells show restriction of Vβ gene usage of TCR (especially interleukin (IL) 2 receptor (R)+ T cells) in comparison with peripheral blood cells from the same patients. The same Vβ gene family transcriptions have been found in different joints from the same patients suggesting that there may be an antigen or superantigen driven expansion of selected T cells in the synovial compartment. Synovial fluid and peripheral blood lymphocytes from children with persistent arthritis have substantial proliferative responses to human heat shock protein (hsp) 60 expressed in *Escherichia coli* whereas no responses to hsp 60 were seen in adult RA or in child controls. Homologues of human hsp 60 have been shown in synovial membranes in patients but not in controls. Heat shock proteins may be important as a T-cell target in persistent arthritis in childhood: it is possible that hsp are expressed during synovial inflammation and become autoantigens.

Serological evidence of immunological activation

A number of indicators of immunological activation are seen in JRA. It has been suggested that cytokines produced during inflammation may be contributory to the anorexia and growth changes seen in paediatric rheumatic diseases. Serum IL-2R and IL-2 concentrations are elevated in pauciarticular and polyarticular JRA, the elevated levels correlating with parameters of clinical activity, whereas interferon γ has not been detectable in some studies. Serum IL-6 concentrations correlate with fever, joint involvement, and thrombocytosis in systemic onset JRA. Serum sCD8 concentrations are also elevated in serum in severe JRA. In contrast, sCD4 levels are normal and are independent of disease activity. A strong correlation between active disease and C4d and Bb plasma levels has been described in JRA.

Antibodies in serum

A variety of serum antibodies against autoantigens have been described in JRA. The most widely described have been ANAs, seen most commonly but not exclusively in young girls with pauciarticular onset disease and often associated with a higher risk of uveitis.

ANA and histones

ANA positivity has been reported in 58% of pauciarticular, 42% of polyarticular, and 17% of systemic JRA patients in a recent study. Percentage positivity has been higher in recent studies with the use of HEp-2 cells. However, it is important to recognize that a significant number of normally healthy children may also have ANA positivity, although often in relatively low titre. Most ANA are IgG, and the pattern of immunofluorescence is usually speckled or homogeneous. Patients with JRA do not have a common extractable nuclear antigen (ENA). Immunoblot positive sera from patients with JRA detect up to 10 proteins on HeLa nuclear sonicates. Overall, the antibody profiles are highly individual and do not correlate with disease subtype of activity.

Antibody to recombinant high-mobility group nonhistone chromosomal proteins or to DNA free histones is common in pauciarticular JRA and RF-positive polyarticular JRA. In EOPA-JRA, 75% have been found to have IgM antibody to histone, the highest values being anti-H3 and-H4 antibody. Antibody to H3 peptides tended to be seen in patients with chronic anterior uveitis and antibody to a 15 kDa nuclear antigen has been shown by immunoblotting in 45% of pauciarticular patients with chronic anterior uveitis compared with 14% of patients without uveitis.

Granulocyte-specific antibody has been described in JRA but the significance is unknown. In a recent study, granulocyte-specific ANA were found in 17% of children with JRA: 80% of these patients had polyarticular disease. Granulocyte-specific ANA were not found in systemic onset disease. None had ANCA or antibody to elastase by enzyme immunoassary (EIA).

Rheumatoid factors

JRA is characterized by the absence of IgM RF, except in the small group with polyarticular onset, usually older girls, who have disease characteristics similar to adult RA. However, hidden 19S IgM RF is seen in up to 75% of children with JRA, mainly in those with active polyarticular or active pauciarticular disease. One-third of patients with JRA who are RF negative express the Wa idiotype (rheumatoid factor crossreactive idiotype, RFCRI, defined by prototypic monoclonal IgM RFs from Waldenströms macroglobulinaemia patient, Wa) in high titre in their sera. This is not associated with hidden RF. The RFCRI concentrations correlate weakly but significantly with the duration of morning stiffness and functional class, but not with the number of active joints. The expression of RCFRI has been reported to be higher in patients with systemic onset disease.

Other antibodies

A number of other antibody specificites have been described in JRA. Over 50% of sera from children with JRA have been reported to be positive for IgG or IgM anticardiolipin antibody (ACA), in comparison with 28% of adult patients with RA. No child controls had IgG ACA; 5% of child controls had IgM ACA. There was no correlation between the presence or titre of ACA and clinical or laboratory variables and none had any features of the anticardiolipin syndrome. The presence of these antibodies is not associated with specific major histocompatibility complex antigens. It is of interest that ACA also was found in 26% of children with JPsA.

Antibodies to human and mycobacterial hsp have been described in relatively high frequency in persistent childhood arthritis, with higher titres in children with chronically active disease. Antiperinuclear factor antibody has been noted in a high proportion of children with JRA, possibly as a cross-reacting antibody with antistreptococcal cell wall peptidoglycan. Antibodies also have been described to DNA topoisomerase II, collagen components and to iris and retinal antigens in children with pauciarticular disease and uveitis.

Human leucocyte antigen/major histocompatibility complex associations

General

A number of HLA associations have been noted in JRA and its subtypes. These associations differ in most instances from those seen in adult RA, and eventually may give insights into the pathogenesis of disease. An increased frequency of A2, DR5, and DR8 is well recognized in JRA, particularly in pauciarticular-onset disease. The frequency of DR4 is decreased in most JRA in comparison to the non-arthritic population, in contrast to RA. HLA-B27 is expressed with higher frequency in late-onset pauciarticular disease. More recent studies have emphasized the importance of the DQA1 gene locus and its even stronger primary association with JRA overall than the DR locus. Two DQA1 alleles (DQA1*0401 and DQA1*0501) are strongly associated with seronegative JRA. The amino acid sequences in exon 2 of DQA1 show a sequence common to all the disease-associated alleles. Thus there may be a functional role for DQ molecules in the pathogenesis of JRA; it is possible that arthritogenic peptides are bound specifically by DQ molecules, and even that some of the arthritogenic peptides may be derived from self histocompatibility antigens, such as A2.

Human leucocyte antigen associations with subtypes of juvenile rheumatoid arthritis

Systemic onset

Systemic onset disease is associated with an increased frequency of DR4, the frequency tending to be greater in patients with less severe disease. B27 has been found to be increased in those in whom relapses were associated with intercurrent infections.

Early-onset pauciarticular disease (EOPA-JRA)

The frequency of A2, DR5, and DR8 is increased. The strongest associations for pauciarticular arthritis are with DRB1 alleles. The critical nucleotides among the HLA genes are not known; however, disease specific mutations have not been shown. The DQA1*0101 allele is found in more than 50% of those with pauciarticular onset who progress to persistent polyarticular disease, the relative risk in comparison with controls being fourfold or more. There is also an increased frequency of DPB1*0201.

In EOPA, PCR amplified DNA has shown a hierarchy in the DRB1 system:

(1) susceptible   DRB1*08; DR5;

(2) permissive   DRB1*01;

(3) moderately protective DR2; DRB1*04;

(4) protective   DRB1*07.

In contrast, in the DPB1 system, there is no hierarchy, and DPB1*0201 appears susceptible. Associations with DPB1*0201, DR5, and DRB1*08 are independent of each other, i.e. they are not due to linkage disequilibrium. It is possible that interactions may exist between DPB1*0201 and a common DQ factor associated with both DR5 and DRB1*08.

EOPA and uveitis

In patients with EOPA and iridocyclitis, DR5 is associated with eye disease, while DR1 is associated with the absence of eye disease. In a recent study of 164 patients with EOPA-JRA, of whom 78 had chronic iridocyclitis, there was only one split of DR5 (DRB*1104) that showed a significant association with a risk of chronic iridocyclitis. DQA1*0501 and DQB1*0301, which are both in linkage disequilibrium with DRB1*1104, were also associated significantly with eye disease. Patients with both DRB1*1104 and DPB1*0201 genes had a 7.7 times increased risk for chronic iridocyclitis compared with other patients. DRB1*1104 is four times as specific but only one-third as sensitive as ANA in identifying patients at risk for eye disease.

In patients without ANA and chronic iridocyclitis, there is an increase in DRB1*0101/02 and DQA1*0101.

Polyarticular onset disease

Polyarticular disease with early onset (<4 years) is associated with DR5 and DR8; polyarticular disease with late onset (>4 years) is associated with DR4 largely because DR4 is associated with RF-positive polyarticular JRA. The main susceptibility factor for RF-negative polyarticular juvenile arthritis is DRB1*0301, as is also seen in adult patients with RF-negative arthritis. A recent study of 94 Caucasian children with polyarticular JRA showed that DRw8, DQw4, DQA1*0401, and DQB1*0402 were increased in seronegative patients, with the highest frequencies in patients with young onset (<5 years).

Presentation and early differential diagnosis of juvenile rheumatoid arthritis

The presentation of arthritis in childhood will usually be with alteration of joint function, for example a limp, refusal to weight bear, or difficulty in running or climbing; pain in the affected joints; joint swelling; and warmth of the affected joint. Occasionally, in the very young child, the presentation will be with a fixed joint deformity. A history of early morning stiffness is often obtained on careful questioning. The diagnosis of JRA is usually one of exclusion. The child with a monoarthritis presents greater diagnostic difficulty in differentiating an acute infective process from non-infective inflammatory disorders. However, children with involvement of more than one joint at presentation need to have a wide range of disorders considered during the early stages of disease. These will include acute rheumatic fever and other forms of reactive arthritis, the arthritis of inflammatory bowel disease,

systemic lupus erythematosus (SLE), and the other connective tissue disorders. Children with systemic onset disease will usually present as a fever of unknown origin and often require investigation for infection and for malignant disorders, e.g. leukaemia or neuroblastoma.

Investigation of the child with suspected juvenile rheumatoid arthritis

The initial investigation of a child with possible JRA depends on the nature of the presentation and the potential differential diagnoses. Useful initial investigations are listed in Table 29.3. In addition, a bone scan may be indicated to identify other areas of inflammatory change; a Mantoux test may be required; ANA characterized (ENA) and antibody to dsDNA measured; and the joint aspirated in those with a monoarthritis at presentation. It is important to note that the ESR and CRP may not be elevated in a number of children with chronic arthritis, that a hypochromic microcytic anaemia is common, and that significant numbers of children without arthritis will have a positive ANA result. The usual changes seen on X-rays of affected joints are soft tissue swelling, effusions, and perhaps an alteration in the joint space but erosions are relatively uncommon, especially early in the disease process.

Management

The principles of management are: the maintenance of joint function; the relief of pain; and the prevention of deformity. The management programme involves medical, physiotherapy, orthotic and nursing skills; education of the child, family and school, and wider community in the many aspects of the disorder; assistance

∎ **Table 29.3** Initial investigations in suspected juvenile rheumatoid arthritis

Complete blood examination
Erythrocyte sedimentation rate
C-reactive protein
Rheumatoid factor
Antistreptolysin-O test, DNase B
Immunoglobulins G, A, and M
Antinuclear antibody
X-ray of involved joints (may X-ray contralateral joints for comparison)
Ophthalmological assessment using a slit lamp

with schooling; consideration of local and systemic effects on growth; nutritional assessment; awareness of the potential side-effects of pharmocological therapies; and support for the child and family for the psychological aspects of a chronic and potentially disabling disease. All of these must be provided in a co-ordinated programme with the close involvement and understanding of the child and her/his family.

The part of the paediatric physiotherapist is of major importance. Passive and active exercises are needed to maintain the range of movement of affected joints and to maintain muscle strength. Splinting in an appropriate rest position is important in preserving the range of movement and preventing deformity. Warmth assists in modifying morning joint stiffness.

Pain relief can be obtained with paracetamol used as needed. Aspirin has been a very useful anti-inflammatory agent, but its use has been supplanted by other non-steroidal anti-inflammatory agents, particularly those available in syrup form such as naproxen. Methotrexate (10 mg/m^2 per week) has an important place relatively early in the management of progressive joint disease, and is well tolerated by the majority of children. Higher doses may prove to be safe and even more efficacious, and need to be evaluated in appropriate trials. Other drugs in common use are sulphasalazine and hydroxychloroquine. Parenteral gold may be useful in a few children unresponsive to other therapies, but has significant toxicity and requires close supervision.

Corticosteroids have a place in topical management of uveitis; as intraarticular injections (using triamcinolone hexacetonide) in selected joints, e.g. in the knee in pauciarticular disease if satisfactory responses to non-steroidal agents are not obtained; and systemically in some patients with systemic onset disease. Pulse doses of intravenous methylprednisolone have been used in some patients with severe progressive uveitis. Intravenous immunoglobulin has been shown to have an effect in some children with systemic onset disease by controlling fever and other systemic features, although this is not maintained and there is no clear evidence of any effect on later joint outcome. Cyclosporin has been used in a few centres for children with arthritis unresponsive to other therapies, but its use should be considered experimental at present.

Surgical approaches are confined largely to consideration of release procedures in joints with fixed deformities and joint replacement, particularly hip replacement, in the late stages of disease.

Outcome

The usual course of JRA is one of a variable period of disease activity, followed by remission of active arthri-

tis. Approximately 80% will have eventual remission without significant disability long term. Those with early-onset disease have a particularly good prognosis, provided that uveitis in managed appropriately in conjunction with good management of the joint disease. Aproximately two-thirds of of those with systemic onset have a good outcome with little late residual disability; approximately one-third will progress to severe polyarticular disease with long-term significant functional impairment. RF positive polyarticular disease is much more likely to have a poor prognosis, with the development of destructive joint disease and associated deformity.

Other chronic arthritides of childhood

The principles of management of the other chronic arthritides of childhood are dependent on the underlying disorder and its treatment. Juvenile ankylosing spondylitis and juvenile psoriatic arthritis require an approach similar to that for JRA. The disease course tends to be longer and more persistent. The arthropathy of inflammatory bowel disease, SLE, and other connective tissue disorders will respond to treatment of the primary disorder in most.

Future developments

The most significant developments in the future for persistent arthritis in childhood will be delineation of aetiology, clarification of the role of genetic susceptibility factors, identification of specific disease markers which will allow early and accurate diagnosis, understanding of the nature of uveitis, and the development of anti-inflammatory agents with greater efficacy and lower toxicity. TCR identification offers promise for the detection of possible aetiological agents, as does careful PCR analysis of joint fluid samples. It may be possible to provide more selective immunomodulation once the role of cytokines such as tumour necrosis factor α is understood more completely.

Further reading

Ansell, B. M. (1992). Juvenile rheumatoid arthritis, juvenile chronic arthritis, and juvenile spondyloarthropathies. *Current Opinion in Rheumatology*, **4**, 706–12.

Ansell, B. M., Rudge, S., and Schaller, J. G. (1991). *A colour atlas of paediatric rheumatology*. Wolfe, London.

Cabral, D. A., Petty, R. E., Fung, M., and Malleson, P. N. (1992). Persistent antinuclear antibodies in children without identifiable inflammatory rheumatic or autoimmune disease. *Pediatrics*, **89**, 441–4.

Cabral, D. A., Petty, R. E., Malleson, P. N., Ensworth, S., McCormick, A. Q., and Schroeder, M. L. (1994). Visual prognosis in children with chronic anterior uveitis and arthritis. *Journal of Rheumatology*, **21**, 2370–5.

Cassidy, J. T. and Petty, R. E. (1994). *Textbook of pediatric rheumatology*. Churchill Livingstone, New York.

De Graeff Meeder, E. R., van Eden, W., Rijkers, G. T., Prakken, B. J., Zegers, B. J., and Kuis, W. (1993). Heat-shock proteins and juvenile chronic arthritis. *Clinical and Experimental Rheumatology*, **11**(Suppl. 9), S25–8.

De Graeff-Meeder, E. R., van Eden, W., Rijkers, G. T., *et al.* (1995). Juvenile chronic arthritis: T cell reactivity to human HSP60 in patients with a favourable course of arthritis. *Journal of Clinical Investigation*, **95**, 934–40.

Donn, R. P., Thomson, W., Pepper, L., *et al.* (1995). Antinuclear antibodies in early onset pauciarticular juvenile chronic arthritis (JCA) are associated with HLA-DQB1*0603: a possible JCA-associated human leucocyte antigen haplotype. *British Journal of Rheumatology*, **34**, 461–65.

Epplen, C., Rumpf, H., Albert, E., Haas, P., Truckenbrodt, H., and Epplen, J. T. (1995). Immunoprinting excludes many potential susceptibility genes as predisposing to early onset pauciarticular juvenile chronic arthritis except HLA class II and TNF. *European Journal of Immunogenetics*, **22**, 311–22.

Fantini, F. (1993). Future trends in pediatric rheumatology. *Journal of Rheumatology*, **20**, 49–53.

Fernandez-Vina, M., Fink, C. W., and Stastny, P. (1994). HLA associations and juvenile arthritis. *Clinical and Experimental Rheumatology*, **12**, 205–14.

Fink, C. W. (1995). Proposal for the development of classification criteria for idiopathic arthritides of childhood. *Journal of Rheumatology*, **22**, 1566–9.

Fink, C. W., Fernandez-Vina, M., and Stastny, P. (1995). Clinical and genetic evidence that juvenile arthritis is not a single disease. *Paediatric Clinics of North America*, **42**, 1155–69.

Haas, J. P., Nevinny-Stickel, C., Schoenwald, U., Truckenbrodt, H., Suschke, J., and Albert, E. D. (1994). Susceptible and protective major histocompatibility complex class II alleles in early-onset pauciarticular juvenile chronic arthritis. *Human Immunology*, **41**, 225–33.

Haas, J. P., Truckenbrodt, H., Paul, C., *et al.* (1994). Subtypes of HLA-DRB1*03, *08, *11, *12, *13 and *14 in early onset pauciarticular juvenile chronic arthritis (EOPA) with and without iridocyclitis. *Clinical and Experimental Rheumatology*, **12** (Suppl 10), S7–S14.

Gare, B. A. and Fasth, A. (1992). Epidemiology of juvenile chronic arthritis in southwestern Sweden: a 5-year prospective population study. *Pediatrics*, **90**, 950–8.

Horneff, G., Hanson, M., and Wahn, V. (1993). T cell receptor V beta chain expression in patients with juvenile rheumatoid arthritis. *Rheumatology International*, **12**, 221–6.

Jacobs, J. C. (1992). *Pediatric rheumatology for the practitioner*. Springer-Verlag, New York.

Lawrence, J. M., Moore, T. L., Osborn, T. G., Nesher, G., Madson, K. L., and Kinsella, M. B. (1993). Autoantibody studies in juvenile rheumatoid arthritis. *Seminars of Arthritis and Rheumatism*, **22**, 265–74.

Leak, A. M., Tuaillon, N., Muller, S., and Woo, P. (1993). Study of antibodies to histones and histone synthetic peptides in pauciarticular juvenile chronic arthritis. *British Journal of Rheumatology*, **32**, 426–31.

Life, P., Hassell, A., Williams, K., Young, S., Bacon, P., Southwood, T., and Gaston, J. S. (1993). Responses to gram negative enteric bacterial antigens by synovial T cells from patients with juvenile chronic arthritis: recognition of heat shock protein HSP60. *Journal of Rheumatology*, **20**, 1388–96.

Lipnick, R. N., Tsokos, G. C., and Magilavy, D. B. (1991). Immune abnormalities in the pathogenesis of juvenile rheumatoid arthritis. *Rheumatic Disease Clinics of North America*, **17**, 843–57.

Muller, K., Pedersen, F. K., Wiikm, A., and Bendtzenm, K. (1992). Lymphokines and soluble interleukin-2 receptors in juvenile chronic arthritis. Clinical and laboratory correlations. *Rheumatology International*, **12**, 89–92.

Nepom, B. (1991). The immunogenetics of juvenile rheumatoid arthritis. *Rheumatic Disease Clinics of North America*, **17**, 825–42.

Ploski, R., Vinje, O., Ronningen, K. S., Spurkland, A., Sorskaar, D., Vartdal, F., and Forre, O. (1993). HLA class II alleles and heterogeneity of juvenile rheumatoid arthritis. DRB1*0101 may define a novel subset of the disease. *Arthritis and Rheumatism*, **36**, 465–72.

Prieur, A. M. (1992). Prospects in pediatric rheumatology. *Journal of Rheumatology*, Suppl. **37**, 2–4.

Pugh, M. T., Southwood, T. R., and Gaston, J. S. (1993). The role of infection in juvenile chronic arthritis. *British Journal of Rheumatology*, **32**, 838–44.

Silverman, E. D., Laxer, R. M., Greenwald, M., Gelfand, E., Shore, A., Stein, L. D., and Roifman, C. M. (1990). Intravenous immunoglobulin therapy in systemic juvenile rheumatoid arthritis. *Arthritis and Rheumatism*, **33**, 1015–22.

Silverman, E. D., Isacovics, B., Petsche, D., and Laxer, R. M. (1993). Synovial fluid cells in juvenile arthritis: evidence of selective T cell migration to inflamed tissue. *Clinical and Experimental Immunology*, **91**, 90–5.

Sioud, M., Kjeldsen Kragh J, Suleyman, S., Vinje, O., Natvig, J. B., and Forre, O. (1992). Limited heterogeneity of T cell receptor variable region gene usage in juvenile rheumatoid arthritis synovial T cells. *European Journal of Immunology*, **22**, 2413–18.

Southwood, T. R., and Malleson, P. N. (1991). Antinuclear antibodies and juvenile chronic arthritis (JCA): search for a specific autoantibody associated with JCA. *Annals of Rheumatic Disease*, **50**, 595–8.

Thompson, S. D., Grom, A. A., Bailey, S., *et al.* (1995). Patterns of T lymphocyte clonal expression in HLA-typed patients with juvenile rheumatoid arthritis. *Journal of Rheumatology*, **22**, 1356–64.

Tucker, L. B. (1992). Heritable disorders of connective tissue and disability and chronic disease in childhood. *Current Opinion in Rheumatology*, **4**, 731–40.

Tucker, L. B. (1993). Juvenile rheumatoid arthritis. *Current Opinion in Rheumatology*, **5**, 619–28.

Wallace, C. A., Sherry, D. D., Mellins, E. D., and Aiken, R. P. (1993). Predicting remission in juvenile rheumatoid arthritis with methotrexate treatment. *Journal of Rheumatology*, **20**, 118–22.

White, P. H. and Ansell, B. A. (1992). Methotrexate for juvenile rheumatoid arthritis. *New England Journal of Medicine*, **326**, 1077–8.

Woo, P. (1993). Cytokines in childhood rheumatic diseases. *Archives of Disease in Childhood*, **69**, 547–9.

<u>30</u> Vasculitides

C. M. Lockwood

Introduction

The primary systemic vasculitides are characterized by the presence of inflammation and necrosis of the blood vessels themselves, with disease outside the vasculature being subordinate to this. As such they are distinct from the secondary forms of vasculitis, which arise in the context of other pathology, for example close to a necrotic tumour or downstream from an abscess cavity. According to the site and size of vessel involved, a number of eponymously defined primary vasculitic syndromes have been recognized. Their classification, however, has been difficult because so little was known about either their aetiology or pathogenesis and much confusion has arisen. The simple classification used here, reached by recent consensus, is largely a morphological one, based on the size of vessel involved and the presence or absence of granulomas near the vasculitic lesions (see Table 30.1). It is worth reviewing briefly the way in which the difficulties with classification arose, as these led to different terminologies being used for the same vasculitides in Europe and the USA, which are still widely used in literature on both sides of the Atlantic.

The first vasculitic syndrome to be identified was in a case report by Kussmaul and Maier in 1866 which contained a classical description of a patient with polyarteritis nodosa. The autopsy revealed widespread nodular inflammation in muscular arteries which had the calibre of coronary and hepatic vessels. In 1948 Davson drew attention to two types of polyarteritis that could coexist, especially in the kidney. The first was the typical arteritis of large vessels found in polyarteritis nodosa, the second was a necrotizing glomerulonephritis or microscopic polyarteritis. How frequently polyarteritis nodosa is accompanied by microscopic polyarteritis is still debated, but the latter became recognized as a separate entity also affecting extrarenal sites; as such it was given the name 'hypersensitivity angiitis' by Zeek in 1953, who considered it might be caused by an abnormal response to drugs or infections. This approach is understandable, given that systemic vasculitis frequently presents with a fever for which antibiotic treatment is ineffective, therefore leading to the suggestion, as the clinical vasculitis developed clinically, that the treatment was causal. Subsequently, the term 'hypersensitivity angiitis' was used to describe idiopathic small vessel vasculitis of the microscopic polyarteritis variety. More recently, Cupps and Fauci in 1982 used the same term to describe a cutaneous leucocytoclastic vasculitis in which visceral involvement was absent or occurred only rarely: present day assessment would probably

∎ Table 30.1 Pathology of vasculitides

Vessel size	Granulomatous	Non-granulomatous
Small	Wegener's granulomatosis	Kawasaki disease Micoscopic polyangiitis (hypersensitivity vasculitis) Henoch–Schönlein syndrome
Medium	Churg–Strauss syndrome	Polyarteritis nodosa
Large	Giant cell arteritis Takayasu arteritis	

consider the latter as an example of microscopic polyarteritis with predominantly skin involvement. Consensus has now been reached that the term 'microscopic polyangiitis' should be used to indicate that a venulitis and capillaritis may be present as well as inflammation of the small arteries, in those conditions previously described as microscopic polyarteritis or hypersensitivity angiitis.

As well as the identification of polyarteritis nodosa and microscopic polyangiitis as separate syndromes, other small vessel vasculitides emerged as individual entities, based largely on the pattern of organ involvement and, to a varying extent, distinctive associated pathology. Thus Henoch–Schönlein purpura (Schönlein 1837; Henoch 1874) was characterized by its gastrointestinal, kidney, joint, and skin symptomatology with distinctive immunoglobulin (Ig) A deposition in kidney, gut, and skin; Wegener's granulomatosis (1936) by the granulomatous involvement of the upper respiratory tract, lungs, and kidneys and Churg–Strauss syndrome (1952) by its asthma and peripheral eosinophilia. Most recently, Kawasaki disease (1967) has been recognized as a childhood vasculitis in which aneurysmal dilation of affected medium-sized arteries, particularly the coronaries, can have substantial clinical pathological consequences.

Aetiology and pathogenesis

The aetiology of the small vessel vasculitides is poorly understood. A genetic predisposition, virus or bacterial infectious agents, as well as abnormal responses to drugs, have been suggested as important factors. A weak genetic linkage of systemic vasculitis with DQw7 has been reported but not yet confirmed by other studies. Hepatitis B infection has been associated with polyarteritis nodosa and the virus identified in both circulating immune complexes as well as in vasculitic lesions, although whether, because of the infectious load, the virus is deposited ubiquitously in any immune complex has yet to be determined. That environmental factors, such as microbial pathogens, may be important is suggested by the seasonal incidence of vasculitis, with a peak in winter in the North American population. However, whether these environmental factors are initiators or amplifiers of injury is uncertain as, for example, there is a well documented association of vasculitis relapse after episodes of intercurrent infection. Better evidence supports the role of drugs in producing vasculitis. Both hydralazine and propyl thiouracil have been reported to cause a microscopic polyarteritis characterized by the associated development of autoantibodies to neutrophil cytoplasm antigens. Withdrawal of the drugs was accompanied by disappearance of the vasculitic lesions. Experimental models to study the aetiology of vasculitis have been difficult to develop but in both the Kinjoh mouse and the Brown Norway rat the role of genetic factors in predisposing to vasculitic injury is now emerging and in the latter the part of infection in exacerbating the vasculitis has been found to be closely analogous to the situation in humans.

Humoral autoimmunity in systemic vasculitis

A major advance in our understanding of the small vessel vasculitides has come with the identification of circulating autoantibodies, antineutrophil cytoplasm antigens (ANCA) in a variety of the syndromes which make up the spectrum of vasculitis. They can be found in the majority of untreated patients with Wegener's granulomatosis, microscopic polyangiitis, and Kawasaki disease, as well as to a variable extent in Churg–Strauss syndrome and polyarteritis nodosa. Their immunochemical properties and pathophysiological effects have led to the belief that they are important in pathogenesis.

Initially, these autoantibodies were characterized by the pattern of indirect immunofluorescence which was produced when sera from patients were overlaid on to immobilized normal human polymorphonuclear leucocytes. Two binding specificities were recognized: the first a cytoplasmic granular immunofluorescence with an interlobular accentuation (c-ANCA) and the second a perinuclear (p-ANCA) pattern. Subsequently, the molecular nature of the ligands was identified, the target of c-ANCA being one molecule, a neutral serine proteinase, proteinase 3 (Pr3), those giving p-ANCA comprising a number of different molecules including myeloperoxidase (MPO), the most frequent, as well as elastase, lysozyme, lactoferrin, and cathepsin G. Careful clinical correlation has shown that anti-Pr3 antibodies are closely associated with the development of Wegener's granulomatosis. However, although anti-MPO antibodies are associated with the development of microscopic polyangiitis, the association is not so close as for anti-Pr3 antibodies and Wegener's granulomatosis: anti-MPO antibodies have been described in a number of conditions, particularly chronic inflammatory gastrointestinal lesions, such as sclerosing cholangitis, chronic active hepatitis, ulcerative colitis, and Crohn's disease. In none of these is a primary vasculitis a dominant component. Furthermore, conditions indistinguishable from microscopic polyangiitis have been described in association with ANCA with specificity for elastase, cathepsin G, and lactoferrin.

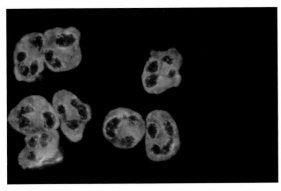

(a)

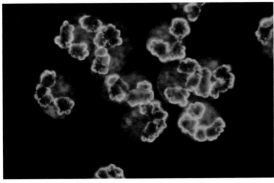

(b)

∎ **Fig. 30.1** Anti neutrophil cytoplasmic antibody (a) cytoplasmic (c-ANCA) and (b) perinuclear (p-ANCA) antinuclear cytoplasmic cytoplasmic antibody in vasculitic diseases.

ANCA in diagnosis and management

Approximately 85% of patients with untreated Wegener's granulomatosis will have anti-Pr3 antibodies. It appears that those with limited disease are less likely to have positive serology. The presence of anti-Pr3 antibodies in conditions other than vasculitis is exceptionally rare and thus the presence of anti-Pr3 antibodies has come to be recognized as highly specific for Wegener's granulomatosis. Approximately 70% of patients with microscopic polyangiitis have circulating MPO antibodies; as mentioned above, other antigenic specificities have been identified, notably to elastase, cathepsin G, and lactoferrin. Thus the presence of anti-MPO antibodies is a less valuable aid to diagnosis in conditions suggestive of vasculitis than is the case for anti-Pr3 antibodies, particularly as the presence of anti-MPO antibodies is increasingly being noted in a variety of inflammatory gastrointestinal conditions. Anti-MPO antibodies have also been recorded in a number of patients with other forms of vasculitis

such as the Churg–Strauss syndrome and polyarteritis nodosa, perhaps reflecting a component of microscopic polyangiitis in these conditions. When indirect immunfluorescence was the only diagnostic test available, false positive ANCA tests were recorded rarely in acquired immune deficiency syndrome (AIDS) and other chronic infections such as subacute bacterial endocarditis (SBE). However, such false positive results have not been substantiated in studies using molecularly defined antigens.

Levels of ANCA have been shown to correlate with disease activity and in many centres their value as a guide to management has been established. Hence, in individual patients, rising titres have often been found to be reliable predictors of relapse. Thus, in management, many physicians use ANCA as a better guide to disease activity than measurements of the acute phase response, such as erythrocyte sedimentation rate (ESR) and C-reactive protein (CRP), which were hitherto the only indices available but which are relatively non-discriminatory, varying with other intercurrent events such as infection. Nevertheless there are certain patients in whom high ANCA levels persist, despite little evidence of disease activity being apparent clinically and there are others in whom vasculitis activity seemingly continues, in the absence of detectable ANCA. Thus, rising titres of ANCA should be viewed with caution and alert the physician to extra vigilance and readiness to treat early, rather than dictate treatment escalation.

ANCA in pathogenesis

Several studies have suggested that ANCA can stimulate polymorphonuclear leucocytes directly, by binding to membrane expressed Pr3 and MPO. As a consequence, neutrophil adhesion is increased through upregulation of the expression of the adhesion molecule CD18 and eventual activation brings about the release of injurious oxygen-free radicals. Thus in inappropriate sites, for example, within the microvasculature the neutrophil may mediate endothelial cell injury and so initiate vasculitis. *In vitro* studies have confirmed the toxic effects of purified ANCA and polymorphonuclear leucocytes on cultured endothelial cells, suggesting that this is indeed a route by which vasculitic damage may occur. Other work has focused on the ability of cytokines, particularly tumour necrosis factor (TNF), to orchestrate the expression of Pr3 on the surface of the endothelial cell. This ligand is then the target for ANCA-mediated cytolysis. Finally, another school of thought has suggested that ANCA may inhibit the complexation of neutrophil enzymes with their physiological inactivators, such as α_1-antitrypsin. Thus tissue destruction may take place wherever inactivation of these enzymes is impeded by the autoantibodies.

Wegener's granulomatosis

Definition

Wegener's granulomatosis is a necrotizing granulomatous vasculitis which involves both the upper and lower respiratory tracts. Typically, this is accompanied by a small vessel vasculitis affecting the kidney and to a variable extent by a vasculitis in other organs. Circulating autoantibodies to neutrophil cytoplasm antigens, usually to Pr3, can be found in most untreated patients at presentation.

Clinical features

Many patients develop clinical evidence of their vasculitis against a background of non-specific symptoms such as malaise, weight loss, fever, and night sweats, reflecting a constitutional disturbance, together with evidence of multisystem disease, reflecting the pattern of vasculitic involvement. The disease has an equal sex incidence and no ethnic group is exempt. The course is variable: some patients have indolent disease which takes months or years to declare itself, during which long periods occur when the patient is relatively symptom-free; other patients develop fulminating life-threatening organ failure within weeks. Because any organ system may be involved the patient may be seen first by a wide range of specialists, so that a varying spectrum of clinical involvement may be reported. However, with the predilection of the vasculitis to affect the airways, usually respiratory tract symptoms and signs predominate.

Upper respiratory tract

Bloody foul smelling nasal discharge, paranasal sinus pain, nasal ulceration, and septal perforation, as well as eventually a saddle nose deformity, may be present. URT involvement includes the development of chronic suppurative otitis media, due to eustachian tube blockage and occasionally painless deafness, due to eighth nerve involvement. Hoarseness or stridor may also be a feature due to granulomas developing on the vocal chords or vasculitis in the trachea producing tracheal stenosis, respectively. Granulomatous space occupying lesions in the sinuses may erode locally leading to fistula formation and bacterial superinfection may be a significant clinical problem wherever the mucosal epithelium is breached (see below).

Lower respiratory tract and lungs

Chronic non-productive cough, dyspnoea, pleurisy, and haemoptysis may all reflect vasculitic injury and/or granuloma development in the airways or lung parenchyma. Occasionally, formation of exuberant endobronchial granulomatous tissue can occlude the airways and lead to segmental collapse, or more rarely an obliterative bronchiolitis may spread sleeve-like along the bronchi or bronchioles. The extension of this into the alveolar spaces either as a capillaritis or as a necrotizing granulomatous pneumonic process may bring about a rapid deterioration in pulmonary function and is an ominous development when it is accompanied by lung haemorrhage, this being particularly resistant to treatment. Although on X-ray characteristically there are pulmonary nodules which may cavitate, transient pulmonary infiltrates or more permanent changes of pulmonary fibrosis may also be found.

Renal involvement

This is dealt with in detail elsewhere and has particular importance because until renal replacement therapy became widely available the prognosis of the disease was determined by the nature of the renal injury and its response to treatment. Even in the presence of normal renal function, early renal involvement may be suspected from the findings of asymptomatic proteinuria and haematuria. Renal biopsy at this stage may only show a minor focal proliferative glomerulonephritis. The tempo of the renal disease is unpredictable and the sudden deterioration in renal function, in the presence of red cell casts in the urine, may indicate the development of an acute focal necrotizing glomerular capillaritis with crescent formation, the histological hallmark of rapidly progressive nephritis. Although the glomerulus usually bears the brunt of the vasculitic injury, capillaritis may be found elsewhere in kidney, for example in the peritubular vessels, so that occasionally the histological picture may be that of a granulomatous tubulo-interstitial nephritis.

The eye

Conjunctivitis, uveitis, and scleritis may all occur in Wegener's, but the finding of proptosis, due to retro-orbital development of granulomatous vasculitis forming a pseudo-tumour, is particularly important. First, in the context of respiratory tract disease or nephritis it is strongly suggestive of Wegener's; second, in approximately 50% of patients it causes loss of vision because of optic nerve ischaemia and third, due to involvement of the extra-ocular muscles, it may be responsible for the loss of conjugate gaze and diplopia.

Other manifestations

Most patients experience generalized myalgias and arthralgias at some stage in the disease, less frequently a symmetrical polyarthritis may develop. Occasionally, the arthritis may be restricted to one or few joints. However, joint deformity is not a feature of arthritis in Wegener's granulomatosis. A variety of lesions can be found in the skin. These may vary from nail fold infarcts and purpuric rashes to isolated ulcers, vesicles, and papules. Biopsy occasionally discloses granulomas typical of Wegener's. Nervous system involvement is unusual but can be severely debilitating. Mononeuritis multiplex is the commonest neurological lesion; occasionally, central nervous system abnormalities are found, including isolated lesions of the cranial nerves, meningeal involvement, and stroke.

Wegener's granulomatosis affecting the heart is rare but pericarditis and coronary arteritis have been reported as well as arrhythmias attributed to granulomas in the conducting bundles of Hiss. Very rarely biopsy-proven Wegener's granulomatosis has been described in the breast, ureter, vagina, cervix, and parotid gland.

'Limited' Wegener's granulomatosis is the term given to the condition where there is only restricted involvement evident clinically and in most patients it describes disease limited to the upper respiratory tract. Sometimes this situation may persist for many years before progression to other organ involvement occurs; occasionally subclinical disease is only discovered at autopsy. There was an impression that limited Wegener's ran a more benign course and was easier to treat, but with the advent of serological tests to diagnose the condition more readily it has become evident that milder, generalized forms of the disease also exist and so the prognostic and therapeutic distinction is no longer evident.

Diagnosis

The diagnosis may be suspected clinically from the combination of upper or lower airways disease together with renal involvement. Usually, there is evidence of constitutional disturbance producing malaise, fever, night sweats, and weight loss. Biopsy confirmation may prove to be frustrating as histological evidence of granulomatous vasculitis is often hard to obtain. Usually, the kidney provides the most suitable tissue, although transbronchial biopsies are also useful. In the kidney the diagnostic requirement is the demonstration of focal necrosis of the glomerular capillary wall in the absence of any other primary glomerular pathology. The differential diagnosis then lies between other small vessel vasculitides such as microscopic polyangiitis and Henoch–Schönlein purpura, systemic lupus erythematosus (SLE) or Goodpasture's syndrome associated with antiglomerular basement membrane (GBM) antibodies. Immunofluorescence of the renal biopsy may be helpful in this differential as mesangial deposits of IgA are characteristic of Henoch–Schönlein disease, glomerular and extraglomerular capillary immunoglobulin deposits of any, and sometimes each, isotype, as well as complement, are found in lupus nephritis and linear deposits of IgG along the GBM are the hallmark of anti-GBM nephritis. Glomerular immunoglobulin deposits, if found at all, are typically scanty in Wegener's granulomatosis or microscopic polyarteritis, accounting for the term 'pauci-immune nephritis' often used to describe the renal lesion in both diseases. Because granulomas are rarely found in the kidney, further distinction between these two disorders has to depend on the clinical context and ANCA specificity.

Until recently, there was no diagnostic laboratory test for Wegener's granulomatosis. However, growing evidence now suggests that ANCA with specificity for Pr3 are closely associated with the development of the disease; rarely have autoantibodies with this specificity validated by accepted criteria (immunoblotting, immunoprecipitation, and competitive inhibition studies using pure molecular species) been reported in other conditions and in none consistently. Thus anti-Pr3 antibodies are proving to be valuable for the diagnosis of Wegener's granulomatosis, frequently alerting the physician to the need for careful evaluation of multisystem symptomatology and close supervision during follow-up of a suspected case. As mentioned above, they can be found in 85% of untreated patients with generalized disease and in approximately 60% of those with limited Wegener's granulomatosis. Other abnormal laboratory findings, characteristic of any small vessel vasculitis in the untreated acute phase, include, almost invariably, normochromic normocytic anaemia, neutrophil leucocytosis, thrombocytosis, and evidence of an acute phase response (raised ESR and CRP), as well as in 80% of patients, a polyclonal increase in immunoglobulins and, in 50%, a positive rheumatoid factor.

Differential diagnosis

The clinical presentation with pulmonary renal involvement and distinctive serology has made the differential diagnosis of the patient with Wegener's granulomatosis relatively straightforward. Atypical forms either with limited disease expression or negative serology may still cause problems. In such circumstances lung tumours or other causes of granulomatous change, such as tuberculosis (TB) or sarcoid may be suspected. Differentiation from other vasculitides or connective tissue diseases may be troublesome and distinction from the pulmonary renal presentation of Goodpasture's syndrome may be difficult because the two can coexist and is important because the implications for treatment are different. The presence of circulating anti-GBM antibodies in patients with Goodpasture's syndrome is usually helpful here.

Idiopathic 'lethal' mid-line granuloma may present with features suggestive of Wegener's limited to the head and neck. This condition is now thought to be a variant of a T-cell lymphoma, which is locally invasive and not found elsewhere other than the head and neck. Unlike Wegener's it may produce destructive ulceration of facial tissues, although both can erode through upper airways. In idiopathic mid-line granuloma laboratory tests reflect the absence of inflammatory vasculitis with near normal ESR or CRP and absence of neutrophilia or thrombocytosis.

Lymphomatoid granulomatosis is extremely rare but closely resembles Wegener's granulomatosis in the multisystem distribution of tissue involvement, where it can affect lungs, kidney, upper respiratory tract, and central nervous system. It differs from Wegener's in the nature of the blood vessel involvement, with an absence of an inflammatory infiltrate; instead the vessel destruction appears to be mediated by infiltrates of lymphocytes of either T- or B-cell lineage. In approximately half the patients lymphomatous transformation eventually occurs. In keeping with absence of the inflammatory component a raised CRP, ESR, and neutrophilia are usually not found.

Microscopic polyangiitis

Definition

Microscopic polyangiitis is a small vessel vasculitis which may affect any organ in the body, either individually or in multisystem fashion. However, disease limited to a single organ is not uncommon, being well described for kidney, gut, and skin, although evolution to a multisystem disease may occur up to several years after presentation. Circulating autoantibodies to a variety of neutrophil cytoplasm antigens, predominantly MPO, can be found in many patients.

Clinical features

The disease has an equal sex incidence and is not restricted by age or race. Constitutional disturbance manifested by fever, night sweats, weight loss, and profound malaise is common and it may not be for some weeks before organ-specific symptoms arise. In one-third of the patients a 'flu'-like prodromal illness may occur prior to presentation.

Renal involvement

The kidney is almost always involved in microscopic polyangiitis and up to 100% of patients have proteinuria and haematuria during their illness. Although occasionally mild at first, more frequently there is a glomerulonephritis of moderate severity which may run a rapidly progressive course. However, it is not possible to predict the outcome, based on the level of creatinine at referral. Renal biopsy usually but not always reflects the severity of the vasculitis, the presence of focal necrosis of glomerular capillary walls supporting the diagnosis. For some time nephrologists have recognized idiopathic rapidly progressive nephritis as a form fruste of microscopic polyangiitis limited to the kidney, which should be treated in the same way as generalized polyangiitis.

Lung involvement

This may present with cough, pleurisy, dyspnoea, or haemoptysis. Radiologically, there may be transient infiltrates or segmental atelectasis. The most serious complication is lung haemorrhage which can be profuse and occasionally fatal.

Other manifestations

Purpuric rashes are common and splinter haemorrhages may be found. Arthralgias are a frequent complaint, the joint involvement usually being symmetrical; however, arthritis is less usual and joint deformation is not a feature of this vasculitis. Mononeuritis multiplex is a particularly debilitating complication of microscopic polyangiitis. Gastrointestinal symptomatology may include non-specific abdominal pains, diarrhoea, or gastrointestinal haemorrhage. Although sometimes present, patients with microscopic polyarteritis do not frequently have upper respiratory tract or ocular symptoms, in contrast to patients with Wegener's granulomatosis, nor do they have asthma and flitting pulmonary infiltrates in contrast to the Churg–Strauss syndrome, nor do they present with severe hypertension and large viscus perforation or organ infarction as may occur in polyarteritis nodosa.

Diagnosis

This may be suspected clinically in a patient in whom constitutional symptoms of malaise, fever, weight loss, and night sweats have failed to be accounted for by an infective and neoplastic aetiology, and in whom there is evidence of multiple organ dysfunction. Confirmation of the diagnosis may come from biopsy of the affected organ, of which the best is usually the kidney, although segmental vascular necrosis with an inflammatory cell infiltrate at any site may provide a useful clue to the diagnosis. However, it must be remembered that these pathological changes may be seen near epithelial surfaces which have been breached due to a variety of causes, infective, traumatic, or neoplastic, or in association with other pathologies such as tumour, abscess cavity formation, or in other connective tissue diseases such as rheumatoid arthritis and SLE. The finding of focal segmental necrosis of glomerular capillary walls does, however, restrict the diagnosis to microscopic polyangiitis or to other small vessel pathologies, such as found in Wegener's granulomatosis, SLE, Goodpasture's syndrome, cryoglobulinaemia, or Henoch–Schönlein disease. The first four of these have distinctive circulating immunoglobulins: autoantibodies to Pr3, DNA, GBM or cryoglobulins, respectively. All have characteristic deposits of immunoglobulin in the renal biopsy except microscopic polyangiitis and Wegener's granulomatosis, where such deposits are not found.

The detection of circulating antibodies to neutrophil cytoplasm antigens has contributed greatly to the laboratory diagnosis of microscopic polyangiitis. Usually these have specificity for MPO but occasionally identical clinical syndromes present with autoantibodies to other neutrophil cytoplasmic antigens such as lactoferrin, elastase, and cathepsin G. In the right clinical context the detection of these antibodies is very helpful but it must be remembered that autoantibodies with similar specificities may be found in a number of other conditions which are not primary vasculitides, for example, inflammatory gastrointestinal diseases, such as chronic active hepatitis, sclerosing cholangitis, Crohn's disease, and ulcerative colitis. Other laboratory investigations which are almost invariably abnormal as in other vasculitides, include a normochromic normocytic anaemia, raised ESR or CRP, and a neutrophilia. Frequently, there is thrombocythaemia as well as hyperglobulinaemia, and occasionally positive rheumatoid factors may be found.

Differential diagnosis

This usually has to be considered among three categories of patients: those presenting with pyrexia of unknown origin, with malignancies, and with covert infection. The differential diagnosis may be particularly difficult as vasculitis may be evident as rash in patients from any of those, for example associated with sarcoid or SBE in those with pyrexia of unknown origin, with carcinoma or leukaemia in those with malignancy or with TB or syphilis in those with infection. All of these disorders may also show additional multisystem involvement due to the underlying disease. Hence the diagnostic problems, underscoring the importance of ANCA detection, as in none of the preceding conditions have ANCA consistently been found.

Polyarteritis nodosa

Polyarteritis nodosa is a vasculitis of medium-sized arteries in which aneurysm formation is a frequent occurrence. The clinical manifestations reflect the size of vessel involved: major organ infarction may affect the gut, renal, or cerebral vasculature. Moderate to severe hypertension is common. In many patients an overlap with microscopic polyangiitis is apparent clinically and at biopsy. Circulating ANCA are rarely found and when present may indicate the coincident development of the smaller vessel vasculitis. An association with hepatitis B antigenaemia is evident in certain patient populations.

Clinical features

The disease may present at any age and is commoner in men, with a male to female ratio of 2:1. Constitutional disturbance with tachycardia, fever, and weight loss is frequent and may be accompanied by striking clinical signs, such as an acute abdomen, myocardial infarction, stroke, or severe hypertension.

Renal involvement

Extraglomerular arteritis rarely occurs alone and often a glomerular capillaritis similar to microscopic polyarteritis is found. Thus proteinuria, haematuria, and urinary casts are evidence of renal involvement, additional clinical findings such as malignant hypertension or frank haematuria may reflect the contribution of arterial ischaemia or infarction due to larger vessel vasculitis. Progressive renal failure was an important cause of death before renal replacement therapy was available.

Cardiac involvement

Coronary arteritis is an important cause of intractable heart failure or death due to myocardial infarction in polyarteritis. The cardiac involvement may be compounded by renovascular hypertension and other cardiac complications include the development of an acute vasculitic pericarditis.

Gastrointestinal tract

Typically, the presentation may be with severe abdominal pain or gastrointestinal haemorrhage due to mucosal ulceration or perforation. Polyarteritis may also affect single organs mimicking acute cholecystitis, pancreatitis, or appendicitis. Liver involvement may produce a hepatitic presentation or even hepatic necrosis. However, there is no distinctive clinical entity associated with hepatitis B polyarteritis.

Skin

Cutaneous involvement may vary from vasculitic purpura or urticaria to subcutaneous haemorrhage with gangrene. The presence of palpable nodules which may occur near to the course of superficial arteries is a distinctive feature of polyarteritis nodosa. These may reach the size of a large pea, and can persist from days to months. Rarely these small 'nodosed' aneurysms may cause the surrounding skin to ulcerate.

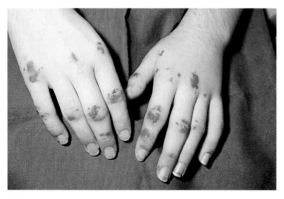

(a)

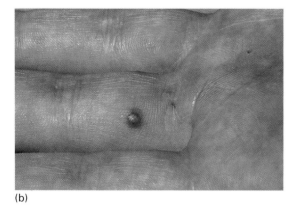

(b)

▌**Fig. 30.2** Forms of cutaneous involvement seen polyarteritis nodosa.

Other manifestations

Arthralgias and myalgias are frequently present in polyarteritis nodosa. Neurological manifestations are rare with stroke due to cerebral vasculitis or visual disturbance due to retinal aneurysms and haemorrhage (visible fundoscopically) being the most striking. Mononeuritis multiplex secondary to arteritis of the vasa nervorum may also produce peripheral neurological signs. Rarely, polyarteritis nodosa may be found to affect ovaries, testes, epididymis, and bladder.

Diagnosis

It is unusual for the disease to present without clinical features to suggest a microscopic polyarteritis but a superimposition of substantial dysfunction of any of the major organs, together with hypertension, are useful pointers to a diagnosis of polyarteritis nodosa. The diagnosis may be confirmed by angiography or by histology of affected tissue.

There are no specific laboratory tests for polyarteritis nodosa. However, almost all patients have a normochromic normocytic anaemia, raised ESR or CRP, and neutrophilia.

Differential diagnosis

As well as the differential diagnosis for microscopic polyarteritis the size of vessel involved in polyarteritis nodosa makes it worth excluding two other multisystem vascular occlusive diseases. The first, thrombotic thrombocytopenic purpura is readily identified by the

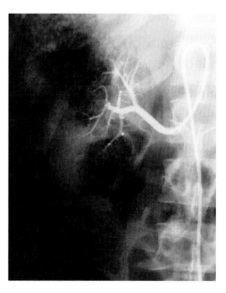

▌**Fig. 30.3** Renal angiogram revealing presence of aneurysms on renal vessels in polyarteritis nodosa

presence of thrombocytopenia and intravascular haemolysis; the second, Degos disease which is an occlusive arterial disease affecting skin, gastrointestinal tract, and brain is distinguished by its skin lesions which are distributed centrifugally towards the extremities and undergo a typical course starting as pink grey papules which then develop a depressed scaly centre surrounded by an elevated red margin.

Churg–Strauss syndrome

Definition

This is probably a polyarteritis variant in which there is a granulomatous necrotizing vasculitis predominantly affecting the lungs and to a lesser extent other organs. Typically, patients present with asthma and eosinophilia with clinical evidence of multisystem vasculitis.

Clinical features

As with other vasculitides marked constitutional disturbance is frequently found at presentation.

The lungs

Asthma is the clinical feature which distinguishes the patient with Churg–Strauss syndrome from the other vasculitides, it is often severe and usually pre-dates the development of the systemic vasculitis. Transient pulmonary infiltrates may be seen radiologically.

Gastrointestinal tract

There may be disturbance of bowel habit and abdominal pain due to gut vasculitis. Biopsy usually shows an eosinophilic infiltrate which may be present extensively throughout the gastrointestinal tract.

Occasionally, involvement of other organs similar to that seen with microscopic polyarteritis occurs. When present, mononeuritis multiplex and coronary vasculitis may prove particularly refractory to treatment.

Diagnosis

This may be suspected on clinical grounds in a patient with asthma and evidence of multisystem vasculitis. Confirmation comes from demonstration of vasculitis on biopsy in which frequently the affected tissues show eosinophilic infiltrates. Moderate, $<20 \times 10^9/l$ peripheral eosinophilia is common. In occasional patients ANCA, with specificity for MPO, are to be found.

Differential diagnosis

The main disorder to consider in the differential diagnosis is the hypereosinophilic syndrome that accompanies endomyocardial fibrosis (Loeffler's endocarditis). In this condition hypereosinophilia may be intense (usually $>20 \times 10^9/l$) and the eosinophils are morphologically abnormal, displaying loss of granules and vacuole formation. Asthma is rare in the hyperoesinophilic syndrome and although involvement of other organs with eosinophilic infiltrates may occur, rarely is there evidence of overt vasculitis.

Henoch–Schönlein purpura

Definition

This is a childhood necrotizing vasculitis which involves the skin, gastrointestinal tract, and kidneys. Immunofluorescence studies of skin and kidneys show deposits of IgA in dermal capillary walls and in the mesangium of the glomerulus. Total serum IgA levels are frequently raised. In childhood the triad of characteristic rash, gastrointestinal involvement, and renal disease, together with fever and arthralgia make the diagnosis of this systemic vasculitis.

Clinical features

Children between 2 and 10 years are predominantly affected with a seasonal incidence which peaks in winter. Adult forms of the disease are well documented, the mean age of onset being 43 years. Usually, the first manifestations are fever and a palpable purpuric rash, followed by joint pain, abdominal pain, and haematuria in that order. However, arthralgias or abdominal pain may precede the appearance of the rash, making the diagnosis less easy to secure clinically. In almost all patients the course is self-limiting within weeks, although relapses may occur.

Skin

Initially, the rash may be urticarial but this usually evolves into the typical slightly elevated purpuric rash affecting the extensor surfaces of the limbs and buttocks. The purpura, typically non-thrombocytopenic, may vesiculate or coalesce before gradually fading.

Gastrointestinal tract

Colicky abdominal pain may be severe, particularly after meals ('bowel angina') and intussusception can complicate haemorrhage or oedema in the gut wall; gastrointestinal bleeding and melaena may occur, and the presentation may resemble that of an acute abdomen. Any bowel segment may be involved but the small bowel usually predominates.

Renal involvement

Proteinuria and haematuria occur in 40% of patients. The renal disease is usually mild in children and heals spontaneously in all but 10%, in whom the nephritis may be progressive. There is some evidence to suggest the nephritis is more severe in the adult.

Other manifestations

There is frequently a characteristic mono- or oligo-arthritis affecting large joints, which is transient and which may produce severe pain, disproportionate to the evident synovitis. Notable by absence is involvement of nervous or respiratory systems, although rare examples of pulmonary vasculitis or mononeuritis multiplex have been recorded.

Diagnosis

The triad of characteristic rash, gastrointestinal involvement, and renal disease, together with fever and arthralgia make the diagnosis of this systemic vasculitis, when it occurs in childhood, relatively straightforward on clinical grounds. Biopsy shows a necrotizing vasculitis of small vessels, predominantly post-capillary venules with deposits of IgA and C3 in their walls. A stippled pattern of vascular IgA deposition may be seen in vessels throughout the skin, gut, or kidney and in the latter additionally there are deposits in the mesangium of the glomerulus indistinguishable from those found in IgA nephritis. Dermal IgA deposition may be present, even in skin biopsies taken from areas unaffected by rash. The presence of IgA and fibrinogen in vasculitic lesions distinguishes Henoch–Schönlein purpura from other necrotizing vasculitides where deposits of IgG, IgM, and early complement components are more usual. There is no specific laboratory test for Henoch–Schönlein purpura. The normochromic normocytic anaemia and neutrophil leucocytosis typical of the other small vessel vasculitides are not invariably present. Raised IgA levels, circulating IgA containing immune complexes, and IgA rheumatoid factors are further evidence that in Henoch–Schönlein purpura disturbance of IgA homeostasis underlies the disease. However, it must be remembered that the IgA deposition in the kidney in IgA nephritis is identical to that in Henoch–Schönlein purpura, thus necessitating further clarification of the factors producing the multisystem involvement of the latter disease.

Differential diagnosis

In a case with an atypical rash, Crohn's disease may enter the differential diagnosis. However, the skin lesions of Crohn's disease present slowly and are painful: they include pyoderma gangrenosum, erythema nodosum, aphthous ulceration, and metastatic granulomatous infiltration. Usually, the differential is from other forms of small vessel vasculitis among which Wegener's is usually excluded by its predominant upper respiratory tract involvement and anti-Pr3 serology, polyarteritis nodosa by hypertension and aneurysms demonstrable on arteriography and microscopic polyarteritis by its pronounced and usually prolonged constitutional disturbance of fevers, night sweats, and weight loss as well as the presence of circulating anti-MPO antibodies.

Relapsing polychondritis

This is a very rare condition in which a small vessel vasculitis appears predominantly to affect cartilaginous structures such as the pinna of the ear, nasal cartilage, larynx, and trachea.

Clinical features

Males and females are equally affected and the onset is most frequent in the seventh decade; untreated it carries a poor prognosis. Fever, weight loss, and malaise are common at the onset.

Cartilage

Tenderness, inflammatory swelling, and eventual destruction of the cartilage, often in cyclical fashion, is the main feature of relapsing polychondritis. Thus there may be gross deformation of the pinna of the ear, a saddle nose, and stridor due to collapse of the larynx or trachea. Involvement of the heart valves or aorta may produce heart failure or aneurysm, respectively.

Other manifestations

There may be episcleritis and monoarticular arthropathy as well as infrequently evidence of small vessel vasculitis in other organs.

Diagnosis

The diagnosis is usually made on clinical grounds with biopsy showing necrotizing vasculitis and cartilage destruction in affected tissue. There is no specific laboratory test but normochromic anaemia, marked acute phase response, and leucocytosis are frequently found.

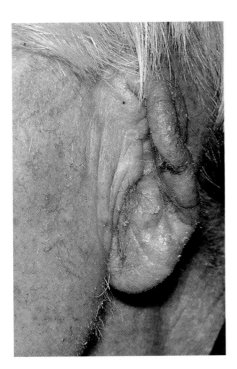

▌ **Fig. 30.4** Relapsing Polychondritis showing involvement and destruction of ear.

Treatment of systemic vasculitis

Cytotoxic drugs and steroids are the main stays of treatment for the small vessel vasculitides. Usually these are combined, at high dose, in an induction regimen to gain effective control of the disease activity at presentation which is followed after 2 months by a lower dose, maintenance regimen for the longer term, in which other immunosuppressive agents may substitute for the cyclophosphamide.

Induction therapy

Empirically, it has been determined that doses of cyclophosphamide at 3 mg/kg body weight (rounded down to the nearest 50 mg) are suitable for the induction regimen to control the disease at the outset. This dosage should be lowered or discontinued temporarily if the total white cell count falls to less than 4.0 $\times$ 10^9/l, or the neutrophil leucocyte count falls to less than 2.0 $\times$ 10^9/l. Cytotoxic therapy should also be modified if severe infection occurs. In the older patients, aged 55 years or over, a lower induction dose of 2

mg/kg is often given because of the greater susceptibility of the elderly to bone marrow immunosuppression and infection. Steroids are given at high dose, initially prednisolone 60 mg/day, tapering at weekly intervals until at 2 months the patient is receiving 10 mg/day.

Maintenance therapy

Usually cyclophosphamide can be substituted by the same dose of azathioprine at 2 months and at the same time steroid treatment may be converted to an alternate day regimen. Both drugs may then gradually be withdrawn at 12 months.

Monitoring disease activity

Standard tests of organ function should be used to monitor the effect of treatment on disease activity. Serial measurements of the ESR and CRP are a useful guide as to whether the vasculitis has been brought under control but are relatively non-specific, being elevated during intercurrent infection or by other causes of inflammation as well as by vasculitic injury. Many centres now use serial ANCA measurements to help monitor treatment with an aim to reduce levels to background during induction therapy, withdrawing treatment at an earlier stage if control of the autoimmune response can be demonstrated in this manner. However, it must be noted that certain patients have persistently raised ANCA levels despite no evident disease activity and also that vice versa a very small number of patients apparently have undetectable ANCA but continuing vasculitis.

Other therapeutic strategies

Use of pulse dose (0.75–1 g intravenously) cyclophosphamide or prednisolone has been advocated by some. However, recent evidence suggests that pulse cyclophosphamide is less effective at maintaining remission than oral cyclophosphamide. Furthermore, as the active metabolites of cyclophosphamide are in part renally excreted, then, in patients with nephritis, lower dose oral therapy should allow more accurate titration of dose effect. It remains to be demonstrated whether pulse dosage of prednisolone is superior for the management of systemic vasculitis.

For patients who are intolerant of cyclophosphamide perhaps the most useful drug is azathioprine. Where disease activity if not controllable by either drug, then other immunomodulatory agents such as methotrexate or cyclosporin A have been tried. Although some patients benefit, as yet there is no substantial evidence to warrant their use as first line agents in management.

The use of trimethoprim–sulphamethoxazole has enjoyed a vogue for the management of systemic vasculitis, particularly Wegener's granulomatosis. However, with the advent of better diagnostic criteria, careful exclusion of intercurrent infections (particularly a problem in Wegener's affecting the upper respiratory tract), and study of controls given trimethoprim–sulphamethoxazole alone, doubts have been cast over the efficacy of this agent.

In patients who have fulminating vasculitis, threatening vital organ function, then intensive plasma exchange may be beneficial. There is now evidence from several studies that such an approach may benefit patients with severe renal vasculitis (requiring dialysis support), lung haemorrhage, due to pulmonary vasculitis, or in a coma due to cerebral vasculitis.

Finally, for patients with intractable vasculitis, resistant to conventional immunosuppression, a few reports now point to the value of more specific forms of immunotherapy such as high-dose intravenous immunoglobulin, 0.4 g/kg per day for 5 days, believed to exert one of its immunomodulatory effects through anti-idiotypic control of B-cell function, or humanized monoclonal antibody therapy which targets T cells.

Response to treatment

Wegener's granulomatosis and microscopic polangiitis

Approximately 75% of patients with Wegener's granulomatosis and microscopic polyangiitis treated with cytotoxic drugs and steroids will achieve complete remission. However, the rate varies in that 60% of patients with microscopic polyangiitis gain complete remission by 2 months compared with only 50% of patients with Wegener's granulomatosis, who gain remission by 12 months. Although the data are difficult to compare from different series of patients the rate of relapse does not appear to differ between the two disorders. These occurred in approximately 50% of patients, although in patients followed for long periods the remission interval could amount to several years before relapse was identified.

Henoch–Schönlein purpura

Most cases of childhood Henoch–Schönlein purpura resolve spontaneously within 2–3 weeks, although relapses do occur within the first 2 years these are usually also self-limiting and permanent sequelae are rare. For patients with progressive disease induction of remission may be effected by short courses of steroids alone or, for resistant cases, then similar regimens used for the other small vessel vasculitides may be employed.

▮ **Table 30.2** Causes of vasculitis

Infective agents	
Viral	Hepatitis B
	Epstein–Barr virus
	Hepatitis C
Bacterial	Streptococcus
	Bacterial endocarditis
	Mycobacterium
	Gonococcus
Autoimmune disease	
	Systemic lupus erythematosus
	Rheumatoid arthritis
	Chronic active arthritis
	Wegener's granulomatosis
	Ulcerative colitis
	Kawasaki disease
Drugs	
	Xenogeneic serum
	Sulphonamides
Cryoglobulinaemia	
	Hepatitis B or C
	Lymphoproliferative disorders

Polyarteritis nodosa and Churg–Strauss syndrome

As well as the identification of polyarteritis nodosa and microscopic polyangiitis as separate syndromes, other small vessel vasculitides emerged as individual entites collectively with sufficient evidence that a similar autoimmune diathesis underlies their development. Consequently, treatment for both polyarteritis nodosa and Churg–Strauss syndrome generally follows a similar pattern to that for small vessel vasculitis with the minor variation that high-dose steroids, prednisolone 40–60 mg/day, may be effective when given alone initially. These are then tapered according to disease activity. Cyclophosphamide should be added if there is a slow response, or in any case where small vessel vasculitis may also play a prominent part.

Further reading

Hoffman, G. S., Kerr, G. S., Leavitt, R. Y., Hallahan, C. W., Lebovics, R. S., Travis, W. D., *et al.* (1992). Wegener's granulomatosis: an analysis of 158 patients. *Annals of Internal Medicine*, **116**, 488–98.

Savage, C. O. S. and Lockwood, C. M. (1993). Systemic vasculitis. In *Clinical aspects of immunology* (ed. D. K. Peters and P. J. Lachmann), Vol. II, pp. 1205–16. Blackwell Scientific, Oxford.

Savage, C. O. S., Winearls, C. G., Evans, D. J., Rees, A. J., and Lockwood, C. M. (1985). Microscopic polyarteritis: presentation, pathology and prognosis. *Quarterly Journal of Medicine*, **56**, 467–83.

J. Bradley

Giant cell arteritis

Definition

GCA is a generalized panarteritis which affects large to medium arteries with a well-defined elastic lamina. The extracranial branches of the carotid are most frequently involved and the disease rarely occurs below the neck. In the past it was also known as temporal arteritis, but this is not as appropriate because any artery of that size may be involved.

Introduction

Incidence

Overall ~16 per million are affected but the incidence increases with age being 30 times greater at 80 years. It is rare in those <50 years old.

Genetic factors

The incidence is greater in Caucasians, females (M–F=1:3–4) and those with HLA DR4.

Pathology

Histologically, there is segmental involvement especially of the media with mononuclear infiltrate due to many CD4+ T cells, some macrophages, and giant cells. Smooth muscle necrosis occurs in the media, with disruption of internal elastic lamina and variable intimal proliferation which may progress to occlude the vessel (Fig 31.1).

Clinical features

The typical symptoms are those of a systemic disease with headache, localized scalp tenderness, anorexia, fatigue, fever, and weight loss. However, the symptoms vary and headache may only be present initially in ~50% patients. Weight loss, shoulder pain, anaemia, and throat discomfort may be the presenting

symptoms. In addition, there may be jaw claudication, i.e. jaw pain on chewing or talking. Of great concern is the presence of any visual symptom or impairment, due to involvement of the retinal artery, which occurs in one-third of untreated cases. This requires immediate treatment if sight is to saved.

Examination may be unhelpful, but may reveal thickened or tender arteries; localized scalp tenderness, or hair loss in the distribution of the extracranial branches of the carotid artery. An elevated erythrocyte sedimentation rate (ESR) or C-reactive protein (CRP) is invariably present.

Polymyalgia rheumatica (PR) is an associated disease in which there is proximal myalgia especially of the neck and shoulder muscles. Of all the patients with PR ~50% also have giant cell arteritis (GCA).

Diagnosis

This is made on a typical clinical history and examination. It may be confirmed by an arterial biopsy, usually of temporal artery, which may shows a mononuclear infiltrate in all layers of the artery with giant cells sometimes visible. Other laboratory findings are non-specific: a normochromic, normocytic anaemia of ~11–12 g/dl; an elevated CRP; and an ESR usually >100 mm.

Treatment

It is important to establish the diagnosis as soon as possible and commence therapy because the most serious problem is irreversible visual loss. This can be avoided by prompt administration of corticosteroids, 40–60 mg/day, which usually brings a quick relief of symptoms. Headache, shoulder girdle or scalp pain, and fever lessen within a few days of treatment. After 4–6 weeks the dose of corticosteroids is gradually reduced to 5–10 mg/day. Falling CRP levels and resolution of symptoms are a good guide to reduction of the dose of corticosteroids. The mean duration of the disease is about 2 years and corticosteroids are needed to cover this period. If upon reducing the dose symptoms or signs reappear the dose of corticosteroid will need readjusting but rarely needs to go back to the levels used initially. However, sometimes a low dose of corticosteroids may be needed for some years; and in some cases cytotoxic drugs, e.g. azathioprine or cyclophosphamide, may be necessary.

Takayasu arteritis

Definition

A rare form of arteritis affecting young adults of 15–20 years who are predominantly female (M–F=1:9), which histologically is similar to GCA. It occurs typically in three phases. The incidence in the USA is ~2.6 per million but is much greater in Asia, particularly Japan. Genetic factors appear to be important and it occurs in monozygotic twins. There is an increased incidence in some HLA types.

Clinical features

Three phases are recognized:

1. A *systemic*, pre-pulseless, phase which resolves over several weeks. Clinically, this presents as fever, malaise, fatigue, headache, weight loss, night sweats, joint, and/or muscle pain. There are findings of chronic inflammation: anaemia, leucocytosis, increased platelet count, and an elevated CRP/ESR.

2. An *arteritic* phase develops. There may be pain and tenderness over the affected vessels. The subclavian, carotid, renal, and descending aorta may be involved in >40% cases whereas the abdominal and ascending aorta, mesenteric, pulmonary, and iliac arteries are less frequently (10–40%) involved. This then resolves and an asymptomatic period of ~8 years follows.

3. A *vaso-occlusive* phase with absent or decreased pulses of aorta or its major branches. The pulmonary vessels are involved in ~50% cases.

Laboratory results that are important are: an elevated CRP or ESR, anaemia, and a polyclonal hypergammaglobulinaemia. During the inflammatory stages CRP (or ESR) is elevated and is a good indication of disease activity. Angiography reveals the presence of vessel obstruction and/or narrowing, and is important in establishing the diagnosis and following the course of the disease.

Treatment

Corticosteroids may be helpful but their place in decreasing morbidity and mortality is not known. Cytotoxic drugs are used when corticosteroids are not sufficient to control the disease.

Kawasaki disease

Definition

An acute febrile, multisystem illness with vasculitis in the recovery phase occurring mainly in children. The aetiology is unknown, although infectious agents and autoimmune response to vascular endothelial cells have been suggested. The incidence is ~60 per 100 000 but can be as high as ~200 per 100 000

Clinical features

The features occur in four phases.

1. In the first 10 days there is a high fever accompanied by cervical lymphadenopathy.

2. From 2–4 weeks general systemic symptoms are accompanied by vasculitis and myocarditis; this phase resembling polyarteritis nodosa.

3. From 4 to 6 weeks the vasculitis regresses and fibrosis occurs.

4. From 40 days to 4 years scar formation and thrombus organization take place.

Death may occur any stage from days after the onset to years later due to formation of coronary artery aneurysm. About 25% develop arteritis of the coronary arteries which produce aneurysm, and 2% die suddenly as a result of this pathology.

Treatment

The disease responds dramatically to immunoglobulin preparations given intravenously, and this reduces risk of coronary artery aneurysm. The mechanism of action of immunoglobulin is not known but may be to decrease of acute inflammation and acute phase reactants; neutralization of unidentified agents; or blockade of Fc receptors.

Behçet's disease

A multisystem disease of unkown origin characterized by recurrent oral and genital ulcers, and some of the following: cutaneous vasculitis, synovitis, uveitis, and meningoencephalitis. It has been associated with HLA-B51.

Clinical features

The diagnosis is based on clinical features only. Various sets of criteria have been established for this purpose, e.g. the presence of recurrent oral aphthous ulcers and two of the usual features: genital ulcers, synovitis, cutaneous vasculitis, uveitis, and meningoencephalitis. Other diseases that may cause these features must be excluded, i.e. Reiter's disease, inflammatory bowel disease, and systemic lupus erythematosus. Cutaneous lesions should be biopsied to exclude non-vasculitic causes. See section Behçets, Chapter 19, p. 227.

Therapy

Disease that involves only the skin, mucous membranes, and joints is treated with colchicine. Colchicine, a plant alkaloid has an anti-inflammatory activity due probably to its effect on neutrophils by its action on microtubule function and neutrophil migration. A dose of 0.6 mg twice to three times daily. Dapsone also may inhibit neutrophil migration and may be used. For more severe cases non-steroidal anti-inflammatory drugs and occasionally steroids or methotrexate are used. Involvement of the central nervous system and eye are usually treated with high-dose steroids and, if there is not a satisfactory response, immunosuppressive agents, e.g. methotrexate 5–15 mg/week. Elderly patients are treated with lower doses.

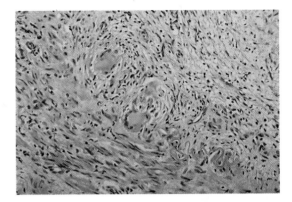

∎ **Fig. 31.1** Infiltrate in vessel wall: giant cell seen just below centre.

Section V

Transplantation

32 The human leucocyte antigens and clinical medicine

James McCluskey

Introduction

Human leucocyte antigens (HLA) were first recognized in the early 1950s by blood bank scientists who noticed agglutination of white cells mixed with serum from polytransfused patients. We now know that alloantibodies in the patient serum were recognizing inherited structural differences (polymorphisms) present on the HLA molecules expressed by the allogeneic white cells. Since then, there have been many international workshops and conferences as well as countless scientific papers describing the structure and function of HLA molecules. Such is the genetic complexity of this system that it sends a shudder down the spine of every medical student and is ultimately understood by only a very small proportion of clinicians. This chapter reviews some of the basic features of the HLA system and attempts to simplify what is otherwise a very complex field.

Genetics of human leucocyte antigens

The HLA molecules are encoded by a cluster of genes, linked on the short arm of chromosome 6 (6p) in a region known as the major histocompatibility complex (MHC) Fig. 32.1. The MHC spans approximately 4 Mb and contains numerous genes only some of which are related to histocompatibility. This genetic region is the major determinant of graft acceptance or rejection between genetically distinct individuals, and so is known as the *major* histocompatibility complex in contrast to other genetic loci, which exert only relatively minor effects on histocompatibility. The naming of these molecules as histocompatibility factors has constrained a proper understanding of their function by many medical students and scientists. Ironically, the key role of the HLA molecules has nothing to do with transplantation. Rather these molecules are receptors

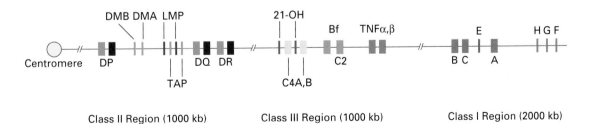

Fig. 32.1 The human major histocompatibility complex (MHC) on the short arm of chromosome 6.

which capture fragments of antigen for presentation on cell surfaces to T cells. In presenting foreign antigen to T cells, HLA molecules evoke cytotoxic T-lymphocyte (CTL) and helper T-cell responses which orchestrate specific immunity.

There are six major HLA genes encoded within the MHC. These are divided into HLA, class I and class II molecules which differ in their tissue distribution, source of peptide antigen, and in the function of responding T cells. The class I HLA molecules are encoded by three distinct genetic loci known as HLA-A, -B, and -C. The class II molecules include HLA-DR, -DQ, and -DP, each of which is encoded by a distinct genetic locus. Therefore the MHC located on each chromosome 6p contains 6 linked loci each of which encodes a distinct HLA product (Fig. 32.2).

Class I molecules comprise a single heavy chain complexed to a smaller molecule known as β_2-microglobulin. Although the gene structure and overall shape of the HLA-A, -B, and -C molecules are very similar the primary amino acid sequence of these molecules differ from each other. None the less, the HLA-A, -B, and -C class I heavy chains all associate non-covalently with a single molecule of β_2-microglobulin, which is non-polymorphic and encoded on chromosome 17. The excess of β_2-microglobulin produced by most cell types means there is plenty of this to go around for all the class I molecules. There are between 10^4 and 10^6 class I molecules on most nucleated cell types and all three locus products are expressed in a co-dominant fashion (i.e. the products of both maternal and paternal MHC loci are simultaneously expressed by all cells) (Fig. 32.2). Within human populations HLA-A, -C, and -B loci are highly polymorphic. Indeed, the degree of polymorphism is more striking than in any other genetic system within the human genome. For example there are more than 150 allelic variants of HLA-B class I molecules. The dif-

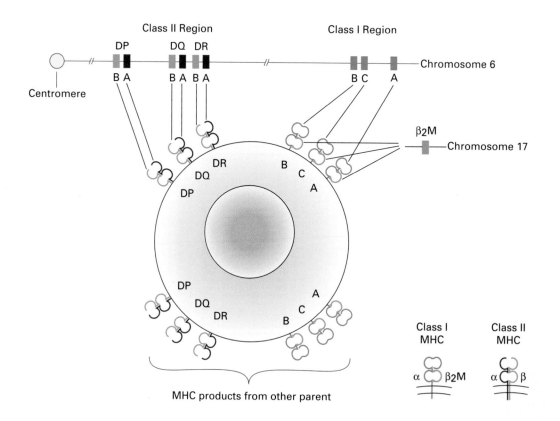

∎ **Fig. 32.2** Co-dominant expression of HLA A, B, C, DR, DQ, and DP gene products on the surface of antigen presenting cells (APC).

ferent alleles currently known for each locus and their serological identity is shown in Table 32.1. The location of polymorphic residues in MHC class I and class II molecules is shown in Fig. 32.3.

The structure of a class I molecule is ideally suited to capture short peptides for presentation to T cells. The relatively conserved membrane-proximal structure of the class I molecule is capable of interacting with CD8 molecules on T cells. However, the outermost domains comprise two long α helices separated by a cleft with a floor composed of β-pleated sheet, Fig. 32.3. This cleft is the antigen binding pocket of HLA class I molecules and is the major site of the structural polymorphism, which occurs at each of the loci. Thus, different alleles of HLA-A can differ from each other by 20–30 amino acids (aa) and these differences are virtually all concentrated in the antigen-binding cleft. This polymorphism has the effect of changing the electrostatic charge and shape of the cleft between different class I alleles. This in turn changes the peptide binding properties of allelic class I molecules, so that each of them will bind a unique repertoire of peptides with distinct sequence properties. These peptides are constitutively derived

from endogenous self proteins (so they are being continuously presented) and might include as many as 20 000 different peptides being simultaneously presented by any one set of class I products (e.g. HLA-A2) on the cell surface.

The overall protein structure adopted by class II molecules is similar to class I, but is achieved by the association of two membrane bound chains known as α and β. These chains assemble non-covalently to create an antigen-binding cleft located above a conserved membrane proximal structure, which can interact with CD4 on T cells. The MHC class II α and β chains are each encoded by distinct loci, which are closely linked as pairs of α and β genes (i.e. DRα/DRβ DQα/DQβ, and DPα/DPβ). The HLA-DR, -DQ, and -DP loci are all highly polymorphic. The polymorphisms are confined largely to the antigen-binding pocket of these molecules but in HLA-DR they are confined to the DR β chain (DRB gene) with the DR α chain (DRA gene) being essentially monomorphic. However, HLA-DP and -DQ contain polymorphisms in both the α and β chain genes (DPA, DPB, DQA, and DQB). The number of alleles at each

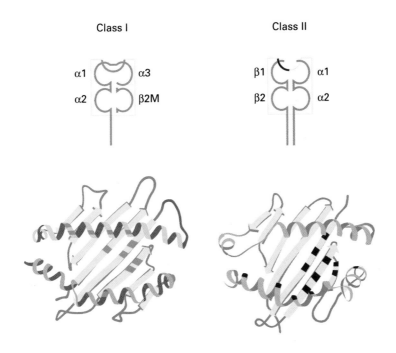

▋**Fig. 32.3** The location of polymorphic sites in the antigen binding cleft of HLA class I and class II molecules.

■ **Table 32.1**

(a) Listing of HLA class I alleles

HLA-A		HLA-B		HLA-C	
Serology	**Alleles**	**Serology**	**Alleles**	**Serology**	**Alleles**
A1	A*0101, 0102	B7	B*0702–0706	Cw1	Cw*0102, 0103
A2	A*0201–0217	B8	B*0801–0803	Cw2	Cw*0202
A3	A*0301, 0302	B13	B*1301–1303	Cw3	Cw*0302–0304
A11	A*1101–1103	B14	B*1401, 1402	Cw4	Cw*0401–0403
A23(9)	A*2301	B15	B*1501–1531	Cw5	Cw*0501
A24(9)	A*2402–2410	B18	B*1801–1803	Cw6	Cw*0602
A25(10)	A*2501	B27	B*2701–2710	Cw7	Cw*0701–0705
A26(10)	A*2601–2608	B35	B*3501–3518	Cw8	Cw*0801–0803
A29(19)	A*2901, 2902	B37	B*3701, 3702	–	Cw*1202, 1203
A30(19)	A*3001–3004	B38(16)	B*3801, 3802	–	Cw*1301
A31(19)	A*31012	B39(16)	B*3901–3909	–	Cw*1402, 1403
A32(19)	A*3201	B40	B*4001–4008	–	Cw*1502–1505
A33(19)	A*3301–3303	B41	B*4101, 4102	–	Cw*1601, 1602
A34(10)	A*3401, 3402	B42	B*4201, 4202	–	Cw*1701, 1702
A36	A*3601	B44(12)	B*4402–4407		
A43	A*4301	B45(12)	B*4501		
A66(10)	A*6601, 6602	B46	B*4601		
A68(28)	A*6801–6803	B47	B*4701		
A69(28)	A*6901	B48	B*4801, 4802		
A74(19)	A*7401	B49(21)	B*4901		
–	A*8001	B50(21)	B*5001		
		B51(5)	B*5101–B*5107		
		B52(5)	B*5201		
		B53	B*5301		
		B54(22)	B*5401		
		B55(22)	B*5501–5503		
		B56(22)	B*5601, 5602		
		B57(17)	B*5701–5704		
		B58(17)	B*5801, 5802		
		B59	B*5901		
		B67	B*6701		
		B73	B*7301		
		B78	B*7801, 7802		
		–	B*8201		

of these loci is growing steadily as anthropological and workshop studies around the world unearth unsuspected new alleles in extant populations.

T cells, through their specific antigen receptors, are designed constantly to scrutinize the array of different HLA-peptide complexes which are continuously present on cellular surfaces, shown schematically in Fig. 32.4.

The class II region contains many pseudogenes (ψ; non-expressed genes) which represent genetic tombstones derived from ancestral gene duplication and mutation. A knowledge of these pseudogenes can be important in HLA typing by DNA methods. The total number of class II loci, including pseudogenes, varies between different HLA haplotypes as shown in Fig. 32.5.

The alleles at each of the HLA class I and class II loci are numbered, although not always in a logical order (e.g. HLA-A1, -A2, -A10, etc.). The original detection system for identification of alleles was based on the reactions of specific antisera with human cells. Human alloantisera have been invaluable tools in

∎ **Table 32.1** *Continued*

(b) Listing of HLA class II alleles
MARCH 1996

HLA DR		HLA DQ		HLA DP	
Serology	**Alleles**	**Serology**	**Alleles**	**Specificity**	**Alleles**
α-Chain		α-Chain		α-Chain	
	DRA*0101–0102	—	DQA1*0101–0105	—	DPA1*0103–0104
			DQA1*0201		DPA1*0201–0202
			DQA1*0301–0303		DPA1*0301
			DQA1*0401		DPA1*0401–0402
			DQA1*0501–0503		
			DQA1*0601		
β-Chain		β-Chain		β-Chain	
DR1	DRB1*0101–0104	DQ5(1)	DQB1*0501–0504	DPw1	DPB1*0101
DR15(2)	DRB1*1501–1505	DQ6(1)	DQB1*0601–0611	DPw2	DPB1*0201–0202
DR16(2)	DRB1*1601–1605	DQ2	DQB1*0201–0203	DPw3	DPB1*0301
DR3	DRB1*0301–0308	DQ3	DQB1*0301–0306	DPw4	DPB1*0401–0402
DR4	DRB1*0401–0423	DQ4	DQB1*0401–0402	DPw5	DPB1*0501
DR11(5)	DRB1*1101–1127			DPw6	DPB1*0601
DR12(5)	DRB1*1201–1204				
DR13(6)	DRB1*1301–1312			—	DPB1*0801–4101
	DRB1*1314–1324				
DR14(6)	DRB1*1401–1425			—	DPB1*4401–6501
DR7	DRB1*0701				
DR8	DRB1*0801–0813				
DR9	DRB1*0901				
DR10	DRB1*1001				
	DRB3*0101				
DR52	DRB3*0201–0205				
	DRB3*0301				
DR53	DRB4*0101–0103				
	DRB4*0101102N				
DR51	DRB5*0101–0105				
	DRB5*0201–0203				

HLA lists of alleles, monthly updates and aligned sequences can be accessed from the TAL Homepage at: http://www.icnet.uk/axp/tia
The serological assignments of HLA class II molecules do not always correlate with the DNA nomenclature. Serological assignment of HLA DR alleles is largely determined by the DRB1 gene product, whereas assignment of DQ alleles reflects contributions from the DQA1 and DQB1 gene products. As new alleles of DQ were identified DQ was split, eg. DQ5 and DQ6 are splits of DQ1 whereas DQ7, 8, and 9 are splits of DQ3. DPw refers to workshop assignments of DP alleles which in general are poorly defined serologically.

defining many allelic HLA variants, but are rather insensitive at detecting allelic variation located deep within the cleft of the HLA molecules, which is inaccessible to antibodies. Consequently, many polymorphisms in HLA molecules can be serologically silent or undetectable by allotypic antisera or monoclonal antibodies. A great expansion in the characterization of new alleles in the HLA system has come with polymerase chain reaction (PCR) DNA based gene typing methodology. For example, the HLA-A2 allele appears indistinguishable in cells from different individuals when tested with a restricted panel of antibodies. However,

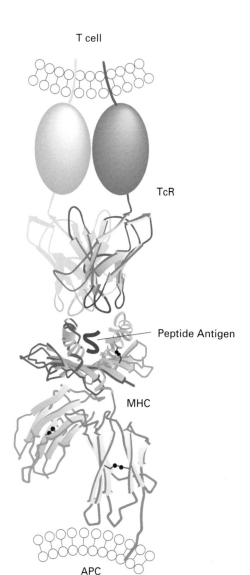

T cell

TcR

Peptide Antigen

MHC

APC

▮ **Fig. 32.4** A model of the antigen-specific T cell receptor (TCR) co-recognising peptide antigen bound to HLA receptors on the surface of APC.

there are now known to be at least 14 HLA-A2 subtypes (i.e. alleles; HLA-A*0201–0214) distinguished by polymorphisms in their antigen-binding pocket. The same principle of serologically silent variation applies to many of the polymorphisms located at other HLA loci including the class II gene products. The

naming of new HLA alleles is decided by an international nomenclature committee; however, the workshop prefix 'w' and local names such as DR 'Bon' often precede formal naming so deciphering the literature is a minefield for the uninitiated. The current naming system retains remnants of previous naming so for example alleles of the serological specificity A2 are called A*0201, 0202, etc. Annual HLA nomenclature reports with additional frequent updates are published in the journals *Tissue Antigens* and *Human Immunology*.

The function of human leucocyte antigen molecules

HLA class I molecules are expressed on most nucleated cell types, whereas class II molecules are confined to specialized antigen-presenting cells (B cells, dendritic cells, macrophages). The level of expression of both sets of HLA molecules can be enhanced by cytokines such as interleukin (IL) 4, α interferon (IFN), and tumour necrosis factor. These cytokines act on regulatory elements mostly in the 5′ region of the HLA genes and can induce expression of HLA class II molecules on cells which normally do not express these proteins, such as vascular endothelial cells. The distribution of HLA class I and class II molecules reflects their different roles in immune surveillance. Class I molecules capture endogenous peptides created in the cytoplasm. These peptides are largely derived from molecules synthesized within the cell and exogenous proteins are not presented very efficiently by class I molecules. This means that peptide loading of HLA class I molecules requires cellular infection or gene transcription leading to cytoplasmic translation of proteins for presentation to the immune system. The peptides presented by class I molecules are generally recognized by antigen-specific T cells of the CD8 phenotype. Thus, class I molecules are mostly used to present antigen to killer T cells (CTL).

Major histocompatibility complex class I peptides

Peptides presented by class I molecules are apparently derived from the small fraction of all translated proteins which are degraded by a multicatalytic protease known as the proteasome. The proteasome is an evolutionarily ancient barrel-like structure which degrades polypeptides into short 8–10 aa long peptides. The proteasome is composed of 12–14 subunits, at least two of which, known as LMP2 and LMP7 are

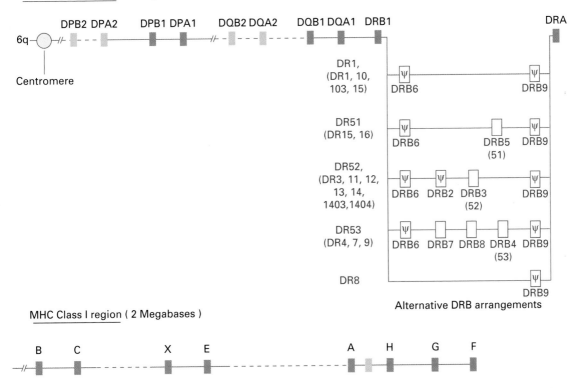

▌Fig. 32.5 The organisation of gene loci within the MHC class II region varies in different haplotypes.

encoded within the class II region of the MHC (see Fig. 32.1). These MHC-linked subunits are also induced in their expression by cytokines such as IFNγ. Peptides created by the proteasome have a very short half-life in the cytoplasm unless they are protected from further degradation. Many of these peptides are actively transported across the membrane of the endoplasmic reticulum and into the lumen of that organelle. This transport is facilitated by a dimeric molecular pump known as the TAP molecule (TAP = transporter associated with antigen presentation). The TAP genes are also encoded within the class II region of the MHC, closely linked to the genes encoding LMP2 and 7 (see Fig. 32.1). The TAP 1 and TAP 2 gene products form a multidrug resistance-like pump which is adenosine triphosphate dependent. This pump apparently associates with peptides on the cyto-

plasmic side of the endoplasmic reticulum (ER) membrane and with class I molecules on the lumenal surface and so is capable of delivering peptides directly to the class I molecules.

Major histocompatibility complex class II peptides

Class II molecules also acquire a large fraction of the peptides they present from an endogenous source; however, the majority of these peptides are created in the endocytic compartment and not the cytoplasm. Endosomes are membrane bound vesicles which shuttle proteins between various vacuolar compartments of the cell and are separated from the cytoplasm by a lipid bilayer. Therefore only a small fraction of the peptides presented by class II molecules are derived from the cytoplasm. Class II molecules assemble in the ER and are escorted to the endosomal compartment by a monomorphic protein known as invariant chain. Once the endosomal compartment has been reached, invariant chain is degraded and the class II cleft becomes competent for binding to antigenic peptides. Most antigenic peptides (8–15 aa in length) are derived from the activity of endosomal/lysosomal proteases on endogenous proteins; however some peptides are created by the endocytic uptake and proteolysis of exogenous proteins. The loading of class II molecules with peptides generally requires a function carried out by the HLA-DM molecule. HLA-DM comprises two gene products HLA-DMA and B which are both encoded in the class II region of the MHC (Fig. 32.1). The exact function of HLA-DM is still uncertain, however, it is believed to catalyse the dissociation of invariant chain peptides from class II molecules and therefore promote loading of peptide into class II molecules. The pathways of antigen presentation exploited by class II molecules means they can present both endogenously and exogenously derived antigenic peptides. Thus, T-cell responses to toxins, phagocytic material, and non-infectious virions are all quite efficient via the class II pathway. The T cells which recognize class II molecules are generally CD4 positive T-helper cells; however, some responses to viral envelope proteins can involve class II-restricted, CD4 positive killer T cells. The role of T-helper cells is to augment B-cell differentiation and proliferation of cytotoxic T cells.

Human leucocyte antigens and the transplant response

Processed foreign antigen complexed to HLA class I or class II molecules is recognized by a specific membrane bound receptor (T-cell receptor: TCR) on the surface of T cells (see Fig. 32.4). The TCR appears capable of co-recognizing the structure of the HLA molecule itself as well as exposed parts of the peptide antigen. This exquisite co-recognition event means that T cells are highly specific and usually genetically restricted to the individual from which they were derived. Thus a killer T cell raised against an influenza virus peptide in an individual expressing HLA-A2 will not confer any influenza immunity when passively transferred to an individual expressing HLA-A1. This concept is known as MHC restriction. Because T cells are MHC restricted it is difficult to understand why

they should ever recognize a foreign HLA type. However, in practice they do and indeed they do so with alarming frequency. Thus somewhere between 1/10 and 1/1000 activated clonally distinct T cells will be capable of recognizing any given allogeneic HLA molecule. Given the number of T cells in the human lymphoid system, this represents a striking tendency for T cells to cross-react on foreign or allogeneic HLA molecules. This cross-reaction usually depends on the peptide antigen as well as the allogeneic HLA molecule. In the normal course of events this alloreactivity is quite irrelevant, however, the transplantation of organs from one individual to an HLA incompatible second individual exposes the host immune system to at least six and usually 12 non-self HLA alleles expressed by the allograft. Moreover, the 'self peptides' selected for presentation by allogeneic HLA molecules are likely to be quite distinct from those presented by syngeneic HLA molecules, further diversifying the array of unfamiliar ligands expressed by allograft cells. These allogeneic HLA–peptide complexes naturally stimulate powerful allogeneic T-cell responses which results in cellular rejection of organs. For this reason HLA matching is required, or desirable, in many forms of transplantation. The degree of HLA matching required for various types of transplantation is shown in Table 32.2.

In addition to the allogeneic cellular response, the antibody response to HLA molecules and ABO blood groups can cause rejection of certain grafts especially where these antibodies are preformed and therefore present at the time of organ transplantation. Antibodies to ABO blood group antigens react with these determinants on vascular endothelium and therefore ABO-incompatible solid organs can be rapidly rejected by humoral mechanisms. In patients who have been transfused or previously transplanted; or in multiparous females, exposure to allogeneic HLA molecules can also result in the production of anti-HLA class I antibodies. These preformed antibodies can lead to acute and hyper-acute rejection of grafts expressing the particular HLA molecules recognized by these antibodies. Therefore for solid organ transplants, individuals are matched as closely as possible for their HLA types to avert cellular rejection, but it is also necessary to ensure ABO compatibility and to exclude preformed antidonor HLA antibodies in the host.

Ironically, patients who have received multiple blood transfusion prior to transplantation appear to develop some form of T-cell tolerance to allogeneic donor HLA alleles and renal graft survival is actually enhanced in these individuals. This is known as the 'transfusion effect' and in many centres pretransplant transfusion and even donor-specific transfusions are

▌ **Table 32.2** Human leucocyte antigen (HLA) testing in organ transplantation and platelet transfusion

Clinical situation	Test	Comment
Bone marrow transplantation, sibling or related	HLA-A, -B type DR, DQ	A single major mismatch is allowed at most centres.
Bone marrow transplantation unrelated	HLA-A, -B type DR, DQ	A complete match is required at most centres. A single minor mismatch is allowed at some centres.
Renal transplantation	HLA-A, -B type DR, DQ	Various degrees of mismatch permitted, but matching is optimized by organ sharing.
	Anti-HLA class I antibody crossmatch	A positive crossmatch contraindicates transplantation.
	ABO blood group	ABO compatibility is necessary (blood group O donors into A, AB, or B recipient are acceptable).
	Anti-HLA class II cross match	Controversial, transplantation often proceeds even if crossmatch is positive.
Heart/lung transplantation	HLA-A, -B, -DR, -DQ type	For use retrospectively (level of compatibility can influence type of immunosuppression).
	Anti-HLA class I crossmatch	Positive crossmatch contraindicates transplantation.
	Anti-HLA class II crossmatch	Controversial, usually ignored.
Liver transplantation	HLA-A, -B, -DR, -DQ	For use retrospectively to assist monitoring.
	Anti-HLA class I crossmatch	Controversial, ignored at most centres.
	Anti-HLA class II crossmatch	Controversial, usually ignored.
Corneal transplantation	HLA-A, -B	Matching is only carried out for grafts at high risk of rejection, e.g. previous graft rejection; vascularized graft bed.
Pancreatic transplantation	ABO blood group	ABO compatibility necessary.
	Anti-HLA class I crossmatch	A positive crossmatch contraindicates transplantation.
Platelet transfusion	HLA-A, -B.	For use in identification of HLA-matched platelet donors.
	Anti-HLA class I antibodies	Screening for presence and specificity of anti-HLA class I antibodies in alloimmune refractory thrombocytopenia.

carried out routinely. Transfusion of potential renal transplant recipients does run the risk of inducing undesirable anti-HLA antibodies in the patient.

Testing for anti-HLA antibodies is known as the 'cross-match'. In practice it is only important to carry out the cross-match seeking anti-HLA class I antibodies. However, there is a school of thought which believes that anti-HLA class II antibodies might be responsible for some forms of early graft rejection. Cross-match compatibility to exclude anti-HLA-antibodies is essential for renal and important in heart/lung transplantation. Patients awaiting renal transplantation are usually monitored for anti-HLA class I antibodies because the level and specificity of these antibodies can change with time. When carrying

out a cross-match between a patient serum and donor cells, many centres test the current as well as 'historical peak' serum from the patient. The 'historic peak' is defined as the serum giving a positive cross-match on the highest proportion of random donor cells from allogeneic individuals.

Cross-matching is also used to detect anti-HLA antibodies causing refractoriness to platelet transfusion with random platelets. The class I cross-match does not appear to be critical in liver transplantation, although some controversy still surrounds this issue. It is possible that the low level of expression of class I molecules on liver cells, and the secretion of class I molecules by the liver, protects this organ from the damage caused by anti-HLA class I antibodies. The role of antibody cross-matching in bone marrow transplantation is unclear and most centres do not take the class I or class II cross-match into account when identifying a bone marrow transplant donor.

Pedigree analysis in compatibility testing

The linkage of HLA loci on chromosome 6 means that individuals will usually inherit a set of non-recombined HLA alleles encoded at linked HLA loci from each parent. This set is often identifiable in family studies where all the alleles present on one chromosome cosegregate. The set of HLA alleles found on one chromosome is known as the haplotype. In identifying donors for bone marrow transplantation, family studies are essential to determine haplotypes accurately because very careful matching is required to

avoid graft-versus-host disease (GVHD). An example of haplotyping is shown in Fig. 32.6.

Doubts about the role of HLA-DP in transplantation mean that testing for this locus is rarely carried out clinically. Typically an HLA typing laboratory would test for HLA-A, -B, -DRB1, -DRB3, -B4, -B5, and -DQB1 loci. In the family study shown in Fig. 32.6 the mother and father are mismatched at both haplotypes. Among the children, John and Andrew are haploidentical (and therefore phenotypically identical). Jane and Jim share a single haplotype as do Tom and Jim. Jane's paternal haplotype is a recombinant involving a cross-over event between HLA-A and -B. Recombination is observed between HLA-A/B and independently between B/DR in about 1% of meiotic events. The implications of this family study are that Andrew and John would be ideal bone marrow donors for each other. However, none of the other siblings would be suitable. Even though there is haplotype sharing between some of these siblings the complete

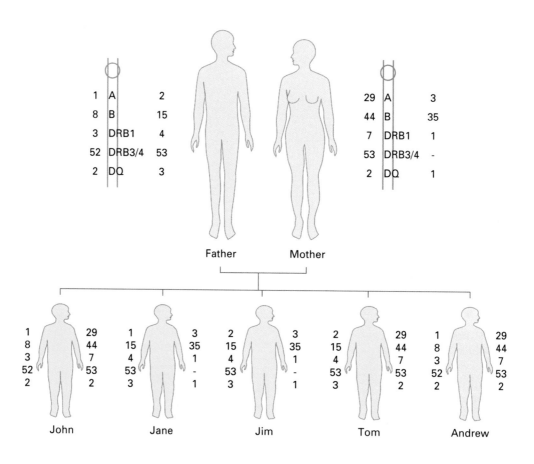

▌**Fig. 32.6** Segregation of HLA haplotypes in a family study.

mismatch in the second haplotype would make them unsuitable donors for bone marrow transplantation which requires very close matching of HLA. On the other hand they might still be suitable donors for renal transplantation where perfect HLA matching is not required. However, for renal and other solid organ transplantation, ABO blood group compatibility is essential because these determinants are expressed on vascular endothelium where recognition by iso-haemagglutinins leads to rapid vascular coagulation and organ failure.

Where a matched sibling donor does not exist for a patient requiring allogeneic bone marrow transplantation (70% cases) searching of the extended family or unrelated bone marrow registries is indicated as discussed in the chapter on allogeneic bone marrow transplantation.

Functional tests of human leucocyte antigen compatibility

Testing for HLA identity at all HLA loci is a daunting task for most laboratories because of the very large number of alleles present in the population. Therefore there has been a great deal of interest in developing functional or *in vitro* cellular tests of overall donor–recipient compatibility. This is especially important in selecting suitable unrelated donors for bone marrow transplantation. Unfortunately, none of the tests so far developed provides convincing predictability of impending graft rejection or more importantly GVHD. Among the most widely used functional compatibility tests are the mixed lymphocyte reactivity (MLR) test and allogeneic T-helper or CTL precursor studies. The MLR or MLC (C = culture) involves measuring T-cell proliferation of host T cells in response to donor lymphocytes and vice versa. In a one-way MLR the stimulating lymphocytes are irradiated to inhibit their proliferation whereas in the two-way MLR both stimulator and responder cells are allowed to proliferate. The proliferation of responding T cells is normalized as a percentage of the maximal response achieved by the same T cells when stimulated by the lectin phyto-haemagglutinin or by a pool of histoincompatible (i.e. HLA non-identical) stimulator cells usually derived from three or more unrelated individuals (lab staff!). This is known as the relative response (RR). Interpretation and reproduceability of the MLR is problematic and there is now limited enthusiasm for this test as a predictor of GVHD or HLA incompatibility. It is necessary to include controls showing that

responder cells can all respond and that stimulator cells can all stimulate across an appropriate barrier such as third-party donor cells. Relative responses can vary widely and individual laboratories use their own cut-off values defining negative (i.e. non-reactive) and positive (reactive) MLR results. Unfortunately, known HLA mismatches can be present in a negative MLR, and a positive MLR can be obtained between pheno-typically HLA-identical individuals. In general, a relative response of ≤7% is generally consistent but not diagnostic of HLA identity; relative responses between 7 and 30% are non-predictive and a relative response of ≥30% is suggestive of HLA non-identity. These values vary between laboratories. As the MLR is biased towards measuring HLA class II discrepancies many laboratories have abandoned this test with the implementation of high-resolution PCR-based HLA class II typing.

Measurement of allogeneic CTL or helper T-cell precursor frequencies is carried out at specialized bone marrow transplant centres but is not universally accepted as being predictive of GVHD. The test is very labour intensive and requires a skilled technician for its reproduceability. Precursor frequencies are estimated by limit dilution analysis of donor versus host lymphocytes (i.e. GVHD vector only). High precursor frequencies (up to 1 in 10^4 cells) are thought to be associated with a greater risk of acute GVHD. It is possible that precursor studies detect major and minor incompatibilities and so theoretically at least might give a broad measure of the transplant barrier but technical improvements will be required before this test is widely adopted in clinical practice.

Human leucocyte antigen and disease

Alleles of HLA molecules are frequently strongly associated with certain diseases. In particular the autoimmune diseases are well known to be associated with alleles of HLA class II loci. For instance, insulin-dependent diabetes mellitus is strongly associated with HLA-DR3 and-DR4. Indeed this association may be secondary to an association with HLA-DQ2 and -DQ3. Many of the systemic rheumatic diseases also have a strong association with HLA-DR3 and -DQ2. The mechanism underlying these associations is not known, but one possibility is that these allelic forms of class II molecules can selectively present autoantigens to T cells. This might confer susceptibility to those individuals possessing these particular HLA alleles. A related example of this is coeliac disease. Coeliac disease is

■ Table 32.3 Human leucocyte antigen (HLA) testing in disease diagnosis

Clinical situation	Test	Comment
Paternity testing	HLA-A, -B, -C, -DR, -DQ, -DP, -C4, -C2 Family study	Superseded at most centres by newer polymorphic gene markers.
Narcolepsy	HLA-DR2 (HLADQBI*0602)	DR2, DQBI*0602 is present in nearly all patients with nar colepsy but is also found in ~ 25% of normal Caucasians. Therefore the presence of DR2 is not diagnostic of narcolepsy but the absence of DR2 virtually excludes narcolepsy.
Ankylosing spondylitis (AS)	HLA-B27	B27 is found in >98% of patients with AS but is also found in 7% of Caucasian populations. Therefore the presence of B27 is not diagnostic. The absence of B27 virtually excludes AS.
Insulin-dependent diabetes mellitis) (IDDM	HLA-DQ2	DQ2 and related DR alleles containing unique amino acids around position 57 of the DQ β chain are strongly associated with IDDM. This association may be used to assess the clinical risk of IDDM in first-degree relatives of patients at specialized centres but is of no value in routine testing of patients.
Recurrent abortion/ infertility	Anti-HLA class I antibodies	Recurrent abortion or infertility associated with anti-paternal HLA class I antibodies. Used only at special centres in conjunction with full assessment of individual cases.
Familial haemochromatosis	Family study HLA-A, -B	Familial haemochromatosis is associated with HLA-A3, but this is not diagnostic. Prediction of affected individuals is based on cosegregation of the haemochromatosis gene with the linked HLA-A haplotype of the affected individual.
Rheumatoid arthritis (RA)	HLA-DRB1 typing	HLA-DR4 is found in approximately 70% of patients with RA and 25% of normals. DR4 subtypes B1*0402, 0403 and 0407 may not be associated with increased risk of RA in Caucasians. In some studies DR1 is also associated with RA. DR4 is associated with more aggressive erosive disease and a gene dosage effect has been observed in some studies. Interpretation needs great care and may be more prognostic than diagnostic.
Antenatal diagnosis	HLA-A, -B, -DR phenotype	Very rarely used to predict affected fetus where a sibling has congenital adrenal hyperplasia. Relies upon cosegregation of HLA haplotypes with genetically linked 21-hydroxylase enzyme defect.

strongly associated with HLA-DQA1*0501 and DQB1*0201. The DQA1*0501 and DQB1*0201 alleles may be linked on the same chromosome (*cis*) or be present on opposite chromosomes (*trans*) suggesting the primary susceptibility to coeliac disease is conferred by the selective antigen presentation properties of the DQA1*0501/DQB1*0201 class II dimer.

Some HLA disease associations are of diagnostic importance (Table 32.3). The best example is the asso-

ciation of HLA-B27 with ankylosing spondylitis. More than 98% of patients with ankylosing spondylitis in virtually all ethnic groups will express HLA-B27. However, the presence of HLA-B27 does not diagnose ankylosing spondylitis as this allele is also found in approximately 7% of normal Caucasians. Thus the use of HLA-B27 testing in ankylosing spondylitis is largely to rule out this diagnosis. If a patient has rheumatic back pain and is HLA-B27 negative they are extremely unlikely to have ankylosing spondylitis. On the other hand if the patient was HLA-B27 positive this would make the diagnosis of ankylosing spondylitis tenable, but would not prove the case.

The association of HLA-DR2-DQB1*0602 with narcolepsy falls into a similar category. More than 90% of patients with narcolepsy carry these alleles; however, this combination is also found in approximately 30% of healthy normal Caucasians. Thus, the presence of either of these alleles does not diagnose narcolepsy, but their absence makes a diagnosis of narcolepsy extremely unlikely.

The presence of certain HLA alleles can raise the risk of developing certain disorders and in specialized situations this information can be helpful. Thus, in a family with multiple individuals affected with insulin-dependent diabetes mellitus, cosegregation of HLA-DR3 or -DR4 haplotypes with the disease phenotype is quite common and can be used to predict which unaffected individuals have the greatest risk of developing the disease. The strong association of HLA-DR4 with rheumatoid arthritis (70% of patients, 25% of normals) may have some prognostic implication. For instance, several studies have shown that patients who are homozygous for certain DR4 alleles are more likely to develop aggressive rheumatoid disease (erosions, rheumatoid factor, etc.) than those who are heterozygous or do not carry the DR4 allele at all. Not all DR4 subtypes are associated with rheumatoid arthritis (e.g. DRB1*0402, 0403, 0407) and so some laboratories will subtype DR4 for disease susceptibility testing. Those DR4 subtypes associated with rheumatoid arthritis and HLA-DR1 which is also increased in patients with rheumatoid arthritis are similar in the third hypervariable region of the DRB1 β chain leading to the suggestion that a shared structure (aa67–86) might confer selective peptide binding and susceptibility to rheumatoid arthritis in individuals with these alleles. Homozygosity for high-risk DR4 subtypes may be of prognostic relevance in predicting more severe disease and worse outcome than DR4 heterozygosity and DR4 negative phenotypes. The use of HLA typing for these latter purposes is generally confined to specialist situations, as the interpretation of this information requires great care.

There are several known disorders which are inherited in a simple Mendelian fashion which are associated with particular HLA alleles. These include haemochromatosis, the congenital form of 21-hyroxylase deficiency (leading to congenital adrenal hyperplasia) and complement C2 deficiency. HLA typing is occasionally used to assist in the diagnosis of these disorders. However, this usually occurs in the context of a family study where there is at least one diseased individual and the question involves identifying other potentially affected siblings or relatives. In this situation cosegregation of HLA haplotypes with the disease phenotype is used to assign probable affected family members. The weak population association of the allele HLA-A3 with familial haemochromatosis is of no diagnostic relevance.

Further reading

Germain, R. N. and Margulies, D. H. (1993). The biochemistry and cell biology of antigen processing and presentation. *Annual Review of Immunology*, **11**, 403–50.

Hansen, T. H. and Sachs, D. H. (1989). The major histocompatibility complex. In *Fundamental immunology* (ed. W. E. Paul), pp. 445–87. Raven Press, New York.

Klein, J. (1986). *Natural history of the major histocompatibility complex*. John Wiley, New York.

Mandel, T. E (ed.) (1993). *Transplantation. An effective therapy*. Australian Medical Publishing Company, Kingsgrove NSW, Australia.

Terasaki, P. I. (ed.) (1900). *History of transplantation: 35 recollections*. CLA Tissue Typing Laboratory, Los Angeles, California.

Tsuju, K., Aizawa, M., and Sasazuki, T. (ed.) (1992). *HLA 1991*. Oxford University Press, Oxford.

33 Renal, cardiac, and lung transplantation

P. D. Mason and R. Lechler

Introduction

Early attempts to transplant kidneys in the early 1950s used no immunosuppression, and as the human leucocyte antigen (HLA) system was uncharacterized, were unmatched. Although several kidneys did survive a short period, (probably due to uraemic immunosuppression) and some patients did receive cortisone, the results were poor. Total body irradiation was used as immunosuppression from 1959, and 6-mercaptopurine and then azathioprine were introduced in the early 1960s. Since then renal transplantation has become a routine treatment and the one of choice for most patients with chronic renal failure. Clinical heart transplantation began in 1967, although it took until the 1980s for it to become established as a routine operation. Similarly, despite some early attempts at heart–lung transplantation in the late 1960s, this operation did not become an established therapeutic procedure until the late 1980s. Hamilton (1994), and Lansman *et al.* (1989) have reviewed the history of transplantation.

The immunological barrier(s) to transplantation have been discussed in Chapter 32 on histocompatibility, and so the focus here will be on the clinical issues pertaining to renal, cardiac, and lung transplantation.

Immunosuppression

The ideal immunosuppressive regimen for transplantation, irrespective of the organ(s) involved, would be one that is donor-specific, does not impair the host's ability to deal with infection or malignancy, and which has no side-effects. Although several strategies have proved successful in inducing and maintaining donor-specific tolerance in rodent models of transplantation, it has to date proven impossible to reproduce such tolerance in humans (see below). Clinical transplantation therefore currently relies on a combination of non-specific immunosuppressive drugs, resulting in an increased susceptibility to infection and malignancy.

There is no clear consensus as to the optimal immunosuppressive regimen, either for the prevention or the treatment of acute rejection episodes. Most centres now use cyclosporin, usually in combination with one, or a combination of, steroids, azathioprine, and anti-T-cell antibody preparations.

Cyclosporin

The introduction of cyclosporin, originally isolated from a soil fungus, resulted in a significant improvement in graft survival of vascularized solid organ transplants. Its mechanism of action involves formation of a complex with a cytosolic protein, cyclophilin. This then binds calcineurin (a calcium/calmodulin-dependent phosphatase) and the complex prevents the expression of genes, including interleukin (IL) 2 and IL-2 receptor, normally associated with T-cell activation. Although the major effects of cyclosporin are on T cells it does also have effects on B cells and macrophages, both directly as well as via inhibition of T-lymphocyte-derived cytokines such as IL-3, IL-4, interferon (IFN) γ, tumour necrosis factor (TNF) α, and granulocyte–macrophage colony-stimulating factor (GM-CSF) which act on these cells.

Azathioprine

Azathioprine was the first widely used immunosuppressive drug. It is metabolized to 6-mercaptopurine by the liver, and then intracellularly to active metabolites, particularly thioinosinic acid, which inhibit DNA and RNA synthesis by interfering with purine metabolism. The effect of the drug is to reduce both the numbers and function of lymphocytes, monocytes, and natural killer cells, and the toxic effects include neutropenia and thrombocytopenia.

Steroids

Corticosteroids have a large number of anti-inflammatory and immunosuppressive effects, the latter probably mainly the result of inhibition of cytokine production. Steroids are commonly given during transplantation, and continued at least in the first few weeks afterwards. It is clear that high-steroid doses do not improve transplant survival but are associated with a high incidence of side-effects, particularly infection. Pulses of methlyprednisolone are effective treatment for acute rejection episodes (see below).

Antilymphocyte antibodies

Polyclonal sera from animals, usually horse or rabbit, raised against human-cultured lymphocytes (antilymphocyte globulin: ALG) or human thymocytes (antithymocyte globulin: ATG) are available. They are used by some centres as prophylaxis against rejection, and also for treatment of acute rejection, especially when steroid resistant. Currently only one monoclonal antibody (MoAb), OKT3, an anti-T-cell MoAb, has a clinical licence. Polyclonal antibodies and MoAbs have similar efficacy and long-term side-effects, although first dose and early reactions occur more frequently with OKT3. The use of these preparations results in profound immunosuppression with a high incidence of herpes reactivation, opportunistic infections especially with cytomegalovirus (CMV) and fungi, and Epstein–Barr virus (EBV)-associated lymphoproliferative disorders and B-cell lymphomas.

Other immunosuppressive agents

There are a large number of newer immunosuppressive agents currently under intensive investigation.

FK 506 binds to FK506 binding protein (FKBP), which is distinct from cyclophilin, but the complex binds to and inactivates calcineurin in a similar manner to cyclosporin–cyclophilin. Although FK506 may be superior to cyclosporin for liver transplantation, most data suggest that it has no advantages over cyclosporin for renal, heart, or lung transplantation.

Rapamycin also binds to FKBP, but this complex neither binds calcinerin nor blocks the expression of T-cell activation genes. It inhibits the cellular events triggered by IL-2 and other cytokines.

Mycophenolic acid, which is likely to be widely available very soon, blocks purine synthesis and preliminary studies suggest that it may be a promising alternative to azathioprine because of its relative specificity for lymphocytes. It also inhibits glycosylation of adhesion molecules and prevents smooth muscle proliferation. This latter property is of interest as this may ameliorate the vascular changes seen in chronic graft rejection.

15-deoxyspergualin is particularly potent at suppressing B-cell proliferation and the development of

humoral responses, and may also influence the expression of the HLA molecules.

Brequinar sodium is an inhibitor of pyrimidine synthesis and leflunomide inhibits both B and T cells by an unknown mechanism.

Further work to confirm efficacy and safety of these newer agents is required. As the 1 year graft survival rates typically exceed 80% with current regimens, it is likely to be some time before the optimum dosage and combination of the newer immunosuppressive drugs is established. Thomson and Starzl (1993) have recently reviewed the mechanisms of actions and clinical data on the newer immunosuppressive drugs.

Total body irradiation

This was the first effective immunosuppressive therapy in renal transplantation, but was associated with a high incidence of serious side-effects. More recently some centres have used total body irradiation (TLI), with inverted Y-mantle irradiation, which is effective and relatively well tolerated. Experimentally, TLI has been successful at inducing donor-specific tolerance, although the mechanisms are unclear. A few units do use TLI, especially for sensitized patients. However, there are concerns about the long-term results, the fact that other immunosuppressive drugs are still necessary, and the difficulties in finding a donor within 1 month of TLI when efficacy is greatest.

Monoclonal antibodies

As already discussed the anti-T-cell MoAb, OKT3, already has an established place in clinical transplantation. There are many other MoAbs currently under investigation including those directed against CD4, CD25, CD7, CD54 (ICAM-1), CD34, CD6, CD45, CD69 (CAMPATH-1), CD2, CD8, and the T-cell receptor. Many of those that have been used clinically are effective as prophylactic agents and for the treatment of acute rejection, although when compared with ALG/ATG, most appear to have a similar efficacy. However, in preliminary studies, MoAb against CD25 (the IL-2 receptor) and CD54 (ICAM-1) appear to be particularly promising. Antibodies against CD45, the leucocyte common antigen present on B and T cells, monocytes, and neutrophils, has been used to deplete grafts of 'passenger' donor-derived leucocytes by *ex vivo* perfusion prior to transplantation. The rationale for this proposed by Lechler and Batchelor (1982) is that donor bone marrow-derived leucocytes are crucial to the development of acute rejection in experimental models of transplantation. Pilot studies have suggested that anti-CD45 treatment of human allografts is associated with a lower incidence of early rejection, and a larger randomized controlled trial is in progress. O'Connell *et al.* (1993) review details regarding MoAb therapy.

Mouse MoAb have several disadvantages. Many, particularly, those directed against T cells have a 'first dose' effect with pyrexia, rigors, 'flu-like' symptoms, and occasionally hypotension and pulmonary oedema, which are due to cytokine release. Secondly, they are immunogenic, and the development of neutralizing antimurine antibodies nullifies their effects. However, their immunogenicity can be reduced or eliminated by genetically or chemically manufacturing hybrid immunoglobulin molecules, comprising the antigen-binding domains from the original mouse sequence, and the constant, Fc portion of human origin. Substitution of alternative Fc fragments has also been shown to greatly influence the *in vivo* effects of the antibodies, e.g. immunoglobulin (Ig) G3 neither stimulates nor results in cell death, while IgG1 efficiently fixes complement and directs antibody-dependent cellular cytotoxicity (ADCC) resulting in cell depletion. Other approaches to immunotherapy include the use of combinations of MoAb, the generation of MoAb conjugates with cellular toxins and the use of cytokines, e.g. IL-2, to direct killing.

Blood transfusion effect

Recommendations regarding blood transfusion of potential transplant recipients has changed cyclically over the last 20 years. Until the late 1970s every effort was made to avoid blood transfusion because 30% of transfused patients develop anti-HLA antibodies which may preclude transplantation. However, it was then noted that rejection episodes were less frequent, and graft survival was substantially improved, by 20–30%, compared with non-transfused patients. Although part of the explanation may be that 'high responders' are screened out, due to the formation of alloantibodies, and are thus excluded from transplant statistics, this is not the whole explanation. The immunological mechanisms responsible for the blood transfusion effect remain unclear, although the induction of some form of allo-specific tolerance may be involved. The introduction of cyclosporin, led to a 15–20% improvement in 1 year graft survival, and the additional beneficial value of transfusion is minimal, while the risk of allosensitization remains substantial. Consequently, most units no longer recommend pre-transplant transfusion, although there are data suggesting that transfusions may be beneficial in patients who develop early rejection but such patients cannot reliably be predicted in advance. More recently, attention has again been focused on the beneficial effects of blood transfusion following reports that receipt of blood sharing one DR antigen with the recipient is associated with fewer rejection episodes, an improved 1 year graft survival in renal and heart transplant recipients and a low incidence of sensitization. Further studies are, however, necessary before this can be widely recommended.

Potential strategies for the induction of donor-specific tolerance

Much of the morbidity and mortality of transplant recipients is associated with the direct and side-effects of the non-specifically acting immunosuppressive drugs which are currently necessary to prevent rejection. Induction of donor-specific tolerance would be the ideal solution. There are documented patients with renal allografts who have stopped all immunosuppressive drugs but maintain stable, normal kidney function, suggesting that tolerance can occur. The challenge is to determine how this could be induced deliberately in all solid organ transplant recipients.

Central tolerance can be induced by neonatal exposure to alloantigen, but this is an unrealistic approach for clinical transplantation. In rodents, whole body irradiation followed by T-cell-depleted bone marrow transplantation results in tolerance to the alloantigens expressed by the transplanted bone marrow-derived cells. Unfortunately, this is too dangerous and impractical in humans. However, a modification of this approach involving elimination of recipient T cells with ATG and infusion of T-cell-depleted donor-derived bone marrow cells has been tried in renal transplant recipients, but so far without success. Another strategy, successful in rats, is to inject donor cells directly into the thymus. It is uncertain as to whether this would be successful in adult humans who have involuted thymuses.

A large series of observations, *in vitro*, have demonstrated that specific recognition by T cells, in the absence of costimulatory signals, can lead to T-cell inactivation. Recapitulation of this phenomenon *in vivo* may account for the induction on donor-specific tolerance in many *in vivo* models of transplantation. Given that the parenchymal cells of the transplanted tissues lack costimulatory properties the crucial requirement is to prevent acute rejection with some form of immunosuppression during the first few weeks while donor, specialized, antigen-presenting cells are present. Once these are eliminated, the allograft itself will favour the induction of tolerance. The necessary short-term immunosuppression with long-term graft survival can be achieved by several methods in rodents. These include a variety of drugs, including cyclosporin, and a multitude of monoclonal antibodies, especially against CD4 and/or CD8, but also those against LFA-1 (CD18/CD11a), ICAM-1 (CD54) or the high-affinity

IL-2 receptor (CD25). An alternative approach involves pretreating recipients with alloantigens on cells lacking costimulatory molecules. This can induce a non-responsive state prior to placing an allograft. It appears to be much more difficult to achieve these goals in larger animals or humans. This may be due to more effective indirect pathway processing, resulting in the efficient presentation of alloantigens by recipient antigen-presenting cells. This route of allorecognition may be more difficult to suppress without impairing immune responses more generally.

The concept of donor micro-chimerism being central to long-term tolerance has been promoted recently by Starzl *et al.* (1992, 1993). They argue that donor bone marrow-derived leucocytes, transferred to the recipient with solid organ transplants, are responsible and necessary for the establishment of donor-specific tolerance. Donor bone marrow-derived leucocytes have been detected in long-term recipients, although it is unclear whether this is the cause of donor-specific tolerance or merely a consequence of it. However, as mentioned above, kidney transplantation carried out at the same time as donor bone marrow transplantation has not resulted in improved renal graft survival.

Risk of malignancy

Recipients of organ transplants and, indeed, patients receiving long-term immunosuppressive drugs for any reason have an increased risk of developing malignancies. The explanation is likely to be multifactorial but many hypotheses implicate the immunosuppressive regimens used. Some of these are supported by experimental and clinical data, and are not mutually exclusive. They include impaired immune surveillance, increased susceptibility to oncogenic viruses (especially EBV and papillomaviruses) and direct mutagenic effects of the drugs themselves. The overall increase in the relative risk of developing tumours is 5–10 but is greater for particular types of tumour, especially lymphoma and skin cancers, and the latter are considerably more frequent in sunny regions. The effects are cumulative and a high proportion of long-term survivors can be expected to be affected, with an actuarial incidence of 20–35% at 20 years for non-skin tumours, with rates for skin tumours which may exceed 50% at 20 years in sunny countries (Sheil 1986).

Renal transplantation

Patient selection

Renal transplantation is generally the treatment of choice for patients with chronic renal failure, irrespective of the underlying cause. Age is a relative contraindication (especially under 2 and over 70 years) as are serious co-morbid conditions such as heart failure, psychiatric illness, and chronic infection. Patients with urological problems and peripheral vascular disease, especially diabetics, need careful assessment before acceptance on to transplant programmes. Some forms of glomerulonephritis recur in the allograft but loss of function as a consequence is fortunately uncommon.

In Europe, North America, and Australia the demand for renal transplantation is about 60 patients per million population. Cadaver donation rates have been falling, probably as a result of seat belt and crash helmet legislation, and are currently running at less than half of that required to meet the demand. Nowadays, cadaver donors often provide kidneys, liver, heart, lungs, and sometimes pancreas. For kidney transplantation, live-related donors are suitable and provide 15–20% of kidney transplants in Europe and the USA, although live donation is much commoner in the Middle East and Asian subcontinent. Better results are obtained with live-related donors' organs especially if donor and recipient have identical HLA antigens (see below), but it is important that the potential donor is suitable on medical, psychological, and ethical grounds.

Tissue matching of transplants

Kidneys must be ABO blood group compatible. The huge polymorphism of the HLA genes means that unrelated individuals are very unlikely to be identical at all or even most HLA loci. Beneficial matches can only be obtained by organ sharing on a national or even international level. The advent of cyclosporin has meant that 1 year graft survival is good even for HLA-mismatched organs and this had led some to advocate transplantation without attention to HLA type. However, long-term follow-up suggests that the risk of graft loss is related to the degree of HLA mismatch between donor and recipient especially at the DR locus (see below). It is also clear that traditional serological DR typing is frequently missing subtype differences and may even be incorrect up to 25% of the time, although since genetic methods of tissue typing (especially polymerase chain reaction based) have been introduced, this has become less of a problem. A direct cross-match is always performed prior to transplantation in order to detect any preformed anti-HLA allo-antibodies. The traditional lymphocytotoxicity test involves mixing recipient sera with donor lymphocytes and a source of complement. The presence of lympho-cytotoxic antibodies results in lysis of donor lymphocytes and almost always predicts hyperacute rejection, so that a positive cross-match generally precludes transplantation. Patients awaiting transplantation should be regularly screened for lymphocytotoxic alloantibodies using a panel of typed third-party cells. Serum samples should be stored for sensitized patients and tested, together with a current serum sample in the direct cross-match prior to transplantation. The presence of donor-reactive IgG alloantibodies in an earlier sample, even if the current serum is non-reactive should be regarded as a contraindication to transplantation. Occasionally, such antibodies appear to be autoantibodies, low-affinity anti-class I or anti-class II antibodies and there is controversy as to their influence on the outcome of transplantation. A variety of other more sensitive cross-match techniques have been described. In particular, flow cytometry is allegedly exquisitely sensitive at detecting antibodies bound to donor lymphocytes and is not dependent on complement fixation. It seems likely that this flow cytometric cross-match is sometimes predictive of outcome, especially in sensitized patients (Mahoney *et al.* 1990).

Surgical aspects

The surgical techniques of organ retrieval and reimplantation are relatively straightforward and have been described by Morris (1984). During removal, the kidney is perfused with cold preservation fluid. The time between cessation of blood flow and cold perfusion is known as the *warm ischaemic time* and should preferably be less than 30 min. The time the kidney is stored on ice before reperfusion in a recipient (the *cold ischaemic time*) should be as short as possible and preferably less than 24 h, although may be up to 48 h. The graft is usually placed extraperitoneally in one iliac fossa with anastamosis of the renal to iliac vessels, and implantation of the ureter into the bladder directly or via a submucosal tunnel.

The early postoperative period

For most live-related and more than one-half of cadaver transplants urine is produced immediately following reperfusion. It is important that the patient's fluid volume is well maintained and carefully monitored in order to detect signs of blood loss and changes in urine output. A sudden early fall in urine output, in the absence of hypotension, is most commonly due to a blocked urinary catheter. Primary non-function occurs in up to 20% of first cadaver transplants and a greater percentage in regrafts. Registry data suggest that overall, although >95% of transplant recipients with primary non-function eventually do work, they have a significantly lower 1 year graft survival (64%) than patients whose transplants work immediately (83%) (Lim and Terasaki 1991). Factors predisposing

▌ **Table 33.1**   Causes of renal transplant dysfunction during the first 3 months

Common
  Rejection
  Acute tubular necrosis
  Cyclosporin nephrotoxicity
  Obstruction
  Combination of causes

Uncommon
  Renal vein thrombosis (usually with rejection)
  Renal artery thrombosis
  Infection
  Recurrent renal disease
  Drug nephrotoxicity (other than cyclosporin)
  Urine extravasation

to primary non-function include prolonged warm and cold ischaemic times, donor hypotension, high doses of cyclosporin, and previously failed grafts especially in sensitized patients. In this latter group hyperacute or accelerated rejection (see below) are more likely to occur. More rarely, arterial or venous thrombosis, ureteric obstruction or external compression may be responsible for primary or early non-function.

The first 3 months following transplantation are critical, and the 1 year and long-term outcome are possibly dependent on optimal management during this period. The major causes of graft dysfunction during the first 3 months are shown in Table 33.1. It is important to remember that more than one cause may be responsible. In particular, rejection can develop in a kidney with proven acute tubular necrosis (ATN) and so regular biopsy of a transplant with known ATN is essential. Cyclosporin toxicity which, acutely, is due to vasoconstriction of the afferent glomerular arterioles resulting in reduced renal blood flow and glomerular filtration may become an important differential diagnosis several days after transplantation. Continued administration of cyclosporin prolongs the period of primary non-function and some units therefore omit it until renal function recovers. Recurrent renal disease is an occasional cause of graft dysfunction.

Differentiation of the causes of early graft dysfunction

The ideal test is one that is sensitive (and will give an early indication of rejection), specific (and will reliably differentiate rejection from ATN, cyclosporin toxicity, and infection) and preferably cheap, simple, and reproducible. The wide variety of tests that are routinely used in different units is a testament to the inadequacy of all of them. Most of the available tests are good at predicting the presence or absence of clear-cut established rejection, but are insensitive in cases of early or mild rejection. Others are very sensitive and may be positive up to 2 days before rejection is evident by conventional criteria, but these often give false positive results, especially with infection.

Rising serum creatinine, fluid retention, and hypertension are all non-specific. However, in the context of progressive improvement in renal function, therapeutic cyclosporin levels, the absence of obstruction, and good graft perfusion these features are suggestive of rejection. The main value of ultrasound is to exclude obstruction and to confirm perfusion (with Doppler) of the kidney. More recently, derivation of a pulsatility (or resistivity) index has been found to be helpful, particularly when serial measurements have been made. Isotope imaging to detect flow, uptake, and excretion also has its proponents, but is a relatively crude indicator, especially when function is poor. The gold standard remains, for most units, the renal biopsy. However, early rejection is often focal and may be missed with a small sample. Furthermore, even stable well functioning grafts often have a mild and focal increase in interstitial cellularity making the diagnosis of mild early rejection difficult. For these reasons, the decision to treat for rejection must be based on an integration of the clinical picture together with other test results and histopathology. Fine needle aspiration (FNA) is a valuable technique, but requires considerable expertise. In centres where this is available it is probably at least as good as a needle biopsy for detecting acute cellular, but not vascular, rejection. FNA has the advantage of a lower complication rate, and can be performed more frequently.

Acute rejection

Allogeneic organs normally stimulate an early vigorous host response resulting in acute rejection which is, at least in experimental models of transplantation, induced principally by donor-derived antigen presenting, especially dendritic, cells carried as 'passenger leucocytes' within the organ. The effector limb of the alloresponse has several components. Antibodies undoubtedly mediate hyperacute rejection, but have also been implicated in graft loss in other situations. However, most experimental data suggest that it is the T cells that are central to the induction of acute graft rejection, although controversy remains as to the major effector cells responsible for graft destruction. For instance, although cytotoxic T cells are capable of lysing donor cells *in vitro*, these cells are neither nec-

essary nor augment graft rejection in most experimental models of transplantation. It appears, rather, that CD4+ 'helper' T cells orchestrate the alloimmune response *in vivo* and probably lead to graft destruction by the delayed-type hypersensitivity (DTH) response with recruitment of monocyte–macrophages and other effector cells. A minor role for B cells, CD8+ 'cytotoxic' T cells, eosinophils, and natural killer cells has been suggested, although their effects are probably CD4+ T-cell-dependent.

Clinical of types of acute rejection

Hyperacute rejection

This is due to rapid graft destruction as a result of pre-formed antibodies reactive with donor cells. These may be directed against ABO blood group antigens in the case of an ABO incompatible graft, or anti-HLA class I antigens in sensitized patients. With appropriate ABO matching and a negative direct cross-match, hyperacute rejection is rare. When it occurs it is usually evident within a few minutes of organ perfusion with cyanosis and infarction. If delayed slightly, it is characterized by primary non-function with absence of perfusion as ascertained by diethylene triamine pentacetic acid (DTPA — ^{99}Tc) scanning or Doppler ultrasound. Histologically, the major feature is intrarenal coagulopathy with thrombus formation within small arteries and glomerular capillaries, usually accompanied by interstitial haemorrhage, and an intense neutrophil infiltrate with widespread necrosis.

Accelerated rejection

In sensitized patients, accelerated rejection can develop within the first 5 days after transplantation. In those receiving a re-graft, it may be associated with a positive cross-match by flow cytometry despite a negative lymphocytotoxic cross-match. The kidney does not work but the diagnosis requires a biopsy which reveals severe interstitial and/or vascular rejection. Patients considered to be at high risk of accelerated rejection, regrafts, especially in sensitized patients, should therefore be biopsied early (days 2–5).

Acute rejection

Episodes of acute rejection affect one-half or more of all kidney transplants, the incidence depending on multiple factors including the degree of HLA mismatch, the background level of immunosuppression used, and the patients' sensitization history. The definition of rejection is imprecise, and although the histopathology is often regarded as the 'gold standard', renal dysfunction may respond to 'anti-rejection' treatment in the absence of convincing evidence on renal biopsy.

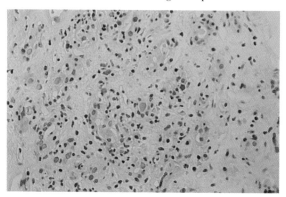

▌ **Fig. 33.1** Photomicrograph of a transplanted kidney showing acute parenchymal rejection. There is a mononuclear infiltrate with invasion of tubules, so-called 'tubulitis'. (Kindly supplied by Dr Mary Thompson, Hammersmith Hospital, London.)

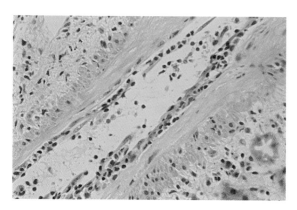

▌ **Fig. 33.2** Photomicrograph of a transplanted kidney showing acute vascular rejection. There is endothelial cell lifting with invasion of the intima by mononuclear cells. (Kindly supplied by Dr Mary Thompson, Hammersmith Hospital, London.)

Acute cellular rejection (also referred to as interstitial or parenchymal rejection) is characterized by an interstitial mononuclear infiltrate, often with eosinophils, and with invasion of tubules (so called tubulitis) (Fig. 33.1). The tubules are often separated indicating interstitial oedema and the changes, although initially focal, become diffuse. The intensity of the infiltrate does not always correlate with the clinical severity, except that extensive damage with disruption of capillaries and interstitial haemorrhage carries a poor prognosis. Immunohistology reveals the presence of macrophages and T cells. Although most studies report that CD8+ cells outnumber CD4+ T cells, others have reported the exact opposite, a result probably explained by the type of rejection and the timing of the biopsy.

The pathology of acute vascular rejection is characterized by endothelial swelling and the 'lifting off' of cells from the basement membrane, with lymphocytic infiltration (Fig. 33.2).

More severe changes, often predictive of irreversibility, include fibrinoid necrosis and fibrin and platelet thrombi. Similar changes may be seen in larger vessels and cortical necrosis may occasionally occur. Clinically, cellular and vascular rejection cannot be distinguished and often a mixed picture is present.

Early treatment is essential. High-dose steroids, usually as three or four daily pulses of 0.5 g methylprednisolone, is the most widely used treatment and this is effective in approximately 80% of episodes of acute rejection. Response to steroids generally occurs within 2–4 days, during which time the patient should be monitored and treated for hypertension and hyperglycaemia. ALG and OKT3 (anti-CD3 MoAb) are

effective in more than 90% of rejection episodes, but are more expensive and have a higher incidence of short-and long-term side-effects (see above). They are therefore generally used after failure of two courses of methylprednisolone unless the histology and clinical picture are particularly severe. It has been suggested that anti-T-cell antibody treatments are more effective than steroids for acute vascular rejection, but the data are not convincing. Similarly, a role for plasma exchange has not been demonstrated.

Acute tubular necrosis

This is the commonest cause of delayed graft function. It is more likely to occur if the donor kidney comes from a hypotensive or an elderly patient, or following a prolonged warm ischaemic (>30 min) or cold ischaemic (>24 h) time. Although ATN is usually associated with primary non-function, oliguria is sometimes delayed for several hours. Sensitized patients, and those who develop accelerated or early acute rejection are more likely to have ATN suggesting that the aetiology may sometimes have an immunological component. Although essentially a diagnosis of exclusion, the renal biopsy may reveal dilated tubules with a desquamated or swollen epithelium and sometimes mitoses, suggestive of recovery. However, a mononuclear interstitial infiltrate is seen more often than the typical appearance of ATN in native kidneys, making differentiation from early rejection difficult. It is important to remember that acute rejection can develop in a kidney affected by ATN (when urine output and creatinine are uninformative), and in order not to miss this, most units have a policy of biopsying regularly during the period of non-function.

Cyclosporin nephrotoxicity

Cyclosporin in high doses results in vasoconstriction of the glomerular afferent arterioles resulting in a 'pre-renal' reduction of glomerular filtration. Dose reduction is then associated with a fall in creatinine and cyclosporin nephrotoxicity may be diagnosed retrospectively. Nephrotoxicity may be suspected if the cyclosporin levels are high and other causes of a raised creatinine level have been excluded. The presence of histological features of cyclosporin toxicity is controversial. Tubular epithelial swelling and vacuolation, arteriolar hyalinosis, focal interstitial infiltrate, and fibrosis have all been associated with toxicity, but most studies have not been able to confirm these features as diagnostic, or even occurring more frequently in patients whose graft function improves following dose reduction. High doses of cyclosporin used in the early days, especially in heart transplantation probably do result in chronic cyclosporin toxicity. However, there is accumulating evidence regarding the long-term safety of cyclosporine in renal transplant patients.

Chronic rejection

There has been a huge improvement in the 1 year graft survival rates over the last 30 years, particularly since the introduction of cyclosporin. However, there has been no reduction in the rate of graft loss after the first 12 months, which continues at 3–5% per annum, with a half-life (after the first year) of 7–8 years for all non-HLA-identical cadaver transplants (Takemoto *et al.* 1992). The major cause of this graft loss, which now accounts for a significant proportion of patients commencing dialysis, is 'chronic rejection'. The entity is poorly defined and its aetiology uncertain (Tilney *et al.* 1992). Clinically, it is associated with a progressive deterioration of function often with increasing proteinuria and hypertension.

Pathologically, the most constant feature is a vasculopathy which is common to chronic rejection of all solid organs. Medium and small arteries became thickened with myointimal proliferation and subintimal accumulation of connective tissue with disruption and reduplication of the internal elastic lamina (Fig. 33.3). The lumen eventually becomes occluded. Medial necrosis with fibrin deposition may also occur and the changes are similar to those of atherosclerosis. Characteristic glomerular changes also develop. The glomerular capillaries become thickened and the basement membrane may develop a double contour. These features, together

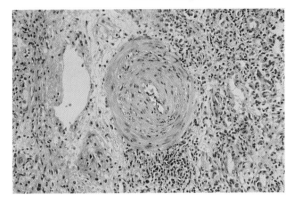

∎ **Fig. 33.3** Photomicrograph of a transplanted kidney showing chronic rejection. There is marked fibrointimal proliferation of the arteriole resulting in near obliteration of the vessel lumen. (Kindly supplied by Dr Mary Thompson, Hammersmith Hospital, London.)

with an enlarged lobular appearance results in a pattern similar to type I mesangiocapillary glomerulonephritis. Progressive glomerulosclerosis eventually develops. Tubular atrophy, often with fibrosis, is apparent in the interstitium but there is rarely much cellular infiltrate.

The aetiology of these chronic changes, is unknown and non-immunological mechanisms such as scarring initiated by early rejection episodes, or as a result of reperfusion injury, have been proposed. However, support for an immunological a etiology is several-fold. The incidence of chronic rejection is lower in HLA well-matched kidneys and progresses rapidly in patients who stop their immunosuppressive drugs. A number of studies have identified risk factors for the development of chronic rejection (Table 33.2). The

∎ **Table 33.2** Proposed risk factors for chronic rejection of renal transplants

---

Number of early acute rejection episodes (within 1 year of transplantation)

Acute rejection episodes after 1 year

Degree of human leucocyte antigen matching

Maintenance of cyclosporin dose <5 mg/kg per day

Non-compliance

Hypertension

Hyperlipidaemia

Documented episodes of infection

Retransplants

Prolonged organ ischaemic times

---

incidence appears to be particularly strongly associated with the number of early rejection episodes and in one report chronic rejection was detected in 1 and 2% (at 1 and 5 years, respectively) of patients experiencing no acute rejection episodes compared with 13 and 48%, respectively, for patients who had had one or more episodes (Almond *et al.* 1993). Cyclosporin toxicity has also been implicated but most data actually suggest that lower cyclosporin doses and levels are associated with a greater risk of chronic graft loss.

Long-term results of transplantation

Despite the improvements in the 1 year graft survival rates that have occurred over the last 20 years there have not been any changes in the subsequent rate of graft loss. The causes are mainly chronic rejection and patient death. Long-term survival is related to the degree of HLA matching, especially at the DR locus, with a smaller effect at the HLA-A and -B loci. The effect of preferential matching improving graft survival is apparent by 12 months and is magnified especially for completely matched organs (Fig. 33.4), The half-life of first renal transplants surviving the first 12 months has been estimated to be 17 years for completely matched grafts and overall about 8 years for

non-matched kidneys (Takemoto *et al.* 1992). However, within the latter group graft survival is related to the degree of matching (Opelz 1992; Fig. 33.5). These data argue strongly for the beneficial matching of cadaver organs, and outweigh the effect of increasing the cold ischaemic time which inevitably results. A programme based entirely on beneficial matches would disadvantage ethnic minorities and patients with special problems and the 'correct' balance remains controversial (Takemoto *et al.* 1994). Events early in the transplant course also appear to have a major influence on longer-term outcome (Cecka *et al.* 1992), possibly by affecting the incidence of chronic rejection (see above). Recurrence of the original renal disease sometimes recurs but is not a frequent cause of graft loss (Ramos and Tisher 1994).

Heart transplantation

The success of heart transplantation improved dramatically following the introduction of cyclosporin. Nevertheless, with no satisfactory artificial heart, failure of a heart transplant will result in patient death unless immediate retransplantation can be undertaken. Consequently, to reduce the risk of failure from acute rejection, heart transplant recipients are more heavily

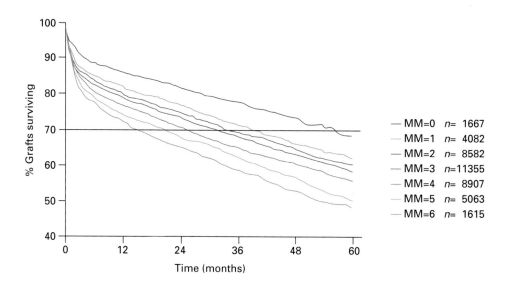

— MM=0	*n*=	1667
— MM=1	*n*=	4082
— MM=2	*n*=	8582
— MM=3	*n*=	11355
— MM=4	*n*=	8907
— MM=5	*n*=	5063
— MM=6	*n*=	1615

∎ **Fig. 33.4** Renal transplant survival. The effect of matching for HLA-A, -B, -DR on survival of the first cadaveric kidney transplant. MM = mismatched antigens.

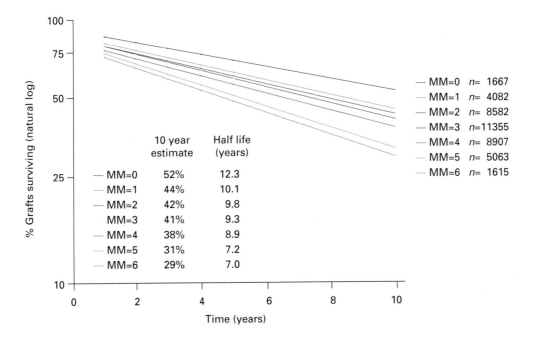

∎ **Fig. 33.5** Half-life and long-term graft survival in first cadaveric kidney graft in those in whom the graft has survived one year. The effect of the degree of HLA-A, -B, -DR match. MM = mismatch.

immunosuppressed than their renal counterparts, and as a result have a higher incidence of infective complications.

Patient selection

Heart transplantation is generally reserved for patients whose risk of death is greater without transplantation, although some advocate transplantation as a means to improve dramatically the quality rather than quantity of life. As the 1 and 5 year survival figures are now 85 and 75% respectively (Fig. 33.6), a substantial number of patients are eligible even if those over 50–55 years of age are excluded. In addition to severe refractory heart failure at rest (New York Heart Association NYHA class IV) some units use the maximum uptake of oxygen (VO_2 as an additional objective parameter of prognosis (a value of 10–14 ml/kg per min is of grave significance) but this needs careful interpretation in the context of the patient's clinical condition and age. The major contraindications are pulmonary hypertension, infection, malignancy, and significant peripheral and cerebrovascular disease. Relative contraindications include

age >50–55 years, diabetes, liver disease (especially alcohol related), and renal impairment.

HLA matching

HLA matching has in the past been considered to be impractical because of the constraints of the limited myocardial preservation times and the availability of donor organs. However, by HLA typing of donors before organ removal and recent advances in DR typing this may be possible routinely. Several studies have suggested that better DR matching is associated with fewer early rejection episodes, although most have so far failed to demonstrate benefit in terms of accelerated atherosclerosis (see below) or 1, 3 or 5 year patient survival.

Surgical aspects and immunosuppression

The myocardium cannot be preserved for long and the total ischaemic time should be less than 4–6 h. The recipient should be in theatre and on cardiopulmonary bypass by the time the donor organ arrives. In general orthotopic transplantation is performed but the details are beyond the scope of this chapter.

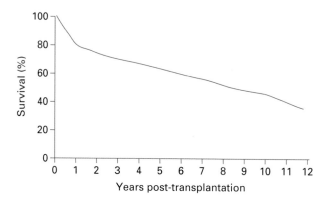

■ Fig. 33.6 Heart transplant survival.

Prior to the introduction of cyclosporin patients generally received azathioprine, steroids, and a 14 day course of ATG with additional ATG and steroids for rejection episodes (see below). Most centres now use relatively high-dose cyclosporin (15 mg/kg per day) combined with steroids, azathioprine and usually a shorter course of ATG. Some units have recently advocated the use of low-dose or even the omission of routine steroids.

Acute graft rejection

The immunological mechanisms involved in heart and lung transplant rejection are believed to be the same as for renal transplants. More than 85% of heart transplant recipients have at least one acute rejection episode and most have several episodes. A number of non-invasive tests have been proposed as methods of detecting rejection. These include subset analysis of peripheral blood lymphocytes, complex analyses of the ECG and echocardiograms, radionuclide scans, and the measurement of a variety of circulating factors associated with immune activation (e.g. neopterins and IL-2 receptors). However, endomyocardial biopsy is relatively straightforward, has a low complication rate, and is the most reliable means of diagnosing acute rejection, although several biopsies must be taken to minimize the risk of missing rejection due to sampling error. The precise timing of routine biopsies varies between units, but in general are performed weekly for the first 6 weeks, with a gradually reducing frequency over the following months, and annually thereafter. Other indications include dysrhythmias, low ECG voltage, and signs of heart failure which may be due to rejection. Biopsies

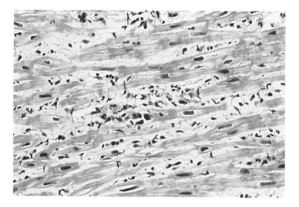

■ Fig. 33.7 Photomicrograph of an endomyocardial biopsy taken from a heart transplant. Acute rejection is characterized by a moderate infiltrate of mononuclear cells with myocytolysis. (Kindly supplied by Drs Marlene Rose and Margaret Burke, Harefield Hospital, London.)

are also usually repeated after a few days if there are equivocal changes of rejection.

The pathological features of acute cardiac rejection are focal interstitial lymphocytic infiltrates, especially around vessels. More severe damage is characterized by damage and necrosis of single and then groups of myocytes culminating in neutrophil infiltration and haemorrhage (Fig. 33.7). Increased steroid dose is the mainstay of treatment for acute rejection, and ATG/OKT3 (often given for shorter periods than in renal transplant rejection) are reserved for particularly severe or steroid-resistant episodes. There is some evidence that intravenous cyclosporin may also be effective.

Infection

In view of the heavy immunosuppressive regimens used, infection is common and responsible for two-thirds of the deaths within 3 months of transplantation. The lungs are the most commonly affected site and opportunistic infections, especially CMV and fungi are relatively frequent.

Longer-term problems

Accelerated atherosclerosis affects up to 40% of patients at 5 years and is a major cause of mortality in heart transplant recipients. Overall, it is the third commonest cause of death after rejection and infection, and the commonest cause after the first 12 months. Histologically, it is characterized by myointimal cell proliferation followed by infiltration with lipid-laden macrophages and subsequent intimal fibrosis (Fig. 33.8). The vascular features are similar to those typical of chronic rejection in renal and liver transplants.

Several features suggest that the aetiology of accelerated atherosclerosis is different from that of primary coronary artery disease. These include the diffuse nature of the condition, the often rapidly progressive course, the lack of development of a collateral circulation, and the fact that it occurs in patients with underlying non-ischaemic cardiomyopathies. Although the cause of this lesion is unknown it is believed to result from endothelial injury, possibly immunologically initiated. However, the number of acute rejection episodes does not correlate with accelerated atherosclerosis, although some data suggest that MHC class I mismatches and alloantibody formation are predictive. Serum triglyceride levels, but not cholesterol, may also

be an independent risk factor. Affected patients may develop heart failure, silent myocardial infarctions and arrhythmias, but do not develop angina as cardiac allografts are denervated. Unfortunately, there is no known treatment for accelerated atherosclerosis. Angioplasty or bypass grafting are not usually options as focal lesions are unusual, and retransplantation offers the only realistic solution. Antiplatelet drugs are often given as they have proved valuable in animal models but their efficacy has not been demonstrated in clinical trials.

Lung and heart–lung transplantation

The introduction of cyclosporin and the development of surgical techniques for combined heart–lung transplantation (HLT) have resulted in a marked improvement in the success of lung transplantation (Fig. 33.9).

The major advantage of HLT over isolated lung transplantation is the conservation of the tracheal blood supply that results in improved healing of the tracheal anastomosis, which can be a major problem in isolated lung transplants. HLT is obligatory in patients with pulmonary hypertension, but often extended to patients with chronic lung disease including cystic fibrosis. The latter patients, whose hearts are normal, may have the 'domino' procedure in which the recipient receives a HLT and the recipient's heart is retransplanted into a second patient who requires a heart only. Single lung transplantation is used for interstitial lung disease, but is unsuitable for patients with cystic fibrosis as infection spreads from diseased to transplanted lung. In these patients HLT or the less frequently performed double lung transplant is indicated.

Surgical aspects and immunosuppression

The donors have to be carefully selected and size-matched with the recipient. Until improved cold preservation techniques are developed, the organs should be transplanted within 4 h of procurement, although the inclusion of prostacyclin in the perfusion protocol, which dilates the pulmonary vasculature, extends the acceptable ischaemic time slightly to 6 h. The details of the operative procedure can be found elsewhere (Baumgartner *et al.* 1990).

Immunosuppressive regimens usually include cyclosporin, azathioprine, and often ATG. Steroids were previously omitted as they were believed to compromise the healing of the tracheal anastamosis. However, more recent studies have not confirmed

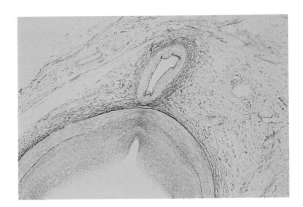

▌**Fig. 33.8** Photomicrography from a heart transplant showing chronic rejection. The vascular changes are similar to those seen in chronic renal rejection. (Kindly supplied by Drs Marlene Rose and Margaret Burke, Harefield Hospital, London.)

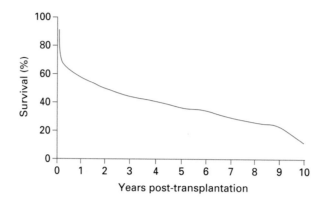

▮ **Fig. 33.9** Heart–lung transplantation survival.

these fears and steroids are now generally included in both induction and maintenance regimens.

Acute rejection

Rejection and infection are the commonest causes of death in lung transplant recipients. The lungs are large and very vascular organs with a well developed intrinsic immune system and large numbers of antigen-presenting cells. It is therefore not surprising that they are highly immunogenic and successful transplantation requires heavy immunosuppression. The immunological mechanisms are presumably similar to those of other organ transplants but less research has been done on lung than renal and heart transplants. Although rejection may be suspected from hypoxia, new or altered infiltrates on the chest X-ray and a fall in forced expiratory volume in 1 s (FEV_1), the transbronchial biopsy (TBB, taken via a fibreoptic bronchoscope) is the most sensitive. Bronchoalveolar lavage may be helpful to diagnose infection, but it cannot reliably distinguish this from rejection.

In keeping with rejection in the heart and kidneys, the histological features are of a mononuclear infiltrate which has a predilection for perivascular areas. Alveolar exudates which are often fibrinous are also seen, progressing, if untreated, to severe alveolar pneumocyte damage, necrosis, and infarction.

Acute lung rejection occurs early and invariably precedes heart rejection in HLT, such that endomyocardial biopsies are not routinely performed. Antirejection treatment given for the lung effectively prevents acute rejection of the heart. Despite the risk of infection and deleterious effects on healing, steroids are the treatment of choice, reserving ATG/OKT3 for severe, recurrent or steroid-resistant episodes.

Long-term outcome

Long-term survival of lung transplant recipients is limited by infection and obliterative bronchiolitis. The latter complication affects up to 50% of recipients and is believed to be the manifestation of chronic rejection of the lung and most commonly develops 8–12 months after transplantation. Physiologically, it is associated with progressive airflow limitation. The histological features are a denuded epithelium with inflammatory cells within the bronchioles followed by replacement with fibrous tissue. There is an associated vasculopathy of the pulmonary vessels with concentric intimal fibrosis, strikingly similar to the vascular changes seen in chronic rejection of hearts and kidneys. The reliability of TBB for making the diagnosis is variable, but open lung biopsy is undertaken only if the clinical features and physiological measurements leave doubt as to the diagnosis. Obliterative bronchiolitis is more likely to occur in patients who have frequent and severe acute rejection episodes, and it has also been linked with pulmonary infection particularly with CMV. As the condition is almost invariably progressive with a grave prognosis and it is believed to have an immunological basis, most patients are treated with steroids and antilymphocyte preparations. Despite reports that such treatment stabilizes or improves clinical and lung function parameters, relapse and death, which may be hastened by infection, is almost inevitable.

Further reading

Almond, P. S., Matas, A., Gillingham, K., Dunn, D. L., Payne, W. D., Gores, P., Gruessner, R., and Najarian, J. S.

(1993). Risk factors for chronic rejection in renal allograft recipients. *Transplantation*, **55**, 752–6.

Baumgartner, W. A., Reitz, B. A., and Achuff, S. C. (ed.) (1990). *Heart and lung transplantation*. W. B. Saunders, Philadelphia, PA.

Burke, J. F. Jr, Pirsch, J. D., Ramos, E. L., *et al.* (1994) Long-term efficacy and safety of cyclosporine in renal-transplant recipients. *New England Journal of Medicine*, **331**, 58.

Cecka, J. M., Cho, Y. W., and Terasaki, P. I. (1992). Analyses of the UNOs scientific renal transplant registry at three years — early events affecting transplant success. *Transplantation*, **53**, 59–64.

Hosenpud, J. D., Novick, R. J., Breen, T. J., and Daily, O. P. (1994). The registry of the international society for heart and lung transplantation: eleventh official report. *Journal of Heart and Lung Transplantation*, **13**, 561–50.

Lansman, S. L., Ergin, M. A., and Griepp, R. B. (1989). History of cardiac transplantation. In *Heart and heart–lung transplantation*, (ed. J. Wallwork), pp. 3–19. W. B. Saunders Co., Philadelphia.

Lechler, R. I. and Batchelor, J. R. (1982). Restoration of immunogenicity to passenger cell-depleted kidney allografts by the addition of donor strain dendritic cells. *Journal of Experimental Medicine*, **155**, 31–41.

Lim, E. C., and Terasaki, P. I. (1991) Early graft function. In: *Clinical transplants* (ed. P. I. Terasaki), p. 401. UCLA Tissue Typing Laboratory, Los Angeles.

Mahoney, R. J., Ault, K. A., Given, S. R., *et al.* (1990). The flow cytometric crossmatch and early renal transplant loss. *Transplantation*, **49**, 527–35.

Morris, P. J. (1994) *Kidney transplantation: principles and practice*. Grone & Stratton, New York, NY.

O'Connell, P. H., Corpier, C. L., Steele, A., and Strom, T. (1994). Monoclonal antibody therapy. In *Immunology of renal transplantation* (ed. A. W. Thomson and G. R. D. Catto), pp. 281–302. Edward Arnold, London.

Opelz, G. For the Collaborative Transplant Study (1992). 10 year report. (1992). *Transplantation Proceedings*, **24**, 2342–55.

Ramos, E. L. and Tisher, C. C. (1994). Transplantation for the nephrologist. Recurrent diseases in the kidney transplant. *American Journal of Kidney Diseases*, **24**, 142–54.

Schreiber, S. L. and Crabtree G. R. (1992). The mechanism of action of cyclosporin A and FK506. *Immunology Today*, **13**, 136–42.

Sheil, A. G. R. (1986). Cancer after transplantation. *World Journal of Surgery*, **10**; 389–96.

Starzl, T. E., Demetris, A. J., Murase, N., Ildstad, Ricordi, C., and Trucco, M. (1992). Cell migration, chimerism, and graft acceptance. *Lancet*, **339**, 1579–82.

Starzl, T. E., Demetris, A. J., Murase, N., Thomson, A. W., Trucco, M. and Ricordi, C. (1993). Donor cell chimerism permitted by immunosuppressive drugs: a new view of organ transplantation. *Immunology Today*, **14**, 326–32.

Takemoto, S., Terasaki, P. I., Cecka, J. M., Cho, Y. W., and Gjertson, D. W. (1992). Survival of nationally shared HLA-matched kidneys transplants from cadaveric donors. *New England Journal of Medicine*, **327**, 834–9.

Takemoto, S., Terasaki, P. I., Gjertson, D. W., and Cecka, J. M. (1994). Equitable allocations of HLA-compatible kidneys for local pools and for minorities. *New England Journal of Medicine*, **331**, 760–4.

Thomson, A. W. and Starzl, T. E. (1993). New immunosuppressive drugs: mechanistic insights and potential therapeutic advances. *Immunology Reviews*, **136**, 71–97.

Tilney, N. L., Whitley, W. D., Diamond, J. R. *et al.* (1991). Chronic rejection — an undefined conundrum. *Transplantation*, **52**, 389–98.

Waer, M. (1994). Total lymphoid irradiation. In *Kidney transplantation: principles and practice*, 4th edn, (ed. P. J. Morris), pp. 244–9. W. B. Saunders, London.

Wecker, H. and Auchincloss, H. (1992). Cellular mechanisms of rejection. *Current Opinion in Immunology*, **4**, 561–6.

34 Allogeneic bone marrow transplantation

F. T. Christiansen and C. S. Witt

Introduction

Bone marrow transplantation (BMT) is being increasingly used in clinical medicine and in many cases is the only treatment offering long-term cure for otherwise fatal diseases. In 1957 Thomas and co-workers from Seattle first showed that large quantities of bone marrow could be obtained and safely infused into humans. In 1965 Mathe *et al.* reported the first sustained allogeneic graft, although the patient subsequently died of chronic graft-versus-host disease (GVHD). The first successful allogeneic BMTs were performed in 1968 for three children with severe congenital immunodeficiencies. All three were alive and well 25 years later. With the recognition and the development of techniques for typing for genes within the major histocompatibility complex (MHC) in humans through the 1960s and 1970s the application of BMT using human leucocyte antigen (HLA) identical sibling donors rapidly expanded. By 1993 some 50 000 allogeneic bone marrow transplants had been performed and at least 6000 are now carried out each year in over 300 centres.

Clinical immunologists may be involved in BMT in a number of ways: in the identification of suitable allogeneic donors; in the development of immunosuppressive and immunomodulating therapies for the prevention and treatment of rejection and GVHD; in the management of the infections associated with the severe immune deficiency present in the post-transplant period and in the evaluation of the restitution of immune function. This chapter will review the procedure of BMT, its indications, results and complications, and the identification of suitable donors. New developments and future challenges are also discussed.

The clinical procedure

The principle

BMT uses normal bone marrow to replace marrow in the patient which has failed either due to the disease process or the potentially corrective chemotherapy and radiotherapy given for various malignancies. Two major sources of marrow are available.

1. *Autologous* marrow in which 'healthy' marrow is collected from the patient during disease remission or in which the diseased cells are removed by *in vitro* manipulation.

2. *Allogeneic* marrow from a healthy individual of the same species but genetically different. Allogeneic transplantation requires appropriate donor/recipient histocompatibility and suitable patient conditioning and immunosuppressive therapy to prevent rejection and GVHD.

The marrow harvest

BMT is a relatively simple procedure. Once a suitable donor is identified, 10–15 ml of bone marrow per kilogram of donor body weight (i.e. 500–1000 ml) is obtained through multiple marrow punctures, usually of the iliac crest, performed under general anaesthetic. The donor usually receives an autotransfusion using blood collected a few weeks previously to replace blood lost during harvest and is usually hospitalized overnight. The procedure is safe with a very low rate of complications. There may be some bruising and a dull ache over the harvest site. The donor marrow is reconstituted within 1–2 weeks and there are no long-term sequelae.

Once harvested, the marrow is filtered to remove bone and tissue fragments, cell numbers determined and then infused via a peripheral intravenous line into the recipient. Infusion is performed as soon as possible after donation, although it is possible for the marrow to be maintained for up to 24 h at 4°C. Alternatively, the marrow can be aseptically frozen for infusion at a later date. This approach allows the shipment of marrow from donors at centres distant from the patient.

Some groups have applied various *in vitro* manipulations of the marrow such as lectin binding or treatment with monoclonal antibodies to remove mature immunocompetent cells, particularly T cells. The value of this procedure remains controversial; while it undoubtedly reduces the severity of GVHD, it does result in an increased likelihood of graft rejection and tumour relapse. Very few studies have shown a long-term benefit of T-cell-depleted marrow in terms of increased patient survival.

Conditioning and supportive care

Prior to transplantation the patient undergoes an intensive conditioning regimen to: (i) prevent allograft rejection by the ablation of the recipient's immune system, particularly when it is not affected by the disease process; (ii) completely destroy malignant cells in the patient thereby reducing the likelihood of disease relapse; and (iii) eradicate normal marrow not affected by the disease process thereby creating space for the donor marrow. The latter is particularly important in those disorders such as thalassaemia major, which are associated with normal or increased marrow cellularity.

Various conditioning regimens have been used depending upon the disease present and the likelihood of graft rejection. In patients with a severe combined immunodeficiency no conditioning is usually required. For diseases such as aplastic anaemia conditioning usually consists of cyclophosphamide 200 mg/kg body weight given intravenously over 4 days followed by transplantation some 24–36 h later. In patients with metabolic disorders, myeloablative therapy such as busulphan (4 mg/kg per day orally for 4 days) is also added. In leukaemia high doses of chemotherapy (usually cyclophosphamide) followed by 10–15.75 Gy total body irradiation (TBI) (given either in a single dose or increasingly in fractionated doses over several days in an attempt to reduce toxicity) are given. New regimens which contain drugs such as busulphan, cytarabine, melphalan, etoposide, and thiopeta as well as new radiation protocols have been used but without convincingly superior results. Several non-radiotherapy regimens have also been successfully used: the most common consisting of high-dose busulphan plus cyclophosphamide with others consisting of cylophosphamide/etoposide and cyclophamide/melphalan.

Following suitable conditioning the bone marrow is given in a dose of at least 2×10^8 cells/kg of body weight. Increasing cell numbers results in a reduced incidence of rejection but may result in an increased severity of GVHD. The donor stem cells lodge within the recipient's bone marrow where subsequent differentiation to the various mature cellular components occurs. Engraftment is considered to have taken place when the peripheral blood neutrophil count reaches greater than 0.5×10^9/l and the platelet count greater than 30×10^9/l. This usually occurs within 14–32 days (median about 25 days).

In this period patients require considerable supportive care. They are particularly vulnerable to infection and haemorrhage and complications from irradiation such as interstitial pneumonitis. The patient is therefore usually kept in isolation often involving laminar flow or positive pressure rooms. Erythrocyte transfusions and platelet transfusions, using wherever possible HLA-matched platelet donors, are given as required. In patients with severe infections or fevers not responding to antibiotics, granulocyte transfusions maybe given. Blood should be irradiated to prevent GVHD. Recently various haemopoietic growth factors, such as granulocyte colony-stimulating factor (G-CSF), have been shown to hasten granulocyte cell count recovery and reduce the risks of infection. When afebrile, tolerating an adequate oral diet, and showing evidence of adequate engraftment the patient is discharged from hospital — usually within 21–35 days.

Haemopoietic recovery

Following engraftment there is a continuing improvement in haematological parameters over time such that granulocyte and platelet counts and haemoglobin level usually return to normal within 40–50 days and 60–90 days, respectively. Cellularity of bone marrow takes 3–6 months to normalize. However, assays of various colony forming units show long periods of depression, suggesting diminished reserve. Neutrophil and phagocytic cell function returns to normal relatively quickly. However, complete immune reconstitution takes considerably longer.

The rate of haemopoietic recovery is dependent on a variety of factors which include prior chemotherapy, radiotherapy, and the conditioning regimen; the dose of bone marrow cells infused; the presence of acute GVHD; the drugs used in GVHD prophylaxis; the presence of infectious complications, particularly cytomegalovirus (CMV) infection; the use of antibiotics such as trimethoprim — sulphamethoxazole and ganciclovir; and donor/recipient compatibility.

Immune reconstitution

In the immediate post-transplant period some immunity may be provided by residual host cells and by the passive transfer of mature immunocompetent T and B cells within the infused marrow. However, these cells are short lived and recipients have a profound immunodeficiency during the first 3 months after BMT. The ultimate restitution depends upon the development of differentiated immunocompetent cells of donor origin.

Total lymphocyte and natural killer (NK) cell counts usually return to normal within 2–3 months. CD4+ cell numbers take 6–12 months to recover and there is generally a reversal of the normal CD4/CD8 ratio due to a 6–12 month delay in CD4+ cell recovery. Functional assays of T-cell function such as responses to mitogens and alloantigens usually recover within 6 months. Delayed-type hypersensitivity responses to intradermal recall antigens are usually slower to recover and may or may not return to normal within 12 months. Recovery is delayed by the presence of GVHD.

While it has generally been considered that B-cell numbers normalize within 2–6 months, more recent studies using CD19 or CD20 B-cell markers have suggested this may take 4–8 months or even longer. Total immunoglobulin levels fall in the immediate post-transplant period, although never to zero, probably due to the presence of recipient plasma cells that survive the conditioning regimen. Immunoglobulin (Ig) M normalizes within 2–6 months, IgG within 3–9 months (IgG1 and IgG3 earlier than IgG2 and IgG4) with IgA being the last to normalize taking 6 months to sometimes much longer than 1 year.

The ability to develop antibody responses is severely impaired post-transplant and recovery is considerably delayed. Responses to recall antigens such as tetanus toxoid and hepatitis B surface antigen cannot usually be elicited until at least 1 year post-transplant, while responses to T-independent antigens such as pneumococcal polysaccharide may take even longer. The ability to make antibody responses should be determined and appropriate reimmunization courses, using killed virus and toxoid vaccines, given once there is evidence of immune reconstitution.

Bone marrow donor selection

Patient

Allogeneic BMT is rarely considered as an option in patients over 50 years of age and in some centres even younger patients might be excluded because of the higher complication rate especially involving GVHD. In general children fare significantly better than adults. Transplantation is best carried out during disease remission where possible; however, in the relapsed acute leukaemias BMT may be the only option. BMTs should only be carried out by specialized centres because of the complexity of the management and need for sophisticated infrastructure. The relative roles of stem cell transplantation, allogeneic transplantation, and chemotherapy in the acute leukaemias is still the subject of debate. None the less allogeneic BMT is acknowledged as a curative treatment for leukaemia and related disorders.

Donor

Donors up to 65–70 years have been successfully used for BMT. Cord blood has also been used because of its relative enrichment for CD34 stem cells. Donors need to be in good general health and free from chronic viral infections.

Histocompatibility requirements

The major genetic determinants which influence allograft outcome are encoded within the MHC, a region of approximately 4000 kb on the short arm of chromosome 6 (Ch6 p21). Nearly 100 genes are encoded within the MHC and these include the class I HLA genes (including HLA-A, HLA-B, and HLA-C) and the class II HLA genes (HLA -DRA, -DRB, -DQA, -DQB, -DPA, and -DPB), which are both known to be directly involved in immune recognition. The other polymorphic genes include various complement components, cytokines, heat shock proteins, determinants of NK allorecognition, and other genes whose function is not understood. The genes within the MHC are closely linked and usually inherited *'en block'* within a family as a haplotype with recombination between genes within the MHC occurring infrequently. Each individual has two MHC haplotypes, one inherited from each parent and therefore any offspring can inherit one of four possible combinations of parental haplotypes. Within a family, siblings who have inherited the same two parental haplotypes are identical for all of the genes within the MHC.

Matching for genes within the MHC is particularly important in BMT. Some of the evidence for this is shown in Table 34.1 in which the influence of MHC compatibility on the risks of graft rejection, acute GVHD, and patient survival are summarized. Decreasing compatibility results in poorer outcome.

There are also a number of other genes outside the MHC, the minor histocompatibility loci, which

∎ **Table 34.1** Major histocompatibility complex (MHC) matching is a major determinant of success of bone major transplantation

MHC compatibility	Risk of graft rejection	Risk of acute graft-versus-host disease	Survival (3 years)
Share two haplotypes (HLA identical sibling)	2%	40%	50%
Share one haplotype plus			
phenotypically identical	7%	40%	50%
1 HLA mismatch	9%	70%	50%
>2 HLA mismatches	21%	80%	15%
Share zero haplotypes (unrelated)			
'Matched'	3%	80%	35%
'Mismatched'	5%	95%	35%

HLA, human leucocyte antigen.

influence BMT outcome and particularly the development of GVHD. Apart from the H–Y locus these have not been identified in humans. While monozygous twins will be completely matched for these genes, HLA identical siblings will on average only be 25% matched. GVHD and graft rejection in HLA identical siblings is at least in part, due to immune responses against these antigens.

Haplotype versus phenotype match

The ideal allogeneic bone marrow donor is a MHC genotypically identical sibling, i.e. one who shares with the patient both parental haplotypes which are identical by direct descent. In this case the donor and recipient are matched at the genomic level for the entire MHC complex, i.e. two-haplotype match. On the other hand unrelated donors are generally only phenotypically matched for the class I and class II alleles using serological and more recently DNA-based techniques. This level of matching does not necessarily mean that the donor and recipient are matched for all of the possible epitopes on the class I and class II molecules nor for the numerous other polymorphic genes within the MHC. Within families it is also possible to identify individuals (e.g. parent and child or some siblings) who share one haplotype which is identical by descent and who are phenotypically matched on the non-shared haplotype.

In two unrelated individuals where both haplotypes are matched at multiple markers identifying genomic 'blocks' these individuals may be equivalent to HLA identical siblings, i.e. identical by descent. It is possible that this approach to MHC matching of donor recipients might reduce the immunological complications of unrelated BMT. The relationships of MHC haplotypes are outlined diagrammatically in Fig. 34.1 and a summary of the degree of matching achieved using different donors is shown in Fig. 34.2.

Donor identification

The outline of a strategy for the identification of a suitable bone marrow donor is given in Fig. 34.3. Initially, HLA typing of the nuclear family is undertaken. Testing across two generations, e.g. parents or offspring enables the assignment of HLA haplotypes within the family and confirmation of allele segregation. While in many cases it is possible to determine haplotype sharing simply from class I typing, in our experience it is preferable to also undertake class II typing at this stage.

If a sibling sharing two HLA-A to HLA-DR/DQ haplotypes identical by descent is identified (see Fig. 34.1(a)) then transplantation can proceed. Generally, repeat testing should be undertaken to ensure that there has been no error in sample labelling, and a cross-match at this stage may also be useful, particularly if the patient has received multiple blood transfusions. A positive cross-match indicates a higher likelihood of graft rejection, although it is not a contraindication to transplantation. If more than two HLA identical siblings are identified some investigators suggest additional testing including HLA -DP typing or CTLp or HTLp assays to assist in deciding between these alternate donors. However, there is no good evidence that such assays provide additional useful information in these circumstances.

Given that there is a 25% chance that any one sibling will share two haplotypes with another, the probability of finding at least one matched sibling is $1-(3/4)^n$ where n is the number of siblings. Because of

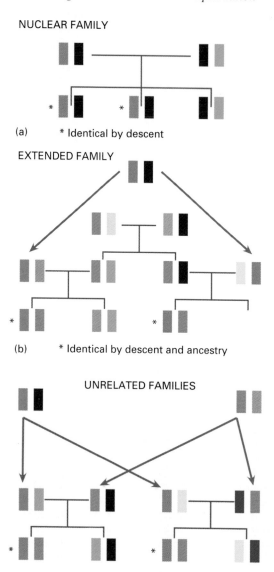

(a)   * Identical by descent

(b)   * Identical by descent and ancestry

(c)   * Identical by ancestry only

■ **Fig. 34.1** Matching donors in nuclear, extended, and unrelated families.

the small size of modern families, on average only 30–35% of patients will have an HLA identical sibling. Alternative donors are required for the other 65–70% of patients.

For those patients without a sibling-matched donor, a donor within the extended family should be sought in the first instance. This is particularly feasible if there is a history of consanguinity in the family, there is homozygosity or sharing of antigens between the

parents, or if the patient has one or two common haplotypes. By this approach it may be possible to identify a donor who shares with the patient one haplotype identical by descent and a second haplotype which is at least phenotypically identical at all MHC loci and possibly identical by more remote descent (see Fig. 34.1b). This approach is successful in 5–10% of cases. Many centres will accept a single HLA mismatch in a related donor and there are data indicating that these transplants will fare at least as well as matched-unrelated donor (MUD) transplants, and are perhaps indistinguishable from phenotypically identical family donors.

If the patient has no family available, or no suitable donor can be identified within the family, then the only alternative is an unrelated donor. The indications for transplantation in these circumstances should be reviewed and if BMT is still considered appropriate then a search of the various unrelated donor registries undertaken. Through electronic communication these searches can be undertaken very quickly. Panels have now been established in North America, Europe, Asia, and Australasia and in excess of 3 million potential donors have been registered. Generally, the panels consist of volunteers who have been serologically HLA-A and HLA-B typed and, in an increasing proportion of cases, DR typed by serology or DNA-based methods. If an HLA, -B, -DR matched donor is identified then further detailed typing should be undertaken. Generally, the best available matched donor should be used. Ideally, the donor should be matched at HLA-A and HLA-B serologically and at the class II DRB loci using DNA-based techniques. However, there is now some evidence that successful transplantation can be achieved using unrelated donors who are mismatched at one of these loci particularly if the mismatch occurs within a broad or cross-reactive antigen group. More data are required to define the minimal matching requirements and determine which assays best define graft outcome. However, the first aim should be to identify unrelated donors who are as near possible the equivalent of HLA identical siblings.

Laboratory tests

Details of some of these tests are described in Chapter 32 on HLA compatibility. The role of these assays in donor/recipient matching will be briefly reviewed.

Class I and class II allele typing

Typing for the class I antigens by serological techniques remains the most widely applied and useful assay. The development of DNA based techniques has proved quite difficult, primarily due to the large

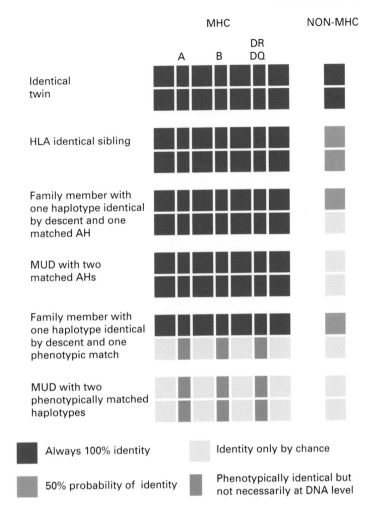

∎ **Fig. 34.2** The degree of major histocompatibility complex (MHC) and non-MHC matching achieved using different donors.
MUD; Marrow unrelated donor.
AH; Ancestral haplotype.
HLA, human leucocyte antigen.

number of class I genes within the MHC complex. However, these problems are now being overcome and class I DNA techniques are likely to be more widely applied in the future. The biochemical analysis of class I alleles by isoelectrofocusing has allowed the identification of additional heterogeneity which, at least on some occasions, has been shown to be relevant in BMT. However, this technique does not lend itself to routine application and in most cases provides little additional information.

Class II typing has previously been performed by serology but now increasingly various DNA-based techniques are being used. Details of these methods are described elsewhere. These methods utilize smaller quantities of blood and allow the more complete definition of the alleles at the DRB1, DRB3, DRB4, DRB5, DQA1, DQB1, and DPA1 and DPB1 loci. HLA-DP typing using DNA-based methods can now be undertaken but, matching for DP has not been shown to influence outcome.

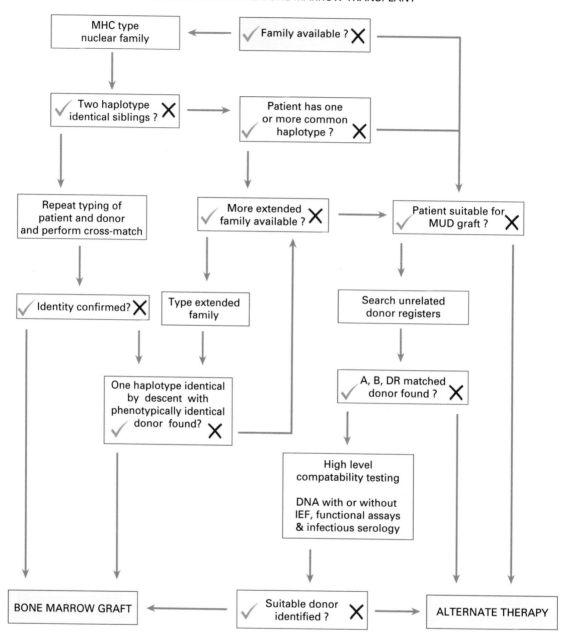

Fig. 34.3 An approach to the identification of a bone marrow donor.
MUD; Marrow unrelated donor.
IEF;
MHC; major histocompatibility complex.

Block matching and other DNA matching techniques

Amplification of anonymous duplicated polymorphic genomic sequences within the MHC can distinguish between allelic blocks based around HLA-B (beta block) and around HLA-DR, -DQ (delta block). The electrophoretic profiles obtained from each individual acts as a surrogate marker of the genomic sequence within these MHC blocks. Block matching of unrelated donor-recipients for BMT is still under evaluation.

Several other methods to directly compare the DNA sequence of the donor and recipient have been developed. These include heteroduplex formation and temperature gradient gel electrophoresis. However, their efficacy in BMT remains to be determined. It is likely that direct automated sequencing of HLA class I and II alleles will become the standard method of identifying HLA alleles. This method is not widely used at present.

Cellular assays

Mixed lymphocyte reaction (MLR)

For many years this assay was considered essential prior to transplantation. However, the assay is difficult to standardize and in spite of its widespread application has not been shown to provide any useful information additional to that provided by HLA typing. MLC responses are low between HLA identical siblings and do not predict GVHD. In unrelated BMT this assay has been used to confirm class II identity but does not predict outcome. With the availability of DNA-based class II typing this assay is unnecessary.

Cell-mediated lympholysis

The ability of T cells of the recipient to recognize and lyse allogeneic target cells of the donor has been applied by several groups in the assessment of donor/recipient pairs both prior to and following transplantation. The test can detect minor histocompatability antigen mismatches in addition to MHC mismatches but no clear correlation with clinical outcome has been demonstrated.

T-cell precursor frequency

Assays to measure the frequency of T-helper (HTLp) and T-cytotoxic cell (CTLp) precursors recognizing alloantigens on a target cell have been recently applied to BMT. While these assays are time-consuming and difficult to standardize, recent studies have suggested that high T-helper cell precursor frequencies in the donor against the recipient's cells are predictive of the development of severe acute GVHD, although these findings have not been confirmed by all groups.

Further studies are required to determine their part in donor selection.

Indications and results of bone marrow transplantation

Indications

The numbers of diseases for which BMT has been successfully applied is continually expanding. While extensive prospective controlled trials comparing BMT with other therapeutic modalities are not available for all diseases, a consensus is now emerging on those diseases for which BMT is the treatment of choice. These are listed in Table 34.2 together with some specific indications.

Factors influencing outcome

There are many factors known to influence the outcome of BMT. The effects of some of these are complex and involve multiple interactions. Factors which have shown to be associated with poor patient survival include increasing patient age, relapse at the time of transplantation and acute leukaemia and advanced disease. Severe acute GVHD is also associated with poorer outcome.

Outcome of bone marrow transplantation in specific diseases

Acute leukaemia

The prospects of achieving long-term cure using allogeneic BMT in acute leukaemia largely depends upon the likelihood of disease relapse in the post-transplant period. This is influenced by the effectiveness of the antileukaemia therapy, the presence of graft-versus-leukaemia response (see below) and particularly the disease status at the time of transplantation. Generally, the best results are obtained when transplantation is performed during the first complete remission (CR) with poorer outcome in second and subsequent CRs and the worst results during disease relapse. The results from the International Bone Marrow Transplant Registry (IBMTR) in acute lymphoblastic leukaemia (ALL) and acute myelogenous leukaemia (AML) stratified according to the disease status at the time of transplantation are shown in Figs. 34.4a and b, respectively. The outcomes for both are similar with 5 year leukaemia-free survival (LFS) probabilities of approximately 50 and 20% when the transplant is performed

■ **Table 34.2** Diseases in which the benefit of allogeneic bone marrow transplantation is established

Disease	Indications
Haematological malignancies	
Acute lymphocytic leukaemia	Failed induction
	First remission with high-risk criteria
	After first relapse — especially if occurred during or within 6 months of stopping therapy
	Extramedullary leukaemia except possibly CNS
Acute myeloid leukaemia	Primary induction failure
	Especially first remission or later stages
Chronic myeloid leukaemia	Any stage specially chronic phase
Non-Hodgkins' lymphoma	Relapse with high-grade disease at or beyond second remission — in absence of CNS disease. Possibly other poor prognosis groups
Multiple myeloma	<60 years old and chemotherapy responsive
Myelodysplasia	<40 years old — before disease progression or complications. Older — life-threatening cytopenias or blast transformation.
Disorders of haematopoiesis	
Severe aplastic anaemia	Especially prior to multiple transfusions
Fanconi's anaemia	Early in disease if symptomatic
β-thalassemia major	Effective but timing uncertain — before hepatomegally and portal fibrosis
Sickle cell anaemia	Effective-timing uncertain.
Immunodeficiencies	
Severe combined immunodeficiency	Treatment of choice — before complications
Wiscott–Aldrich syndrome	Treatment of choice — before complications
Genetic disorders	
Mucopolysacchidosises Hurler's disease, multifocal leucodystrophy and Maroteaus - Lamy syndrome	Before onset of neurological complications
Adrenoleucodystrophy syndrome	With early radiological signs of involvement

during CR and in relapse, respectively. The results are better in children with a probability of LFS at 5 years of approximately 60% when transplanted in first CR.

A long-term cure of AML is rarely achieved using standard chemotherapy. For this reason, given the availability of an HLA identical sibling, BMT is the treatment of choice and should be undertaken during first CR. With lesser matched donors the situation is less clear and transplantation is usually only undertaken in poor risk patients or in patients in relapse. Alternatively, an autologous transplant during second remission using marrow collected during first CR may be considered, although there are no good data on the relative merits of autologous versus unrelated allogeneic transplantation.

In children with ALL the best time to perform marrow transplants is still not completely determined.

Cure rates with chemotherapy of between 80 and 90% can be achieved for children in low and intermediate risk groups and may even be as high as 70% in the high-risk groups. Therefore, transplantation in first CR is not usually undertaken except in children who are at particularly high risk including those less than 6 months of age, those with t(9;22) chromosomal translocation, and those with hybrid (lymphoid/myeloid) leukaemias. A BMT is indicated in those who have failed to respond to the first cycle of chemotherapy or in those with extramedullary leukaemia or if relapse occurred during therapy or within 6 months of ceasing therapy. Data from non-randomized studies in children and adolescents have shown LFS of 30% in those who received allogeneic marrow transplants during second or later remissions when compared with those given chemotherapy with a LFS of 10%.

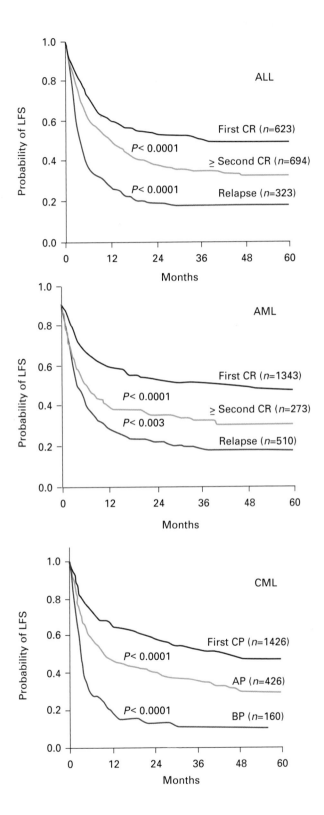

Fig. 34.4 The outcome as leukaemia-free survival (LFS) of allogeneic bone marrow transplantations from human leucocyte antigen identical siblings.

ALL, Acute lymphoblastic leukaemia; AML, Acute myeloblastic leukaemia; CML, Chronic myeloid leukaemia; CR, Complete remission; CP, chronic phase; AP, acute phase; BP, blast phase.

Chronic myeloid leukaemia (CML)

The results of BMT using HLA identical siblings for CML, stratified according to disease status, are shown in Fig. 34.4c, with LFS probabilities of 45% in chronic phase, 30% in accelerated phase, and 6% in blast phase. By treating younger patients in earlier stages of their disease, particularly within the first year of diagnosis, long-term LFS of approximately 80% has been achieved. Therefore BMT is widely accepted as the treatment of choice for CML. The critical issues remain the availability of a suitable donor and the timing of the transplant. Given the availability of a matched family donor, transplantation should be undertaken immediately following the diagnosis especially in patients less than 60 years of age and otherwise in good health. With an unrelated donor the situation is less clear, although with the improving results, transplantation is increasingly being undertaken earlier in the chronic phase, especially in younger patients (less than 45–50 years of age).

Other haematological malignancies

BMT has been used successfully in the treatment of non-Hodgkin's lymphoma in patients who have relapsed following initial chemotherapy. Cure is more likely when transplantation is undertaken early in the course of the disease, while the tumour is still sensitive to chemotherapy. Long-term disease-free survival of between 20 and 40% can also be achieved in patients who do not have an initial CR but lack other adverse prognostic indicators. The source of marrow (autologous or allogeneic) does not influence survival, although autologous transplants are most commonly performed. Current interest is focused on the use of peripheral blood stem cells or the purging of autologous marrow to remove lymphoma cells, but there is no clear consensus on the best approach.

Multiple myeloma is a disease which affects primarily the elderly and has therefore only recently been considered for BMT. In a recent study of 90 patients conducted by the European Group for Bone Marrow Transplantation an actuarial survival of 40% at 76 months was achieved. Survival was longer in those with stage 1 disease at diagnosis and in those who were responsive to treatment prior to transplantation. Further studies are required to determine the long-term results of BMT and its ultimate role in this disease.

The myelodysplastic syndrome is a group of haemopoietic disorders with a variable but inevitably fatal prognosis. Allogeneic BMT offers a potentially curative treatment. Recently, a disease-free survival at 4 years of 41% has been achieved, with a survival of 61% of among patients less than 40 years of age without excess blast cells. Allogeneic BMT can cure some patients with myelodysplasia and it should be considered, in younger patients, prior to disease progression or the development of life-threatening cytopenias.

Severe aplastic anaemia

BMT has now been shown to be a very effective therapy for severe aplastic anaemia. A major retrospective analysis by the European Group for Bone Marrow Transplantation has shown transplantation results in superior survival probability than treatment with antilymphocyte globulin, with an actuarial survival at 12 years of 56% for a group of patients transplanted with an HLA identical sibling between 1976 and 1990. An analysis from the IBMTR of 737 recipients (1985–91) has shown a 5 year probability of survival of 64%. Recently, the Seattle group have reported 90% survival for patients who have received a pregraft conditioning regimen of cyclophosphamide plus antithymocyte globulin (ATG) together with postgraft methotrexate and cyclosporin (CyA) GVHD prophylaxis, with a total incidence of GVHD of no more than 15% and no associated deaths. In the absence of an HLA identical sibling, the role of BMT is less clear. Generally, a trial of immunosuppressive therapy is given particularly in the older patients with the use of unrelated donors reserved for those in whom this therapy fails.

Factors which have been shown to result in a less favourable outcome include the absence of CyA treatment, the presence of GVHD, the presence of infection prior to transplantation, the use of a parous or transfused female donor, a history of multiple transfusions prior to transplantation, and a period of greater than 1 month between diagnosis and the time of transplantation. A number of factors have been shown to contribute to the likelihood of graft rejection including prior blood and platelet transfusions, a low number of donor cells infused, and the use of donor peripheral blood buffy coat cells at the time of transplantation. The incidence and severity of acute GVHD has been significantly reduced by the use of a short course of methotrexate and CyA in the post-transplant period. In contrast, the incidence of chronic GVHD has remained relatively unchanged over the years and remains a significant cause of morbidity.

Haemoglobinopathies

BMT is being successfully applied in the treatment of homozygous β thalassaemia trait. More than 450 transplants in this condition by one Italian group have shown that it offers at least an 80–90% chance of success if performed with an HLA identical sibling early in life and before complications of the disease occur. They have identified three risk factors which correlate with poor outcome: degree of portal fibrosis; liver size; and inadequate previous chelation therapy. Patients who had none of these three risk factors had a survival of 98% and an event-free survival of 94% compared with a survival of 91% and event-free survival of 60% for those with all three adverse prognostic factors. Those who survive do particularly well with very infrequent chronic GVHD. These results suggest that when an HLA identical sibling donor is available BMT should be considered.

BMT has also been shown to treat sickle cell anaemia successfully. Generally, the results have been good with negligible mortality and surprisingly little acute or chronic GVHD. Graft failure is emerging as the major complication but this rarely results in patient mortality. The indications for transplantation are unclear but may include frequent crises, cerebrovascular disease, osteonecrosis, and acute chest syndrome. However, more information about the natural history of the disease and ability to predict those with a more severe course are required.

Genetic diseases

Severe combined immunodeficiency (SCID) is a clinical syndrome caused by a series of primary defects, including adenosine deaminase (ADA) deficiency, which result in an absence of antigen-specific T-and B-cell immunity. BMT is the treatment of choice and results in permanent T-lymphocyte and, in most cases, B-lymphocyte antigen-specific immunity. Transplantation can be undertaken without the need for pre-transplant conditioning and GVHD is uncommon. Generally, 70% success has been achieved and failure is often related to pre-existing infections. If patients are transplanted without pre-existing infections success approaching 90% can be achieved. For those patients without an HLA identical sibling, transplantation of T-cell-depleted marrow from a parent has resulted in successful immunological reconstitution in 50–70% of patients. Unrelated donors have also been used with similar success.

BMT has been successfully applied in the treatment of other primary immunodeficiencies. In a recent review of the European experience of transplants performed since 1985, 1 year survivals of >80% using an HLA identical sibling donor and 50% using other donors have been obtained. In Wiscott–Aldrich syndrome more than 90% of patients of transplanted with an HLA identical sibling have complete remission of their disease. However, GVHD has been a particular problem when unrelated donors are used and such donors probably should only be used for patients with

clinically significant thrombocytopenia and/or for immunodeficiency.

BMT has also been applied to the treatment of a number of inborn errors of metabolism. Gaucher's disease was the first to be successfully treated with BMT, but the efficacy of BMT versus alternative replacement therapy is unknown. The most experience has been in the mucopolysaccharidosis Hurler's syndrome. Patients transplanted early in their disease (less than 18 months of age) seem to have an improvement in their intellectual function but it is unclear whether this improved function will be maintained in later life. Other diseases which have been treated with BMT include osteopetrosis, Maroteaux–Lamy syndrome, adrenoleucodystophy and metachromatic leucodystrophy, and Lesch–Nyhan syndrome but there is insufficient experience for the role of BMT to be defined. In all metabolic diseases it is likely that the best results will be obtained when transplantation is undertaken early in the disease.

Complications of bone marrow transplantation

The final outcome of BMT is influenced by multiple interrelated factors which act at different stages in the post-transplant period. The four most important factors are:

(1) graft rejection;

(2) graft versus host disease;

(3) immunodeficiency;

(4) disease relapse.

These cause both mortality and morbidity and are the major limitations to the application of BMT.

Graft failure and graft rejection

Successful bone marrow engraftment has occurred when the bone marrow of the host has been replaced with marrow cells of donor origin. Sometimes poor graft function may be due to suppression of donor marrow function, due, for example, to drug toxicity (e.g. methotrexate) or infections (e.g. CMV) and function returns once these factors are removed. More importantly, however, failure may be due to rejection of the allogeneic marrow by residual immunocompetent host cells. Attempts at a second graft are usually unsuccessful.

Successful engraftment depends upon both recipient and donor factors. Adequate conditioning is required for ablation of the recipient's haemopoietic stem cells to prevent the subsequent regeneration of host marrow-derived blood cells which mediate graft rejection. This is particularly important in aplastic anaemia where the host's immune system is relatively intact.

Several cell types are thought to mediate graft rejection. There is good evidence CD8+ positive cells can mediate allograft rejection probably through cytotoxicity directed against MHC class I disparity or through minor antigens presented by class I molecules. In mice treatment with CD8+-specific antibodies can prevent graft rejection and CD8+ positive cytotoxic and suppressor cells can be isolated from the blood of humans with graft failure. While CD4+ positive cells may also be involved in experimental models, there is less direct evidence for a role in humans.

NK cells have been known to be capable of mediating bone marrow allograft rejection in mice since the early 1970s. Lethally irradiated F_1 hybrid mice could reject parental bone marrow, a phenomenon called 'hybrid resistance', which was at variance with the laws of transplantation. These NK cells recognize a set of functionally recessively inherited 'haemopoietic histocompatibility' (Hh) target antigens expressed on donor haemopoietic cells and encoded within the MHC. Strains homozygous for these alleles express determinants which are lacking in heterozygous F_1 hybrids. The nature of these antigens and the mechanism by which NK cells mediate allorecognition remains to be determined, although recently it has been suggested that NK cells are triggered to kill by the absence of a self-determinant on their target rather than the presence of a specific foreign antigen.

There is now good evidence that NK allorecognition can occur in humans and that the genes encoding this recognition are within the human MHC between HLA-A and complement factor Bf. Particular NK allodeterminants are associated with particular ancestral haplotypes and will be matched in HLA identical sibling transplants. However, these NK allodeterminants may be mismatched in unrelated transplant situations in which graft rejection occurs. Direct evidence that NK cells can mediate allograft rejection in humans has not yet been provided, possibly due to the extensive conditioning precluding NK activity, or, the presence of alloreactive T cells, which may also have a major role in graft rejection.

Among the donor factors which influence engraftment, stem cell numbers are important particularly in sensitized recipients. Mature donor lymphoid cells can facilitate engraftment, at least in part through the presence of alloreactive cells directed against the residual immunocompetent cells in the host, which might otherwise mediate graft rejection. However, there is

experimental evidence that donor cells which do not recognize host alloantigens may also facilitate engraftment through mechanisms which are not understood. Enrichment of marrow for such cells may improve engraftment without the concomitant risk of GVHD.

Graft rejection is uncommon in leukaemia patients but has been a problem in patients with aplastic anaemia with failure rates as high as 30–60%. This has been overcome by intensive conditioning including antithymocyte globulin or the use of donor peripheral blood buffy coat cells. Sensitization by prior transfusion is also associated with an increased risk of graft rejection, and this effect is now managed by avoiding transfusion whenever possible, the use of neutrophil-depleted blood, and earlier transplantation. Rejection frequency is also dependent on the HLA disparity between donor and recipient (see Table 34.1).

Graft-versus-host disease

Definition and pathogenesis

GVHD is classified as acute, occurring within 100 days of transplantation, and chronic disease. It is the major cause of morbidity and mortality following BMT occurring in 30–80% of allogeneic grafts between HLA identical siblings resulting in a mortality as high as 50%. It represents a reaction of immunocompetent cells in the donor against target cells of the recipient.

In 1966 Billingham established three prerequisites for the development of GVHD: (i) the presence of immunocompetent cells in the graft; (ii) histocompatibility differences between the recipient and donor; and (iii) an inability of the recipient to reject the immunocompetent donor cells.

GVHD is mediated by T cells present in the donor marrow. In animals treatment with heterologous antithymocyte globulin or specific T-cell antibodies abrogates GVHD, while in humans removal of T cells from the donor marrow results in a marked reduction in GVHD. However, there is still no consensus on the relative contribution of T-cell subsets. Depending upon the model, both CD4+ and/or CD8+ cells have been shown to initiate GVHD. GVHD can occur after the transfer of lymphoid cells from athymic mice which lack mature T cells. Other cell populations have been implicated including NK cells and large granular lymphocytes. The precise effector mechanism and target molecule of the reaction are still unclear. Cytokines are also involved. These may be of both host and donor origin and act either directly or to amplify the inflammatory response with the recruitment and activation of effector cells. Some evidence for the importance of the cytokine cascade has been provided by showing a relationship between cytokines in the circulation and the presence of GVHD and the ability of antagonists to either the cytokine or its receptor to modify GVHD. Thus tumour necrosis factor (TNF) levels have been associated with GVHD, while TNF antibodies and interleukin (IL) receptor antagonists can modify GVHD. Such findings have important implications for future therapy of GVHD.

Clinical features of acute graft-versus-host disease

The commonest manifestation of acute GVHD is a maculopapular rash which usually develops between days 7 and 50 (median day 20). The palms, soles, and ears are frequently involved early but the rash may spread to involve the trunk, face, and extremities. The liver may also be involved, first reflected in abnormal liver function tests. Because of the many potential causes of liver dysfunction following BMT, the diagnosis of hepatic GVHD usually requires a biopsy which demonstrates a lymphoid infiltrate with bile duct atypia and degeneration. The gut is also a commonly involved organ resulting in diarrhoea which is often severe, watery, and sometimes bloody. Biopsy of the gut shows crypt cell necrosis and subsequently diffuse loss of crypts and in severe GVHD total loss of the gut epithelium. Gut involvement is the most serious complication of GVHD and the most difficult to treat. Acute GVHD is usually graded I–IV for each of the three major organs involved. Multiorgan involvement is particularly serious especially with stage III or IV involvement of the liver and gut.

Incidence and predictors of graft-versus-host disease

Even in most recent studies it is likely that 30–50% of patients receiving an HLA identical sibling transplant will develop at least some degree of GVHD. The major predictor GVHD is MHC disparity between the donor and recipient (see Table 34.1). Sex disparity between donor and recipient is important with male recipients of female donors having a higher risk especially if the female donor has been previously pregnant or transfused. Increasing patient age is associated with increased frequency and severity of acute GVHD, an effect which may in part reflect reduced tolerance of prophylactic therapy. Infection may also play a part in GVHD. In animal models, decontamination of the gut and the use of a germ-free free environment have been shown to reduce the incidence and severity of GVHD while one study in patients with aplastic anaemia has shown a benefit of a germ-free environment. HLA-B7, HLA-DR 2, and HLA-B12 may be associated with a

reduced and increased incidence of GVHD, respectively, but confirmatory studies are required. Recently, a number of minor antigens have been identified as influences in GVHD between HLA identical donor-recipient transplant pairs. These minor antigens represent peptides derived from endogenous polymorphic self-antigens. Genetic typing for these antigens may be a possibility in the near future.

Prevention and treatment of acute graft-versus-host disease

The mainstay of prevention of GVHD involves the use of immunosuppressive drugs with methotrexate (MTX) and CyA the two most commonly used. Several randomized trials have shown that they are comparable. Studies from Seattle have shown that combined therapy with MTX and CyA is more effective than monotherapy in preventing GVHD, a finding also shown in a study from the IBMTR of 2286 recipients of HLA identical sibling transplants with early leukaemia. The probability of grade II–IV acute GVHD was 29% in the MTX plus CyA group compared with 50 and 43% in the MTX and CyA groups, respectively, while leukaemia-free survival was higher in the combined therapy group. Other prophylactic regimens have included CyA and prednisolone, CyA, and cyclophosphamide or triple therapy including MTX, CyA, and various regimens of prednisolone, but none have shown a clear advantage over combined CyA and MTX therapy. A number of new therapeutic approaches are currently been evaluated in experimental models or pilot clinical studies. These include new immunosuppressive agents such as rapamycin, FK506, deoxyspergualin, the use of monoclonal antibodies against IL-2 receptor (CD25), or campath1-G, and the use of pentoxitylline, an agent shown to inhibit the production of TNF by monocytes and macrophages.

The second common approach to prevent GVHD is T-cell depletion of the donor marrow. However, while this is a most effective form of prophylaxis, it also results in a high rate of non-engraftment and relapse with no subsequent improvement in survival. Therefore the use of more intensive conditioning regimens or alternatively more selective methods of T-cell depletion are currently being evaluated. Among the latter are the use of partial T-cell depletion by counter flow elutriation, selective T-cell depletion using anti-CD8, anti-CD6, or anti-CD25 antibodies or T-cell depletion *in vivo* using a monoclonal antibody to CD5 linked to the ricin-A chain toxin.

Therapy for acute GVHD remains unsatisfactory. Steroids have been the mainstay of therapy. Trials comparing ATG plus steroids versus steroids alone have been disappointing as have various regimens of

ATG, CyA, and steroids. Several monoclonal antibodies specific to various lymphocyte effecter cell populations such as anti-CD2, anti-CD25, anti-CD5, or campath I-G, or directed against specific cytokines (e.g. TNFα), or cytokine receptors (e.g. IL-2 receptor) are under evaluation. However, it is not possible at this stage to know whether any of these approaches will result in improved outcome.

Chronic graft-versus-host disease

Chronic GVHD occurs after the first 100 days following BMT and is the commonest late complication occurring in 20–80% of patients. It is a multisystem disease with manifestations ranging from mild and transient to severe, permanent, and debilitating. Patients may die from the disease or its complications. The clinical manifestations include scleroderma-like skin changes, loss of sweat glands and areas of hyper- and hypopigmentation, oral ulcers, alopecia, keratoconjunctivitis and sicca syndrome, polyserositis, photosensitivity, oesophageal and vaginal strictures, chronic liver disease, intestinal involvement, and generalized wasting. Many of the features are those seen in progressive systemic sclerosis, lichen planus, systemic lupus erythematosus, and primary biiary cirrhosis. Biopsy of the skin shows either lichen planus-like skin changes early or sclerotic changes late in the disease. A variety of autoantibodies have been detected, and the patients reveal a variable immunodeficiency.

Most risk factors for acute GVHD also predict chronic GVHD and there is substantial concordance between the two diseases. A recent multivariate analysis identified preceding acute GVHD as the predominant risk factor for chronic GVHD. Whether acute and chronic GVHD are different forms of the one disorder or distinct cannot be determined at present. Several factors have been shown to predict poor outcome with chronic GVHD. These include the disease evolving from acute GVHD, hepatic disease, and thrombocytopenia. The incidence of chronic GVHD may be reduced by the use of an extended course of CyA prophylaxis.

Little information is available on the natural course and progression of chronic GVHD as immunosuppressive therapy was instituted empirically shortly after its description. Therapy has been based on the use of steroids. Among patients with standard risk (as defined by an absence of thrombocytopenia) prednisolone alone has been shown to be as effective as prednisolone plus azathioprine with less toxicity and lower non-relapse mortality. More recently, the addition of CyA to prednisolone has been shown to result in a complete remission in more patients but post-treatment mortality resulted in similar patient survival. Among those with high risk, the addition of CyA to prednisolone has resulted in improved survival, and there are recent data that CyA alone may be as effective as combined therapy.

Other approaches reported to be useful in chronic GVHD include thalidomide, oral immunoglobulin, FK506, antibodies to IL-2 receptor, and PUVA therapy. However, these studies have been uncontrolled and involve small numbers of patients with advanced disease so the role of these agents has not been adequately evaluated.

Leukaemia relapse and graft-versus-leukaemia reaction

Recurrent malignancy is a major cause of failure of BMT. Almost always it is the original malignant cell population which reappears suggesting failure of the conditioning regimens to eliminate all the leukaemic cells. Most conditioning regimens utilize drugs with non-specific activity against metabolically active cells with consequent extensive non-haempoietic toxicity. Therefore alternative approaches involving the use of specific tumoricidal agents such as tumour-specific antibodies linked to toxins such as the ricin-A chain, or short-lived radioactive isotopes have been developed. These approaches have been tested in mice and dogs with some success but experience in humans remains limited.

There are now considerable clinical and experimental data suggesting that allogeneic BMT is associated with a clinically significant immunological antitumour effect — graft-versus-leukaemia response (GVLR) — which results in a reduction in leukaemia relapse. Such evidence includes:

(1) the association of acute and particularly chronic GVHD with a reduced incidence of disease relapse;

(2) higher relapse rates following syngeneic and autologous transplants compared with HLA matched allogeneic transplants;

(3) higher relapse rates following T-cell-depleted grafts and following intensive post-transplant immunosuppression; and

(4) the effective use of infusion of donor lymphocytes to induce haemotological and cytogenetic remission of relapse of CML following transplantation.

The mechanism of GVLR is not fully understood. The target molecules may be leukaemia-associated antigens or minor histocompatibility antigens present on malignant cells. While the alloreactive T cells that initiate GVHD may be involved, there is increasing evidence that GVLR can be separated from GVHD and that the effector cells mediating these two reactions may be different. For example, depletion of CD8+ positive cells has been shown to abolish severe chronic GVHD in CML without increasing the risk of leukaemia relapse. Approaches which could stimulate GVLR without affecting GVHD would likely be potentially beneficial but little progress has been achieved to date. Currently, there is a counterbalance between the harmful effects of GVHD and the beneficial effects of GVLR and regimens aimed at reducing GVHD will also need to provide additional antitumour therapy.

Opportunistic infections

Just prior to and following BMT the patient has a profound immune deficiency resulting in predisposition to a variety of infections. The nature of the defect varies depending upon the time following transplant and results in a characteristic pattern of infections.

The first phase of aplasia, characterized by the presence of severe neutropenia, lasts until marrow recovery occurs. These patients are at risk of infection primarily with bacteria or fungi particularly *Candida* and somewhat later *Aspergillus*. Bacterial infections include Gram-negative enteric flora, Gram-positive cocci, and Gram-positive skin commensals and other more unusual bacterial isolates. The common occurrence of Gram-positive organisms may relate to the use of central venous lines and the presence of mucositis. Gram-negative sepsis probably arises from the gut. Viral infections other than herpes simplex (HSV) are uncommon. HSV infection after transplantation is virtually always a reactivation of prior infection and occurs within the mouth or genitals. Its occurrence has been dramatically reduced by the regular use of prophylactic acyclovir.

With haematological recovery the patient undergoes a phase lasting up to 4–6 months of gradual immune reconstitution but profound defects, particularly of cellular function, remain. The presence of acute GVHD and its therapy also profoundly influence immune function. Bacterial infections are less common though they still occur. *Aspergillus* and other filamentous fungal elements are a particular problem and cause of mortality during this phase. *Pneumocystis carinii* infection, previously a common cause of pneumonitis, is now uncommon with the regular use of trimethoprim/sulphamethoxazole prophylaxis.

The major infectious problem during this phase is CMV infection usually occurring 40–50 days after transplantation. Infection is usually the result of reacti-

vation of endogenous virus occurring in up to 80% of seropositive individuals, but can also occur in seronegative individuals who receive unscreened CMV positive blood. CMV infection may result in pneumonia, gastroenteritis, hepatitis, encephalitis and, rarely, retinitis. Risk factors for CMV pneumonia include recipient seropositivity, the use of TBI, increasing age of the recipient, and the development of acute GVHD. Successful treatment of CMV infections has been achieved with ganciclovir and foscarnet, and the use of ganciclovir plus high-dose CMV immunoglobulin has been shown to be effective in some cases of CMV pneumonitis.

Primary CMV infection is prevented by the use of seronegative blood and blood products. High-dose acyclovir given immediately after transplantation and for the first 100 days has been shown to reduce the incidence of CMV infection significantly. Ganciclovir is a bone marrow suppressant and is therefore not used until haematological recovery occurs but has also been shown to be an effective prophylaxis. Regular screening for CMV using buffy coat and urine cultures and prompt early treatment with ganciclovir has been recommended.

The last phase of immune recovery begins about 5–6 months post-transplant and lasts until complete restoration of the immune system occurs, usually within 1–2 years. In the absence of GVHD life-threatening infections are uncommon. These patients are similar to asplenic individuals in their predisposition to infection with encapsulated organisms such as *Streptococcus pneumoniae*, *Neisseria meningitides*, *Haemophilus influenzae*, and *Klebsiella pneumoniae*. This has led to the long-term usage of penicillin or trimethoprim/sulphamethoxazole. The most common viral infection in this period is varicella/zoster occurring in up to 40–50% of cases. High-dose acyclovir has proven effective therapy, although its role in prophylaxis is less well established.

Future challenges

BMT has developed over the past 20 years from an experimental treatment only used in patients with end-stage disease to the treatment of choice for a large number of diseases, and offers the chance of a long-term cure for otherwise fatal diseases. A number of challenges, however, remain and a number of new innovations are being assessed.

The ideal allogeneic bone marrow donor remains an HLA identical sibling. However, in only about one-third of patients is such a donor available and alternative donors are required. To provide suitable unrelated donors large panels of HLA-typed volunteers have been established in many Western countries, with over 3 million donors recruited. Transplantation using unrelated donors is being increasingly utilized and recent results from the Seattle group suggest survival similar to that obtained between identical siblings can be achieved. However, only a little over a half of patients will find a HLA-A, -B, -DRB1 matched donor on the initial search and these proportions are unlikely to rise dramatically even if the panels are considerably enlarged.

Current matching strategies are inadequate. There are long delays in providing a suitable donor and unrelated transplantation is still associated with increased morbidity. What are the critical matching requirements and can some mismatches be accepted without compromising outcome? Recent studies from the Seattle group suggest that transplants using an unrelated donor with a minor mismatch at one HLA locus can result in good long-term outcome, although there is somewhat more GVHD and transplant-related mortality and overall poorer survival. Thus it may be possible to accept some degree of mismatch and this would result in the availability of donors for an increased number of patients. New matching methods may also allow better prediction of graft outcome.

Recently, alternative sources of stem cells have been used obviating the need for bone marrow harvest. More efficient stem cell mobilization using haemopoietic growth factors and modern automated continuous flow cell separators have led to the use of peripheral blood stem cells in allogeneic transplantation. There are potential advantages for both the donor, with reduced morbidity, and the recipient with accelerated engraftment and reduced risk of graft rejection. It may also be particularly preferable to a second bone marrow harvest from the donor following rejection or delayed engraftment. Cord blood has also been shown to be a good source of stem cells and has been successfully used for haemopoietic reconstitution of children with lethal haemopoietic disorders. Panels of stored cord blood could provide a readily available source of allogeneic stem cells which may be less alloreactive than normal adult bone marrow. Panels are currently being established and these will allow the role of cord blood stem cells to be evaluated.

Better drugs and prophylaxis for GVHD; earlier reconstitution of the haemopoietic system using CSFs and other growth factors; and improved management of infectious complications are likely to play an equally important part in cementing BMT as a cost-effective treatment for leukaemia and other diseases

Further reading

Reviews

Armitage, J. O. (1994). Bone marrow transplantation. *New England J Medicine*, **330**, 827–38.

Forman, S. J., Blume, K. G., and Thomas, E. D. (ed) (1994). *Bone marrow transplantation*. Blackwell Scientific Publications, Oxford.

Hansen, J. A., Petersdorf, E. W., Yoon Choo, S., Martin, P. J., and Anasetti, C. (1994). Marrow transplants from HLA partially matched relatives and unrelated donors. *Keystone Symposia* (in press).

Storb, R. (1992). Marrow transplantation. *Current Topics in Microbiology and Immunology*, **177**, 169–86.

Histocompatibility matching

Anasetti, C., Amos, D., Beatty, P. G., Appelbaum, F. R., Bensinger, W., Buckner, C. D., *et al.* (1989). Effect of HLA compatibility on engraftment of bone marrow transplants in patients with leukemia of lymphoma. *New England Journal of Medicine*, **320**, 197–204.

Ansetti, C., Beatty, P. G., Storb, R., Martin, P. J., Mori, M., Sanders, J. E., *et al.* (1990). Effect of HLA incompatibility of graft-versus-host disease, relapse and survival after marrow transplantation for patients with leukemia or lymphoma. *Human Immunology*, **29**, 79–91.

Christiansen, F. T., Witt, C. S., and Dawkins, R. L. (1991). Questions in marrow matching: the implications of ancestral haplotypes for routine practice. *Bone Marrow Transplantation*, **8**, 83–6.

McGinnis, M. D., Conrad, M. P., Bouwens A. G. M., Tilanus M. G. J., and Kronich M. N. (1995). Automated solid phase sequencing of DRB region genes using T7 sequencing chemistry and dye-labelled primers. *Tissue Antigens*, **46**, 173–9.

Mickelson, E. M., Guthrie, L. A., Etzioni, R., Anasetti, C., Martin, P. J., and Hansen, J. A. (1994). Role of the mixed lymphocyte culture (MLC) reaction in marrow donor selection: Matching for transplants from related haploidentical donors. *Tissue Antigens*, **44**, 83–92.

Moreau, P. and Cesbon, A. (1994). HLA-DP and allogeneic bone marrow transplantation. *Bone Marrow Transplantation*, **13**, 675–81.

Petersdorf, F. E. W., Longton, G. M., Anasetti C., Martin, P. J., Mickelson E. M., Smith, A. G. and Hansen, J. A. (1995). The significance of HLA-DR B1 matching on clinical outcome after HLA-A, B, DR identical unrelated donor marrow transplantation. *Blood*, **86**, 1606–13.

Petersdorf, E. W., Stanley, J. F., Martin, P. J., and Hansen, J. A. (1994). Molecular diversity of the HLA-C locus in unrelated marrow transplantation. *Tissue Antigens*, **44**, 93–9.

Santamaria, P., Reinsmoen, N. L., Lindstrom, A. L., Boyce-Jacino, M. T., Barbosa, J. J., Faras, A. J., *et al.* (1994). Frequent HLA class I and DP sequence mismatches in serologically (HLA-A, HLA-B, HLA-DR) and molecularly (HLA-DRB1, HLA-DQA1, HLA-DQB1)HLA identical unrelated bone marrow transplant pairs. *Blood*, **83**, 280–7.

Tay, G. K., Witt, C. S., Christiansen, F. T., Charron, D., Baker, D., Herrmann, R., *et al.* (1995). Matching for MHC haplotypes results in improved survival following unrelated bone marrow transplantation. *Bone Marrow Transplantation*, **15**, 381–5.

Uhrberg, M., Enczman, J., and Wernet, P. (1994). Rapid DNA crossmatch analysis of HLA class II genotypic polymorphisms by temperature gradient gel electrophoresis in unrelated bone marrow donor selection. *European Journal of Immunogenetics*, **21**, 313–24.

Indications and outcome of bone marrow transplantation

Apperley, J. F. (1993). Bone marrow transplant for the haemoglobinopathies: past, present and future. *Ballieére's Clinical Haematology*, **6**, 299–325.

Beatty, P. G. and Hansen, J. A. (1993). Bone marrow transplantation for the treatment of haematologic disease: status in 1992. *Bone Marrow Transplantation*, 1123–9.

Bortin, M. M., Horowitz, M. M., Rowlings, P. A., Rimm, A. A., Sobocinski, K. A., *et al.* (1993). Progress report from the International Bone Marrow Transplant Registry. *Bone Marrow Transplantation*, **12**, 97–104.

Fischer, A., Landais, P., Friedich, W., Gerritsen, B., Fasth, A., Porta, F., *et al.* (1994). Bone Marrow transplantation in Europe for primary immunodeficiencies other than severe combined immunodeficiency: a report from the European Group for BMT and the European Group for Immunodeficiency. *Blood*, **83**, 1149–54.

Gratwhal, A., Hermans, J., Niederwieser, D., Frassoni, F., Arcese, W., Gahrton, G., *et al.* (1993). Bone marrow transplantation for chronic myeloid leukemia: long term results. *Bone Marrow Transplantation*, **12**, 509–16.

Horowitz, M. M. and Bortin, M. M. (1993). Results of bone marrow transplants from human leukocyte antigen-identical sibling donors for treatment of childhood leukemias. *American Journal of Pediatric Haematology/Oncology*, **15**, 56–64.

McCann, S. R., Bacigalupo, A., Gluckman, E., Hinterberger, W., Hows, J., Ljungman, P., *et al.* (1994). Graft rejection and second bone marrow transplants for acquired aplastic anaemia: a report from the aplastic anaemia working party of the European Bone Marrow Transplant Group. *Bone Marrow Transplantation*, **13**, 233–7.

Somani, J. and Larson, R. A. (1995). Reimmunization after allogeneic bone marrow transplantation. *American Journal of Medicine*, **98**, 389–98.

Storek, J. and Saxon, A. (1992). Reconstitution of B cell immunity following bone marrow transplantation *Bone Marrow Transplantation*, **9**, 395–408.

Vase, J. M. and Armitage, J. O. (1993). Bone marrow transplantation for Hodgkin's disease and lymphoma. *Annual Reviews of Medicine*, **44**, 255–63.

Complications of bone marrow transplantation

Antin, J. H. and Ferrara, J. L. M. (1992). Cytokine dysregulation and acute graft-versus-host disease. *Blood*, **80**, 2964–8.

Chao, N. J. (1992). Graft-versus-host disease following allogeneic bone marrow transplantation. *Current Opinion in Immunology*, **4**, 571–6.

Hiemenz, J. W. and Greene, J. N. (1993). Infectious complications in the immunocomprised host: special considerations for the patient undergoing allogeneic or autologous bone marrow transplantation. *Haematology/Oncology Clinics of North America*, **7**, 961–1002.

Jadus, M. R. and Wepsic, H. T. (1992). The role of cytokines in graft-versus-host reactions and disease. *Bone Marrow Transplantation*, **10**, 1–14.

Martin, P. J. (1992). Determinants of engraftment after allogeneic marrow transplantation. *Blood*, **79**, 1647–50.

Mehta, J. (1993). Graft-versus-leukemia reactions in clinical bone marrow transplantation. *Leukemia and Lymphoma*, **10**, 427–32.

Nash, R. A., Sullivan, G., Pepe, M., Storb, R., Longton, G., Pettinger, M., *et al.* (1992). Acute graft-versus-host disease: analysis of risk factors after allogeneic marrow transplantation and prophylaxis with cyclosporine and methotrexate. *Blood*, **80**, 1838–45.

Ochs, L. A., Miller, W. J., Filipovic, A. H., Haake, R. J., McGlave, P. B., Blazar, B. R., *et al.* (1994). Predictive factors for chronic graft-versus-host disease after histocompatible sibling donor bone marrow transplantation. *Bone Marrow Transplantation*, **13**, 455–60.

Parkman, R. (1991). Graft-versus-host disease. *Annual Reviews of Medicine*, **42**, 189–97.

Schiller, G. and Gale, R. P. (1993). Is there an effective therapy for chronic graft-versus-host disease? *Bone Marrow Transplantation*, **11**, 189–92.

Smyth, L. A., Witt, C. S., Christiansen, F. T., Herrmann, R. P., Hollingsworth, P. N., Townend, D. *et al.* (1993). The MHC influences acute graft versus host disease in MHC matched adults undergoing allogeneic bone marrow transplantation. *Bone Marrow transplantation*, **12**, 351–5.

Unrelated transplantation and stem cell transplantation

Anasetti, C., Etzioni, R., Petersdorf, E. W., Martin, P. J., and Hansen, J. A. (1995). Marrow transplantation from unrelated volunteer donors. *Annual Reviews of Medicine*, **46** (in press).

Bearman, S, I., Mori, M., Beatty, P. G., Meyer, W. G., Buckner, C. D., Petersen, F. B., *et al.* (1994). Comparison of the morbidity and mortality after marrow transplantation from HLA gene typically identical siblings and HLA phenotypically identical unrelated donors. *Bone Marrow Transplantation*, **13**, 31–6.

Beatty, P. G., Hansen, J. A., Longton, G. M., Thomas, E. D., Sanders, J. E., Martin, P. J., *et al.* (1991). Marrow transplantation from HLA matched unrelated donors for treatment of haematologic malignancies. *Transplantation*, **51**, 443–7.

Beatty, P. G., Anasetti, C., Hansen, J. A., Longton, G. M., Sanders, J. E., Martin, P. J., *et al.* (1993). Marrow transplantation from unrelated donors for treatment of haematologic malignancies: effect of mismatching for one HLA locus. *Blood*, **81**, 249–53.

Howard, M. R., Gore, S. M., Hows, J. M., Downie, T. R., and Bradley, B. A. (1994). A prospective study of factors determining the outcome of unrelated marrow searches: report from the International Marrow Unrelated Search and Transplant Study working group on behalf of collab-

orating centres. *Bone Marrow Transplantation*, **13**, 389–96.

McGlave, P., Bartsch, G., Anasetti, C., Ash, R., Beatty, P., Gajewski, J., *et al.* (1993). Unrelated donor marrow transplantation therapy for chronic myelogenous leukemia: initial experience of the national marrow donor programme. *Blood*, **81**, 543–50.

Nicol, A. J., Hows, J. M. and Bradley, B. A. (1994). Cord blood transplantation: a practical option. *British Journal of Haematology*, **87**, 1–5.

Russell, N. H. and Hunter, A. E. (1994). Peripheral blood stem cells for allogeneic transplantation. *Bone Marrow Transplantation*, **13**, 353–5.

35 Pancreatic transplantation

C. J. Simeonovic and K. J. Lafferty

Introduction

The impetus for clinical pancreatic tissue transplantation as a treatment for insulin-dependent diabetes has come from the failure of exogenous insulin treatment to prevent the development of severe secondary complications including blindness, renal disease, neuropathy, heart disease, and gangrene. The basic pathological defect associated with these complications is micro-angiopathy, a small blood vessel disorder which probably arises from erratic blood glucose control. Pancreatic tissue transplants on the other hand offer the advantages of a physiological means of replacing endocrine function, precise blood glucose control, and the arrest of progressive vascular disease.

Pancreas transplantation

The vast majority of clinical experience in pancreatic tissue transplantation has involved implantation of immediately vascularized grafts consisting of either the whole pancreas organ or a segment of pancreas. Surgical techniques have been developed to control hydrolytic exocrine secretions in the recipient, for example, enteric drainage, urinary drainage via the ureter or bladder and, in the case of segmental transplants, occlusion of the main pancreatic duct by polymer injection. Although technical problems associated with graft thrombosis, exocrine leakage, and pancreatic fibrosis (following duct occlusion) remain potential hazards, graft rejection represents the major obstacle to this surgical approach. While human leucocyte antigen (HLA) matching of the donor and recipient, and simultaneous kidney transplantation have shown some beneficial effects on pancreas graft outcome, the success of clinical pancreas transplants is ultimately dependent on long-term immunosuppressive therapy. In the case of the juvenile-onset diabetic, long-term immunosuppression cannot be justified as the associated risk of opportunistic infections, neoplasia, and nephrotoxicity can result in more immediately life-threatening conditions than the disease-related complications, which develop chronically over a long period of time.

Pancreatic cell transplantation

The passenger leucocyte concept

Experimental animal studies in the 1970s identified pancreatic islet cell transplantation as a potential alternative to whole pancreas transplants and as an approach which offered the major advantage of obviating the need for recipient immunosuppression. This advance resulted directly from a major breakthrough in the understanding of transplantation immunobiology. The classical Medawarian view that major histocompatibility complex (MHC) antigens expressed on the parenchymal cells of a graft constitute the major barrier to transplantation was challenged by studies which showed that transplantation antigens when isolated from living cells were weakly immunogenic and did not evoke a strong allograft response. A solution to this conflict was provided by Lafferty's two-signal model for the activation of T lymphocytes or T cells: foreign antigen binding to the T-cell receptor provides signal 1 and the second inductive signal or 'co-stimulator' (CoS) is produced by an antigen-presenting cell (APC) or 'stimulator (S⁺)' cell. In the inductive phase of the immune response, recognition of MHC antigens on stimulator cells triggers expression of CoS activity; thereafter, MHC antigens on all graft cells act as targets for recognition by the immune response. *In vitro* experiments of T-cell activation showed that only metabolically active lymphoreticular cells, e.g.

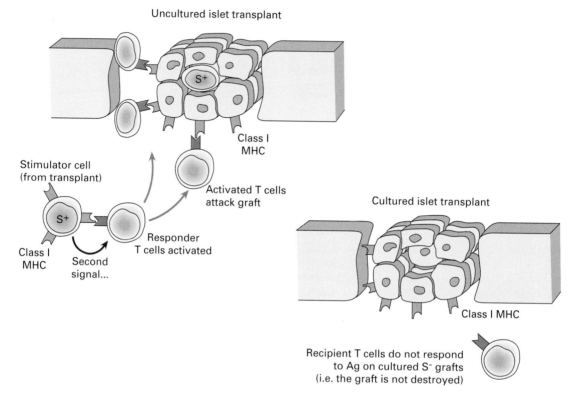

∎ Fig. 35.1 (a) Passenger leucocytes represent the major barrier to tissue allotransplantation because they function as S+ cells which can directly activate recipient T cells. Graft destruction results from activated T cells recognizing transplantation (major histocompatibility complex: MHC) antigen (Ag) on the graft tissue. (b) Removal of passenger leucocytes from tissue before grafting prevents allograft rejection. Transplantation antigen carried on parenchymal graft cells is not immunogenic.

macrophages and dendritic cells displayed the S+ phenotype. As a consequence, major histocompatible antigens expressed on the surface of graft parenchymal cells are antigenic (recognized by the immune system once it has been activated) but not immunogenic; these cells cannot provide the second signal and thus express the S− phenotype. Tissue immunogenicity therefore, is a property determined by the load of S+ cells, 'passenger leucocytes', passively carried in graft tissue (Fig. 35.1). This concept was confirmed by the experimental observation that pretreatment of mouse thyroid lobes in high oxygen culture prior to transplantation prevented thyroid allograft rejection in non-immunosuppressed hosts. Furthermore, the allograft rejection response was reconstituted by immunizing recipient mice with donor-type lymphoreticular cells (S+ cells) at the time of transplantation. This study provided indirect evidence that passenger leucocytes were removed during organ culture and verified that the graft tissue remained antigenic after culture, that is, it retained the capacity to be recognized by the immune response.

Islet transplantation

The approach of *in vitro* modulation of graft immunogenicity has been successfully applied to pancreatic islet cell transplants. Allografts of untreated adult islets transplanted to mice with drug-induced diabetes initially restore normoglycaemia but subsequently result in a rapid reappearance of hyperglycaemia due to graft rejection. However, following organ culture in 95% oxygen for 7 days, islet allografts survive (Fig. 35.2) and permanently reverse diabetes in non-immunosuppressed recipient animals. Additional pretreatment procedures which have also facilitated long-term islet allograft acceptance include: low temperature culture, anticlass II MHC or antidendritic cell

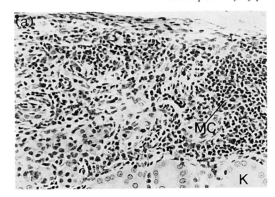

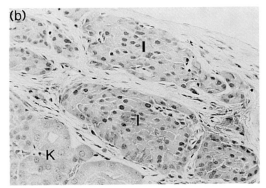

❚ **Fig. 35.2** (a) Histological appearance of an allograft of uncultured mouse adult islets at 2 weeks after transplantation under the capsule of the kidney (K). The rejection response is characterized by mononuclear cells (MC) which infiltrate the graft and destroy the islet tissue. (b) Cultured islet allograft at 4 weeks post-transplant shows the presence of intact islet tissue (I) and no cell infiltration. Haematoxylin and eosin, × 450.

antibodies, ultraviolet irradiation, and low pH media. Fetal pancreas represents an alternative source of donor tissue for pancreatic islet cell transplantation. Fetal mouse pancreas explants are highly immunogenic due to contaminating lymphoid tissue. *In vitro* cultivation techniques have been used to isolate fetal proislets (islet precursors) which are more weakly immunogenic than fetal pancreas; perinatal rat islets have also been isolated in culture and have been shown to survive in non-immunosuppressed allogeneic recipients. In addition to *in vitro* immunomodulation, islet cell transplants offer other potential advantages over the use of vascularized whole pancreas organ transplants: microencapsulation of isolated islets is currently being assessed as a barrier technique to avoid immune cell recognition, neovascularization of cellular transplants by host vascular endothelium limits susceptibility to damage by anti-

donor antibody, cryopreservation of islets permits subsequent storage in tissue banks, and the flexibility of transplant site provides the option for minimal surgical intervention or placement in 'privileged' transplant sites which intrinsically afford protection from rejection mechanisms. Experimental studies have also demonstrated that long-term surviving islet cell transplants can result in allograft tolerance, i.e. lack of graft-specific reactivity following subsequent *in vivo* challenge of host animals with donor-specific lymphoid cells or an unmodified secondary donor-specific allograft. Further analysis of the underlying mechanisms of such tolerance will be required to identify protocols which may be potentially useful for the acute or immediate induction of tolerance to clinical pancreatic tissue transplants. Overall, the islet cell transplant approach is attractive because the need for immunosuppressive therapy can be eliminated or minimized.

Despite advances in experimental pancreatic islet cell transplantation, clinical islet transplants to date have enjoyed limited success. Although major developments in islet isolation techniques have vastly improved the yield of islets harvested from human pancreas, graft failure continues to frustrate the clinical application of islet cell technology. The complexity of the clinical hurdle can be attributed to the susceptibility of pancreatic tissue transplants to immune assault via two distinct mechanisms: transplantation immunity and the process of disease recurrence.

Susceptibility of pancreatic tissue transplants to autoimmune disease

Insulin-dependent diabetes in humans and in animal models (NOD mice, BB rats) which develop spontaneous diabetes is due to autoimmune disease which specifically destroys the insulin-producing β cells of pancreatic islets. The disease process is characterized by tissue-specific cell-mediated immunity which activates an inflammatory process in and around the islet tissue (Fig. 35.3). Experimental studies in NOD mice have demonstrated tissue-specific destruction of islet isografts and cultured islet allografts; co-transplanted cultured thyroid allografts remained intact, confirming that allograft immunity was not responsible for islet allograft damage. Selective immune targeting of a human pancreas allograft but not a co-transplanted kidney allograft from the same donor has indicated that the tissue-specificity of the autoimmune disease is a general phenomenon.

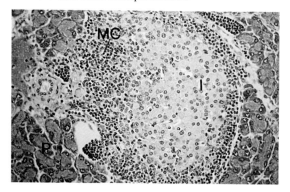

∎ Fig. 35.3 Autoimmune disease in pre-diabetic NOD (non-obese diabetic) mice is characterized by the presence of mononuclear cells (MC) which surround and invade the pancreatic islets (I). The islets are scattered throughout the exocrine tissue of the pancreas (P). Hameatoxylin and eosin, × 324.

Disease transfer studies in NOD mice have shown T cells play a critical part in the pathogenesis of the disease; both CD4 and CD8 T cells are required to initiate disease pathology. In contrast, *in vivo* depletion of T-cell subsets via monoclonal antibody therapy has identified a requirement for only CD4 T cells for expression of disease recurrence. Immunohistochemical analyses of the destructive islet lesions in both diabetic human and animal pancreas have confirmed the local accumulation of both T cells and macrophages. The exact nature of the mechanism of β cell destruction is unclear, but experimental evidence suggests that cytokines and the generation of free radicals may be involved. The cytokines interleukin (IL) 1, tumour necrosis factor (TNF)α, TNFβ, and interferonγ have been found to be expressed in the insulitis lesions in NOD mice and BB rats; such cytokines are also cytotoxic for β cells and inhibit insulin synthesis *in vitro*. IL-1 selectively acts on islet β cells by inducing the formation of nitric oxide, a free radical that inactivates iron-containing enzymes. The contribution of cytokines and free radicals to the inflammatory disease process may therefore be intimately related. Other evidence implicating a role for free radicals includes the protective effect of radical scavengers against disease recurring in NOD islet isografts and the enhanced oxygen radical production by macrophages from diabetes-prone BB rats. Neither immunomodulation nor islet encapsulation procedures protect islet cell transplants from such inflammatory mediators. The success of islet allotransplantation as a routine treatment for insulin-dependent diabetes will therefore depend on the development of benign strategies that prevent reactivation of the autoimmune disease process.

Cross-species transplants

The transplantation approach to treating insulin-dependent diabetes is restricted by the limited availability of cadaver human pancreases. Use of pancreatic tissue from other animal species represents a possible solution to the problem of supply. Immediately vascularized whole organ xenografts classically suffer hyperacute rejection due to the interaction of preformed antidonor antibody with donor antigens present on the graft's vascular endothelium. This process would be expected to occur in the case of whole pancreas xenografts but not with islet cell xenografts which require recipient neovascularization. Cellular xenografts nevertheless are subject to T-cell-mediated rejection. Unlike the activation of T cells by allogeneic APCs, xenogeneic APCs cannot directly activate a T-cell response. This difference appears to be due to the species specificity of the second signal (CoS). As a result, peptides of xenoantigens are processed by recipient APCs, presented in association with host class II MHC and thereby, preferentially activate a CD4 T-cell response. In support of this notion, animal studies have demonstrated that short-term treatment of host mice with anti-CD4 monoclonal antibody can prevent the acute rejection of pig and human pancreatic islet tissue xenografts. Such xenografts have demonstrated the capacity to reverse experimentally induced diabetes in recipient mice. Microencapsulation of xenogeneic islets has also facilitated long-term graft survival and function. As yet the susceptibility of xenogeneic islet tissue to autoimmune disease, for example, in NOD mice, has not been resolved. If the disease process is shown to be species specific, xenogeneic islet cell transplants might offer the advantage of disease resistance in insulin-dependent diabetic humans.

Further reading

Lafferty, K. J., Prowse, S. J., Simeonovic, C. J., and Warren, H. S. (1983). Immunobiology of tissue transplantation: A return to the passenger leukocyte concept. *Annual Review of Immunology*, **1**, 143–73.

Rabinovitch, A. (1994). Immunoregulatory and cytokine imbalances in the pathogenesis of IDDM. Therapeutic intervention by immunostimulation? *Diabetes*, **43**, 613–21.

Ricordi, C. (ed.) (1992). *Pancreatic islet cell transplantation*. R. G. Landes Company, Austin, Texas.

Shehadeh, N. N. and Lafferty, K. J. (1993). The role of T-cells in the development of autoimmune diabetes. *Diabetes Reviews*, **1**, 141–51.

Sutherland, D. E. R. (1994). State of the art in pancreas transplantation. *Transplantation Proceedings*, **26**, 316–20.

36 Corneal transplantation

K. A. Williams

Introduction

Corneal transplantation, or penetrating keratoplasty, involves the replacement of a full-thickness thickness disc of central corneal tissue, typically 7–8 mm in diameter, with normal tissue harvested from a human donor eye. Lamellar keratoplasty, in which the anterior portion only of the cornea is replaced, is also sometimes performed. Currently, no 'artificial cornea' suitable for clinical use exists, and corneal xenografts are not performed except in experimental animals, so that transplantation depends upon the availability of donated human corneas. Most corneas are procured and stored within eye banks, which are responsible for arranging the process of consent for donation, enucleation of the globes, serological testing of the donor, corneal assessment and preservation, and equitable distribution. Once collected, corneas can be stored in any one of a number of specialized tissue culture media containing colloidal osmotic agents for periods of 4–28 days, depending on the medium.

Tissue typing for corneal transplantation

Some corneas are harvested from brain-dead multiorgan donors. However, most corneas are collected within 12 (and preferably within 6) h of death, from donors who typically have died from myocardial infarction or other cardiac or circulatory system failure, cerebrovascular accident or cancer, and who are not donors of other tissues or organs. Peripheral blood collected prior to death, or lymphoid tissue collected at the time other transplantable organs are harvested, is thus seldom available. Tissue typing (human leucocyte antigen, HLA typing) can be performed on post-mortem blood, usually collected (albeit sometimes with difficulty) from the external jugular vein. Typing of retinal pigment epithelial cells cultured from the back of the donor eye has also been employed.

Any method of typing can be used, and because corneas can be stored for up to 3 weeks in the eye bank, a really rapid method of typing is not essential. Potential recipients can, of course, be HLA typed whenever convenient.

Effect of human leucocyte antigen matching on corneal transplantation

The influence of HLA matching on corneal graft outcome is unclear. There is little or no evidence that HLA matching benefits recipients who are at low risk of graft failure. Such patients include those receiving a first graft for keratoconus or a corneal dystrophy. A number of studies have reported that matching for major histocompatibility complex class I antigens improves corneal graft survival in high-risk cases. The effect of matching for class II antigens appears less certain, but beneficial results have been reported. However, a recent multicentre trial reported from the USA failed to find any effect of matching for HLA class I or II antigens in high-risk patients and furthermore, a study from Bristol in the UK found a *negative* influence of matching for class II antigens when failures due to irreversible corneal graft rejection were examined. The case for matching thus remains an open question.

Indications for corneal transplantation

Corneal grafts are generally performed to improve visual acuity, to relieve pain, or to repair a damaged globe. The main indications for corneal transplantation from one large registry series are shown in Table 36.1.

The relative importance of these indications differs only slightly from one developed country to another.

∎ **Table 36.1** Indications for corneal transplantation in a developed country

Indication for graft	Percentage
Keratoconus	31%
Bullous keratopathy	25%
Failed previous graft	14%
Corneal scar or opacity	11%
Corneal dystrophy	7%

Within developing countries, the patterns of corneal blindness may vary significantly, with the sequelae of vitamin A deficiency and of infectious diseases such as measles keratitis, trachoma, and river blindness being more important. Recipient age is usually unimportant in considering whether a potential recipient will benefit from corneal transplantation and grafts are performed in both infants and nonagenarians.

Contraindications for corneal donation

In developed countries, the relatively few absolute contraindications for corneal donation include seropositivity for, or suspicion of infection by, human immunodeficiency virus (HIV), hepatitis B or C, and death from, or possible infection with, rabies or Creutzfeldt–Jakob disease. Transmission of hepatitis B, Creutzfeldt–Jakob disease, and rabies by corneal transplantation has been confirmed. Serological testing for HIV and hepatitis B and C are performed on serum collected at the time of enucleation. Many eye banks refuse to collect corneas from potential donors with a history of dementia or any neurological disorder including multiple sclerosis, from donors who have died of unknown causes, from unstable diabetics, from those with haematological malignancies, disseminated carcinoma, septicaemia, jaundice, a history of radiotherapy to the head and neck, or with a history of major ocular disease or intraocular surgery. Corneas are not collected from individuals who have undergone cataract extraction, but refractive errors are irrelevant. It is important to stress that age is not a contraindication to donation, although many eye banks prefer not to harvest material from children under the age of 2 years or from very elderly donors.

Monitoring and immunosuppression

Practices vary widely, but a corneal graft recipient might typically be hospitalized for 1–3 days postoperatively, seen weekly in out-patients for the first month, and then at 3 monthly intervals until after removal of the graft sutures. Graft sutures are usually left in place for approximately 12–18 months post-graft. In the absence of any complications, recipients will then usually be seen once per year. Patients are advised to seek urgent attention, should the grafted eye become red or painful, or should they notice a decrease in visual acuity.

Most corneal graft recipients receive topical corticosteroids postoperatively to prevent corneal graft rejection, but there is no standard regimen of therapy. A typical regimen might involve the topical administration of 0.5% prednisolone phosphate to the grafted eye once daily for 1 year postoperatively. Occasional patients, usually those considered to be at a high risk of corneal graft rejection, may also be prescribed systemic immunosuppression, usually low-dose cyclosporin A. Topical cyclosporin A has not proved to be particularly useful for prevention of corneal graft rejection. Ongoing corneal graft rejection may be treated with more frequent administration of a topical steroid, usually on an in-patient basis, or with bolus intravenous methylprednisolone.

Graft and visual outcome after corneal transplantation

Kaplan–Meier graft survival is of the order of 90% at 1 year and 70% at 5 years. These figures can be broken down further, depending on the indication for graft. Grafts performed for keratoconus exhibit 5 year survivals approaching 98%, whereas those performed in eyes with a history of inflammatory eye disease, corneal neovascularization, or failed previous graft show much poorer survival rates. The most common cause of graft failure in most series is irreversible rejection.

Corneal transplantation is frequently successful in restoring vision in people with corneal opacities, provided the visual potential of the eye concerned has not otherwise been compromised. Some blinding co-morbidities such as cataract can be readily managed, but coexisting vitreoretinal disorders are not always amenable to treatment and may limit the final visual acuity able to be achieved. Fully 70% of graft recipients may expect to use some form of refractive correction, usually spectacles, and approximately 50% of recipients will achieve a Snellen acuity of 6/18 with this correction.

Further reading

Batchelor, J. R., Casey, T. A., Werb, A., Gibbs, D. C., Prasad, S. S., LLoyd, D. F., and James, A. (1976). HLA matching and corneal grafting. *Lancet*, **i**, 551–4.

Baumgartner, I., Asenbauer, T. T., Kaminski, S. L., Grabner, G., and Mayr, W. R. (1992). Retinal pigment epithelial cells in post mortem HLA typing of corneal donors. *Investigative Ophthalmology and Visual Science*, **33**, 1940–5.

Boisjoly, H. M., Roy, R., Dubé, I., Laughrea, P. A., Michaud, R., Douville, P., and Hébert, J. (1986). HLA-A, B and DR matching in corneal transplantation. *Ophthalmology*, **93**, 1290–7.

Collaborative Corneal Transplantation Studies Research Group. (1992). The collaborative corneal transplantation studies (CCTS). Effectiveness of histocompatibility matching in high-risk corneal transplantation. *Archives of Ophthalmology*, **110**, 1392–403.

Hill, J. C. (1992). The use of cyclosporine in high-risk keratoplasty. *American Journal of Ophthalmology*, **107**, 506–10.

Hill, J. C., Maske, R., and Watson, P. G. (1991). The use of a single pulse of intravenous methylprednisolone in the treatment of corneal graft rejection. A preliminary report. *Eye*, **5**, 420–4.

Hoffman, F., von Keyserlingk, H-J., and Wiederholt, M. (1986). Importance of HLA DR matching for corneal transplantation in high-risk cases. *Cornea*, **5**, 139–43.

Lee, P. P., Yang, J. C., McDonnell, P. J., Maumenee, A. E., and Stark, W. J. (1992). Worldwide legal requirements for obtaining corneas. 1990. *Cornea*, **11**, 102–7.

Mamalis, N., Anderson, C. W., Kreisler, K. R., Lundergan, M. K., and Olson, R. J. (1992). Changing trends in the indications for penetrating keratoplasty. *Archives of Ophthalmology*, **110**, 1409–11.

Pepose, J. S., Buerger, D. G., Paul, D. A., Quinn, T. C., Darragh, T. M., and Donegan, E. (1992). New developments in serologic screening of corneal donors for HIV-1 and hepatitis B virus infections. *Ophthalmology*, **99**, 879–88.

Rakoczy, P., Garlepp, M., and Constable, I. (1992). HLA DQA tissue typing of cadaveric eye bank donor material with polymerase chain reaction. *Current Eye Research*, **11**, 445–52.

Rinne, J. R., and Stulting, R. D. (1992). Current practices in the prevention and treatment of corneal graft rejection. *Cornea*, **11**, 326–8.

Sanfilippo, F., MacQueen, M., Vaughn, W. K., and Foulks, G. N. (1986). Reduced graft rejection with good HLA-A and B matching in high-risk corneal transplantation. *New England Journal of Medicine*, **315**, 29–35.

Vail, A., Gore, S. M., Bradley, B. A., Easty, D. L., Rogers, C. A., Armitage, W. J., on behalf of Corneal Transplant Follow-up Study Collaborators (1994). Influence of donor and histocompatibility factors on corneal graft outcome. *Transplantation*, **58**, 1210–16.

Völker-Dieben, H. J., D'Amaro, J., Kok-van Alphen, C. C. (1987). Hierarchy of prognostic factors for corneal allograft survival. *Australia and New Zealand and Journal of Ophthalmology*, **15**, 11–18.

Williams, K. A. and Coster, D. J. (1993). Clinical and experimental aspects of corneal transplantation. *Transplantation Reviews*, **7**, 44–64.

Williams, K. A., Muehlberg, S. M., Wing, S. J., and Coster, D. J. (1993). The Australian Corneal Graft Registry, 1990–1992 report. *Australia and New Zealand Journal of Ophthalmology*, **21** (Suppl.), 1–48.

Section VI

Immunology and infection

37 Immunology of infectious diseases

K. J. Christiansen and F. T. Christiansen

Introduction

Micro-organisms cause disease in humans by a variety of mechanisms. Bacteria can colonize an epithelial surface and by the elaboration of enzymes or toxins lead to local or distant tissue damage. They can also invade directly into the body with some organisms remaining in the extracellular spaces while others are found in an intracellular location, often within an endosome. Viruses are obligate intracellular parasites requiring host cell functions for replication. Translation and transcription of the viral genome occurs from within the cytoplasm of the host cell. Parasites such as protozoa can also be in the extracellular spaces or within cells whereas the much larger organisms like nematodes and trematodes are extracellular. The immune system must therefore deal with organisms in a number of sites within the body and with a variety of toxins and enzymes produced by them. Although the immune response is usually successful in eradicating or controlling the infectious agent, in some instances the response itself may give rise to tissue damage and sometimes death of the host.

Two separate but interrelated systems are used by the host in the defence against infectious diseases. The initial protective system is termed innate immunity. This system requires no prior exposure to the organism and is responsible for the prevention of invasion by many organisms. Adaptive immunity is employed if the initial defences are breached. The response is organism specific and becomes incorporated into immunological memory enabling a rapid response on re-exposure to the agent.

Innate immunity

There are many factors involved in the initial defence of the host when exposed to an infectious agent. The

Table 37.1 Components of innate immunity

Physical barrier	skin
	mucous membranes
	cilia
	motility
Soluble factors	lysozyme
	fatty acids
	Iron binding proteins
	C-reactive protein
	complement
Cellular factors	phagocytes, e.g. neutrophils, monocytes
	tissue macrophages
	natural killer cells
Other	commensal flora

components of innate immunity are outlined in Table 37.1.

Physical barrier

The body surfaces such as skin and mucous membranes provide a mechanical barrier preventing penetration. The breaching of the intact tegument as in burns, lacerations, and transcutaneous devices (e.g. intravenous lines) leads to an increased susceptibility to infection. Motility of the mucous lining of membranes provided by the musculature of the gut or the cilia of the respiratory system transport bacteria out of the body or prevent attachment to underlying host cells.

Commensal flora compete with pathogens for nutrients, occupy the same receptors on host cells, produce bacteriocins which are cidal for other organisms, and of importance for the adaptive immune system provide continual stimulation thus maintaining low, constant levels of major histocompatibility complex (MHC) class II molecule expression on macrophages and other accessory cells.

Soluble factors

Bactericidal soluble factors in secretions are produced in almost every part of the body. One of these, lysozyme, is particularly active against Gram-positive bacteria, lysing the organism by splitting the muramic acid B (1–4)-*N*-acetylglucosamine linkage in the bacterial cell wall. Other soluble factors include fatty acids in sebaceous secretions and iron-binding proteins in all mucosal secretions which act to deprive organisms of this essential nutrient. During the acute phase response to infection serum iron, and zinc levels fall in the serum due to increased release of transferrin and ceruloplasmin. C reactive protein also produced during the acute phase response recognizes and binds to molecular groups present on a large number of bacteria and fungi facilitating their uptake by phagocytes and activating the complement cascade.

The complement pathway is an important component of innate immunity and can be activated by two mechanisms. The classical pathway requires the presence of antibody–antigen complexes and therefore is dependent on the humoral immune system. Activation of the alternative pathway is independent of immune-specific mechanisms. The production and deposition of C3b is central to either of the complement pathways, the difference being in the mechanism of its generation. The alternate pathway relies on the natural low-grade hydrolysis of circulating C3 to C3i. The C3i binds to factor B ultimately leading to the formation of C3 convertase. This cleaves C3 to C3b which is deposited on to any adjacent cell surface. This deposition is non-specific. Bound C3b has two possible outcomes depending on the nature of the cell surface. When the surface is non-self, e.g. a micro-organism, the C3b acts as a binding site for factor B leading to production of the convertase enzyme which focuses deposition of more C3b to the same surface leading to an amplification of the response. On autologous cells C3b is catabolized using factor H thereby inhibiting the cascade.

The presence of *N*-acetyl neuraminic acid or sialic acid in autologous cell membranes facilitates the breakdown of C3b because these compounds favour the binding of factor H rather than factor B. The deposition of C3b on the surface of a micro-organism has three consequences:

1. *Opsonization*. The C3b on the microbe surface binds to C3b receptors on phagocytic cells promoting uptake into endosomes.
2. *Cell activation*. Complement receptors on phagocytic cells when bound to their specific ligand activate the cell promoting chemotaxis and the production of free oxygen radicals.
3. *Cell lysis*. The successive binding of C6, C7 to C5b results in a complex to which C8 and C9 bind. The final form is the membrane attack complex (MAC) which effectively consists of a hydrophobic pore inserted into the lipid membrane layer causing osmotic disruption of the cell to occur.

Micro-organisms have developed various mechanisms for evading complement-mediated uptake and lysis. Such mechanisms include:

1. The direction of C3b and MAC deposition to sites on the bacterial surface where they are unable to mediate opsonization or lysis, e.g. some strains of *Salmonellae* and *Escherichia coli* preferentially deposit C3b on lipopolysaccharide molecules with long *O*-polysaccharide side chains such that the membrane attack complex formed cannot interact with the cell membrane.
2. the possession of a capsule preventing the insertion of the MAC or binding of antibody to a cell wall sited antigen, e.g. the size of the capsule of staphylococci correlates directly with the ability to avoid phagocytosis.
3. Surface components having a high affinity for factor H thereby promoting catabolism of C3b, e.g. streptococcal M protein, a surface fibrillar molecule binds factor H, as does the cell membrane sialic acid of group B streptococci, *E. coli* type K1 and group B meningococci. Group B streptococci and *E. coli* type K1, both of which are part of normal maternal flora, are particularly important causes of neonatal sepsis. Prior to the development of an adequate immunity, infants are dependent on passively transferred maternal antibody to these organisms. If this does not occur the infant is dependent on the alternative complement pathway to contain any invasion. The ability of these two organisms to evade complement- mediated lysis and opsonization after infection results in mortality rates approaching 50%.

Cellular factors

Phagocytosis depends on the binding of the organism to the phagocytic cell via various cell surface receptors. These include receptors for lectins present on the surface of the microbe, for example, the mannose binding lectin on the fimbriae of *E. coli*, or for the C3b component of complement or the Fc component of antibody. Once the organism is internalized in a vacuole, fusion with a lysosome occurs. Microbial killing requires the formation and release of toxic agents that accumulate in the phagosome. These antimicrobial agents can be classified by their requirement for oxygen metabolism.

The oxygen-dependent systems generate reactive oxygen intermediates (ROIs) generated by a burst of oxidative metabolism. These ROIs consist of the superoxide anion, hydrogen peroxide, hypochlorous acid, the hydroxyl radical, and singlet oxygen. Patients with the hereditary disorder chronic granulomatous disease (CGD) have a defective nicotinamide adenine dinucleotide phosphate (NADPH) oxidase system in their phagocytes and do not undergo a respiratory burst. They are therefore unable to kill those organisms whose killing is dependent on this mechanism. The disease is characterized by chronic granulomatous lesions involving pyogenic organisms such as staphylococci. The oxygen-dependent systems also produce reactive nitrogen intermediates (RNI), in particular nitric oxide, which is very toxic to intracellular parasites such as toxoplasma and leishmania.

The non-oxygen-dependent system is probably more important in microbial killing but is less well understood. This system consists of a number of granule-associated proteins such as lysozyme, bactericidal/permeability-increasing protein, defensins, lactoferrin, and cationic peptides.

Adaptive immunity

This specific immune mechanism is effected by either antibody production or by a cell-mediated response. The type of response is dependent on the nature and site of the antigenic stimulation.

Humoral immunity

Specific antibodies are important in the defence against both micro-organisms and their toxic products. Antibodies may immobilize motile organisms, prevent adherence of both bacteria and viruses to host receptor molecules, neutralize toxins, in synergy with complement cause bacterial lysis, and act as opsonins to facilitate phagocytosis. Antibodies are produced by plasma cells following differentiation and clonal expansion of B cells upon antigen stimulation. The antigen/B-cell interaction can occur by two mechanisms, one being T-cell independent and the second requiring the involvement of T cells.

T-cell-independent humoral response

This type of response is determined by the structure of the stimulating antigen which typically is a large polymeric molecule with repeating antigenic determinants. The response to *Streptococcus pneumoniae* infection is a good example of T-cell-independent humoral immunity. (Fig. 37.1). When pneumococci invade the body they escape initial recognition by phagocytes because of the presence of a polysaccharide capsule. This capsule is a high molecular weight polysaccharide with repeating epitopes. Specific immunoglobulin receptors on B cells recognize this antigen and because of the repetitious nature of the antigen numerous receptors on each B cell will bind to them. This 'cross-linking' of receptors gives rise to activation of the B cell with subsequent proliferation and specific antibody production. This response is amplified further by the activation of the complement cascade through the classical pathway with C3b production which when bound to C3b receptors on B cells give rise to added B-cell activation. The initial B-cell activation is independent of T cells or antigen-presenting cells (APCs); however, proliferation of the B-cell clone requires T-cell involvement with the production of interleukin (IL) 6, B-cell growth factor (BCGF), and IL-1.

Pneumococci are opsonized by the antibody and complement thus facilitating uptake by macrophages via Fc and C3b receptors. Evasion of this process is attempted by the organism by the production of pneumolysin, which inhibits lymphocyte proliferation and synthesis of immunoglobulins.

T-cell-dependent humoral response

This type of response accounts for immunity to a very wide range of bacterial infections including disease mediated by toxin production, e.g. diphtheria and tetanus. Each B cell has membrane bound immunoglobulin on its surface specific for a single epitope. This immunoglobulin is generated by somatic recombination of non-contiguous germ-line variable (V), diversity (D), and joining genes (J) to form a continuous variable region gene, thus giving the host the ability to recognize the enormous number of possible antigenic structures of micro-organisms. On binding of an antigen to the specific B-cell receptor, the antigen is internalized in a vesicle where it is broken down to peptides by cellular enzymes. MHC class II molecules manufactured in the endoplasmic reticulum migrate to the vesicle where they bind to the peptide antigen. The MHC–peptide complex then migrates to the cell surface. The MHC class II molecule presents the processed peptide fragment to T-cell receptors (TCR) on CD4+ (subtype Th2) cells. The TCR is generated in a similar way to that of immunoglobulins and B-cell receptors. The CD4+ (Th2) cell is stimulated to produce cytokines Il-4, IL-5, IL-6, and IL-10 necessary to activate B cells to proliferate and produce specific antibody. Opsonization and phagocytosis of the bacteria or toxin then occurs see Fig. 37.2.

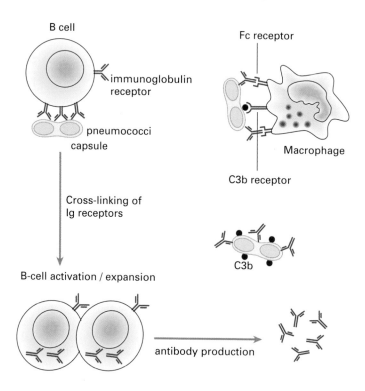

■**Fig. 37.1**   T independent humoral responses.

Evasive mechanisms

Masking

Antibodies directed to antigenic structures on the cell wall are prevented from binding by the possession of a capsule. However, for many organisms the capsule itself is antigenic.

Antigenic mimicry

Some organisms have surface structures that imitate host molecules. Streptococci have antigenic similarity with cardiac muscle, *Yersinia* with HLA-B27 and *Neisseria meningitidis* type B with embryonic brain. This property, however, may play a more important part in inducing an autoimmune reaction than protecting against killing.

Camouflage

The incorporation of host molecules in the organism surface is employed by some organisms. Schistosomes rapidly become covered with host-derived glycoproteins, MHC molecules, and non-specific immunoglobulins and *Treponema pallidum* coats itself with human fibronectin.

Antigenic variation

This is a common evasive mechanism used by a large number of organisms. The African trypanosome, a unicellular flagellate, is covered with a single species of glycoprotein that can be varied enormously. Within the nucleus of the trypanosome there are more than 1000 genes each encoding a different glycoprotein species allowing the progeny of a single trypanosome to make over one hundred different coats having no exposed antigenic determinant in common. Thus the antibody response cannot keep pace allowing chronic infection to be established. Antigenic variation can also be achieved by mutation of the genes encoding the immunodominant antigens or recombination of genes between different strains of the same organism. The former mechanism is employed by the human immunodeficiency virus and both by the influenza virus. Gonococci have the ability to vary their surface properties by altering the expression and sequences of attachment pili and outer membrane proteins. The bacteria, salmonellae and streptococci, and viruses such as adeno- and enteroviruses have evolved a number of

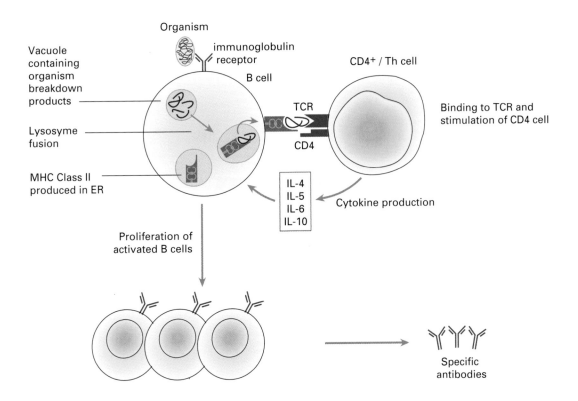

▌Fig. 37.2 T dependent humoral response. MHC, major histocompatibility complex; ER, endoplasmic reticulum; TCR, T cell receptor.

antigenic variants over a long period of time that has led to the coexistence of multiple stable variants to which a specific host response must be made, i.e. serotypes.

Antibody inactivation

Some organisms produce specific proteins active against antibody. *Neisseria gonorrhoeae* and *Haemophilus influenzae* produce an immunoglobulin (Ig) A protease and staphylococci produce protein A which binds to the Fc portion of IgG possibly acting to immobilize the immunoglobulin.

Cell-mediated immunity

This response can be mediated by two different mechanisms. The first involves the CD4+, T-helper cell (usually of the subset Th1) which recognizes antigen in association with MHC class II molecules expressed on APCs. For intracellular pathogens the APCs of particular importance are cells of the lymphoid system such as the monocyte/macrophage series. In the second mechanism, CD8+, cytotoxic T cells (Tc), recognize

antigen in association with MHC class I molecules which are expressed on all nucleated cells. Which of these two mechanisms is employed when an intracellular organism is present depends on its intracellular location, i.e. whether it is present in a membrane bound organelle such as a phagosome or whether it is free in the cytoplasm.

Organisms in membrane bound organelles (CD4+ response)

When infection with organisms such as mycobacteria, leishmania, and leprosy occur the organism is readily phagocytosed but as successful intracellular parasites they have developed mechanisms to prevent their destruction by the macrophage (MP). Mycobacteria gain entry to the MP by endocytosis via C3b receptors, attached to antibody via Fc receptors or by fibronectin receptors as a result of the large amounts of fibronectin-binding molecules produced by these organisms. Once in the endosome the organism is able to survive and replicate by producing ROI detoxifying enzymes, inhibiting phagosome–lysosome fusion and neutralizing

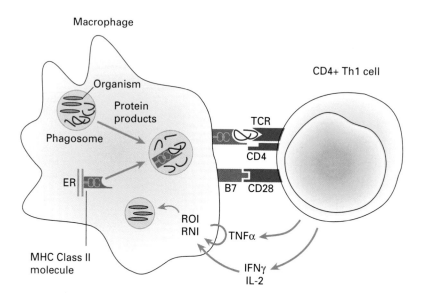

∎ **Fig. 37.3** Cell mediated response: organism in membrane bound organelle. ER, endoplasmic reticulum; TCR, T cell receptor; MHC, major histocompatibility complex.

endosomal acid by the production of NH_4^+. Heat shock proteins (*hsp*) are also produced. These are a group of polypeptides synthesized by cells, both bacterial and host, in response to a variety of insults. Their increased production by intracellular organisms protects them in some way. Defective *hsp* genes in *Salmonella typhimurium* mutants is associated with loss of virulence and greater susceptibility to intracellular killing.

Having survived the initial bactericidal mechanisms of the macrophage the organism replicates in the endosome with the production of a number of peptides. MHC class II molecules produced in the endoplasmic reticulum (ER) are transported to the endosome. A protein, the invariant chain, binds to the MHC molecule during transport to prevent binding to endogenous peptide. Once in the endosome the invariant chain is released and the active MHC molecule binds to any exogenously derived peptides present, including peptides belonging to the *hsp* group. For example in leprosy the MHC class II molecule, DR3 binds to a specific amino acid sequence of the *hsp* produced by the organism, other DR molecules (DR1, DR5, DR2) bind to multiple amino acid sequence areas of this heat shock protein. The MHC–peptide complex migrates to the cell surface where it is recognized and bound by a TCR on a CD4+ Th1 cell. Recognition requires an

additional signal to the T cell, this being provided by B7 expression on the surface of the MP when it is infected. The B7 molecule is recognized by CD28 on the T-cell surface. The CD4 Th1 cell then releases IL-2, gamma interferon (IFNγ) and tumour necrosis factor (TNF). IFNγ and IL-2 act on the macrophage to produce more TNF. IFNγ and TNF act synergistically on the two main macrophage cytotoxic pathways, the superoxide pathway producing ROI and the nitric oxide pathway producing RNI. The nitric oxide production is particularly important in the eradication of leishmania and mycobacteria. TNF plays a part in granuloma formation, is chemotactic for monocytes and induces the expression of adhesion molecules on the surface of endothelial cells thereby enabling leucocyte emigration. The release of TNF by macrophages may lead to a potentially self-amplifying chain with further accumulation of macrophages. The successful containment and eradication of intracellular organisms depends on the production of IFNγ and IL-2 (Fig. 37.3).

The diverse spectrum of disease produced by organisms such as *M. leprae* and *Leishmania* can be explained by the type of cytokines produced by the CD4+ cell when stimulated by the peptide/MHC class II molecule. It has been shown that patients who eliminate *Leishmania* easily and patients with a vigorous response to the leprosy bacillus (as in tuberculoid leprosy) produce predominantly IL-2 and IFNγ. Those with chronic leishmaniasis or with the lepromatous form of leprosy, in which many organisms can be found, produce predominantly IL-4 and IL-10 induced by a Th2 response. These two cytokines inhibit the IFN-induced production of ROI and RNI and hence prevent MP killing of the organism.

Organisms within the cytoplasm (CD8+ response)

The commonest cytoplasmic micro-organisms are viruses, although some bacteria such as *Listeria monocytogenes* can escape from an endosome into the cytoplasmic compartment. Viruses gain entry to the cell often by attachment to specific cell receptors. Some of these are well described such as the CD21 receptor used by the Epstein–Barr virus and those belonging to the immunoglobulin superfamily of proteins such as the CD4 receptor used by the glycoprotein 120 of the human immunodeficiency virus, the intracellular adhesion molecule-1 (ICAM-1) which is the major receptor for rhinoviruses and the more recently described polio

virus receptor. The distribution of specific cell receptors is one of the determinants of tissue tropism. The binding of the rabies virus, for example, to acetylcholine receptors which are present at the neuromuscular junction provide the mechanism for neural uptake and subsequent transfer to the central nervous system. Once entry to the cell has been obtained and transcription and translation started, viral proteins in the cytoplasm are pumped by distinct cellular transporter molecules to the rough endoplasmic reticulum where they are transferred on to MHC class I molecules. From there they are taken to the cell surface in a secretory vesicle and inserted in the outer cell membrane. The MHC class I/peptide complex is recognized by specific receptors on the surface of CD8+ T cells. These cells are cytotoxic effector cells (Tc). The exact mechanism causing death of the target cell is not completely understood; however, two possible mechanisms have been described. The most rapid occurs after binding of the Tc to the MHC class I–peptide molecule on the target cell. The cytotoxic cell releases perforin and other enzymes at close proximity to the target cell membrane. In the presence of Ca^{2+} the perforin is polymerized and inserted into the cell membrane to form

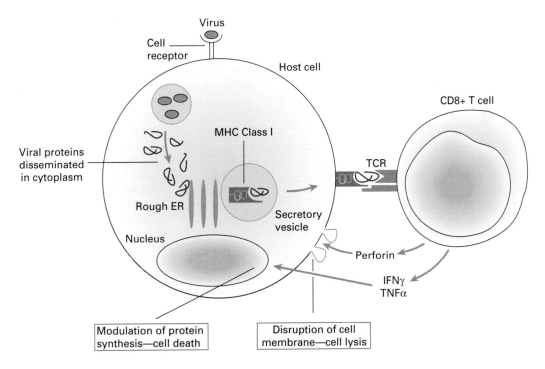

▮ Fig. 37.4 Cell mediated response: organism free in cytoplasm. ER, endoplasmic reticulum; TCR, T cell receptor; MHC, major histocompatibility complex.

channels. These channels allow the other degradative enzymes secreted by the Tc to enter the target. The result is apoptosis or death of the cell. (Fig. 37.4) The cytotoxic cell secretes a protective molecule preventing damage to itself. A slower killing mechanism requires the release of cytokines, $TNF\alpha$ and $IFN\gamma$ from the Tc which modulate protein synthesis in the target cell via receptors eventually causing cell damage and death. If the infected cell is destroyed before the release of new infectious particles, e.g. virions which have not been fully assembled, expansion of the infection can be prevented. However, if the immune response lags behind completed organism replication, immune-mediated cell damage occurs without containment of infection. The pathology seen with some viral infections is mainly due to the immune response.

Evasive mechanisms

Most viruses have not evolved specific mechanisms to avoid or interfere with the immune response, but those organisms that achieve persistent or latent infection have evolved such strategies. For example adenoviruses have two distinct mechanism for downregulating the expression of MHC class I molecules on the surface of infected cells. The first involves the production by the virus of a protein that binds to both the ER and to MHC class I molecules resulting in the retention of the resulting complex in the ER. The second mechanism involves the production of a different protein, which greatly reduces the levels of MHC class I antigen mRNA. This protein is made early during viral gene expression. Later gene products may override this protein indicating its importance in persistent infection when early gene products are expressed in the absence of late gene expression. Similarly, human cytomegalovirus reduces MHC class I expression as a post-transcriptional event.

Combined humoral and cell-mediated response

The response to most organisms is complex and involves varying combinations of the humoral and cellular mechanisms. An example can be seen with the influenza virus. This virus has two major antigenic structures on the capsid, a haemagglutinin and a neuraminidase. These structures undergo frequent change. Major changes, called antigenic shifts, occur infrequently and result in influenza pandemics. Minor changes, called antigenic drifts, occur often and are responsible for the less severe outbreaks seen every year. The neuraminadase and haemagglutinin antigens are recognized by the humoral immune system and the response is MHC class II restricted. Antibodies bind

to the virus preventing cell entry or if taken up by a cell prevent escape from the lysosome into the cytoplasm. Vaccine strategy is aimed at providing an antibody response to the most recent types of haemaglutinins and neurominidases. If the virus escapes the humoral response, it enters the cytoplasm of the infected cell with subsequent transcription and translation of the viral genome leading to new virus production. The viral proteins in the cytoplasm are more likely to be of the more conserved internal nonstructural type. An MHC class I restricted response is generated with cytotoxic T-cell lysis of the infected cells.

The response to parasites that are too large to be phagocytosed also involves both humoral and cell-mediated mechanisms. The features of helminth infections are an elevated IgE serum concentration, eosinophilia, and increased numbers of mast cells. The traditional explanation for these features has been that they confer some degree of immunity. Antigens produced by the parasites result in a T-cell (Th2) dependent humoral response with the production of cytokines IL-4, IL-5, IL-6, and IL-10, with B-cell activation and proliferation. The antibodies produced are of both IgG and IgE classes. Eosinophils are attracted to the worm by parasite-derived chemotactic factors and are stimulated to proliferate by eosinophil stimulation promoter (ESP) produced by the antigen-stimulated Th2 cells. Damage to the parasite is caused by antibody-dependent cellular cytotoxicity (ADCC). Specific antibody bound to the surface of the organism binds to receptors on neutrophils, macrophages, and eosinophils bringing them in close proximity to the parasite integument where they degranulate. The neutrophils and macrophages release toxic oxygen products as described above. The eosinophil granules contain two major toxic products, eosinophil major basic protein (MBP) and eosinophil cationic protein (ECP), the latter protein being a member of the perforin family. The ECP is a more potent product but the MBP is produced in greater concentrations and therefore plays a more important part. The IgE-specific antibodies also sensitize mast cells which release mediators when they come into contact with antigen. These mediators attract more eosinophils as well as promoting a local inflammatory response.

Recent work has questioned this simplistic explanation with some evidence being produced that the eosinophilia and elevated IgE may be immunopathological manifestations of the dominant Th2 response, with immune protection being conferred more by a Th1 response or by some other unidentified cytokine produced by the Th2 cells.

Immunopathology of infectious diseases

In general, the immune response results in clearance of the infecting organism from the body or the maintenance of latency. In some circumstances, however, the disease produced is due to the immune response itself. This may be due to a granulomatous reaction or tissue damage sustained by cell destruction during a cell-mediated response, inappropriate antibody production, immune complex formation, the production of large amounts of cytokines, or the initiation of an auto-immune response (Table 37.2).

Cell-mediated response induced tissue damage

Granulomatous reactions commonly result from the persistent presence within macrophages of micro-organisms which the cell is unable to destroy by a CD4+ T-cell mediated response. *Mycobacterium tuberculosis* and *M. leprae* typically produce granulomas consisting of a core of epithelioid cells and macrophages often with a central area of necrosis surrounded by a cuff of lymphocytes. Multinucleated giant cells are present, the internal structure of which suggests that they are a terminal differentiation stage of the monocyte/macrophage line.

Tissue damage during the course of a normal cell-mediated immune reaction can be seen with many viral diseases, for example, in persistent hepatitis B infection it has been suggested that liver injury results from hepatitis B virus (HBV)-specific cytotoxic lymphocytes lysing virus-infected hepatocytes. The destruction of lung tissue during influenza pneumonia can be attributed to the lysis by Tc of virally infected bronchial and parenchymal cells.

Inappropriate antibody production

The production of antibody can in some circumstances lead to the phenomenon of *antibody-dependent enhancement*. For example a second infection with a differing serotype of the dengue virus can give rise to the dengue shock syndrome (DSS), the enhancement being that non-neutralizing antibody produced to the first serotype infection binds to the second infecting serotype facilitating uptake by macrophages via the Fc receptor. This leads to increased viral replication with high titres. The ensuing shock is mediated by increased cytokine release from the infected cells.

▌ **Table 37.2**   Disease produced by the immune response

Immune mechanism	Tissue damage/disease entity	Initiators
Cell mediated response		
CD4+ helper T cells	Granulomatous disease	Mycobacteria
CD8+ cytotoxic T cells	Destruction of infected cells	
	hepatitis HBV	
	pneumonia Influenza	
Humoral		
Antibody dependent enhancement	Haemorrhagic shock	Dengue virus
Immune complex formation	Glomerulonephritis	Group A streptococci
	Skin rash	HBV, measles virus
Cytokine production	Septic shock	Endotoxins
		lipopolysaccharide of Gram-negative rods
		cell wall components of Gram-positive cocci and yeasts
	Toxic shock syndrome	Superantigens
	Food poisoning	TSST-1 of staphylococci
		enterotoxins of staphylococci
Autoimmune	Rheumatic fever	Group A streptococci
	myocarditis	
	arthritis	
	endocarditis	

Immune complex formation

Immune complex formation resulting in disease has been described for many organisms. Post-streptococcal glomerulonephritis is at least partially the result of immune complex deposition in glomeruli of the kidney. The glomerulonephritis seen with HBV infection is also thought to be due to immune complex deposition as is the rash and arthralgias of this and many other viral infections.

Cytokine production

Septic shock is a particular consequence of the release of large amounts of cytokines after exposure to bacterial components. Septic shock is defined as the presence of clinical infection with fever, tachycardia, tachypnoea, and evidence of inadequate organ perfusion as evidenced by altered mental state, oliguria, or elevated plasma lactate. The mortality is almost 50%. The pathogenesis of septic shock is now understood to be a cascade of inflammatory mediators, which are part of the normal immune response but in this case act in an exaggerated manner resulting in severe endothelial damage, profound haemodynamic impairment, and potentially death.

The cascade of events is initiated most commonly by endotoxins of which the lipopolysaccharide (LPS) of Gram-negative bacilli is the most frequent, although other endotoxins such as Gram-positive cell wall products and yeast components can equally be the cause. The central cells mediating this response are macrophages and endothelial cells. A normal component of serum, LPS-binding protein, binds to the lipid A portion of bacterial LPS enhancing opsonization and hence phagocytosis of intact bacteria. However, when free endotoxin binds to LPS-binding protein there is potent macrophage activation and therefore production of TNF. This production of TNF is due to accelerated transcription of the TNF gene and translation of TNF mRNA as a result of the binding of the LPS/LPS-binding protein complex to CD14 molecule receptors on the macrophage. The activated macrophage also produces other cytokines, IL-1, IL-6, IL-8, and platelet-aggregating factor (PAF). TNF and IL-1 act synergistically on the endothelial cell, which in turn also produces IL-6, IL-8, and PAF. The combined action of TNF and IL-1 produce changes in the cytoskeletal structure of the endothelial cell thereby increasing the permeability of the vascular wall. There is enhanced expression of adhesion molecules on the endothelial cell surface giving increased adhesiveness for both neutrophils and lymphocytes thus potentiating the attraction and accumulation of leucocytes at the site of inflammation. There are a number of different adhesion molecules (GMP-140, ELAM-1, LAM-1, VCAM-1, ICAM-1 and 2) produced to differing stimuli including local inflammatory mediators such as histamine and thrombin as well as to the cytokines. The different molecules are produced at varying times after the initial insult thereby changing the cellular nature of the inflammatory exudate. Neutrophils can induce damage to the endothelium due to the release of ROI and lysosomal enzymes and their adherence to the endothelium gives rise to vasodilatation. The endothelial cell normally has surface anticoagulant properties due to the production of thrombomodulin and protein S, which catalyse the activated protein C pathway. TNF and IL-1 can initiate the extrinsic clotting pathway by inducing the production of tissue factor which binds to factor VIIa and by decreasing the expression of thrombomodulin.

LPS has a direct effect on the endothelial cell, in ways similar to TNF and IL-1, in promoting clotting and leucocyte attraction. In addition LPS and TNF can activate the coagulation cascade and the complement system. C3a and C5a are produced in large quantities leading to activation and degranulation of neutrophils, basophils, and mast cells with resulting further tissue damage by reactive oxygen radicals and lysozymes.

The sequence of events during septic shock is very complex and many of the mediators have multiple functions and negative feedback mechanisms. The tissue damage, increased vascular permeability resulting in hypotension and thus impaired organ perfusion and the coagulopathy are all a result of immune mechanisms with TNF and IL-1 playing a central part. The endothelial cell and its response to these mediators is crucial as well. Numerous therapeutic approaches are being considered to interrupt the cascade. Antibodies to LPS, to LPS-binding protein and to the CD14 receptor are possibilities in the early phase of infection. Antibodies to TNF and IL-1 are being trialled. Most clinical trials so far, however, have shown only partial benefit, probably reflecting the complex pathways with multiple interacting factors.

Toxic shock syndrome and staphylococcal food poisoning are other diseases mediated primarily by the excess production of cytokines. These are thought to be due to the production of superantigens by the causative organism, e.g. the staphylococcal exotoxin, TSST-1, and staphylococcal enterotoxin. Superantigens bind to the variable (V) region of the MHC class II molecule on APCs which is separate to the normal peptide binding site, and to the same region on the TCR, resulting in T-cell activation (Fig. 37.5). Each superantigen may be recognized by a number of V types each having a large range of peptide–antigen specificites. A conventional antigen can activate only those T-helper cells that are specific for that antigen whereas a superantigen can activate an enormous number, the only limitation being the V type. The activation of many T-helper cells is accompanied by the release of large amounts of IL-2 and TNF giving rise to the fever, malaise, nausea, vomiting, and shock seen in these diseases. Autoimmune reactions can also occur due to the activation and multiplication of the small number of T cells that recognize self. Immune suppression can also occur as the T cells may die after activation.

Autoimmune response

Rheumatic fever is thought to arise as a consequence of autoimmune mechanisms initiated by a group A streptococcal infection. Rheumatic fever is characterized by inflammation of cardiac muscle, cardiac valves, synovium, skin, and neurons within the caudate and subthalamic nuclei of the brain, giving rise to a variety of clinical manifestations such as carditis, endocarditis, arthritis, subcutaneous nodules, and Sydenham's chorea. These manifestations arise about 3 weeks following a group A streptococcal infection. It has been suggested that the poststreptococcal sequelae are due to molecular mimicry between streptococcal M proteins, particularly types 1, 5, 6, 12, and 19, streptococcal membrane proteins and host tissue proteins. M proteins are helical coiled-coil proteins, a structure shared with host tissue such as myosin, keratin, tropomyosin, vimentin, and laminin. Cross-reactive antibodies have been demonstrated between streptococcal M protein and human cardiac antigens located in cardiac myosin and sarcolemmal membrane. In addition, myosin and vimentin present in heart valves react with monoclonal antibodies against M protein. Valvular interstitial cells contain large amounts of vimentin and antibody reactions with these cells may result in inflammatory changes leading to collagen deposition seen on valves during the acute phase of rheumatic fever. Antibodies reacting with cytoplasmic antigens of neurons within the caudate and subthalamic nuclei have been described from patients with Sydenham's chorea. These findings support the hypothesis that rheumatic fever is an autoimmune disease initiated by infection with a group A streptococcus of certain M protein type. The limited occurrence of disease despite frequent streptococcal infection requires the involvement of some selective mechanism. A genetic susceptibility would be one explanation and there is some evidence to support this. An increased incidence of rheumatic fever has been associated with HLA-DR2 in black people and HLA-DR4 in Caucasians.

Further reading

Akira, S. and Kishimoto, T. (1992). IL-6 and NF-IL6 in acute-phase response and viral infection. *Immunological Reviews*, **127**, 25–50.

Bradley, J., Wilks, D., and Rubenstein, D. (1994). The vascular endothelium in septic shock. *Journal of Infection*, **28**, 1–10.

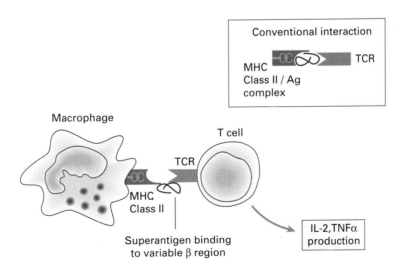

∎ **Fig. 37.5** Interaction of superantigen with the immune system. MHC, major histocompatibility complex; Ag, antigen; TCR, T cell receptor.

Cerami, A. (1992). Inflammatory cytokines. *Clinical Immunology and Immunopathology*, **62**, S3–10.

Doherty, P., *et al.* (1992). Roles of and T cell subsets in viral immunity. *Annual Review of Immunology 10*, 123–51.

Frank, M. (1990). Complement in host defense against bacterial infections. In *Microbial determinants of virulence and host response* (ed. E., Ayoub, G., Cassell, W., Branche, T. Henry), pp. 305–17. American Society for Microbiology, Washington DC.

Giroir, B. (1993). Mediators of septic shock. New approaches for interrupting the endogenous inflammatory cascade. *Critical Care Medicine*, **21**, 780–89.

Janeway, C. (1993). How the immune system recognises invaders. *Scientific American*, **September** 41–7.

Johnson, H., Russell, J., and Pontzer, C. (1992). Superantigens in human disease. *Scientific American*, **April**, 42–8.

Kaufman, S. (1993). Immunity to intracellular bacteria. *Annual Review of Immunology*, **11**, 129–63.

Levi, M., *et al.* (1993). Pathogenesis of disseminated intravascular coagulation in sepsis. *Journal of the American Medical Association*, **270**, 975–9.

Paul, W. (1993). Infectious disease and the immune system. *Scientific American*, **September**, 57–63.

Sher, A., and Coffman, R. (1992). Regulation of immunity to parasites by T cells and T cell-derived cytokines. *Annual Review of Immunology*, **10**, 385–409.

Taub, D., and Blank, K. (1993). Superantigens and microbial pathogenesis. *Annals of Internal Medicine*, **119**, 89–90.

Vassalli, P. (1992). The pathophysiology of tumor necrosis factors. *Annual Review of Immunology*, **10**, 411–52.

38 Mycobacterial infections

W. J. Britton and R. J. Garsia

Introduction

The host immune response is critical to the outcome of infection with mycobacteria. Resurgence of tuberculosis with the development of multidrug resistant (MDR) strains of *Mycobacterium tuberculosis* has refocused efforts to understand mechanisms of host immunity and mycobacterial virulence. The increased prevalence of tuberculosis in industrialized countries since the mid-1980s is related both to coinfection with human immunodeficiency virus (HIV) and the failure of tuberculosis programmes to provide effective control to deprived groups such as the homeless and poor. The disease, however, had never been adequately controlled in non-industrialized countries despite the availability of chemotherapy. Currently, a third of the human race is infected with *M. tuberculosis* resulting in clinical tuberculosis in 8 million and death for 2.8 million individuals each year, making tuberculosis the major fatal infectious disease of adults. Widespread subclinical infection also occurs with *M. leprae* with over 1.2 billion people still exposed to the bacillus. The prevalence of clinical leprosy is falling with the implementation of effective multidrug therapy; however, leprosy remains a major cause of disability in developing countries because of immune-mediated nerve damage. Other mycobacteria, in particular members of the *M. avium–intracellulare complex* (MAC), have emerged as common opportunistic infections in advanced HIV infection.

This chapter will address the host response to mycobacteria as a paradigm of the interaction between intracellular parasites and the immune system. Paradoxically in both tuberculosis and leprosy, cellular immune responses are responsible for both protective immunity and tissue destruction. In most infected individuals the response limits the mycobacterial infection even if the organisms are not completely eradicated. This is at the expense of developing a granulomatous response which damages lung and nerve, respectively.

Mycobacteria are obligate intracellular bacteria with complex cell walls rich in mycolic acid which confers the property of acid fast staining to the bacilli. It is important, however, to realize that there are considerable differences between individual Mycobacterial spp. in their growth characteristics, virulence, route of infection, and persistence in immunocompetent hosts, all of which may influence the host immune response.

Components of the immune response to mycobacteria

The cellular response to mycobacteria depends on the interplay between phagocytic cells of the monocyte lineage and T lymphocytes.

Role of the mononuclear phagocytes

Mononuclear phagocytes, either as circulating monocytes or differentiated tissue macrophages, play a critical part in mycobacterial infections. These cells are the preferred habitat for mycobacteria, but also serve as the chief effector cells for killing mycobacteria. The balance between these functions determines the outcome of infection. As monocytes are mobile, relatively long-lived cells, their infection provides an effective mechanism for the dissemination of mycobacteria throughout the host. Phagocytosis of mycobacteria by macrophages is enhanced by their binding to integrin receptors. This process is independent of Fc receptor binding and so avoids triggering an antimicrobial oxidative burst. Both *M. tuberculosis* and *M. leprae* utilize the macrophage complement receptors CR1 and CR3, which bind to C3 breakdown products fixed by surface phenolic glycolipid. Mycobacteria also bind to fibronectin and vitronectin receptors, the former through fibronectin-binding surface proteins.

The initial response of the macrophage determines whether productive infection ensues. Strains which are avirulent in immunocompetent individuals induce the

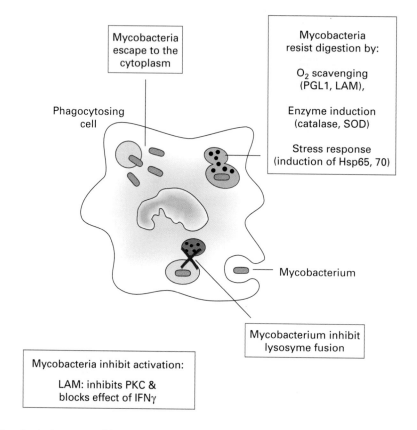

Mycobacteria
escape to the
cytoplasm

Mycobacteria
resist digestion by:

O$_2$ scavenging
(PGL1, LAM),

Enzyme induction
(catalase, SOD)

Stress response
(induction of Hsp65, 70)

Phagocytosing
cell

Mycobacterium

Mycobacterium inhibit
lysosyme fusion

Mycobacteria inhibit activation:

LAM: inhibits PKC &
blocks effect of IFNγ

∎ **Fig. 38.1** Mycobacteria may avoid macrophage-mediated killing in various ways. LAM, lipoarabinomannan; SOD, superoxide dismutase; PKC, protein kinase C; hsp, heat shock protein; IFN γ, interferon gamma.

early activation of macrophages by the direct stimulation of tumour necrosis factor (TNF) α release triggered by the complex cell wall carbohydrate, liparabinomannan (LAM). LAM from virulent strains of *M. tuberculosis* fails to stimulate this early activation, enabling the organisms to multiply within infected macrophages, a necessary step in the induction of disease. Virulent *M. tuberculosis* also partially inhibits the fusion of the infected phagosome with lysosomes through the action of cell wall sulphatides. The organisms secrete ammonium which prevents acidification of the phagolysosome and activation of hydrolytic enzymes. Furthermore, the mycobacterial cell wall retards digestion, in part due to the capacity of LAM and phenolic glycolipid to scavenge oxygen radicals and to the inhibition by LAM of macrophage activation by cytokines.

Infected monocytes/macrophages can thus act as antigen-presenting cells (APCs) in the stimulation of T cells and are particularly important in the local stimulation of CD4+ $\alpha\beta$ T cells at the site of infection.

Although unstimulated monocytes are unable to eradicate pathogenic mycobacteria, sufficient degradation of mycobacterial proteins occurs within them to release peptides which enter the human leucocyte antigen (HLA) Class II or endosomal pathway of antigen presentation. This class II restriction of the T-cell response to mycobacterial peptides underlies the modest association of different HLA phenotypes with some mycobacterial diseases. For example, HLA-linked genes have an influence on the clinical pattern of leprosy, although they do not confer susceptibility to leprosy *per se*. HLA-DR2 and HLA-DR3 are associated with tuberculoid leprosy whereas HLA-DQ1 is increased in patients with lepromatous leprosy. The effect of HLA haplotype on tuberculosis is less clear; however, HLA-DR15 (DR2) is weakly associated with pulmonary tuberculosis.

T-lymphocyte response

The control of mycobacterial infections was the first function attributed to cellular immunity when Chase in

1945 demonstrated that tuberculin reactivity could be transferred between infected and non-infected animals with cell suspensions but not with serum. Subsequently, T lymphocytes and then the CD4+ subset were identified as the principal effector cells. The importance of CD4+ T cells is clinically apparent in HIV infection where their depletion renders the patient exquisitely sensitive to tuberculosis (v.i.). Studies in gene knockout (GKO) mice have confirmed earlier studies indicating that a variety of T-cell subsets contribute to the integrated response to mycobacteria. In GKO mice the genes for single, cell surface glycoproteins or cytokines are disrupted selectively in order to define the role of that molecule. This has revealed that T cells bearing $\alpha\beta$ T-cell receptors (TCR) of both CD4+ and CD8+ phenotype are essential for the control of murine *M. bovis* infection, the expression of delayed-type hypersensitivity (DTH) to mycobacterial antigens and the development of tissue granulomas. In addition, deletion of T cells bearing $\gamma\delta$

TCRs demonstrated that they also participate in the primary response to mycobacteria.

Activation of mycobacteria-specific $\alpha\beta$ CD4+ T cells at the site of infection leads to their proliferation and the release of interleukin-2 (IL-2) (Fig. 38.2). Only the minority of T cells in a tuberculosis or leprosy lesion are antigen-specific and the local inflammatory response is amplified by the recruitment and activation of other CD4+ T cells by IL-2. In addition IL-2 stimulates the expansion of CD8+ T cells and antigen–nonspecific natural killer (NK) cells in leprosy and tuberculosis lesions. The activity of CD4+ T cells is determined by the pattern of cytokines released. Although the clear dichotomy between Th1 and Th2 type T cells observed in mouse T-cell clones is not as apparent in human responses, mycobacteria-reactive CD4+ T cells generally produce an abundance of interferon (IFN) γ and IL-2 and are best classified as Th1 and Th0 phenotype. For example, the infiltrating T cells in tuberculoid leprosy lesions produce both IL-2

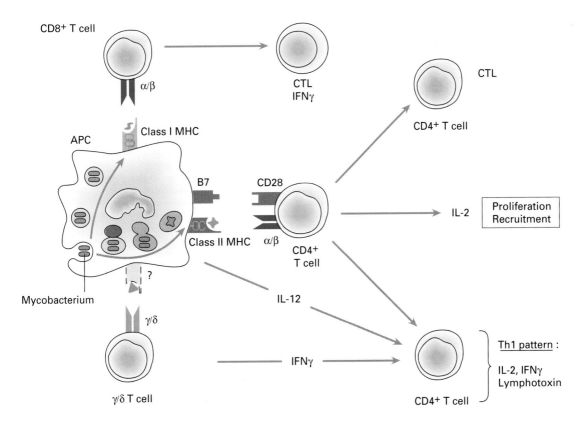

▌**Fig. 38.2** Cellular interactions initiated during mycobacterial infections include activation of CD4+ and CD8+ $\alpha\beta$ T cells and $\gamma\delta$ T cells. MHC, major histocomplatibility complex; APC, antigen-presenting cells; CTL, cytotoxic T lymphocyte.

and IFNγ locally, as do T-cell clones derived from the peripheral blood or pleural fluid of tuberculosis patients. This pattern of cytokine release is determined at the time of activation of the CD4+ T cells, possibly by the cytokine milieu. Mycobacteria-infected macrophages release IL-12, a heterodimeric cytokine first described as NK cell activating factor. A major activity of IL-12 is on T cells undergoing activation, directing them towards the release of IL-2 and IFNγ. Therefore IL-12 plays a critical part in the development of protective immunity towards intracellular pathogens.

The major cytokine triggering mycobacterial killing by macrophages is IFNγ. The essential role of IFNγ is dramatically evident in IFNγ GKO mice which rapidly succumb to a low dose of *M. tuberculosis* with extensive necrosis of infected organs. IFNγ alone, however, is not sufficient to activate the full bactericidal potential of macrophages as this requires at least two separate signals. Experimentally, these have been defined as T-cell-derived IFNγ and monocyte-derived TNFα. However, CD4+ T cells also produce lymphotoxin (TNFβ), granulocyte–macrophage colony-stimulating factor (GM-CSF), IL-3, and the recently cloned macrophage inhibition factor (MIF), all of which may play a part in macrophage activation. An additional activating factor for human macrophages is 1,25 di(OH)-cholecalciferol, which is converted from the inactive circulating form of 25(OH)-vitamin D3 by 1-hydrolase within activated macrophages. This synergizes with IFNγ to stimulate mycobacterial killing. Excessive production of calcitriol during tuberculosis occasionally causes hypercalcaemia.

In addition to releasing cytokines, antimycobacterial CD4+ T cells, particularly those reactive with heat shock protein (Hsp)65 and Hsp70, have direct cytolytic activity against macrophages infected with mycobacteria. Parasitized tissue macrophages eventually lose their bactericidal capacity and lysis of these cells by CD4+ cytolytic T cells releases mycobacteria which are then phagocytosed by fresh monocytes with full bactericidal capacity.

HLA class I-restricted CD8+ T cells also play a part in protective immunity against mycobacteria. These cells accumulate at the site of mycobacterial infections, forming a cuff of CD8+ T cells about epithelioid cell granulomas. Mycobacteria-specific T CD8+ cell lines have been isolated from infected mice and less frequently from patients. The strongest evidence for the participation of this T-cell subset in protection is the failure of β_2-microglobulin GKO mice deficient in CD8+ T cells to control *M. tuberculosis* infection. In addition to their cytotoxic function, mycobacteria-reactive CD8+ T cells secrete IFNγ and IL-4, which may have an immunoregulatory role.

T cells bearing γδ TCR also contribute to the control of mycobacterial infections. γδ T cells accumulate in leprosy skin lesions, particularly during reversal reactions which are marked by an upswing in cellular reactivity to *M. leprae*. They are also prominent in the initial murine T-cell response to mycobacterial infection in the lung and lymph node. Living, but not dead, mycobacteria stimulate the selective expansion of γδ T cells from the blood, skin, and pleural exudate of patients with tuberculosis or leprosy. This expansion is not HLA restricted and is oligoclonal suggesting it is driven by a specific mycobacterial antigen. Initially hsp 65 was implicated as the dominant antigen, but low molecular weight non-protein moieties are now considered to be more important. Mycobacteria-reactive γδ T cells secrete IFNγ, GM-CSF, IL-3, and TNF all of which may contribute to macrophage activation, particularly at mucosal sites early in the course of mycobacterial infection.

Macrophage killing mechanisms

The specific cytokine requirements for activation of macrophages and the bactericidal mechanisms utilized vary for macrophages of different species and different mycobacteria. In human macrophages IFNγ-induced killing of *M. leprae* is accompanied by an oxidative burst, but the generation of reactive oxygen metabolites alone has been an inadequate explanation for macrophage-mediated killing of other mycobacterial species. Non-oxidative mechanisms are also important including digestion by acid hydrolases and other enzymes. Nitric oxide (NO) produced by an IFNγ responsive inducible NO synthase (iNOS) has been implicated as an important mechanism in murine macrophages for killing *M. tuberculosis* and *M. leprae*, but this appears less important in human phagocytes.

Pathogenesis of tissue damage

Persistence of mycobacteria within macrophages provides chronic stimulation to T cells with the local release of cytokines. In this environment macrophages transform into epithelioid cells which may fuse to form multinucleate giant cells (Fig. 38.3). The aggregation of epithelioid cells to form granulomas is dependent on TNFα released by both antigen-reactive T cells and activated macrophages. Typically, granulomas in tuberculosis and tuberculoid leprosy contain a 2:1 predominance of CD4+ to CD8+ T cells with the CD4+ T cells mixed with the epithelioid cells and CD8+ T cells forming a peripheral cuff. In the absence of a specific T-cell response as in lepromatous leprosy or tuberculosis complicating HIV infection, there is a paucity of T cells with equal proportions of CD4+ and CD8+ cells

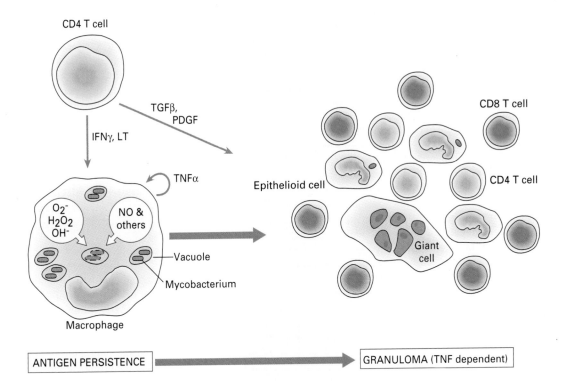

∎ **Fig. 38.3** The mechanisms used by macrophages to kill mycobacteria include generation of reactive oxygen and nitrogen metabolites. Failure to eradicate mycobacteria stimulates the prolonged release of TNF-α and other cytokines and the formation of granulomas. TNF, tumour necrosis factor; LT, leukotriene; PDGF, platelet-derived growth factor; TGF, transforming growth factor.

and the granulomas consist of a loose collection of macrophages laden with mycobacteria and their lipid products (Fig. 38.3).

The accumulation of granulomas leads to destruction of the normal architecture of the infected tissue. In response to transforming growth factor-β (TGFβ) and platelet-derived growth factor (PGDF) the granuloma is walled off with newly synthesized fibrous tissue. The centre of the granuloma may undergo necrosis with the loss of cellular definition and the formation of amorphous caseous or cheese-like material, which may calcify. Residual extracellular mycobacteria replicate poorly in this anaerobic environment but may persist for years as dormant organisms. However, if the host cellular immunity wanes the bacilli may multiply with reactivation of disease. If the necrotic granuloma erodes into the wall of a bronchus, the caseous material containing mycobacteria is spread throughout the bronchial tree and the aerated cavity becomes an ideal environment for the multiplication of organisms.

Therefore the outcome after mycobacterial infection depends on the degree of the macrophage activation. Prompt and adequate stimulation leads to the killing of the intracellular bacteria without tissue damage. Persistence of mycobacteria results in chronic stimulation of T cells, granulomatous inflammation, and tissue destruction. Rather than two distinct mechanisms of immunity and 'hypersensitivity', these represent a continuum of immunological responses with a variety of clinical outcomes in different mycobacterial infections.

Mycobacterial antigens

Developments in immunological analysis and mycobacterial genetics have led to a rapid increase in our understanding of the structural components of mycobacterial cell walls and protein antigens. Over 50 of the estimated 1000 proteins expressed by *M. tuberculosis* have been partially characterized. A collaborative project to sequence the *M. leprae* genome is well established and with similar initiatives for *M. tuberculosis* underway, the genetic structure of both organisms will soon be available. Many mycobacterial proteins were first identified through their immunological reactivity with monoclonal or polyclonal antibodies. Among the first identified were members of the 65 and 70 kDa Hsp families. These ubiquitous proteins are dominant antigens in other intracellular bacteria and protozoa, despite sharing about 50% amino acid identity with their human homologues. This raises the possibility that T and B cells stimulated by mycobacterial Hsps will cross-react with host Hsps and react with stressed cells to induce or perpetuate autoimmune tissue damage. Although this phenomenon occurs in certain experimental models of autoimmune disease, such as adjuvant-induced arthritis, the human cellular response to Hsps is generally restricted to mycobacteria-specific determinants on the proteins. Further, the anti-Hsp 65 or Hsp 70 antibodies reported in rheumatoid arthritis or systemic lupus erythematosus (SLE) are not pathogenic.

Temporal analysis of the T-cell response during murine tuberculosis has demonstrated that proteins secreted by viable mycobacteria are recognized early in the course of infection by IFNγ producing T cells. Cytoplasmic proteins such as Hsps only elicited a T-cell response later in the course of the infection after some mycobacterial degradation had occurred. It has been long recognized that immunization with viable mycobacteria is essential for stimulating protective immunity against tuberculosis in both humans and animals. This may be due in part to the capacity of live mycobacteria to elaborate these secreted proteins. This notion is supported by the observation that immunization with a mixture of secreted proteins protects mice against subsequent infection with *M. tuberculosis*.

Natural history of mycobacterial infections

Tuberculosis

The major route of infection of *M. tuberculosis* is the lung. Aerosol droplets of <5 μm diameter reach the alveoli where the mycobacteria are ingested by alveolar macrophages. Virulent *M. tuberculosis* is able to resist initial macrophage defence mechanisms and the organisms multiply slowly with doubling times of 18–24 h. The infected macrophages enter the interstitium where in response to phagocytosis of *M. tuberculosis* they release proinflammatory cytokines including

TNF, IL-1, monocyte chemotactic protein-I (MCP-I), and other chemokines of the IL-8 family. These induce the expression of adhesion molecules on vascular endothelium and the influx of leucocytes. The initial inflammatory cells are predominantly polymorphonuclear neutrophils which, although activated, are unable to control the infection. During this period infected monocytes may spread through the bloodstream to other organs. Some infected macrophages or antigen-containing dendritic cells migrate to the draining hilar lymph nodes where mycobacteria-specific CD4+ T cells are activated. After 6–8 weeks development of cell-mediated immunity leads to the recruitment of lymphocytes and monocytes to the infected alveoli. The release of cytokines from T cells leads to the activation of mycobacterial killing mechanisms in infected macrophages

In immunocompetent subjects, the majority of mycobacteria are killed and the infection is halted before spread to other organs. Sterilizing immunity is occasionally achieved, but in most infected subjects a small number of organisms persist within the centre of the granuloma. Continuing effective cellular immunity is required to prevent reactivation of the infection. The resulting granuloma within the lung and the draining lymph node is referred to as the primary complex.

Most subjects have no clinical evidence of primary tuberculosis infection apart from the development of a positive skin test to tuberculin, although in a minority of subjects a calcified primary complex is visible on chest radiography. If for a variety of reasons (Table 38.2) the initial T-cell response is unable to control the infection, the infected person may progress to active tuberculosis which may take a variety of clinical patterns. In a general population the lifelong risk of tuberculosis in infected untreated individuals is estimated to be 10%, half of which develops in the first 2 years (Table 38.1).

The first manifestation of tuberculosis is primary pulmonary disease soon after infection, particularly in

▋ **Table 38.1** Properties of *M. tuberculosis* infected subjects who develop clinical tuberculosis

	General population	HIV co-infection
Primary disease	5% in 2 years	37% in 6 months
Reactivated disease	5%	10% per year
Cumulative life-long risk	≤10%	≥50%

those with reduced cellular immunity (Table 38.1). This may take the form of local pneumonia, often in the mid or lower zones. Enlargement of the hilar lymph nodes during a potent antimycobacterial cellular response may obstruct the central bronchi. Involvement of the overlying pleura may cause an exudative pleural effusion with seeding throughout the pleural cavity. In the absence of an effective T-cell response early disseminated disease may result in miliary tuberculosis with haematogenous seeding of mycobacteria throughout the lung and other organs producing small millet-sized inflammatory nodules. The fever and wasting typical of miliary tuberculosis is due to the release of monokines, particularly TNF. Dissemination to other organs, particularly those with high blood flow may result in extrapulmonary disease such as meningitis, bone, and renal tuberculosis.

In the majority of infected subjects, the site of initial infection is walled off by a granulomatous response induced by *M. tuberculosis*-specific T cells; however, some *M. tuberculosis* bacilli persist in most granulomas. During the initial infection seeding commonly occurs to the apices of the lungs where multiplication of *M. tuberculosis* is favoured by the high oxygen tension and low blood flow. Infection is controlled by the onset of the T-cell response, although the granulomatous inflammation with fibrosis often causes tissue damage. Waning of this specific response (Tables 38.1; 38.2) leads to reactivation of dormant bacilli. In response to local cytokine production the caseous necrosis at the centre of the granuloma may liquefy and rupture into a neighbouring airspace resulting in cavitation, a pattern typical of reactivated pulmonary disease. The centre of the cavity surrounded by poorly vascular fibrosis tissue is incompletely penetrated by lymphocytes and fresh monocytes. Extracellular mycobacteria released from necrotic epithelioid cells thrive in the aerobic environment and reach extremely high numbers within the cavity, rendering the subject highly contagious. Mycobacteria may spread via the bronchi to cause tuberculous bronchopneumonia. In addition, reactivation at sites of extrapulmonary spread may cause clinical disease through tissue damage by granulomatous inflammation.

Reduction in protective immunity also renders the individual at risk of reinfection with *M. tuberculosis*. In communities with a declining prevalence of tuberculosis the bulk of pulmonary disease has been attributed to reactivation of past infection rather than reinfection, although until recently it has been impossible to distinguish between the two. Developments in mycobacterial genetics have permitted the characterization of individual isolates with restriction fragment length polymorphism (RFLP) probes. This 'DNA fingerprinting' can identify shared strains which have been transmitted through non-communal or community-acquired infection. The majority of isolates obtained from elderly patients with tuberculosis in European countries are different, confirming that the original infection in these patients was remote. However, 30–40% of successive recent isolates in North American cities demonstrated a limited number of common patterns, indicating that recent active transmission was responsible for the disease. Factors associated with recent transmission were acquired immune deficiency syndrome (AIDS), low socio-economic status and ethnic background.

Leprosy

The dynamic nature of the host response to infection with *M. leprae* is evident in the varied and fluctuating patterns of clinical disease. Subclinical infection by the aerosol route is common in regions of high prevalence, but the gradual development of T-cell-mediated immunity eradicates the infection in over 95% of subjects. In a minority of infected subjects *M. leprae* disseminates to skin and superficial nerves where the bacilli are selectively taken up by macrophages and Schwann cells. Reduced temperatures favour the slow replication of this fastidious bacillus, which is yet to be cultured *in vitro*. Some individuals develop skin lesions of indeterminate leprosy which self-heal in over 50% cases as macrophage bactericidal mechanisms are activated. Cutaneous reactivity to soluble leprosy antigens develops during this subclinical infection and some subjects in regions of high endemicity also mount *M. leprae*-specific serological responses. A further minority progress to unequivocal leprosy of skin or nerves.

The clinical patterns of leprosy form a spectrum which correlates closely with immunopathological responses to the bacillus (Fig. 38.4; 38.5). In tuberculoid (TT) leprosy a vigorous T-cell-mediated response to *M. leprae* is associated with disease limited to a few skin patches or nerve trunks. Few if any bacilli are demonstrable within granulomas in the dermis or peripheral nerves. Cellular immunity is accompanied by strong lymphocyte proliferative responses to *M. leprae* antigens *in vitro*, a positive cutaneous lepromin reaction (*v.i.*) and low-titre anti-*M. leprae* antibody responses. Dominant cytokines expressed within tuberculoid skin lesions include IL-2 and IFNγ and *M. leprae*-reactive T-cell clones secrete similar cytokines of a Th1 or Th0 pattern. By contrast at the lepromatous (LL) pole of the disease spectrum the absence of specific cellular immunity leads to the uncontrolled replication of leprosy bacilli and exten-

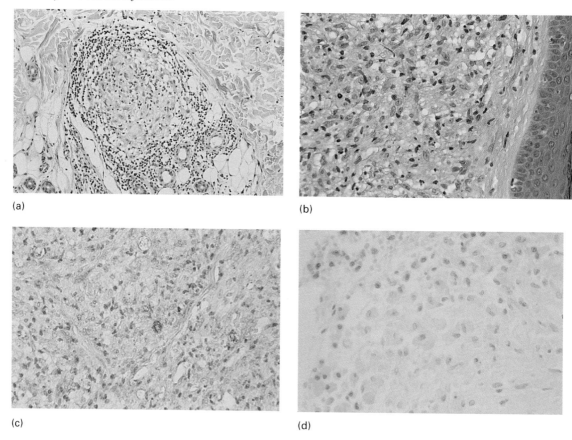

∎ Fig. 38.4 Histological appearance of mycobacterial infections:

Panel (a): Borderline tuberculoid leprosy showing well formed granuloma in the dermis destroying a sweat gland with central epithelioid cells, giant cells and a cuff of lymphocytes. (H&E, ×50).

Panel (b): Borderline lepromatous leprosy with diffuse infiltration of the dermis by lipid laden macrophages and a scattering of lymphocytes, but no epithelioid cell granulomas. (H&E, ×100).

Panel (c): Borderline lepromatous leprosy, section of skin biopsy from patient in Panel B stained for acid fast bacilli showing large numbers of *M. leprae* bacilli within macrophage. Organisms which have been killed become fragmented (H&E, ×100).

Panel (d): Spleen from HIV infected patient with disseminated *M. tuberculosis* infection showing mycobacteria-laden macrophages disrupting the splenic architecture (H&E, ×50).

sive clinical lesions (Fig. 38.6). A high-titre antibody responses to *M. leprae*-specific and cross-reactive antigens is a feature of BL/LL disease. In borderline forms, progressive reduction in cellular immunity is accompanied by more frequent skin and nerve lesions, a greater bacillary load, and increasing antibody levels (Figure 38.5). The polar forms of the disease are stable whereas the borderline forms of the disease tend to downgrade to a more lepromatous form. An enigma in lepromatous leprosy is that cellular reactivity to related mycobacteria is retained even though many of their antigenic components are shared with *M. leprae*. Various explanations for this lepromatous unrespon-

siveness have been proposed including the clonal deletion or anergy of *M. leprae*-reactive T cells or the presence of *M. leprae*-specific suppressor T cells. Both mechanisms are demonstrable in some, but not all, BL/LL patients and the condition is probably heterogeneous in origin. Failure of T-cell recognition is the critical deficit in BL/LL leprosy whereas macrophage function is intact. This is confirmed by the ability of exogenous cytokines IL-2 and IFNγ to activate bactericidal killing in BL/LL patients.

The immunological reactivity of borderline leprosy patients varies with time and results in the different types of leprosy reactions. In reversal or type I reac-

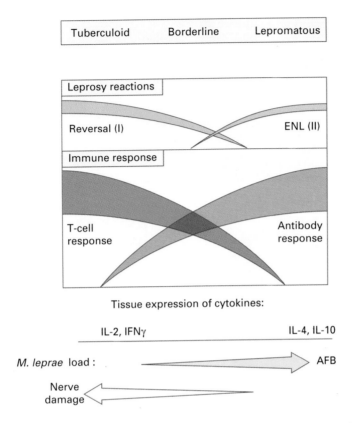

▌ Fig. 38.5 The immunopathological spectrum underlying the clinical patterns of leprosy. ENL, erythema nodosum leprosum; AFB, Acid fast bacilli.

tions there is a spontaneous increase in the cellular reactivity of borderline (BT, BB, BL) patients. This causes influx of IFNγ secreting T cells into skin and nerve lesions leading to macrophage activation and acute inflammation. The skin lesions become raised and erythematous and are marked by increased HLA class II and ICAM-I expression on keratinocytes. Inflammatory swelling within the perineurium of nerve trunks leads to vascular insufficiency and further nerve damage. As a result reversal reactions are a major contributor to nerve function loss in superficial nerve trunks (e.g. ulnar, median, radial, lateral popliteal, posterior tibial, and facial nerves). This results in muscle imbalance, leading to the typical deformities of claw hand and dropped foot, sensory impairment causing trophic ulceration and corneal insensitivity, and facial palsy. Prompt use of high-dose corticosteroids controls the inflammation and prevents or even reverses nerve damage.

Erythema nodosum leprosum (ENL) or type II reactions are restricted to patients with BL or LL disease. This is a model of a type II hypersensitivity reaction with deposition of immune complexes in the skin, eyes, kidney, testis, and nerves manifesting as a 'vasculitis-like' rash, iritis, glomerulonephritis, and orchitis. More recently, T cells have been implicated in the activation of the process. For example, an unwanted effect of IFNγ therapy in BL/LL patients was the induction of ENL in 60% of patients in the first 6 months compared with 15% in control BL/LL patients. The ENL episodes are associated with a rise in serum TNF levels which is responsible for the marked systemic effects of fever, myalgia, and arthralgia. The dramatic effects of thalidomide in controlling ENL have justified its careful use, despite the risks of teratogenicity and neuropathy. The rapid control of inflammation by thalidomide is due to its effects in inhibiting the release of TNF from monocytes.

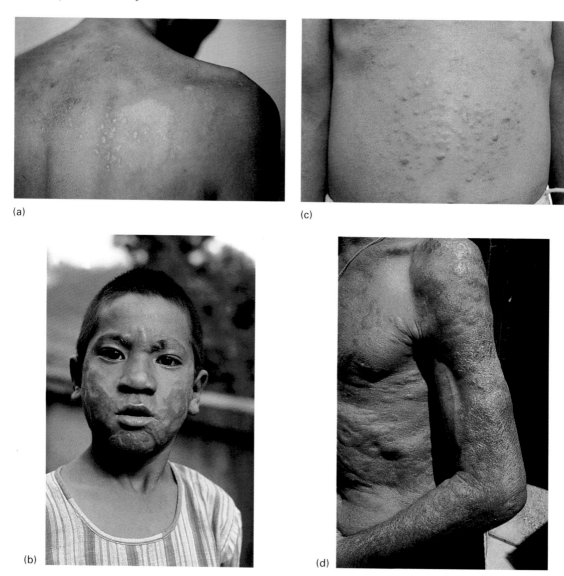

∎ Fig. 38.6 (a) Borderline tuberculoid leprosy. Hypopigmented anaesthetic macule with a raised border typical of BT leprosy. A small adjacent satellite lesion indicates that the cellular immune response to *M. leprae* is not sufficient to prevent extension of the lesion. (b) Mid-borderline leprosy. Several macules with target lesions characteristic of BB leprosy. The lesions show slight loss of sensation and in this subject are raised and erythematous because of an upgrading or reversal reaction. (c) Lepromatous leprosy. Nodular lesions typical of LL leprosy. There is no loss of sensation over the lesions or hypopigmentation. The lesions and adjacent, apparently normal skin are infiltrated by macrophages laden with acid-fast bacilli. (d) Borderline lepromatous leprosy in reversal reaction. The multiple symmetrical lesions are raised and desquamating because of an active, severe reversal reaction. The same process occurring in the infected nerve trunks of this man caused multiple nerve palsies.

Mycobacteria and HIV infection

M. Tuberculosis

With the spread of HIV infection in populations with high rates of underlying *M. tuberculosis* infection, tuberculosis has emerged as the major single opportunistic infection in AIDS. Worldwide there are over 4 million people co-infected with HIV and *M. tuberculosis* at risk for reactivation of tuberculosis. Moreover, HIV-infected immunodeficient children and adults living in communities with active tuberculosis transmission carry both a greatly increased susceptibility to primary infection with *M. tuberculosis* and a high risk of exposure to it. Although less than 10% of AIDS patients develop tuberculosis in industrialized countries, in developing countries a third of HIV-infected patients have tuberculosis at initial presentation and a half have evidence of disease at post mortem. In Africa a high proportion of tuberculosis patients (25–67%) are HIV positive and 30–35% of tuberculosis incidence is attributable to HIV infection. The recent outbreaks in the USA of MDR tuberculosis in HIV-infected subjects and their contacts, including health care workers, highlights the urgency of ensuring adequate public health measures to deal with these twin problems.

Interaction between HIV and M. tuberculosis

HIV infection is the strongest single risk factor for tuberculous disease yet observed. In many countries, tuberculosis is the first clinical indication of advancing immunodeficiency and acts as a sentinel disease for HIV infection. Consequently, both pulmonary and non-pulmonary tuberculosis are now included as AIDS-defining illnesses in HIV infection. Mycobacterial infection may also be a co-factor for the progression of HIV disease. The explanation may lie in the observations that mycobacteria-infected macrophages release TNF, which is a potent activator of HIV replication in T cells, and that patients with HIV-associated tuberculosis have significantly higher levels of serum TNF than those infected with HIV alone.

Reactivation of clinical tuberculosis occurs in 8–10% of tuberculin-positive HIV-infected subjects per annum, rates which approximate the lifetime risk of disease in non-immunodeficient populations (Table 38.1). This results in development of tuberculosis in 30–50% of dually infected subjects. Studies of tuberculosis outbreaks in institutions suggest that HIV-infected subjects have increased susceptibility to primary infection with *M. tuberculosis* with rapid progression to disseminated disease (Table 38.1). HIV-infected patients treated for tuberculous may also be reinfected with genotypically distinct strains of *M. tuberculosis*. This emphasizes the fact that tuberculosis is the most contagious of HIV-associated pathogens, both to immunodeficient subjects and the general community.

Clinical patterns of tuberculosis

Typically *M. tuberculosis* disease occurs in HIV-infected subjects at a relatively early stage of immunodeficiency before the emergence of other

∎ **Table 38.2**   Risk factors of development of active tuberculosis following infection with *M. tuberculosis*

1. **Infections**
   co-infection with HIV
   infection with other viruses, e.g. measles
2. **Protein–calorie malnutrition**
3. **Ageing**
4. **Substance abuse**
   alcoholism
   Intravenous drug use
5. **Pregnancy**
6. **Malignancy**
   lymphoma
   Hodgkin's disease
7. **Immunosuppressive therapy**
8. **Other diseases**
   Silicosis
   Diabetes
   Post-gastrectomy
   Chronic renal failure
   Jejuno-ileal bypass

opportunistic infections. This reflects the virulence of *M. tuberculosis* and the need for effective T-cell memory to prevent reactivation. The clinical pattern of tuberculosis is modified by coexistent HIV infection. Cross-sectional studies have revealed a consistent correlation between patterns of disease and the level of immunodeficiency. Pulmonary tuberculosis occurs when the CD4+ T-cell count is relatively maintained in the range of $250–500/\text{mm}^3$. With increasing immunodeficiency, extrapulmonary and lymph node tuberculosis are more common followed by meningeal and disseminated miliary disease at low median CD4 T-cell levels (Fig. 38.7). Extrapulmonary tuberculosis is more frequent in HIV-infected subjects, accounting for 50–75% of disease in African studies compared with 20–25% in HIV-seronegative patients. In early HIV infection, the clinical and radiological features of tuberculosis may be characteristic. However, with advancing immunodeficiency pulmonary lesions are often atypical with half not involving the upper lobes. Histologically, the characteristic well-formed granulomas of tuberculosis in the immunocompetent are replaced by poorly organized aggregations of macrophages lacking T cells and Langhans giant cells. Caseation is often absent and the lesions usually fail to cavitate. Radiologically, the lesions of tuberculosis in HIV infection may be atypical with hilar lymphadenopathy and pleural effusions being more common. In advanced HIV infection a miliary pattern

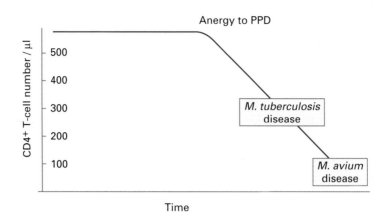

∎**Fig. 38.7** Different patterns of mycobacterial infection develop at different stages of the progressive CD4+ T-cell deficiency in HIV infection. PPD, purified protein derivative.

with bilateral coarse nodular patterns can develop. Therefore, tuberculosis should be strongly suspected in unexplained pulmonary disease in HIV infection, regardless of the radiographic features. Although the demonstration of acid-fast bacilli in the sputum of such patients may be due to infection with MAC rather than *M. tuberculosis*, treatment for tuberculosis is warranted while awaiting the results of culture.

Role of tuberculin and other DTH skin tests

Tuberculin skin testing of HIV-infected subjects is recommended as soon as practicable after the diagnosis of HIV. The results must be interpreted in the knowledge that progressive anergy develops in HIV infection. When the CD4+ T-cell count is in the ranges of <200/mm^3, 200–500/mm^3 and >400/mm^3, 75%, 50% and 20%, respectively of HIV-infected subjects are anergic. Therefore, tuberculin should be tested concurrently with a panel of recall DTH antigens, such as available in commercial multiple antigen devices. Reactivity with other recall antigens but not tuberculin, suggests the subject has not been infected with *M. tuberculosis*, but is susceptible to future infection and suitable for retesting. Tuberculin reactivity of any degree (>5 mm) in bacille Calmette-Guérin (BCG) non-vaccinated subjects warrants prophylactic therapy unless previously treated. Non-reactivity to tuberculin along with anergy to other recall antigens is not a reliable indicator of past exposure. If such an HIV-infected subject comes from a population with >10% tuberculin reactivity, the risk of reactivation may justify prophylactic therapy. Children of HIV-infected mothers demonstrate lower

rates of tuberculin reactivity after BCG vaccination than those of HIV-seronegative mothers, reflecting the difficulty of generating effective DTH responses in seropositive infants.

Response to therapy

Patients with drug sensitive *M. tuberculosis* generally respond well to conventional multidrug antituberculosis therapy. However, the high bacillary load and difficulties in therapy have led to suggestions for more prolonged therapy and some centres continue it lifelong. Infection with MDR-tuberculosis isolates which are resistant to rifampicin and isoniazid and possibly other agents, poses major problems both in therapy for the individual and prevention of spread to others. In developing countries the response to standard antituberculous therapy has been less satisfactory. HIV-infected tuberculosis patients suffer increased mortality (from three to 15-fold) in the first year of treatment. Relapse also occurs more frequently from both reactivation and reinfection. HIV-infected patients also experience increased antituberculosis drug toxicity, and thiacetazone is often associated with severe skin reactions.

Prophylactic therapy in tuberculin-positive HIV-infected subjects ideally should use at least two drugs, usually isoniazid and rifampicin, and be continued for at least 12 months. In developing countries where HIV and tuberculosis commonly coexist, Isoniazid alone has proved a valuable intervention despite the possibility of increased drug resistance. In one Haitian study, 12 months isoniazid prophylaxis in HIV-infected subjects resulted in a 71% reduction in the risk of tuberculosis overall, with the greatest benefit, 83%, in tuberculin-positive subjects. As there was also a delay in the progression to AIDS and death, antituberculosis prophylaxis may represent the single most cost-effective therapy for HIV infection in developing countries with high rates of tuberculosis.

Non-tuberculous mycobacteria

Environmental sampling has established that exposure to atypical mycobacteria of low pathogenicity is common. A variable proportion of healthy subjects in different regions (15% in Canadians) demonstrate skin test reactivity to purified protein derivative (PPD) prepared from 'atypical' mycobacteria. A normal immune system usually prevents these organisms from causing clinical disease. With advancing immunodeficiency in HIV infection, atypical mycobacteria, particularly of the MAC complex become major opportunistic infections. In addition, in countries where bovine tuberculosis has not been eliminated, *M. bovis*, which has intermediate pathogenicity, is also a documented cause of localized and disseminated tuberculosis complicating HIV infection.

Clinical disease from MAC develops only in advanced immunodeficiency, typically when the mean CD4+ T-cell count is below 100/mm³. This usually follows primary infection, probably via the gastrointestinal tract, rather than reactivation. In the late stages of AIDS, sensitive culture techniques have isolated MAC organisms from the majority of patients. The clinical manifestations include fever and wasting, anaemia with increasing dependency on blood transfusion, diarrhoea, hepatic dysfunction, and lymphadenopathy. Some patients may be asymptomatic despite significant bacteraemia. Granulomas are absent from infected tissues which are infiltrated by foamy macrophages laden with acid-fast bacilli (Fig. 38.5). The cachexia and fever typical of MAC bacteraemia are caused by high levels of serum TNF and other cytokines and these are often the first symptoms to respond to effective treatment. In HIV-infected patients with comparable immunodeficiency, the presence of MAC infection is associated with increased mortality.

MAC isolates are often resistant to multiple antibiotics on *in vitro* sensitivity testing and in early studies, treatment appeared ineffective. However, therapy with multiple bactericidal and bacteriostatic drugs has resulted in significant control of symptoms and possibly prolonged survival. In some intensively treated patients who died from other causes, eradication of mycobacteria was confirmed at subsequent autopsy. Short-term prophylaxis studies with Rifabutin, an ansamycin, have supported its use as a single drug to delay the onset of MAC infection. The long-term benefit of such an approach remains to be proven. In MAC and other mycobacterial infection the introduction of antiretroviral therapy may enhance the immune response to the organisms. In its most extreme form this may lead to enlargement of lymph nodes and a scrofula-like syndrome.

Immunological assays and the diagnosis of mycobacteria infections

Immunological assays are widely used to diagnose infection with mycobacteria and to investigate the host response. These assays which generally detect T-cell memory to mycobacterial antigens do not necessarily indicate active disease and are not a substitute for microbiological diagnosis. However, in situations where it is difficult to demonstrate or isolate organisms, such as tuberculoid leprosy or paediatric tuberculosis, clinical decisions may be based on results of immunological assays.

Tuberculin test

The use of tuberculin, the heat-sterilized culture filtrate of *M. tuberculosis*, as a skin test reagent to diagnose *M. tuberculosis* exposure dates to Koch in 1890. Its role as a diagnostic reagent for skin testing has developed to the point where understanding the molecular basis of its immunoreactivity is one of the most pressing issues in mycobacterial research. In 1939, old tuberculin was replaced by PPD, which has been standardized for potency but not for precise molecular content. For *in vivo* quantitative diagnostic use it is generally administered using the intradermal technique of Mantoux.

Tuberculin reactivity indicated by induration at 48–72 h reflects the accumulation of activated chronic inflammatory cells at the site of intradermal injection. The predictive value of the test for measuring *M. tuberculosis* exposure depends on the quantity of tuberculin injected, the cut-off threshold chosen for a positive result and the prevalence of exposure to other mycobacteria, both environmental mycobacteria and BCG vaccine, in the subject population. At the commonly used dose of 10 IU PPD, tuberculosis patients display an unimodal distribution of induration diameter peaking at 16–17 mm with few tuberculosis patients having diameters less than 5 mm. The risk of developing tuberculosis in a BCG naive population is directly correlated with the diameter of the PPD reactivity and this finding forms the rational basis for adjusting the threshold for 'positivity' depending on the population's tuberculosis prevalence and BCG vaccination history.

Tuberculin-negative subjects who convert to positive after exposure to *M. tuberculosis* are at increased risk of developing clinical tuberculosis. In the British Medical Research Council trial of BCG vaccination, 80% of adolescent tuberculin converters developing tuberculosis did so within 2 years of skin test conversion. The risk of subsequent tuberculosis fell significantly after 2 years. Therefore, the benefits to be obtained in immunocompetent tuberculin-positive individuals from isoniazid prophylaxis diminishes with time after infection.

Active tuberculosis is not always associated with tuberculin reactivity. In two studies 17 and 30% of newly diagnosed tuberculosis patients had false negative tuberculin results. This anergy is more common with overwhelming infection as in miliary tuberculosis; however, tuberculin positivity returns with therapy. Anergy also occurs following acute infection with viruses, bacteria and fungi at any age. Chronic illness such as nutritional and metabolic disturbance, recurrent infection and malignancy may also be associated with false negative tuberculin tests. In these conditions tuberculin negativity correlates with increased susceptibility to tuberculosis infection (Table 38.2). Therefore, the implication of a negative tuberculin test depends on the immunocompetence and clinical status of the host.

False positive results with tuberculin in BCG naive are generally due to prior environmental contact with mycobacteria which presensitize the individual to cross-reactive or shared epitopes. These reactions are usually <10 mm and are associated with reactivity to PPD prepared from an environmental mycobacteria, such as *M. intracellulare* (PPD-B). Tuberculin reactivity following BCG vaccination is usually less (<10 mm) than following natural infection with *M. tuberculosis* and wanes more rapidly. None the less a desire to preserve the utility of tuberculin testing as a diagnostic tool has influenced some countries to disband or discourage programmes of universal BCG vaccination.

An important practical consideration in tuberculin testing is the 'booster phenomenon'. Although tuberculin in standard doses does not induce T-cell memory and skin test reactivity, in the booster phenomenon, subjects whose skin test reactivity has waned to subthreshold levels on the first test can be boosted by tuberculin testing. This is demonstrated by a positive DTH response when retested with tuberculin on a second occasion and may be present in about 5% of young adults. As this may be subsequently mistaken for tuberculin conversion after *M. tuberculosis* exposure, it is generally recommended that negative subjects who are being prospectively evaluated for tuberculin reactivity should be retested at 7 days to exclude the booster effect.

Leprosy skin tests

Two forms of skin tests are available to measure cellular reactivity to the leprosy bacillus. Soluble preparations of *M. leprae* elicit DTH reactions at 48–72 h levels, analogous to tuberculin reactivity, in subjects presensitized to *M. leprae* through exposure. As *M. leprae* cannot yet be cultivated *in vitro*, the organisms are obtained from experimentally infected armadillos, a species particularly susceptible to systemic infection with *M. leprae*. The second skin test utilizes whole heat-killed *M. leprae* bacilli injected intradermally. Although a transient DTH response may develop at 72 h in presensitized subjects, this is followed by a granulomatous or 'Mitsuda' reaction at 21–28 days. This consists of a subcutaneous nodule of >3 mm diameter which contains typical non-caseating granulomas on histopathology. The Mitsuda reaction reflects the induction of T-cell reactivity and the capacity to mount a granulomatous response in subjects with and without prior infection with *M. leprae*. A positive Mitsuda reaction is characteristic of tuberculoid leprosy and is absent in lepromatous disease. As such it is an important tool in the classification of leprosy patients both for diagnosis and immunological studies. The lack of reactivity to prolonged antigen challenge in lepromatous leprosy is paralleled by non-responsiveness to *M. leprae* during *in vitro* assays of lymphocyte function.

In vitro assays of T-cell reactivity

Cellular reactivity to mycobacteria can be detected *in vitro* by the stimulation of T-cell proliferation or cytokine release with soluble or particulate mycobacterial antigens. The response of human lymphocytes in the 6 day lymphocyte proliferation assay usually parallels the DTH response; however, the assay is not practicable for large-scale clinical use. Recently, more rapid assays have been developed in which whole blood is stimulated by mycobacterial antigens and IFNγ release measured by enzyme-linked immunosorbent assay (ELISA) after 24 h. This assay proved valuable in the diagnosis of bovine tuberculosis in cattle, and if validated in humans may provide a powerful *in vitro* diagnostic tool. An advantage of *in vitro* assays is that multiple antigen preparations can be tested such as PPD from different mycobacteria or individual recombinant mycobacterial proteins.

Serology in mycobacterial infections

Infection with either *M. tuberculosis* or *M. leprae* stimulates antibody responses to species-specific and shared carbohydrate and protein antigens; however, these antibodies play no part in protective immunity. As both subclinical infection and active disease may be associated with antibodies, serological tests have not proved useful for routine clinical diagnosis. Patients with lepromatous leprosy, however, have high levels of *M. leprae*-specific antibodies and these fall with effective chemotherapy, providing a correlate of clinical response.

Immunoprophylaxis with BCG vaccine

M. bovis (BCG) is the most widely used bacterial vaccine and yet uncertainties persist about its optimal utilization. BCG was developed by serial passage of a virulent strain of *M. bovis* on ox bile enriched potato–glycerin medium and in the process BCG lost its pathogenicity in a wide range of experimental animals. Since its first use in humans in 1921, over 3 billion people, chiefly infants, have been vaccinated with a very low risk of adverse effects. As a live vaccine, a single inoculation of BCG induces multiple immune responses and long-lasting sensitization to tuberculin. BCG is safe, stable, cheap, and can be given at birth; however, its efficacy has varied widely in many different trials.

A recent meta-analysis of 14 prospective trials and 12 case–control studies concluded that BCG vaccine significantly reduced the risk of tuberculosis by 50%. There were higher rates of protection against tuberculosis death (71%), tuberculosis meningitis (64%), and disseminated tuberculosis (78%). Age at vaccination had no effect on protective efficacy. Much of the variation in individual trial results was attributed to differences in the study protocols and the distance from the equator of the study sites. The latter may reflect differences in prior exposure to environmental mycobacteria which provides a degree of protection against tuberculosis and so masks the effect of BCG. Other factors which may have influenced the variable outcomes include differences in the vaccine strains tested, in the genetic composition of target populations and in the virulence of *M. tuberculosis* strains in the trial areas. One important observation from BCG trials is that protection against tuberculosis is not correlated with conversion to tuberculin positivity. As BCG is less effective against the infectious forms of adult tuberculosis, it does not prevent transmission within the community. BCG vaccination also provides about 50% protection against clinical leprosy and may have had a greater impact on the epidemiology of leprosy than of tuberculosis.

The current recommendations for the use of BCG against tuberculosis vary widely. The World Health Organization (WHO) advises vaccination in the first year of life and this is the practice in most developing communities with high rates of tuberculosis infection. Concern has been expressed at risk of BCG vaccination in communities with high prevalence of HIV. Although disseminated BCG infection has occurred in some HIV-infected children, prospective studies have confirmed that children of HIV-seropositive mothers given BCG do not develop increased rates of local or systemic reactions to BCG. Therefore, WHO supports the continuation of BCG vaccination as part of the expanded programme of immunizations except in children with symptomatic HIV infection.

In industrialized countries with low rates of tuberculosis, universal BCG immunization has been replaced by selective use in defined groups with continuing high rates of tuberculosis transmission. In some countries health care workers exposed to tuberculosis are vaccinated with BCG, while in others BCG is withheld in order to permit monitoring with skin tests to detect tuberculin conversion. The recent emergence of MDR-tuberculosis and its transmission to health care workers strengthens the argument for BCG vaccination of health care workers.

Further reading

Barnes, P. J., Le, H. Q., and Davidson, P. T. (1993). Tuberculosis in patients with HIV infection. *Medical Clinics of North America*, **77**, 1369–89.

Bloom, B. R. (1994). *Tuberculosis. Pathogenesis, protection and control*, 1st edn. ASM Press, Washington, DC.

Britton, W. J. (1993). Immunology of leprosy. *Transactions of the Royal Society of Tropical Medicine and Hygiene*, **87**, 508–14.

Britton, W. J, Roche, P. W., and Winter, N. (1994). Mechanisms of persistence of mycobacteria. *Trends in Microbiology*, **2**, 284–8.

Colditz, G. A., Brewer, T. F., Berkey, C. S., et al.–(1994). Efficacy of BCG vaccine in the prevention of tuberculosis. *Journal of the American Medical Association*, **271**, 698–702.

Crowe, S. M., Carlin, J. B., Stewart, K. I., et al. (1991). Predictive value of CD4 lymphocyte numbers for the development of opprtunistic infections and malignancies in HIV-infected persons. *Journal of Acquired Immune Deficiency Syndrome*, **4**, 770–6.

Dunlap, N. E., and Briles, D. E. (1993). Immunology of tuberculosis. *Medical Clinics of North America*, **77**, 1235–51.

Horsburgh, C. R. J. (1991). *Mycobacterium avium* complex infection in the acquired immunodeficiency syndrome. *New England Journal of Medicine*, **324**, 1332–8.

Kaufmann, S. H. E. (1993). Immunity to intracellular mycobacteria. *Annual Review of Immunology*, **11**, 129–63.

Menzies, R., Vissandjee, B., Rocher, I., and St. Germain, Y. (1994). The booster effect in two-step tuberculin testing among young adults in Montreal. *Annals of Internal Medicine*, **120**, 190–8.

Orme, I. M. (1993). Immunity to mycobacteria. *Current Opinion in Immunology*, **5**, 497–502.

Ridley, D. S. and Jopling, W. H. (1966). Classification of leprosy according to immunity. A five group system. *International Journal of Leprosy*, **34**, 255–73.

39 Malaria

M. F. Good

Introduction

Malaria is a disease caused by protozoal parasites of the genus, *Plasmodium*, of which four species infect humans: *P. falciparum, P. vivax, P. malariae*, and *P. ovale. P. falciparum* is responsible for the vast majority of malaria deaths, estimated at between 1 and 2 million per year. Most of these deaths occur in young children and previously immune women during pregnancy.

The parasite is transmitted by female anopheline mosquitoes which inject sporozoites into the host (Fig. 39.1). These enter the circulation and travel to the liver where tens to hundreds of hepatocytes may be infected following the bite of an infected mosquito.

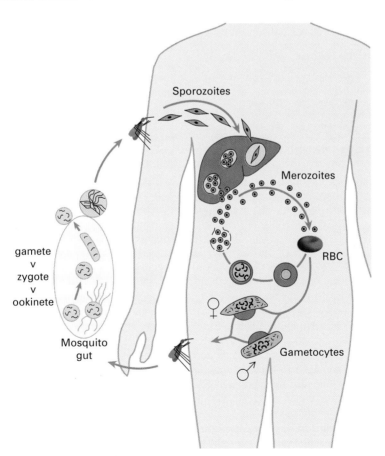

Fig. 39.1 The life cycle of the malarial parasite. RBC, red blood cells.

Over a period of about 1 week these undergo a process referred to exo-erythrocytic schizogony leading to the development of thousands of merozoites within each hepatocyte. No clinical symptoms are associated with the liver phase of the life cycle. However the parasites rupture from the liver cells, probably as a raft of merozoites and red cells are infected. During a red cell cycle which lasts approximately 48 h for *P. falciparum*, *P. vivax*, and *P. ovale* (and approximately 72 h for *P. malariae*), merozoites invade the red cells and develop through the ring stage, the trophozoite stage, and finally the schizont stage before the red cell ruptures to release further merozoites (10–20 per red cell). In a synchronized infection, fever peaks occur just following the rupture of schizont-infected red cells. Eventually, the sexual forms of the parasites (male and female gametocytes) develop in the red cells. These are taken up by the mosquito and in the gut of the mosquito emerge from the red cell to form gametes which fertilize giving rise to zygotes, ookinetes, and then sporozoites which travel to the insect's salivary glands. The different stages of the life cycle are each the target of different types of immune responses and form the basis of different vaccine approaches.

In this section three major issues will be addressed:

(1) the pathogenesis of disease;

(2) current understanding of the development of immunity to malaria; and

(3) progress towards development of a vaccine.

Pathogenesis

This depends on both parasite and host factors. The pathology of malaria is varied and many organs can be affected. Most of the deaths, however, are associated with either cerebral malaria or severe anaemia.

Cerebral malaria

This occurs mostly in areas where the endemicity of malaria is low and children are exposed to infected mosquitoes only infrequently. In African children, it tends to peak at about 3–4 years of age. Visitors from non-endemic areas will also be more likely to develop cerebral malaria. The risk for cerebral malaria increases with the parasitaemia. Histological examination of the brain of people who die of cerebral malaria reveals capillaries and venules which are clogged with parasitized red cells. While the overall blood flow through the brain is maintained in cerebral malaria, levels of lactate are higher in the brain of individuals with cerebral malaria and cerebral oxygen consump-

tion is decreased. There is no evidence of inflammation in the brain.

In recent years, much interest has focused on the role of tumour necrosis factor (TNF) α in the pathogenesis of cerebral malaria. TNFα levels are highest in the serum of children with cerebral malaria and this cytokine may upregulate expression of intercellular adhesion molecule 1 (ICAM-1) on the blood vessels in the brain. This ligand has been shown to bind parasitized red cells. TNFα may also stimulate the endothelium of the blood vessels to produce nitric oxide, which can affect neurotransmission and possibly cause coma. While it is not clear why some children will develop cerebral malaria and others will not, it has recently been shown that individuals expressing a variant of the TNFα promoter region known to increase transcription of TNFα are more likely to develop cerebral malaria.

Severe anaemia

In contrast to cerebral malaria, the severe anaemia (Hb: 3–5 g/dl) that causes death is more commonly found in areas where endemicity is very high and affects children at a younger age. In Africa, surprisingly, severe anaemia is often not associated with a high parasitaemia. In one study, half of those with severe anaemia had a parasitaemia of less than 10 000 parasites/μl. Although these findings might suggest that malaria is not the cause of the anaemia, treatment of children with antimalarials does restore the Hb level. While less severe anaemia associated with malaria (Hb >8 g/dl) is likely to be the result of red cell destruction and occurs at higher parasitaemia, the severe anaemia appears to result from dyserythropoiesis. There is some evidence to suggest that the cytokines, interferon-γ and TNFα, which can be secreted by activated T cells and/or macrophages can suppress haematopoiesis.

Pregnancy

In previously immune women living in falciparum-endemic regions, pregnancy, particularly a first pregnancy, is associated with increased susceptibility to malaria. The mortality rate of mothers is significantly increased and there is retardation of fetal growth and an increased incidence of abortion and stillbirth. The reasons for this are not understood; however, pregnancy is associated with a depressed cell-mediated immunity (CMI) response to a number of antigens, including malaria antigens, and this effect is more marked during the first pregnancy. Antimalaria antibody titres are not affected by pregnancy. Oestrogen is thought to suppress CMI and the uterus contains prostaglandin E_2 and TGFβ, which can inhibit immune responses. This dampening of immune responses, which may be an essential component of normal pregnancy to reduce fetal rejection, would appear to be an important reason for the increased susceptibility to malaria.

Immunity to malaria

This topic could easily fill an entire book and there are a number of journal issues to which it has recently been devoted (e.g. see *Research in Immunology*, 1995). However, the basics of the topic will be covered here with the major mechanisms of immunity to the different stages summarized in Table 39.1. Each stage of the life cycle must be considered separately. Sporozoites, prior to their invasion of liver cells are susceptible to antibodies which bind the sporozoite coat resulting in a precipitin reaction. Sporozoites treated *in vitro* with antibodies to the circumsporozoite protein are non-infectious and it has been shown that mice can be protected against infection with rodent malaria parasites by immunization with peptides from the protein which results in protein-specific antibodies. However, animal studies suggest that very high titres of specific antibody are required for protection. In a number of human vaccine trials (see below), it has been observed that a high titre of antibody is required for protection, but a high titre alone does not guarantee protection. Antibody must be high at the time of infection, as there is no opportunity to boost antibody levels between bite and invasion of hepatocytes. A further important point to remember is that immunity mediated by sporozoite-specific antibodies must be complete — a single sporozoite that invades hepatocytes can give rise to clinical malaria.

Once inside hepatocytes, the host relies on T cells to mediate protection. It was originally thought that only CD8+ T cells could mediate protection against this stage. Mice immunized with irradiated *P. yoelii* or *P. berghei* sporozoites lost their immunity if their CD8+ T cells, but not their CD4+ T cells were destroyed by *in vivo* treatment with specific monoclonal antibodies. Subsequently, CD8+ clones specific for the circumsporozoite protein were shown to be able to adoptively transfer protection. However, CD4+ T cell clones have also been shown to be able to mediate protection. These various clones recognize the liver stage and can be given to the mice after sporozoite challenge. Immunization of mice with recombinant *Salmonella* expressing the CS protein or tumour cells expressing CS protein or another liver stage protein (SSP2/TRAP) has also been shown to induce protection that can be abolished by treatment with anti-CD8+ antibodies. A number of other liver stage proteins which are the target antigens of T cells have also been described and their part in protection is currently being assessed.

The most complex stage with respect to immunity is the blood stage. Here two different types of immunity have been described, antidisease immunity and antiparasite immunity. Antidisease immunity refers to protection from disease symptoms, irrespective of the parasite density, while antiparasite immunity refers to those mechanisms that reduce parasite density. Some studies have suggested that, in endemic situations, antidisease immunity develops initially (manifest by children who are not clinically ill but have significant parasitaemias) and this is followed by antiparasite immunity in which parasites are reduced in number (but often not completely eliminated). Studies in mice suggest that cytokines may be responsible for disease symptoms and parasite molecules have been identified which can induce macrophages to secrete TNFα. Antibodies raised to these parasite products can block the production of TNFα, establishing a vaccine strategy for inducing antidisease immunity. However, cytokines responsible for disease can also be produced by activated parasite-specific T cells. This is particularly relevant to the situation of the non-immune individual. Many children and most adults have malaria-reactive T cells *prior* to initial encounter with malaria. These have apparently arisen as a result exposure to cross-reactive organisms (they express the memory/activation marker CD45RO and often react to one or other of a panel of common environmental organisms). These cells typically secrete interferon-γ and either secrete themselves or direct the secretion of

▌ **Table 39.1** Mechanisms of immunity

Life cycle stage	Effector mechanisms of immunity
Sporozoite	Antibody
Liver stage	CD8+ T cells CD4+ T cells
Blood stage	Cytophilic antibodies CD4+ T cells *Note*: an important accessory role for monocytes and neutrophils
Sexual stage	Antibodies (operative in mosquito) CD4+ T cells (operative in host)

TNFα. These cytokines have been implicated in the aetiology of cerebral malaria, severe anaemia, glomerulonephritis, and other pathological manifestations of malaria. The factors responsible for development of antidisease immunity are not well understood but may involve either the development of antibodies that can block direct activation of macrophages by malarial products, or a change in phenotype of malaria-reactive T cells. It is known, for example, that T cells from malaria-immune individuals are less likely to produce interferon-γ in response to parasite stimulation than T cells from non-immune or semi-immune individuals.

Antiparasite immunity is also complex, but certain crucial observations have been made. Over 30 years ago it was shown that antibodies from immune African adults, but not from non-immune Europeans, could be given to African children with high parasitaemia and reduce dramatically the parasitaemia. This study has been repeated more recently with similar results, but also showing that this antiparasite effect was associated with an antibody-dependent cellular (monocyte) inhibition (ADCI) of parasite growth *in vitro*. It was further shown that ADCI was associated with malaria-specific antibodies of the cytophilic classes (IgG1, IgG3), but not of the non-cytophilic classes. *In vitro* studies suggest that neutrophils can also play an important antiparasite role. The presence of antibodies to agglutinating antigens on the red cell surface has been shown to correlate with clinical immunity. Antibodies to merozoite surface antigens may also play an important part in immunity. In murine models, antibodies to the merozoite-surface protein 1 (MSP-1), can transfer protection to mice, and immunization of mice with this protein can induce immunity.

Malaria-specific CD4+ T cells are also thought to play an important part in protection. As mentioned above, T cells have been implicated in the pathology of malaria. However, human malaria-specific T-cell clones, in association with adherent cells, can inhibit parasite growth *in vitro*, and in murine models clones of malaria-specific T cells can transfer antiparasite immunity to recipient mice. Both Th1-like and Th2-like clones have been shown to be able to transfer immunity, with some studies suggesting that the Th1-like clones mediate protection via induction of nitric oxide. During the course of infection for one rodent parasite, the T cells were shown to switch from being predominantly Th1-like early in infection to being predominantly Th2-like late in infection. It is undisputed that malaria-specific Th1-like cells can be antiparasitic, but a by-product of activation of these cells may be disease symptoms. Evidence suggests that *in vivo* the spleen is a major organ of parasite death

and it is likely that cellular immunity mediated by T cells in association with monocytes operates most effectively in this organ.

Immunity can also develop to the sexual stages of the parasite. In the host, the gametocytes are enclosed within the red cell and are thus not susceptible to attack by antibodies. However, when the gametocytes enter the mosquito's mid-gut, the parasites emerge from the red cell as male and female gametes. Antibodies to the gamete surface can block fertilization and antibodies to the fertilized zygote can prevent development of the parasite inside the mosquito.

About 20 years ago it was shown that immunization of birds with the gametes of an avian malaria induced antibodies in the birds and these antibodies, when taken up by the mosquito during its blood meal, could prevent infection of the mosquito. This is referred to as 'transmission-blocking immunity'. Immunization of mice with gametes of *P. falciparum* can also induce antibodies which when fed to mosquitoes in the laboratory during a blood meal containing *falciparum* gametocytes can also block transmission. A number of genes encoding gametocyte and gamete surface antigens have now been cloned and are vaccine candidates as described below.

Progress towards a malaria vaccine

There are many different approaches to malaria vaccines. These range from attenuated live vaccines to small subunit vaccines containing one or a few epitopes from the malaria parasite. While there will always be a desire for a vaccine to contain as little foreign material as possible, it will be difficult to induce strong immune responses to these very small subunit vaccines in part because of major histocompatibility complex-linked immunological non-responsiveness. On the other hand the subunit vaccines will be least likely to cause side-effects. People have been successfully immunized with irradiated sporozoites, but such a practice is impracticable for large-scale use. Individuals have also been immunized by deliberate infections with blood stage parasites followed by drug cure. Live attenuated blood stage parasites have not yet been tested in humans; however, such parasites have been tested in rodents and monkeys with good results. Most effort today centres on developing subunit vaccines, either recombinant or synthetic.

Each stage of the life cycle can be targeted by vaccines. Vaccine candidates progress through preclinical trials in laboratory animals where immunogenicity is assessed to phase I human clinical trials where safety and immunogenicity is assessed to phase II and III trials where protective efficacy of the vaccine is determined. In this section, the focus will be mostly on the phase I and II clinical trials. However, with respect to preclinical trials, it should be mentioned that the immunogenicity of most of the malaria vaccine candidates has been found to be significantly greater in laboratory animals than in humans.

There is good reason to believe that vaccines against the sporozoite stage must be able to kill all sporozoites in order to be effective, as malaria can be initiated with a single sporozoite. This view has been challenged, however, by a study looking at the effect of certain human leucocyte antigens (HLA) on outcome of malaria. It has been shown that individuals who express a particular HLA class I allele (B53) are at less risk of serious malaria episodes, but not mild malaria episodes. If this relates to development of a specific cytotoxic T lymphocyte (CTL) response that is protective, then it is tempting to speculate that liver stage immunity is responsible as this is the only stage of the life cycle that is thought to be the target of CTL. The observations suggest that a better outcome might result from a reduction in the number of infected hepatocytes (and not necessarily complete elimination of all infected hepatocytes). If the hypothesis is correct, then sporozoite or liver stage vaccines need not kill all sporozoites/infected hepatocytes to have a beneficial effect.

The first malaria vaccine candidate tested in humans (a sporozoite vaccine) was a recombinant protein containing a block of repeat epitopes from the circumsporozoite (CS) protein of *P. falciparum*. This and a similar trial using synthetic peptides linked to tetanus toxoid were published in 1987. Challenge was by the bite of infected mosquitoes. In these trials one from six and one from three individuals were protected and there was a correlation between the development of antibodies and protection. Since then there have been a number of sporozoite vaccine trials in humans based on the induction of antibodies to the CS protein. The strategy has been to increase the immunogenicity of the vaccine by use of different adjuvants. Overall, about 20% of individuals have been protected. A number of trials are still underway and new approaches including the polymerization of multiple epitopes in the immunogen may permit greater success in the future. While liver stage vaccines aimed at inducing specific T-cell responses have been successful in mice, these have not yet been trialled in humans.

Vaccines to inhibit blood stage parasites are currently at an interesting stage of development. A number of antigens have been described and two of the most promising, from the perspective of animal trials, are MSP-1 and AMA-1 (apical merozoite antigen-1). Immunization of mice with rodent malaria homologues of these proteins has led to strong protection following homologous challenge. Trials are currently underway or being planned to test *falciparum* homologues in humans.

Much interest now centres on the synthetic preparation developed by Manuel Pattaroyo and colleagues from Colombia. Initially, three synthetic peptides were administered to monkeys and shown to protect six of six animals. Subsequently, four synthetic peptides were polymerized to form the compound 'SPf66' and administered with alum to human volunteers who were challenged by mosquito bite. Three of five volunteers were shown to be protected, with peak parasitaemia ranging from 0.001 to 0.46%. This phase II trial has now been followed by four large phase III trials involving thousands of individuals where the efficacy of the preparation, in terms of reduction in the number of clinical episodes, has been shown to be approximately 30%. In a trial in Tanzania 600 children between the ages of 1 and 5 years were given either SPf66 or placebo. During follow-up there were five deaths from malaria in the placebo group and only one death in the SPf66 group. One of the enigmas concerning SPf66 is that so far no one has been able to show a correlation between protection and a specific immune response. Individuals who are given SPf66 certainly develop antibodies against both SPf66 and malaria parasites but the extent of this antibody response is not predictive of the protective effect in a given individual.

Transmission-blocking vaccines have now entered clinical trials. These vaccines will not protect the vaccinated individual from malaria but by preventing transmission of malaria, all individuals in the vicinity will be protected. To be effective, nearly all individuals in a given community would need to be immunized. The most promising vaccine candidate is an antigen expressed on the surface of gametes, but not gametocytes, and referred to as Pfs25. As it is not expressed on gametocytes, individuals exposed to malaria do not naturally develop specific antibodies. However, antibodies induced in laboratory animals are highly effective in blocking malaria transmission through mosquitoes.

In the space of little over a decade, there has been enormous progress towards developing a vaccine, from the initial cloning of antigens to preclinical trials and now human trials. It is not unreasonable to predict that the next decade might see a reduction in the incidence of malaria and associated suffering as a result of vaccine intervention.

Further reading

Alonso, P., Smith, T., Armstrong T, *et al.* (1994). Randomized trial of efficacy of SPf66 vaccine against *Plasmodium falciparum* malaria in children in southern Tanzania. *Lancet*, **344**, 1175–88.

Hoffman, S. L. (ed) *Malaria Vaccine Development: a multi-immune response approach.* ASM Press, Washington DC.

Miller, L. H., Good, M. F., and Milon, G. (1994). Malaria pathogenesis. *Science*, **264**, 1878–83.

Nussenzweig, R. and Long, C. (1994). Malaria vaccines: multiple targets. *Science*, **265**, 1381–3.

Section VII

Immunology of malignancy

40 Lymphoma

G. T. Stevenson and D. B. Jones

Introduction

Neoplasms of lymphoid tissue have contributed much to our knowledge of immunology, and have themselves been illuminated by immunological insights. The majority arise from lymphocytes (B, T, and natural killer or NK) and their descendants. Tumours arising from 'histiocytes', a term now often used to refer to cells of either the macrophage or Langerhans lineage, are relatively rare and have been well reviewed by Cline (1994). They have been omitted from the Revised European American (REA) classification of lymphoid neoplasms proposed by the International Lymphoma Study Group (Harris *et al.*, 1994), and for simplicity will not be discussed further.

Despite restricting the discussion to the lymphocytic lineages one is confronted by a complex neoplastic group which is approached in different ways by people with different interests. Clinical oncologists welcome classifications which assist in selecting treatment and assessing prognosis. Immunologists prefer classifications which define lineage and differentiation, and give clues to functional attributes of the cells. Many other scientists find in lymphoma a rich resource for studying tumour viruses, chromosomal translocations, oncogenes, and growth factors and receptors. In the midst of these disparate interests are pathologists, who must convey day-to-day decisions about the nature and likely behaviour of individual tumours.

Table 40.1 sets out the classification of lymphoma to be used in this chapter. It is essentially a simplified version of the REA classification, with rarer varieties of each subdivision gathered under 'others'. It follows the practice of using 'lymphoma' to refer to all lymphoid neoplasms, but clinicians do not usually include the leukaemias and immunoglobulin exporting tumours under this heading. In many centres the leukaemias and solid lymphomas are treated by entirely different people. However, surveys of immunological markers often detect neoplastic lymphoid cells in the blood of patients who present clinically with a mass of solid lymphoma, and a continuum of abnormal lymphocytosis exists between this picture

Table 40.1 A classification of lymphoma

Acute lymphoblastic leukaemias (ALL)
  Pre-B
  Pre-T
  Others

Chronic lymphocytic leukaemias (CLL)
  B cell
  T cell
  Natural killer cell

B-cell non-Hodgkin lymphomas (B-cell NHL)
  Lymphoblastic
  Lymphocytic
  Mantle cell
  Follicle centre-cell
  Diffuse large B cell
  Burkitt
  Mucosa-associated (B-cell MALT lymphoma)
  Others

Immunoglobulin-exporting lymphomas
  Macroglobulinaemia
  Myeloma
  Others

T-cell non-Hodgkin lymphomas (T-cell NHL)
  Lymphoblastic
  Adult T-cell lymphoma/leukaemia
  Enteropathy-associated T-cell lymphoma
  Other peripheral T-cell lymphomas

Hodgkin's disease (HD)
  Lymphocyte-predominant
  Nodular sclerosing
  Mixed cellularity
  Lymphocyte-depleted

and frank leukaemia. These facts have led to the abandoning of a primary distinction between leukaemias and solid lymphomas in the REA classification, which places, for example, chronic lymphocytic leukaemia (CLL) and B-lymphocytic lymphoma under a single major heading. The leukaemias are listed separately in deference to current clinical practice.

A continuum between tumours usually regarded as distinct became apparent also with the realization that most B-cell lymphomas, even without plasmacytoid components, export small amounts of monoclonal immunoglobulin (Stevenson *et al.*, 1980), and that intermediate forms lead from conventionally designated B-cell non-Hodgkin lymphomas (NHL) up to macroglobulinaemia and myeloma.

Those who diagnose or treat lymphoma from day to day must cope with nomenclatures more complex than that in Table 40.1. A detailed clinical subdivision of NHL, the working formulation, is set out in Table 40.2. This has been in wide clinical use since 1982, so that those who would search lymphoma databases must be familiar with it. It has served its clinical purposes reasonably well, but contains no reference to cell lineage and fails to embrace some recently described lymphomas. The designation of low-, intermediate- and high-grade categories of tumour is convenient, but complicates matters by enforcing arbitrary divisions, especially of follicle-centre lymphoma. The present availability of surface and nuclear activation markers (e.g. nuclear Ki-67), supplementing the classical criteria of cell size and appearance, means that a grade of malignancy can be assigned to each individual tumour. Any concomitant need to change its name can be avoided. Table 40.2 sets out the major correlations between the formulation and our classification, but there are many overlaps and uncertainties. Readers are referred to the report by Harris *et al.* (1994) for histological descriptions and lists of synonyms linking the REA, the formulation, and earlier classifications

How far should subdivision of lymphoma be taken? The REA lists some 50 types and subtypes, and one has the impression that it could continue ad infinitum. Experienced clinicians emphasize that each case presents individual features: 'Here comes Mrs Smith with Smith's lymphoma' Croce (1993) suggested that progress in understanding the molecular biology of lymphomas could lead to groupings based on lineage plus oncogenic events. So the terms *{B cell, t(8, 14)}* and *{B cell, t(14, 18)}* may prove more useful than their approximate synonyms, Burkitt's lymphoma and follicle-centre lymphoma.

The neoplasms listed in Table 40.1 are now reviewed, and in Table 40.3 there is a summary linking them with many of the lymphoma markers which are used diagnostically. The markers are best characterized for the B lineage, and in Fig. 40.1 some of them

∎ **Table 40.2**   Non-Hodgkin lymphoma: working formulation

	Predominant correlations with categories in this chapter
Low-grade lymphoma	
Small lymphocytic	B lymphocytic
Follicular, predominantly small cleaved cell	Some follicle centre, some mantle cell
Follicular, mixed small cleaved cell and large cell	Follicle centre
Intermediate-grade lymphoma	
Follicular, predominantly large cell	Follicle centre
Diffuse small cleaved cell	Some follicle centre, some mantle cell
Diffuse mixed small cell and large cell	Mixed correlations
Diffuse large cell	Mixed correlations
High-grade lymphoma	
Large-cell immunoblastic	Mixed correlations
Lymphoblastic	Lymphoblastic (B, T)
Small non-cleaved cell	Burkitt's

▌ **Table 40.3** Phenotypic markers in lymphoma. Characteristic expression by neoplastic cells in biopsies. In all cases heterogeneity may occur within or between biopsies. Less commonly expressed markers are in parentheses

B-lineage neoplasms

ALL/lymphoblastic lymphoma	TdT, CD10, MHC II, (CD19, CD22$_c$, μ chain$_c$)
CLL/lymphocytic lymphoma	CD5, 19, 20, 23, 37, 43, 79a; IgM$_s$, (IgD$_s$)
Hairy cell leukaemia	CD11$_c$, 19, 20, 22, 37, 79a; Ig$_s$
Mantle cell lymphoma	CD5, 19, 20, 37, 79a; IgM$_s$, (IgD$_s$)
Follicle centre lymphoma	CD19, 20, 22, 37, 79a; (CD10, 23); Ig$_s$
Diffuse large B-cell lymphoma	CD19, 20, 22, 37, 79a; (CD5, 10; Ig$_s$, Ig$_c$)
Burkitt's lymphoma	CD10, 19, 20, 22, 37, 79a; IgM$_s$
Mucosa-associated B-cell lymphoma	CD19, 20, 22, 37, 79a; (CD43), Ig$_s$, (Ig$_c$)
Lymphoplasmacytoid lymphoma	CD19, 20, 22, 37, 79a; (CD28), Ig$_s$, Ig$_c$
Myeloma/plasmacytoma	CD38, (CD40, 43, 56, 79a); (EMA), Ig$_c$

T- and NK-lineage neoplasms

T-cell ALL/lymphoblastic lymphoma	TdT, CD10, acid phosphatase, (CD3$_c$, CD7)
T-cell CLL/PLL/lymphocytic lymphoma	CD2, 3, 5, 7, 4, or 8
T-cell large granular lymphocytic leukaemia*	CD2, 3, 8
NK-cell large granular lymphocytic leukaemia*	CD2, 16, 56, 57
Sézary leukaemia/mycosis fungoides	CD2, 3, 4, 5; (CD7)
Adult T-cell leukaemia/lymphoma	CD2, 3, 4, 25; (CD7)
Anaplastic large-cell lymphoma	CD30, (EMA), variable expression of T markers
Other peripheral T-cell lymphomas	(CD2, 3, 5, 7, 4 or 8) — all highly variable

Hodgkin's disease (HD)

Lymphocyte-predominant HD	CD19, 20, 22, 79a; CDw75
HD, other types	CD30, (CD15), occasionally T or B markers

Subscripted s, surface; subscripted c, cytoplasmic; EMA, epithelial membrane antigen; * Sometimes mixed forms of these two phenotypes are seen.
NK, natural killer; ALL, acute lymphoblastic leukaemia; CLL, chronic lymphocyte leukaemia; PLL, prolymphocytic leukaemia.

are aligned against a diagram of a maturing normal B-cell clone. By marking on the maturational path the state of differentiation of a B-cell neoplasm, one obtains a preliminary indication of the markers which that neoplasm is likely to display. After surveying the individual tumours two areas are considered where immunology and molecular biology have major investigative roles — criteria for monoclonality and detection of minimal residual disease.

Lymphoblastic leukaemias

Acute lymphoblastic leukaemias (ALL) are the most common malignancies of childhood. They represent one of the more successful arenas for chemotherapy, with 5 year survivals now approaching 70%. However, such success has been achieved at the cost of considerable toxicity, with particular concerns arising from the measures necessary to prevent relapse in the central nervous system, and from the role of therapy in pro-

moting second malignancies. Treatment of the disease in adults is much less successful, for reasons which are obscure.

Pre-B acute lymphoblastic leukaemias

The most common variant of these leukaemias, with a particular predominance in infants, is *pre-B ALL*. Previously called 'common ALL' this tumour exhibits nuclear positivity for terminal deoxynucleotidyl transferase (TdT), surface positivity for CD10 (common ALL antigen, CALLA), and major histocompatibility complex (MHC) class II. TdT is found also in pre-T ALL, and is regarded as useful in distinguishing lymphoblastic from myeloblastic leukaemias. It is a template-independent DNA polymerase which adds nucleotides to T and B antigen-receptor genes (at junctions of the V, D, and J gene segments) to augment diversity. CD10 is a neutral endopeptidase regarded as an early B-lineage marker, but can be expressed by other early haemopoietic cells as well as various

▮ **Fig. 40.1** The occurrence of phenotypic markers in normal and neoplastic B cells. Depicted at the top of the figure is a diagram of a maturing B-cell clone in which there are three modes of immunoglobulin synthesis: intracellular μ chains, surface immunolgobulin, and immunoglobulin for export packaged in secretory vesicles. Stages of maturation defined partly by these modes are, left to right, a pre-B cell, a small (resting) lymphocyte, a medium or large (activated) lymphocyte, an immunoblast, and a plasma cell. Neoplasms arise throughout the range, with their cellular characteristics more or less frozen. Against each marker is a horizontal line showing the approximate range of cells displaying it; thus surface immunoglobulin is seen to correlate with surface idiotype (on the immunoglobulin molecule) and with CD79a and b (the α and β transducing chains for surface immunoglobulin). Although complicated by the occurrence of B-cell subsets and neoplastic perturbations, one can glean from the scheme the markers which a neoplastic cell of given morphology is apt to display. For example, a typical chronic lymphocytic lymphoma would display all the markers under the small lymphocyte, including CD5 but omitting the two activation antigens.

epithelia. The lineage of pre-B ALL is more clearly indicated by rearranged immunoglobulin gene segments, and the variable presence of other B-cell markers — cytoplasmic μ chains, cytoplasmic CD22, and surface CD19. A study of the immunoglobulin genes in cases of pre-B ALL in children younger that

3 years revealed, in about 90% of cases, an absence of added nucleotides at the DJ junction; this a feature of fetal B cells, and it has been suggested by Wasserman *et al.* (1992) that these leukaemias arose from transforming events *in utero*.

Pre-T acute lymphoblastic leukaemias

In older children, adolescents and adults *pre-T ALL* attains an incidence comparable with that of pre-B. It displays a higher incidence in males, a thymic mass in about 50% of cases, and an aggressive course with frequent involvement of the central nervous system. Some authorities refer to it as 'T-cell' leukaemia, reserving 'pre-T' for its more primitive variants. However, in the majority of cases the phenotype is thymic, with the T-cell receptor for antigen (TCR) rarely expressed. CD7 is generally present on the cell surface, with CD3 (the multichain protein associated with the TCR on T-cell surfaces) in the cytoplasm.

Other forms

Less common lymphoblastic leukaemias include *B-cell* (Burkitt-type) and *NK-cell* variants, and undifferentiated leukaemias where even the question of lymphoblastic or myeloblastic origin is sometimes indeterminate.

Lymphocytic leukaemias

B-cell forms

The common B-cell variant of CLL (*B-cell CLL*) is the commonest of all human leukaemias, with an incidence rising steeply with age. The majority of neoplastic cells resemble mature small lymphocytes with scanty cytoplasm. They are often present in the blood in numbers exceeding 10^{11}/l. Infiltrates progressively enlarge the lymph nodes and spleen, distorting the architecture, and eventually replace the marrow. They display B-cell markers, including sparse surface immunoglobulin (usually IgM, sometimes accompanied by IgD). The light-chain class and idiotype of the immunoglobulin are constant throughout the clone, and characteristically present V regions closely resembling germline sequences, i.e. with little or no somatic mutation (naive immunoglobulin). The surface also reveals CD5, a high ratio of CD19 to CD20, and CD23 (the low-affinity receptor for Fcε). This phenotype is seen on a minority of normal B cells in blood and follicular mantles, but is prominent in fetal primary follicles.

The course of B-cell CLL is usually indolent, and early-stage disease found incidentally on medical examination of elderly subjects is of little actuarial consequence. However, the behaviour of the disease can be more aggressive. Occasionally, a high-grade lymphoma supervenes (Richter's syndrome), with an immunoglobulin genotype confirming progression from the original CLL clone.

Several less common variants of B-cell CLL are recognized. Some authorities describe a particularly benign form as *monoclonal B-cell lymphocytosis*. In contrast *B-prolymphocytic leukaemia* (B-PLL) has a relatively malignant course. The cells are larger than those of common CLL, have prominent nucleoli and more abundant surface immunoglobulin, and show a tendency to infiltrate the spleen rather than lymph nodes.

The cells of *hairy-cell leukaemia* display B-cell markers, but have prominent surface villi and some features characteristic of myeloid and monocytic lineages (surface CD11c and a capacity for phagocytosis). No corresponding normal B-cell population has been identified. This leukaemia is also of interest because it responds well to therapy with α-interferon, although without being cured. Finally, in what are sometimes called 'lymphoma spillovers', one can see CLL-like blood pictures developing in the course of neoplasms which presented as solid lymphomas.

T-cell forms

T-cell lymphocytic leukaemias are much rarer in the Western world than B cell, and there is some confusion regarding their categories. One variety (*T-cell large granular lymphocytic leukaemia*) presents as a lymphocytosis, the cells being in fact medium lymphocytes with cytoplasmic azurophil granules. Unfortunately, there is evidence that large granular lymphocytosis can reflect *three* different conditions: the T-cell large granular lymphocytic leukaemia, in which the cells are of CD8 phenotype and display a clonal rearrangement of TCR genes; an *NK-cell CLL* with CD16 and other NK markers, but often lacking evidence of monoclonality; or a reactive lymphocytic hyperplasia representing a response to chronic infection or other antigenic stimulus. Sometimes the picture is complicated by the presence of cells of mixed phenotype.

Of comparable incidence to the large granular lymphocytoses are chronic leukaemias where the cellular morphologies are intermediate between those of B-cell CLL and B-cell PLL. They have been called *T-cell CLL* or *T-cell PLL*. The cells may be of either CD4 or CD8 phenotype. They are distinguished from those of the Sézary leukaemia by their expression of CD7.

Sézary leukaemia is a rare neoplasm of CD4-positive lymphocytes which circulate in the blood and diffusely infiltrate the epidermis. The cells are predominantly small, with characteristic deeply grooved cerebriform nuclei. The infiltrated skin becomes erythematous, sometimes progressing to generalized erythroderma, and can present plaques and scaling. *Mycosis fungoides* is a related lymphoma of similar CD4-positive cells, similarly skin-seeking, but the clinical course is indolent and frank leukaemia develops only in the terminal stages.

B-cell non-Hodgkin lymphomas

More than 80% of NHL seen in Western society arises from the B-cell lineage. It follows that identifying a tumour by its T or B origin has not been regarded as clinically helpful, and management is still based on conventional histology, particularly through the categories of the working formulation. However, it is likely that more discriminatory typing which reflects lineage and differentiation, and perhaps genetic lesions, will eventually offer superior attractions for clinical use.

B-lymphoblastic lymphoma presents a diffuse distribution of immature cells with cytological features similar to those of pre-B ALL, and the two conditions are regarded as belonging to a single disease spectrum.

Tumours of small or medium B lymphocytes which present a diffuse rather than follicular organization form a difficult group, dissected in different ways under different classifications. We consider just two major types.

B-lymphocytic lymphoma is a tumour which represents a tissue equivalent of CLL, with scattered tumour masses in which infiltrates of predominantly small lymphocytes are effacing normal lymphold architecture (Fig. 40.2). As the name implies the leukaemic component is initially absent or inconspicuous, but both lymphocytic lymphoma and CLL tend to progress slowly to a final mixed leukaemia/lymphoma picture with widespread tumour throughout nodes, spleen, and marrow. Within this group one must include some lymphomas corresponding to B-PLL, with larger cells and a more aggressive course.

Mantle-cell lymphoma is a tumour similar to B-lymphocytic lymphoma, although usually behaving more aggressively. It is composed of small to medium lymphocytes, typically with a diffuse distribution. Sometimes they congregate around normal follicular centres to form striking mantles, an arrangement probably imposed by the presence of the normal cells

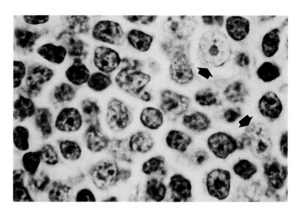

∎ **Fig. 40.2** B-lymphocytic lymphoma/chronic lymphocytic lymphoma. High-power view of a lymph node stained with haematoxylin and eosin. Normal architecture is effaced by infiltrating cells which show a uniform morphology apart from some activated cells (arrowed).

rather than inherent in the neoplasm; it has been suggested that this appearance represents a stage before final destruction of the follicular centres. As in CLL, the cells of this tumour present surface immunoglobulin, commonly IgM ± IgD, and are CD5-positive; however, they are distinguished by being CD23-negative. As the name indicates they are thought to arise from follicular mantles, the same site of origin as has been suggested for CLL. A characteristic (11;14) translocation occurs in the mantle-cell lymphoma, probably disturbing the oncogene *bcl-1* on chromosome 11q.

Follicle-centre lymphomas represent the largest group of NHL occurring in Western society. Their cells resemble cytologically those lymphocytes occurring in the germinal centres of secondary lymphoid follicles, and themselves tend to be organized into follicles (Fig. 40.3). They can be of various sizes and have attracted various names: cleaved follicular centre cells, non-cleaved follicular centre cells, centrocytes/centroblasts, centroblasts, and others. In general, the larger the cells and the more diffuse their organization the more aggressive the tumour. In some tumours, particularly among the large-cell varieties, there is a heavy admixture of normal T cells, sometimes outnumbering and obscuring the neoplastic B cells. Speculation concerning the role of the T cells has varied from immune attack on the neoplastic cells to sustenance of them by release of cytokines. Clinically, no correlation of behaviour with degree of T-cell infiltration has emerged.

Follicle-centre lymphomas express characteristic B-cell markers: surface IgM ± IgD, less commonly

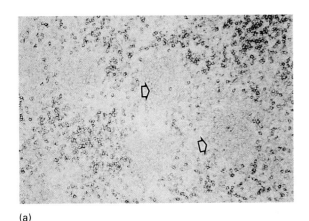

(a)

(b)

■ **Fig. 40.3** Follicle-centre lymphoma. Low-power view of a lymph node with immunoperoidase staining for κ (a) and λ (b) immunoglobulin light chains. In (a) the neoplastic germinal centres show weak membrane staining for κ (open arrows), with stronger staining apparent among the normal B cells in the surrounding mantles. In (b) there is no staining of the germinal centres (open arrows) but strong staining for λ is apparent in the mantles (closed arrows). The monotypic staining for immunoglobulin light chains shows that the follicles are neoplastic rather than reactive.

one of the other immunoglobulin classes, CD19, 20, 21, 22, and 37. The surface densities of these molecules vary considerably from case to case, but the overall pattern is consistent. CD5 is a notable absentee. The tumour immunoglobulin typically shows heavily mutated V regions, as would be expected of B cells which have at some stage undergone physiological clonal expansion following contact with antigen. In many cases this mutation appears to be continuing during the neoplastic clonal expansion, so that the V regions within a single tumour can display microheterogeneity. The contrast with B-cell CLL/

lymphocytic lymphoma, with displays of CD5 and near-germline V regions, is striking.

The characteristic karyotypic abnormality of follicle-centre lymphoma, seen in up to 85% of cases, but less in European and Japanese series, is a (14;18) translocation. This moves the *bcl-2* oncogene from its normal position at q21 on chromosome 18 into the immunoglobulin heavy chain locus at q32 on chromosome 14. There follows an over-production of BCL-2 protein, presumably as a result of influence by immunoglobulin promoter sequences. The protein appears within a variety of intracellular membranes, and acts as a suppressor of programmed cell death. The neoplastic cell thereby resists the apoptotic fate of most normal follicular centre cells. Such a property might be an important contributor to neoplastic autonomy, but is unlikely to be the entire explanation as cells bearing the translocation have been described in normal subjects. Recognized superimposed genomic damage such as mutation of p53 has been associated with more aggressive behaviour.

Diffuse large B-cell lymphomas are an aggressive group accounting for perhaps one-third of B-cell NHL. Patients often present with a single mass at a nodal or extranodal site. The cells are large (larger than B lymphoblastic) with a high proliferative rate. Subdivisions (e.g. centroblastic, immunoblastic, and anaplastic types in the Kiel classification) have been interpreted inconsistently and so for the present are best abandoned; nevertheless, heterogeneity of the group is suggested by the fact that no predominant genomic lesion has been reported. Despite their malignancy these tumours are sometimes cured completely by chemotherapy.

Burkitt's lymphoma is a highly malignant, extranodal tumour composed of B lymphocytes of medium size which resemble follicular centre blasts but are rarely seen to form follicles (Fig. 40.4). Histologically, there is a characteristic 'starry sky' appearance; normal macrophages, engaged in clearing away apoptotic cells, stand out due to their being surrounded by relatively clear areas. The tumour has a high endemic incidence in the tropical uplands of Africa and New Guinea, where it represents some 90% of childhood cancer. The corresponding figure in Western society is about 3%.

In tropical cases of Burkitt's lymphoma the tumour cells regularly contain the genome of the Epstein–Barr virus (EBV), whereas only about 15% of childhood cases in the West reveal the same phenomenon. A constant feature of the tumour is a reciprocal translocation which brings the *myc* gene into proximity with an immunoglobulin gene cluster; in most cases *myc* is translocated from chromosome 8

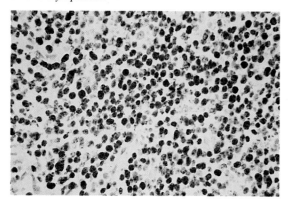

∎ **Fig. 40.4** Burkitt's lymphoma. Low-power view of an extranodal tumour from the neck, with immunoperoxidase staining for the cell-cycle-related marker MIB-1. Strong brown nuclear staining of the majority of cells in the photograph illustrates the high proliferative rate characteristic of this tumour.

to 14, to lie next to immunoglobulin heavy-chain genes; in a minority of cases one or other of the light-chain clusters is translocated from chromosome 2 or 22 to lie next to *myc* on chromosome 8. The result of such translocations is an abnormal activation of the *myc* gene by enhancer elements in the adjacent immunoglobulin gene.

The high incidence of Burkitt's lymphoma in some tropical areas may reflect the following chain of events.

1. Infection with malaria and other parasites leads to lymphoid hyperplasia due to high antigen load.

2. In the societies concerned infection with EBV also occurs very early in life, possibly acquired via the mother's milk or saliva.

3. The virus promotes mitosis in infected B lymphocytes; it is seen to immortalize B cells *in vitro*, but not by itself to confer neoplastic autonomy *in vivo*. Some of the vital genes necessary for promoting mitosis in the host cell have been identified, but the mechanism has not been elucidated.

4. The parasite-preoccupied lymphoid system cannot generate an adequate cytotoxic T-cell response to EBV-infected B cells.

5. Continued B-cell mitosis in an expanded lymphoid system greatly enhances the chances of the chromosomal translocation with *myc* activation which is probably the major determinant of the neoplastic transformation. The translocation occurs apparently in a B cell of early lineage which is rearranging the V, D, and J genes which

will make up the variable region of its immunoglobulin molecules. The breakpoint in chromosome 14 is in a J or less often a D segment. In contrast, in EBV-negative Burkitt's lymphoma the breakpoint is generally in a constant-region switch segment, suggesting that these lymphomas arise from B cells switching heavy-chain class after antigenic stimulation. A third genetic change, a mutation in the p53 suppressor gene, may contribute to oncogenesis in at least some cases of Burkitt's lymphoma, and other genetic lesions have occasionally been described (Klein 1993).

Lymphomas occurring at increased incidence in states of immunodeficiency (including primary immunodeficiencies, acquired immune deficiency syndrome (AIDS), and immunosuppression for organ grafting) are frequently B-cell lymphomas bearing genomic evidence of EBV (Levine, 1994). In some cases a polyclonal immunoproliferation is observed initially, from which a clearly monoclonal tumour may later emerge. The AIDS-associated lymphomas often exhibit also the *myc*-activating translocations and histological appearances typical of Burkitt's lymphoma, but this appears to be uncommon in the more heterogeneous transplantation associated tumours.

Mucosa-associated B-cell lymphomas (B-cell MALT lymphomas) have been described in gut, respiratory tract, salivary glands, thyroid, and ocular adnexa. They usually have a relatively benign course, but may transform to higher malignancy. The histology tends to recapitulate that of normal mucosal lymphoid tissue (MALT), and the neoplastic cells tend to home to mucosal sites. Neoplastic lymphocytes of various sizes are often associated with reactive follicles. Invasion of the overlying epithelium yields characteristic lymphoepithelial lesions. Paradoxically, most of these tumours arise in the stomach, which normally contains no organized lymphoid tissue. It is believed that such tissue is acquired as a result of chronic infection with *Helicobacter pylori*, which is reported to be associated with more than 90% of gastric MALT lymphomas (Isaacson 1994). Low-grade tumours have been seen to undergo regression after eradication of the organism. The association suggests that other causes of chronic inflammation at mucosal sites can also predispose to MALT lymphoma.

Other B-cell lymphomas listed in the REA classification include lymphoplasmacytoid lymphoma (many of which can be classified as macroglobulinaemia), nodal marginal-zone lymphoma, splenic marginal zone lymphoma, primary mediastinal large B-cell lymphoma, and high-grade Burkitt-like B-cell lymphoma.

Immunoglobulin-exporting lymphomas

Consideration of these tumours falls naturally after B-cell NHL, from which they are not sharply demarcated. Their separate grouping reflects their generally distinct clinical pictures, due to secondary effects of secreted monoclonal protein (paraprotein) and, in the case of myeloma, skeletal destruction.

Macroglobulinaemia (of Waldenström)

This is a B-cell lymphoma defined by the presence of exported monoclonal IgM in the plasma. It must be distinguished on the one hand from a persistent monoclonal IgM in the absence of frank neoplasm (a form of 'MGUS' — monoclonal gammopathy of unknown significance), and on the other from lymphomas which export IgM at a level which is not clinically significant. MGUS is more frequent than macroglobulinaemia, and tends to emerge in routine screening of elderly subjects. The standard clinical approach to MGUS is to monitor the patient for ominous biochemical signs, including a rising level of monoclonal IgM, a lowered concentration of other plasma immunoglobulin, and a rising level of urinary immunoglobulin light chains. The other distinction required, from lymphoma (commonly lymphocytic lymphoma) exporting inconsequential amounts of IgM, is arbitrarily dependent on local laboratory practice. Often a sharp IgM band on an electrophoretic strip, representing a concentration in plasma of about 5 g/l or more, will be considered significant.

The common histological picture in Waldenström's macroglobulinaemia is of pleomorphic small lymphocytes, some plasmacytoid, which infiltrate lymphoid tissue extensively. The spleen and lymph nodes are enlarged and normal marrow displaced. The cells are readily detectable in the blood by virtue of their monoclonal surface IgM. Osteolytic lesions as seen in myeloma are rare, although intermediate forms between myeloma and macroglobulinaemia do occur. The secreted IgM is present typically at >10 g/l and at such concentrations can raise plasma viscosity dangerously; possible consequences include retinal haemorrhages with rapid deterioration of vision, and cerebral vascular catastrophes. Such risks sometimes merit emergency plasmapheresis in order to lower the IgM concentration. A bleeding tendency is common, with possible contributions from raised blood viscosity, and interference by the paraprotein with clotting proteins and platelet function. Other problems such as cold haemagglutination and polyneuropathy can follow from autoantibody activities of the IgM.

Myeloma

This is a neoplasm of plasma cells which proliferate in the bone marrow. Commonly, it forms multiple tumour masses (hence 'multiple myeloma') and is highly malignant. Occasionally, it occurs as a solitary osseous or extra-osseous mass (plasmacytoma), which can display relatively benign behaviour.

Myeloma cells usually appear in marrow aspirates or trephines as a mix of normal and atypical plasma cells. They display intracellular but not surface immunoglobulin (Fig. 40.5). Most other surface B-cell markers are also absent, but CD38 is seen regularly, and CD56, CD40, and MHC class II have been reported in some cases. Occasionally, cells with the morphology of small lymphocytes are recognized as belonging to the neoplastic clone, by virtue of a karyotypic abnormality or the synthesis of idiotypic immunoglobulin. The clonogenic role of such cells has been debated, but no good evidence has emerged of their mitotic rate playing a significant part in maintaining the tumour. The malignant plasma cells spread diffusely and form scattered nodules which erode the surrounding bone. The sharply demarcated bony defects are believed to reflect activation of osteoclasts, possibly by cytokines [interleukin (IL) 1β, tumour necrosis factor-β] secreted by the tumour.

In about 75% of cases of myeloma there is an obvious plasma paraprotein, in decreasing order of frequency IgG, IgA, IgD, and IgE. As in the case of IgM, such paraproteins can be seen in MGUS in the absence

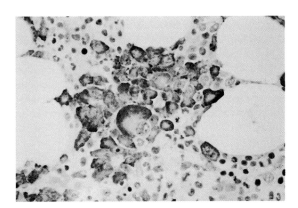

❚ **Fig. 40.5** Myeloma. High-power view of a bone-marrow trephine with immunoperoxidase staining for κ immunoglobulin light chains. The neoplastic cells show a range of morphologies, with strong positive (brown) staining of the cytoplasm.

of obvious neoplasm, and here again the patients must be watched for malignant transformation of the secreting clone, which in the series of Kyle (1994) appeared at an actuarial rate of 33% over 20 years. No case has been made for subjecting patients with MGUS to chemotherapy in the hope of ablating early tumour or delaying its emergence. In about 50% of myeloma patients there is excretion of monoclonal light chains (Bence Jones proteins) in excess of 500 mg/day, the approximate level at which the classical heat test for their presence becomes positive. This test (precipitation at about 50°C at mildly acid pH, followed by variable redissolving during boiling) is rarely positive in MGUS and has historically been useful in diagnosis. In extreme cases excretion of Bence Jones protein can exceed 30 g/day and cause serious nitrogen depletion. In about 25% of patients heavy excretion of Bence Jones proteins occurs in the absence of an obvious plasma paraprotein. In perhaps 10% of patients there is clinically significant light-chain amyloidosis, associated with tissue deposition of the tumour light chains or fragments thereof. There is a limited correlation of the nature of immunoglobulin type with prognosis; patients with an IgD paraprotein, and those with a λ Bence Jones protein as their only abnormality, tend to fare badly.

The common clinical problems in this distressing disease relate to bone destruction, renal failure, and immunodeficiency. A common presentation is bone pain or pathological fracture. The kidney can be damaged by hypercalcaemia associated with bone destruction, by extensive protein deposition in tubules associated with Bence Jones proteinuria, by infection, and by amyloidosis.

Other varieties of immunoglobulin-exporting lymphomas are encountered occasionally. *Heavy-chain diseases* are a group of lymphomas of variable histology which secrete heavy chains, or more often partially deleted heavy chains, not combined with light chains. The light chains are in some cases not secreted at all, while in others they are secreted but are unable to combine with their abnormal partners. The heavy chains can reach a high concentration in serum and/or urine. Gamma γ chain disease is generally accompanied by a lymphoplasmacytic lymphoma. Most cases of μ-chain disease present a pathological picture of CLL. α-chain disease is a small intestinal B-cell MALT lymphoma with plasma cells prominent. Most cases have occurred in the Middle East or Mediterranean littoral. *'Monoclonal immunoglobulin deposition disease'* describes a type of immunoglobulin precipitation which has been observed in association with myeloma, macroglobulinaemia, and MGUS. The deposits lack the staining properties and fibrillar

organization seen in amyloidosis. They consist of light chains, heavy chains, or a mixture of the two.

T-cell non-Hodgkin lymphomas

The first three varieties of T-cell tumour discussed below are well characterized, but the confusing peripheral T-cell lymphomas are a heterogeneous and poorly understood group.

T-lymphoblastic lymphoma is the tissue-equivalent of pre-T ALL, with the cells indistinguishable. There is again a predominance of males and a tendency to involve the thymus, although it may present with peripheral lymphadenopathy. It is rapidly progressive and frequently terminates in acute leukaemia.

In southern Japan and the Caribbean basin, and to a questionable extent in sub-Saharan Africa, there occurs a relatively malignant neoplasm, *adult T-cell lymphoma/leukaemia* (ATLL), associated with the RNA retrovirus HTLV-I (human T-cell leukaemia virus type I). The viral infection is endemic in areas where the tumour occurs. Infection may be present for 30 or more years before the tumour appears. The virus can be spread from mother to child (mainly via milk), by blood transfusion, and (with low infectivity) by sexual activity. The lifetime risk of tumour for carriers of the virus is probably not more than 1%. Another possible consequence of infection is a chronic myelopathy (tropical spastic paraparesis).

The cells of ATLL are of CD4 subtype. They are pleomorphic, often with multilobed nuclei. There is a characteristic high surface density of complete IL-2 receptors, including the CD25 epitope. In its typical malignant form, with median survival of less than 1 year, the disease displays a high leukaemic count, hepatosplenomegaly, skin infiltration, and hypercalcaemia. Less often it is relatively indolent, sometimes with localized nodal involvement and no obvious leukaemic component. The varied clinical course is well described by Catovsky and Foa (1990).

Enteropathy-associated T-cell lymphomas most commonly present as jejunal tumours associated with coeliac disease. The latter is a malabsorptive enteropathy of puzzling pathogenesis, with features of both hypersensitivity (resolving upon elimination of gluten from the diet) and autoimmunity (strong association with MHC class II DQ2 alleles, presence of antireticulin antibodies, and heavy lymphocytic infiltration of the local epithelium). It seems plausible that the tumour is preceded by the enteropathy and arises from the infiltrating lymphocytes, and most cases have a

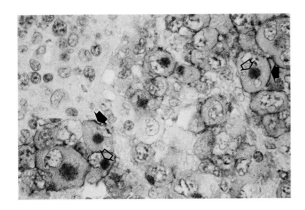

▌ **Fig. 40.6** Anaplastic large-cell lymphoma, a rare peripheral T-cell lymphoma which is notable for its display of the activation marker CD30. High-power view of a lymph node with alkaline phosphatase staining for CD30. Strong staining is apparent on the neoplastic cell membranes (closed arrows), and in the Golgi region of some cells (open arrows).

history consistent with this sequence of events. The behaviour of the tumour is aggressive; the cells are of various sizes, sometimes pleomorphic, and the disease often leads to jejunal ulceration and perforation.

Other T-cell lymphomas are often gathered together as *peripheral T-cell lymphomas*. They are a confusing group. Although uncommon they occur in considerable morphological variety, and both the lineage and clonality of individual tumours can present problems. *Angioimmunoblastic T-cell lymphoma* displays an expansion of high endothelial venules, the specialized vessels of T-cell areas through which lymphocytic migration from blood into lymphoid tissue normally occurs. *Angiocentric lymphoma* has tumour cells which invade and occlude blood vessels, leading to ischaemic necrosis; in some cases NK markers are present as well as or instead of T-cell markers. *Anaplastic large-cell lymphoma* has been delineated by virtue of its consistent and striking display of CD30, an activation antigen first observed in Hodgkin's disease (HD) (Fig. 40.6). The cells are unusually large, and often involve nodal sinuses and extranodal sites. Again the expression of T-cell antigens is variable. The remaining peripheral T-cell (or alleged T-cell) lymphomas can present even greater problems. TCR gene rearrangements have yielded evidence of polyclonality in a surprising number of cases. Occasionally, an apparent T-cell lymphoma is shown subsequently to be a B-cell tumour, confusion having arisen from the masking of inconspicuous neoplastic cells by a heavy infiltrate of reactive T cells.

Hodgkin's disease

Hodgkin's disease (HD) has long been an enigma. For many years workers argued whether it represented chronic infection or neoplasm. With the case for neoplasm conceded, questions have persisted about the nature of the neoplastic cell and the role of a virus in pathogenesis. The current histological subdivision into four types (Table 40.1) has survived in essence since 1966. Moving down through the categories the prognosis worsens as one proceeds from lymphocyte-predominant to lymphocyte-depleted forms. Although the picture is blurred by variations in histological diagnosis, it seems that the most common type, nodular sclerosing, has a peak incidence in young adulthood while the remainder have an increasing incidence with age.

Despite the variation inherent in its four histological types HD has given the impression of being a distinct clinical entity. There is a characteristic axial distribution of involved nodes, and among these the disease can often be seen to spread from an initial focus rather than show dissemination at presentation, as is common in NHL. The mode of spread accounts for the emphasis placed on accurate clinical staging, important in turn for the precisely controlled radiotherapy which has played a large part in making this the most successfully treated of the lymphomas. A general T-cell anergy is another typical feature of HD which is noted clinically. It can be apparent even in early disease, and persist in patients who have been successfully treated.

The neoplastic cell in HD is seen in both binuclear and mononuclear forms, called respectively Reed–Sternberg (RS) and Hodgkin cells (Fig. 40.7).

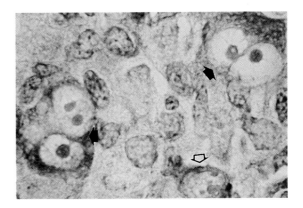

▌**Fig. 40.7** Hodgkin's disease. High-power view of an involved lymph node stained with haematoxylin and eosin. Three neoplastic cells are visible: two are binuclear Reed–Sternberg cells (closed arrows), one a mononuclear Hodgkin's cell (open arrow).

Characteristically, these cells account for only a tiny proportion of the total tumour mass, typically less than 2–3%. Generally, the histology is dominated by a complex and variable inflammatory infiltrate consisting of lymphocytes, macrophages, eosinophils, neutrophils, and fibrous tissue. Cytokines are likely to have a large role in this inflammation and in the patient's T-cell anergy; studies conducted by immunostaining and analysis of gene expression have identified a wide range of cytokines within the tumour tissue.

There is a growing tendency to place lymphocyte-predominant disease, or at least the nodular subtype, to one side of the Hodgkin spectrum. Cells with RS morphology are rarely seen. Commonly one sees germinal centres with a progressive accumulation of atypical cells which have multilobe vesicular nuclei and small nucleoli ('popcorn' cells). These cells show B-cell-associated antigens, such as CD19, 20, 22, and 79a; CD30 is variably present. However, despite the B-cell phenotype, monotypic immunoglobulin is not seen and clonal rearrangements of immunoglobulin genes have rarely been described. Staining for follicular dendritic cells shows prominent networks within the nodules. The evidence suggests that this subtype of HD arises from the B lineage, but one may have to postulate that oncogenesis occurred before rearrangement of immunoglobulin genes, or in cells in which this rearrangement was disabled.

The remaining varieties of HD display Hodgkin and RS cells of typical morphology. The surface antigens are lymphocytic rather than myeloid or monocytic, although the myelomonocytic CD15 is frequently present in a proportion of cells — a useful distinguishing feature from lymphocyte-predominant HD. A variety of lymphocytic activation antigens (CD25, 30, 71, and MHC class II) are apparent, but the expression of markers specific for the T or B lineage has been variable. Clonal rearrangements of the immunoglobulin and TCR genes have often not been detected, and such positive reports as have emerged have not followed any clear pattern. These findings have led to the suggestion that oncogenic transformation has occurred in the lymphocytic lineage before commitment to either the T or B arm has occurred.

Some epidemiological and cellular data suggest that the EBV has a pathogenic role in many cases of HD. A significantly increased risk of the disease exists among those who have a history of symptomatic infectious mononucleosis. The presence of a restricted number of viral antigens, and/or of viral DNA, has been reported in Hodgkin and RS cells in approximately half the cases in the Western world, with the incidence being notably higher among cases classified as mixed cellularity. In AIDS-associated HD the presence of EBV in the neoplastic cells is evident in virtually all cases. The observation that EBV positivity may vary with age of onset of HD, and the existence of a large proportion of EBV-negative cases, complicate our understanding of the role of this virus. Attempts to identify other HD-associated viruses, in particular HHV6, have proved negative.

Criteria for monoclonality

In a suspiciously expanded lymphoid cell population, the demonstration of some monoclonal feature, such as uniformity of its immunoglobulin product, increases the probability that the population is neoplastic in the functional sense of displaying *'progressive, purposeless and parasitic'* growth *in vivo*. Conversely, an obviously heterogeneous immunoglobulin product or other immunophenotypic heterogeneity would suggest that the expanded population is reactive, and unlikely to exhibit neoplastic characteristics.

These are useful generalizations but exceptions are well recognized. One sees in MGUS an apparently monoclonal and sometimes large antibody response, where sometimes the underlying B-cell clone never behaves in a frankly neoplastic fashion. In immunosuppressed patients one is sometimes confronted with a polyclonal B-cell expansion which can display neoplastic aggressiveness, with or without a single monoclonal population emerging as the dominant neoplastic element. Finally, it should be emphasized that polyclonality is to be distinguished from clonal diversification, a common phenomenon associated with mutation in expanding neoplastic clones. We have already alluded to a special example: heterogeneous immunoglobulin variable-region sequences in follicle-centre lymphoma.

Basic immunological phenotyping of a lymphoid population for B, T, and NK markers, usually by flow cytometry and/or immunohistology, will often provide a reasonable basis for judging clonality. A good example is whether or not suspect B cells are exhibiting monotypic surface immunoglobulin, that is with light chains almost exclusively κ or almost exclusively λ. If the immunoglobulin is exported one may resort also to the long-established practice of seeing whether it displays electrophoretic homogeneity.

On some occasions, as when tumour cells are obscured by a heavy infiltration of reactive lymphocytes, one requires more sensitive or stringent criteria of monoclonality. Those available include the homogeneity of variable regions on the antigen receptor (immunoglobulin or TCR), and the presence of a lymphoma-specific chromosomal translocation. These areas, recently reviewed by Aisenberg (1993) are now frequently investigated at the genetic level, usually by the probing of polymerase chain reaction (PCR) amplified material .

When subjected to genetic probing, B-cell neoplasms of mature phenotype will generally reveal uniform rearrangements of the V, D, and J genes encoding their immunoglobulin variable regions, confirming monoclonality. Their TCR genes remain for the most part in non-rearranged (germ-line) configuration. Mature T neoplasms often show the expected converse picture, but a puzzling proportion of what are apparently peripheral T-cell neoplasms present polyclonal TCR gene patterns.

Immature neoplasms (the lymphoblastic lymphomas and leukaemias) reveal B or T gene rearrangements in accord with their other B or T phenotypic features; indeed rearranged immunoglobulin genes were a major factor in establishing the B-cell lineage of common ALL. However, the picture can be complicated by instability, so that new V/D/J combinations emerge: not sufficient to give an appearance of frank polyclonality, but enough to cause problems if probes constructed from PCR-amplified material are used later to search for minimal residual disease. A further complication is the frequent occurrence of double rearrangements, so that T genes are rearranged in B neoplasms and vice versa. Perhaps these instabilities and double rearrangements reflect a neoplastic transformation occurring at about the stage of, and thereby perturbing, the normal shuffling of antigen-receptor gene segments. It is worth noting that the same recombinase enzymes are used to rearrange both T and B genes.

The chromosomal translocations characteristic of some types of lymphoma — t(8;14) or variant in Burkitt's, t(11;14) in mantle cell, and t(14;18) in follicular — offer possibilities for genetic probing across the break-points as a means of establishing monoclonality, of establishing presumptive neoplastic behaviour, and of detecting minimal residual disease. Again PCR promises to be the technique of choice, and a multiplicity of primers and of probes for the amplified material are becoming available. The t(14;18) translocation is receiving particular attention.

Detection of minimal residual disease

The ability to detect small numbers of neoplastic cells in the midst of large normal populations has obvious practical implications for guiding treatment, predicting relapse, and assessing neoplastic contamination of autografts. Investigations of such basic phenomena as tumour dormancy will also be facilitated.

The techniques used to detect minimal disease overlap extensively with those used to define monoclonality. If the neoplastic population has a distinctive set of normal surface markers (for example, monotypic immunoglobulin and CD11c in hairy-cell leukaemia) one can conveniently search for the cells by conventional flow cytometry or immunohistology. For greater specificity one can turn to distinctive features of the antigen receptor. Exported tumour immunoglobulin can be detected at a relatively crude level in serum or urine by virtue of its electrophoretic homogeneity. If in a research setting idiotypic antibodies are available, these can be used to detect the immunoglobulin in body fluids (generally by enzyme-linked immunosorbent assay), on cell surfaces or intracellularly. Again the use of such antibodies is being supplanted by genetic techniques which seek distinctive sequences in the encoding nucleotides for immunoglobulin or TCR, with the use of probes from PCR-amplified material proving particularly useful. In the ALLs where complete clinical response to initial chemotherapy is the norm, there is a strong case for probing for, and dealing with, resurgent tumour at the earliest possible stage. As mentioned earlier the frequent instability of immunoglobulin and TCR gene-segment rearrangements in these tumours means that polynucleotide probes constructed early in the disease might fail to react with cells emerging in relapse. Finally, there is increasing use of probes which will detect the nucleotide sequences brought about by chromosomal translocations such as t(14;18). Such techniques are usually applied to cells from blood or marrow aspirates, with the latter proving the more useful (Gribben *et al.* 1994).

Further reading

Aisenberg, C. A. (1993). Utility of gene rearrangements in lymphoid malignancies. *Annual Review of Medicine*, **44**, 75–84.

Catovsky, D. and Foa, R. (1990). *The lymphoid leukaemias*, pp. 218–52. Butterworth, London.

Cline, M. J. (1994) Histiocytes and histiocytosis. *Blood*, **84**, 2840–53.

Croce, C. M. (1993) Molecular biology of lymphomas. *Seminars in Oncology* **20**, 31–46.

Garand, R., Vannier, R. J. P., Bene, M. C., Faure, G. C., and Bernard, A. (1989) Correlations between acute lymphoid leukemia (ALL) immunophenotype and clinical laboratory data at presentation. A study of 350 patients. *Cancer*, **64**, 1437–46.

Gribben, J. G., Neuberg, D., Barber M., J. Moore, K. W. Pesek, A. S. Freedman, and L. M. Nadler (1994). Detection of residual lymphoma cells by polymerase chain reaction in peripheral blood is significantly less predictive for relapse than detection in bone marrow. *Blood* **83**, 3800–7.

F. G. Haluska, A. M. Brufsky, and G. P. Canellos (1994). The cellular biology of the Reed–Sternberg cell. *Blood*, **84**, 1005–19.

N. L. Harris, E. S. Jaffe, H. Stein, P. M. Banks, J. K. C. Chan, M. L. Cleary, *et al.* (1994). A revised European–American classification of lymphoid neoplasms: a proposal from the international lymphoma study group. *Blood*, **84**, 1361–92.

P. G. Isaacson (1994). Gastointestinal lymphoma. *Human Pathology*, **25**, 1020–9.

T. J. Kipps (1993). Immunoglobulin genes in chronic lymphocytic leukemia. *Blood Cells*, **19**, 615–25.

G. Klein (1993). Multistep evolution of B-cell-derived tumors in humans and rodents. *Gene*, **135**, 189–96.

R. A. Kyle. (1994). Monoclonal gammopathy of undetermined significance. *Blood Reviews*, **3**, 135–41.

A. M. Levine (1994). Lymphoma complicating immunodeficiency disorders. *Annals of Oncology*, **5**, 29–35.

T. Meeker, J. Lowder, M. L. Cleary, S. Steward, R. Warnke. J. Sklar, and R. Levy (1985) Emergence of idiotype variants during treatment of B-cell lymphoma with anti-idiotype antibodies. *New England Journal of Medicine*, **312**, 1658–65.

J. Rodriquez, W. C. Pugh, and F. Cabanillas (1993). T-cell rich B-cell lymphoma. *Blood*, **82**, 1586–9.

M. Seligmann, E. Mihaesco, J. L. Preud'homme, F. Danon, and J. C. Brouet. (1979). Heavy chain diseases: a review. *Immunology Reviews*, **48**, 145–67.

F. K. Stevenson, T. J. Hamblin, G. T. Stevenson and A. L. Tutt (1980). Extracellular idiotypic immunoglobulin arising from human leukemic B lymphocytes. *Journal of Experimental Medicine*, **152**, 1484–96.

E Vandenberghe (1994). Mantle cell lymphoma. *Blood Reviews*, **8**, 79–87.

R. Wasserman, N. Galili, Y. Ito, B. A. Reichard, S. Shane and G. Rovera (1992). Predominance of tetal type D J. joining in young children with precursor lymphoblastic leukemia as evidence for an in utero transforming event. *Journal of Experimental Medicine*, **176**, 1577–81.

B. Wormann (1993). Implications of detection of minimal residual disease. *Current Opinion in Oncology*, **5**, 3–12.

41 Cancer

C. M. Steel, A. G. Dalgleish, and M. J. Browning

Historical background

The concept of tumour immunogenicity is almost as old as the study of immunology itself and so much experimental work had been undertaken by the early years of the twentieth century than in 1916 E. E. Tyzzer commented: *'It is quite impossible to present within reasonable space a comprehensive review of all investigations in tumour immunity'*. Most studies in that era involved attempts to transplant tumours from one animal to another — usually, but not always, of the same species — and sometimes included the observation of accelerated rejection following prior exposure of the recipient to killed cells or cell extracts from the tumour. With hindsight, it is obvious that the immunity so demonstrated was allogeneic or xenogeneic and had little to do with possible tumour-specific antigens. However, that realization dawned only gradually, even after the introduction of inbred strains of mice to the experimental armamentarium. When it finally took hold, it did so with a vengeance and by the 1930s opinion had swung overwhelmingly to the view that tumours were non-immunogenic in the original host or in syngeneic animals.

The experiments that led to such negative conclusions were undertaken largely with spontaneous tumours and the picture began to change again when chemically induced and virally induced tumours became the stock-in-trade of experimental oncology from the 1940s onwards. Ludwig Gross was the first to show clear evidence of tumour-specific immunogenicity with sarcomas arising after exposure to Methylcholanthrene in C3H mice (Gross, 1943). Baldwin (1955), Kripke (1974), Prehn (1976), Old (1981), and others have confirmed and extended his findings so that, by the 1960s, the following concepts were very firmly established:

1. Most virally induced tumours, particularly those associated with polyoma and simian virus 40 (SV40), are quite strongly antigenic. It is possible to confer a measure of protection against inoculated tumour cells by prior exposure to the same tumour or to another tumour caused by the same virus or even to cell-free virus.

2. Tumour cell lines that become infected by virus may then become immunogenic (in syngeneic animals) for the first time, the protective antitumour antigens being virus-coded.

3. Chemically or UV-induced tumours can also show protective immunogenicity in the autologous or syngeneic host but there is rarely any cross-reactivity between the effective antigens of different tumours, whether caused by the same or different agents. This lack of cross-reactivity even extends to separate tumours induced simultaneously by the same chemical in a single animal.

4. Some viral tumours (e.g. those cause by the mouse mammary tumour virus) and virtually all spontaneous tumours show little, if any, evidence of protective immunogenicity in conventional assays. (These involve challenge with an inoculum of viable tumour following excision of a previously growing tumour of the same origin or 'immunization' with killed cells or cell extracts).

One possible conclusion is that tumour immunity, when it is observed, is merely an artefact of a strong oncogenic stimulus that happens to induce alterations in the antigenicity of the target tissue as a side-effect.

Alternatively, altered antigenicity might be a common feature of malignant change so that, in the absence of a powerful carcinogenic influence that causes transformation and rapid growth of large numbers of target cells, the majority of 'spontaneous' tumours are actually eliminated by immune surveillance before they ever become clinically apparent and only rare, unrepresentative, examples survive. Indeed, they do so by virtue of selection for low immunogenicity.

These two conflicting interpretations of the animal data remain the basis for argument to the present day. Both, however, leave open the possibility that levels of immunogenicity too weak to be detected by conventional assays, as described above, may still be displayed by some, or even all, naturally occurring malignancies and that there may therefore be scope for harnessing the immune response in therapy.

Immune suppression and malignancy

If immune surveillance is an important protective mechanism, some correlation might be anticipated between immune suppression and malignancy. Neither animal nor clinical studies, however, provide a clear cut answer. The congenitally athymic 'nude' mouse, and the even more immunocompromised SCID (severe combined immune deficient) mouse, although relatively receptive to transplantation of allogeneic or xenogenic tumours, do not show an abnormally high incidence of spontaneous tumours, apart for those of the lymphoid system. Similarly, human organ transplant recipients receiving large doses of immunosuppressive drugs over prolonged periods are at risk mainly from tumours associated with viruses [Epstein–Barr virus (EBV) and papillomavirus] as well as apparently non-viral lymphomas which may, as suggested by Penn (1988), be attributable to constant stimulation of the lymphoid system rather than to immune suppression. The same is true of patients suffering from human immunodeficiency virus (HIV)-associated or other forms of acquired immune deficiency (Table 41.1). This, of course, does not constitute conclusive evidence against any part for the immune system in protection from cancer as surveillance in the crucial early stage of carcinogenesis could be mediated by some component of the immune apparatus [natural killer (NK) cell or macrophage, for example] that may not be severely impaired in any of these situations.

Indirect evidence for tumour immunogenicity

Given the tenuous nature of direct experimental or observational evidence for immune defences against naturally occurring tumours, it might be questioned why the concept retains such popular appeal. An obvious answer is 'wishful thinking' as if it were valid

▍ **Table 41.1** Tumours characteristic of immunocompromised individuals

---

In primary immunodeficiency states
 Chiefly B-cell lymphomas (often EBV-associated)

In organ transplant recipients
 Lymphomas (EBV-associated and others)
 Basal cell carcinomas of skin
 Squamous carcinomas of skin
 Cervical cancer

In HIV +ve patients
 Kaposi's sarcoma
 Lymphoma: mainly non-Hodgkin's; may be EBV +ve or –ve; often arising in extranodal sites (e.g. CNS or bowel)
 Squamous carcinoma of tongue
 Squamous carcinoma of anorectum

Data from Penn (1988); Hanto *et al.* (1983); *Lancet* (1988); Quinn (1987); Harawi and O'Hara (1989).
EBV, Epstein–Barr virus.

then immune modulation might represent an extra modality of treatment free from many of the disadvantages of conventional therapy. In addition, however, there are some persuasive lines of indirect evidence that lend support to the proponents of tumour immunology.

First, there is the very real phenomenon of spontaneous regression of tumours, rarely complete but often unequivocal, even if temporary or partial, confined perhaps to certain deposits of the disease while others, in the same patient, continue to progress. The classic study of Bodenham (1968) documented simultaneous regression and growth in adjacent cutaneous lesions of malignant melanoma and although non-immunological mechanisms may be proposed for such changes, it does appear that spontaneous regression occurs most commonly in those tumours (melanoma, renal cell carcinoma, lymphoma) in which the other evidence for immunogenicity is strongest, as discussed later.

Second, there is the histological demonstration of tumour infiltration with inflammatory cells, usually most evident within the stroma at the margins of a cancer, although a similar phenomenon can occur more diffusely, for example in acute myeloid leukaemia. These cells, sometimes termed 'tumour infiltrating lymphocytes' (TIL) are, in most cases, a very mixed population, including monocytes, NK cells, and some granulocytes as well as both T and B lymphocytes. There is long-standing controversy about their significance but, as shown by Klein *et al.* (1980)

and many clinical studies, their presence tends to be associated with a more favourable prognosis and regression of individual tumour deposits may be accompanied by a particularly intense local inflammatory response.

Third, in recent years there has been a growing interest in immunogenetic factors and their influence on susceptibility to many diseases, including cancer. Hodgkin's disease was the first malignancy in which both incidence and prognosis were shown to be related to human leucocyte antigen (HLA) type and it remains probably the clearest example, although nasopharyngeal carcinoma, chronic lymphocytic leukaemia, and others have also yielded positive findings (Table 41.2).

Finally, some notice must be taken of the evidence that manipulation of the immune system, usually with the aim of enhancing antitumour activity, can in certain instances cause more aggressive tumour growth. 'Enhancement' or 'facilitation' in this context can evidently be mediated by both humoral and cellular mechanisms. The interpretation of such data, and indeed of many findings in tumour immunology, is complicated by the fact that the presence of tumour can itself disturb immune function, as can surgery, anaesthesia, and almost any experimental procedure designed to measure immunity. Nevertheless, if it is possible by altering immune status to do harm, it can reasonably be argued that other changes may do good.

The nature of tumour antigens

The resolution of all questions about the authenticity of clinically relevant tumour immunity ought to come about through a deeper understanding of the basic mechanisms of carcinogenesis and of immunity. The past two decades have seen enormous advances in both fields but it is still too early to suggest that an end to controversy in tumour immunology is in sight.

One important issue is the extent to which molecular events underlying malignant change can account for altered immunogenicity in the 'transformed' cell. At the DNA level mutations in oncogenes and in tumour suppressors are recognized as being directly responsible for disordered control of growth and differentiation. These 'cancer genes' have protein products and if mutation takes the form of structural alteration (e.g. by mis-sense base substitution, truncation, or translocation generating an in-frame fusion gene) then a distinctive, novel, tumour-specific protein will be generated. Furthermore, if the mutation has been a somatic event, as is usual, there should be no self-tolerance of the altered product. Humoral and/or cell-mediated immunity can be elicited in experimental animals to such mutant proteins as p21*ras*, p53 or *bcr/abl*, and circulating antibodies, for example to c-*myc* or p53 have been demonstrated in some cancer patients. However, it has yet to be shown convincingly that immune responses to these determinants have any influence on the progress of the disease.

It is not necessary for a mutant oncogene product to be a cell surface protein in order for it to be immunogenic. There is very clear evidence that peptides from cytoplasmic proteins can be transported to the membrane and presented there by major histocompatibility complex (MHC) class I or class II antigens. Hence, it may not be unrealistic to contemplate making use of these epitopes as tumour-specific targets in immune-based therapy.

Some causal mutations in tumours result in over- or under-production of a structurally normal gene product. These might be expected to provide less opportunity for protective immune responses but, in at least one example, the *trans*-membrane receptor *erb B 2*, which is over-expressed in a substantial proportion of breast and ovarian cancers, as demonstrated by Slamon *et al.* (1989) infusion of specific antibody may be of therapeutic value. Here the explanation may lie not in direct immune attack on the tumour cells but in blockade of a growth signal normally transmitted via the receptor. Similarly, the unusual but striking examples of response to anti-idiotype antibody in B-cell lymphomas, discussed later in the section on lymphomas, may depend on activation of a regulatory network rather than on antibody-mediated cytolysis.

A number of 'tumour antigens', so termed because they are useful (though not entirely specific) diagnostic markers, such as α-fetoprotein, carcino-embryonic antigen or *Ca125*, are generated by over-production of a protein not normally synthesized in appreciable quantities by mature cells. According to Urban and Schreiber (1992) they are rarely immunogenic in the tumour patient and have no proven value in immunotherapy.

Other, presumably secondary, changes in tumour cell metabolism can result in the synthesis of abnormally modified proteins or lipids. The clearest example is under-glycosylation of the polymorphic epithelial mucin molecule, which can expose the tandem repeat sequence of the core protion, against which specific antibodies can be raised experimentally and may be capable of evoking a specific cell-mediated response in the patient. Once again, it remains to be established how much that response can contribute to tumour rejection.

Antigens with even a modest degree of tumour specificity may be exploited in diagnostic imaging and in therapy, for example by coupling a radioisotope such as astatine-211 to an appropriate antibody. In fact, there are many current proposals based on this concept, often exploiting the biological as well as the immunological characteristics of the tumour-specific antigen. Several of these are at the stage of assessment in animal models. Recent variations on the theme include the design of enzyme/antibody complexes capable of binding selectively to tumour cells. Internalization of the enzyme follows. It can then convert a systemically administered inactive pro-drug to a cytotoxic compound only within the tumour. The technique, 'antibody-directed enzyme pro-drug therapy' (ADEPT) is now entering the stage of clinical trials in humans.

A further technical development of considerable theoretical and practical interest is the use of anti-idiotype as antigen. An antibody (Ab1) is first raised, usually in another species, against the primary tumour antigen, which may belong to any of the above categories. That antibody then becomes the antigen in a second phase of immunization, ideally using a human host. In practice, this round of immunization may be carried out *in vitro* and a human monoclonal antibody (Ab2) derived. The target of Ab2 should be the antigen-combining site of Ab1, i.e. it has anti-idiotype specificity and thus should mimic the original tumour antigen sufficiently closely to stimulate production of antitumour antibody (Ab3) when it is inoculated into the patient. The advantage over purified tumour antigen may be that the match between antigen and anti-idiotype is imperfect so that the latter is actually more immunogenic and, furthermore, modulation of antigen structure is less likely to lead to tumour cell 'escape'. Whether these factors are really of practical importance is controversial but a vaccine of this type is well tolerated and has produced encouraging results in preliminary clinical trials in patients with colorectal cancer.

The antigens of human melanoma cells have been the subjects of particularly intense study and several have been defined which can elicit humoral or cell-mediated responses or both, in the autologous host. These are discussed later in the context of immunotherapy for melanoma.

Paradoxically, for most of the highly immunogenic tumours induced by chemical carcinogens or by UV light, the exact nature of the antigen(s) remains obscure. Virus-induced tumours often have multiple antigens. EBV-transformed lymphoblastoid cells, for example, evoke potent T-cell-mediated rejection responses particularly to EBNAs 3A, 3B, and 3C. The

SV40 and adenovirus each produce proteins functionally associated with transformation, notably 'large T' and 'E1A' respectively, which are strongly antigenic.

Antigen processing and presentation by major histocompatibility complex molecules

Very few antigens will elicit a measurable immune response unless processed and displayed at the surface of the antigen-presenting cell (APC) by molecules encoded in the MHC. MHC class I and class II molecules are highly polymorphic cell surface glycoproteins which present antigen to antigen-specific, T lymphocytes, respectively, of the CD8+ and CD4+ subsets. In broad terms, CD4 T cells act as 'helpers' in the induction and regulation of antibody, cell-mediated, and cytotoxic T-lymphocyte (CTL) responses, while CD8 T cells function principally as CTLs. Both populations play a central part in the cognitive immune response to tumours.

The pathways for processing and presenting antigens to CD8+ and CD4+ T cells by MHC class I and class II, reviewed recently by Germain (1994), are distinct, although both result in antigen being degraded into short peptides, which are bound non-covalently to MHC molecules (see Fig. 41.1).

An MHC class I molecule comprises a heterodimer of heavy and light glycoprotein chains, non-covalently associated with a short, cell-derived peptide. The polymorphic heavy chain spans the cell membrane and is encoded, in humans, by one of the three 'classical' HLA class I genes HLA-A, -B, or -C located on the short arm of chromosome 6. The monomorphic light chain is the non-MHC encoded protein 2-microglobulin (β2m). MHC class I molecules present peptides derived from cytosolic proteins (both self and foreign) to antigen-specific CD8+ T cells. Intracellular proteins which are recognized as 'foreign' in the context of tumour immunology include viral proteins and mutated or aberrantly expressed self proteins. Through the presentation of cell-derived peptides at the cell surface by MHC class I molecules, the array of intracellular proteins, both self and foreign, expressed in somatic cells is continuously surveyed by the immune system.

MHC class II molecules are heterodimers of two MHC polypeptide chains and are encoded in humans by the HLA genes DR, DP and DQ. The overall structure of MHC class I and class II molecules is similar, in

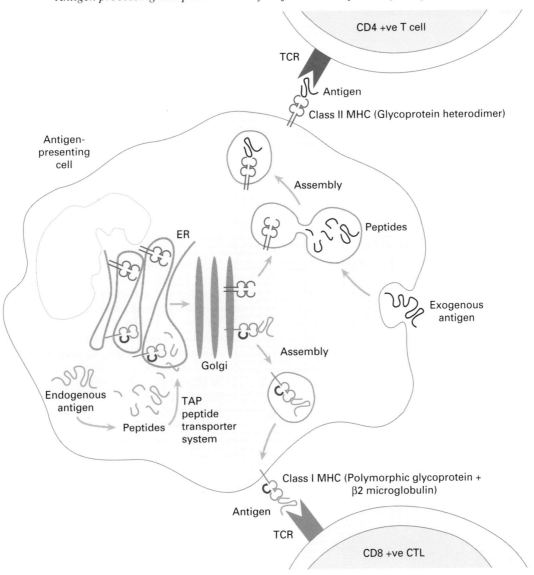

∎ **Fig. 41.1** The processing and presentation of antigens in association with major histocompatibility complex (MHC) class I and II molecules. ER, endoplasmic reticulumn; TCR, T-cell receptor; CTL, cytotoxic T lymphocyte, (after Browning 1995).

spite of their differences in genetic arrangement. Class II molecules present peptides which are derived principally from exogenous proteins to antigen-specific CD4+ T cells. Unlike MHC class I molecules, which are expressed on almost all somatic cells, class II molecules have a restricted distribution, being expressed constitutively only on cells of the immune system which act as APCs in the induction of an immune response (dendritic cells, macrophages, B cells). Class II expression can be induced, however, on a number of cell types at sites of inflammation. The extensive polymorphism of MHC molecules means that, in outbred populations, the majority of individuals will express six different class I and six different class II molecules. The peptides bound and presented by individual MHC class I and class II molecules show distinct structural motifs. Thus the HLA molecules expressed by an individual play a crucial part in determining the range of antigens and peptide epitopes which are presented to the individual's immune system.

∎ **Table 41.2**   Possible mechanisms by which tumours avoid or escape immune responses

Methods of avoidance	Methods of escape
Lack of tumour antigen expression	Loss or modulation of tumour antigen expression
Holes in repertoire of immune recognition	Loss or down-regulation of major histocompatibility complex expression
Poor immunogenicity of tumour cell	Loss of accessory molecule expression
Secretion of inhibitory cytokines	Rapid tumour growth
Secretion of blocking antibodies	

After Browning (1995).

Abnormalities of major histocompatibility complex expression on tumour cells

Loss or downregulation of expression of MHC class I molecules has been described on a wide variety of tumours and has stimulated the theory that this might represent a mechanism of tumour escape from the immune response. Table 41.2 lists the mechanisms by which a tumour might evade rejection by the immune system. Immunohistochemical studies (Fig. 41.2) indicate that abnormalities of HLA expression are relatively common on many tumours including breast, ovarian, lung, colon, melanoma, and cervical malignancies. These abnormalities range from lack of expression of all class I antigens (complete loss) to

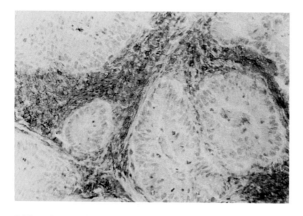

∎ **Fig. 41.2**   Photomicrograph of a section of colorectal carcinoma. The tumour cells show absent expression of HLA class I (as determined by lack of staining with the HLA class I specific monoclonal antibody, W6/32), whilst the intervening stromal cells show strong expression of HLA class I. (Magnification ×200. Photograph courtesy of Dr Loukas Kaklamanis, Oxford.)

selective loss of expression of individual alleles. A number of mechanisms have been implicated in loss of HLA class I expression on tumour cells. Broadly, these mechanisms can be separated into those which involve abnormal regulation of otherwise normal HLA and associated genes, and those which involve structural mutations to HLA and associated genes.

Complete loss of HLA class I expression has been associated in a number of tumour types with mutations or deletions in $\beta2m$ genes. By such a process, complete loss of expression of all HLA class I molecules can be achieved in two genetic steps if each involves the loss of a functional $\beta2m$ gene product. The phenomenon was first observed by Klein *et al.* (1967) in the Burkitt lymphoma cell line Daudi. In colorectal and melanoma tumour cell lines a variety of $\beta2m$ gene mutations have been described, all leading to failure of expression of any functional gene product. Loss of genetic material within the HLA region can also underlie non-expression of HLA alleles in tumours. Deletion of a complete haplotype has been demonstrated in melanoma and in colorectal tumour cell lines. The most likely mechanism is complete or partial chromosome loss through non-disjunction or aberrant somatic recombination, both of which occur with relatively high frequency in malignant cells. Several studies have shown the selective loss of expression of individual HLA determinants on a variety of tumours, by comparing the HLA typing results for tumour and corresponding normal tissue. The basis for the selective silencing of individual alleles has not been identified in most cases. To date, there is no direct evidence for mutations within the heavy chain genes themselves; however, several observations suggest that mutations in the HLA structural genes or in their upstream promoter regions may occur, at least in some instances.

While genetic events at the DNA level account for a proportion of cases of abnormal HLA expression on tumour cells, they do not account for all. Various mechanisms affecting transcriptional control of HLA and related genes may be involved in downregulation of HLA expression. Both the constitutive and inducible levels of HLA class I expression are regulated by *trans*-acting factors binding to *cis*-acting regulatory sequences in the 5′ untranslated portions of MHC genes. Changes which affect chromatin structure or methylation status of these *cis*-acting elements may influence transcription of HLA genes and downregulation of HLA expression has been associated with a decrease in binding of *trans*-acting factors to enhancer regions in MHC genes. Levels of HLA expression in tumour cells have been shown, in a number of studies by Esteban *et al.* (1989), Ruiz-Caballo *et al.* (1991), and others, to correlate with intracellular levels of corresponding mRNA. Alterations of MHC class I expression on tumour cells have been associated also with the expression of certain viral and cellular oncogenes. The transforming E1A protein of adenovirus type 12 is a potent downregulator of MHC class I expression in adenovirus-associated tumours and Rous sarcoma virus infection has been correlated with reduced HLA class I expression in transformed human fibroblasts. HLA class I can also be downregulated in HIV-1 infected cells. The influence of activated cellular oncogenes on HLA expression in tumour cells is less clear, although *v-ras* in transformed murine fibroblasts and N — and c-*myc* genes, in neuroblastoma and melanoma cells respectively, have been associated with downregulation of HLA expression in some studies. While the majority of the mechanisms discussed involve reduced production of HLA antigens, there also are instances of accelerated shedding of these molecules from the surface of tumour cells.

The expression of HLA class I molecules at the cell surface requires not only heavy chain and β2m gene products but also the expression of other gene products such as the peptide transporters (TAP). Absent or deficient TAP expression results in the failure to transport peptides from the cytosol into the endoplasmic reticulum (ER). As a result, MHC molecules fail to bind peptide and are retained within the ER. Recently, lack of HLA expression on tumour cells has been shown to coincide with absence of TAP gene products in a variety of tumours, including non-small-cell lung cancer and cervical carcinoma. In the case of non-small-cell lung cancer cell lines, expression of HLA was restored by treatment of the cells with interferon (IFN) γ, suggesting a regulatory rather than a structural defect constraining TAP gene expression. In spite of the wealth of data accumulated in recent years on the frequency of abnormal HLA class I expression on tumours cells and the mechanisms that underlie the phenomenon, the biological significance of HLA class I deficiency on tumour cells remains obscure. The relatively high frequency of the change suggests that loss or downregulation of HLA is associated with some selective advantage for growth or survival. The most obvious explanation would be that loss of MHC class I expression allows the cell to evade attack by MHC class I restricted CTL, although direct evidence of tumour-specific CTL is lacking in many tumour types, which show loss of HLA expression. An association between HLA loss and poor differentiation has been found for a number of tumour types and a higher incidence of HLA loss on metastatic deposits than on the primary tumour has been reported. A recent study reported that HLA class I loss is rare in benign tumours or in carcinoma *in situ*, suggesting that the loss of HLA expression may be involved in progression of a tumour to invasive carcinoma. Overall, however, there is no clear correlation between lack of HLA expression on tumour cells and patient survival.

The most obvious consequence of HLA loss from tumour cells is that any cell which fails to express appropriate HLA molecules on its surface will be unable to present antigenic peptides to antigen-specific CTL. Regardless of the mechanism of loss of HLA expression, the frequency of HLA loss observed on many tumours may represent a significant barrier to the effective use of immunotherapeutic protocols aimed at stimulating tumour-specific CTL responses in patients. In this respect, the distinction between regulatory and structural genetic mechanisms of HLA loss may be important as the former may potentially be overcome by appropriate upregulatory stimuli, while reversal of structural defects can be achieved only by replacement or repair of the affected gene. However, expression of HLA class I on tumour cells is not obligatory for tumour rejection. Paradoxically, it has been shown that cells which lack HLA expression are more susceptible to lysis by NK cells than HLA class I positive counterparts. Thus the loss of HLA expression from a tumour may permit escape from a tumour-specific CTL response but result in increased susceptibility to NK-mediated lysis. The relationship between the tumour cell, MHC class I and the immune system is more complex, therefore, than might at first be apparent.

Most normal epithelia are HLA class II negative. Many pre-malignant tumours acquire *de novo* class II expression or increase pre-existing low levels of expression. The great majority of malignant tumour cells, however, do not express HLA class II molecules, suggesting that this upregulation of MHC class II is a transient event during tumour evolution. One exception to this general rule is melanoma, in which constitutive HLA class II expression is relatively common.

This may, in part, explain the apparent greater immunogenicity of melanoma in comparison with many other tumour types (see later). The overexpression of cell surface HLA class II in melanomas has been correlated with a more aggressive tumour phenotype, however, and it has been suggested that these molecules may be functionally incompetent.

Major histocompatibility complex expression and tumour immunogenicity

The expression of mutated gene products or the dysregulated expression of normally silent genes in tumour cells potentially gives rise to the association of novel MHC/peptide complexes which the immune system may recognize as foreign. The expression of such complexes on a tumour cell does not equate, however, with its ability to induce a T-cell response. There is a distinction between a tumour cell's antigenicity (i.e. its ability to present an antigen to effector T lymphocytes) and its immunogenicity (i.e. its ability to induce a primary T-lymphocyte response). Several factors may play a part in this distinction, including MHC class I and class II expression, adhesion and co-stimulatory molecule expression and release of inhibitory growth factors and cytokines by the tumour cells. Experiments in laboratory animals have demonstrated that expression of syngeneic MHC class II following transfection of the class II genes can be associated with enhanced immunogenicity of the tumour and rejection of a subsequent challenge with cells of the parent tumour line, suggesting that the expression of MHC class II molecules on the tumour cell allowed it to present antigen directly to tumour-specific CD4+ helper T cells, thus bypassing the need for 'professional' (constitutive MHC class II positive) APCs. This may be something of an over-simplification, as it is now recognized that, in addition to the T-cell receptor interaction with antigen–MHC, costimulatory signals mediated through the interaction of other cell surface receptors on the T cell with their ligand molecules on the APC are required for the induction of the primary T-cell response. The lack of appropriate co-stimulatory signals at the time of first encounter between a T cell and a potentially immunogenic MHC/antigen complex may result in induction of T-cell clonal anergy rather than clonal stimulation.

Quite apart from measures designed to restore or enhance the expression of MHC molecules on tumour cells, there may be possibilities in the use of alternative antigen-presenting 'carrier' molecules, such as heat shock proteins. In theory, these could actually be advantageous for enhancing antitumour imunity as the cytotoxic responses generated appear not to be MHC restricted.

Cell adhesion molecules

Effective presentation and recognition of antigen does not depend only on MHC–T-cell interactions but also on specific cell–cell interactions by a variety of accessory molecules. Broadly, these can be separated into interactions based principally on adhesion of receptor molecules on the lymphocyte to their ligands on the APC, e.g. LFA-1/ICAM-1; CD2/LFA-3, and interactions which provide the 'second, co-stimulatory signal' to the T cell, e.g. CD28/B7 and CTLA-4/B7. Changes in cell adhesion molecule expression on cancer cells have been recorded and their significance assessed in relation to metastatic spread and immune surveillance. Recent studies in mice of poorly immunogenic tumour cells transfected with B7 have emphasized the role of these second signals in priming the immune response, and suggested new approaches to cancer immunotherapy. In humans immunogenic lymphoblastoid cells, for example, often differ from the non-immunogenic lymphoma-derived counterparts in the range of EBV antigens expressed; the levels of MHC class I and II and in the amounts of LFA1, LFA3, and ICAM-1 on the cell membrane. However, as all these differences often coexist it is uncertain what functional importance can be attributed to the adhesion molecules. Similarly, deficits or excesses of adhesion molecule expression in epithelial tumours may coexist with changes in MHC antigens. They may contribute to 'evasion' but formal proof is lacking.

The complexities of cell adhesion molecules, the interactions between them and the signals that they generate are only just beginning to be unravelled and it seems likely that this will prove to be a topic of considerable importance in the field of tumour biology, including its immunological aspects.

Potential mechanisms of immunological attack on tumours

References has already been made to humoral and T-cell-mediated tumour specific responses. Conventionally, a clear distinction is made between these two mechanisms; in practice, however, neither experimental nor clinical findings support a complete

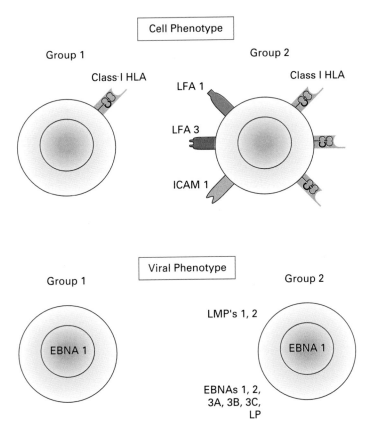

▌Fig. 41.3 Group I versus group II lymphoblastoid cells: cellular and viral phenotypes able to influence immunogenecity for cytotoxic T lymphocytes. Group I are lymphoma derived and show low immunogenecity. Group II are typical of EBV transformed non tumorigenic lymphoblastoid cell lines which elicit a strong autologous cytotoxic T cell response.

separation. The generation of specific antibody requires cooperation between APCs, 'helper' T cells and B lymphocytes and, while T-cell cytotoxicity appears, in most cases, to afford the most effective attack on target cells, including tumours, it rarely if ever occurs in isolation.

Antitumour antibodies can be demonstrated in the serum of some patients and are readily inducible in many experimental animal systems. There is evidence for the cytotoxic effectiveness of such antibody *in vitro* but, except in the special cases (anti-idiotype and anti-*erb B 2*) already mentioned, it is difficult to show that they contribute directly to tumour containment *in vivo*. Antibody-dependent cellular cytotoxicity (ADCC) is, likewise, a significant element of the tumour rejection response in some experimental models and may also be effective clinically, although the evidence is limited.

Indeed it appears that the role of tumour cell-specific antibody may sometimes be to block or inhibit the potentially beneficial effect of cytotoxic T cells.

NK cells, comprising large granular lymphocytes and probably other components, such as monocytes, have been proposed as major elements of the 'immune surveillance' mechanism, in which case their operations should be mainly covert. Their activity, demonstrated by killing of specific target cell lines such as K562 and VAC1 *in vitro*, is increased well above background level in some preparations of TILS. This is so particularly when activated by cytokines such as interleukin (IL) 2 or IFN, but their protective role is inferred mainly from the finding that depletion of circulating NK cells from animals renders them highly susceptible to the establishment of metastatic deposits after intravenous injection of tumour cells.

CTLs, which are mainly but not exclusively CD8, were demonstrated by McMichael (1992) and others to be the principal antitumour arm of the immune system. Much current effort is devoted to definition of the antigenic determinants recognized by effector T cells, for example those isolated from tumour biopsies and encouraged to proliferative *in vitro* in the presence of tumour tissue, APCs, and IL-2. This approach has been particularly fruitful in the case of melanoma as discussed later, but is being studied in relation to many other tumour types. It has been shown by Rooney *et al.* (1995) that EBV-associated lymphoproliferative disease in immunocompromised subjects can be controlled by re-infusion of mixed populations of CD4 and CD8 autologous T cells first activated and expanded *in vitro* by co-culture with EBV-transformed lymphoblasts, then grown in the presence of IL-2. Attempts have also been made to generate tumour-

specific cytotoxic T cells from allogeneic donors, and even from other species such as pig, for use in the management of bladder cancer. However, most current protocols favour autologous TILs as the source of 'lymphokine-activated killer' (LAK) cells in adoptive immunotherapy procedures.

The role of cytokines

Over a century has passed since Coley (1893) first advocated exploitation of the observation that sepsis and acute infections were sometimes associated with temporary remission of malignant disease. He injected streptococci into the tissues around tumours of the head and neck in 10 patients, causing severe erysipelas and recording some reduction in tumour size.

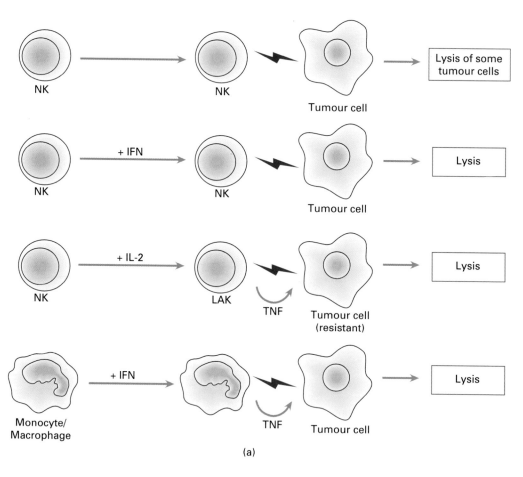

▐ Fig. 41.4a Innate responses to tumour. NK, natural killer cell; TNF, tumour necrosis factor; IFN, interferon; LAK, lymphokine-activated killer.

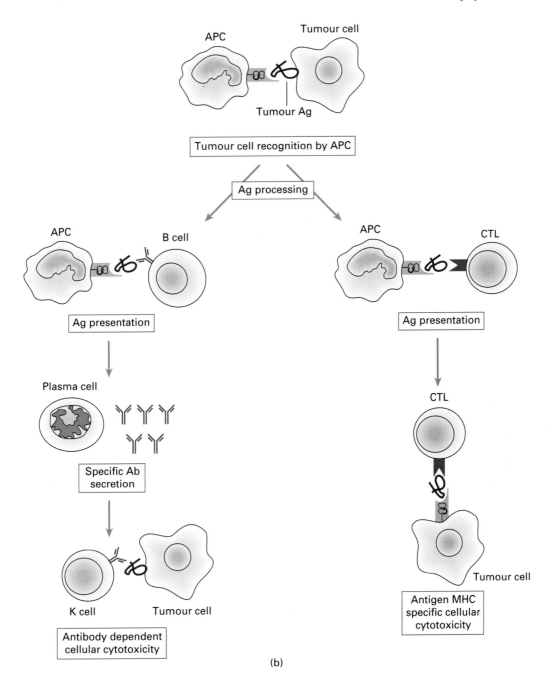

(b)

▌**Fig. 41.4b** (b) Adaptive responses to tumour.

Subsequent development of this work led to the extraction of 'Coley's toxins' from bacterial cultures. These crude mixtures were certainly toxic to the patients and probably caused the release of a variety of cytokines, including tumour necrosis factor (TNF) and IFN. It is still unclear which cytokines, singly or in combination, may have antitumour effects in particular situations and the full range of possible combinations, some of

▮ **Table 41.3** Cytokine enhancement of immunity to experimental mouse tumours

Cytokine	Experimental tumour system	Responding cells
IL-1	NIH 3T3 transformed fibroblasts	Not determined
IL-2	B16 melanoma; fibrosarcoma; colon Ca; bladder Ca; lung Ca; breast Adeno Ca	CD8 CTL (also natural killer cells and neutrophils)
IL-4	Plasmacytoma; renal Ca; hamster Ovary Ca; breast–adeno Ca. (Not melanoma)	Eosinophils, T cells, macrophages
IL-6	B16 melanoma; lung Ca; sarcoma	Monocytes, neutrophils, T cells
IL-7	Plasmacytoma; breast–adeno Ca; fibrosarcoma. (not melanoma).	CD4 cells, macrophages, eosinophils
IL-12	B16 melanoma; carcinomas; lymphomas; sarcomas	CD8 (also CD4)
IFN α	Friend leukaemia	Not determined
IFN γ	Neuroblastoma; fibrosarcoma; carcinomas (colon, bladder, lung, breast)	CD8 CTL (+macrophages)
TNF α	Plasmacytoma; sarcomas	CD4, CD8, macrophages
G-CSF	colon Ca	Neutrophils
GM-CSF	B16 melanoma	Not determined

The data in this table are derived mainly from experiments in which a cytokine gene has been transfected into the tumour cells before inoculation. Growth rate and immune response were compared for cytokine expressing versus sham-transfected tumours. GM-CSF, granulocyte-macrophage colony-stimulating factor; IFN, interferon; TNF, tumour necrosis factor; CTL, cytotoxic T lymphocyte.

Adapted from Colombo, M. P. and Formi, G. 1994 *Immunology Today*, **15**, 48–51. Added data from Trimchiari, G. and Scott, P. (1994). *Immunology Today*, **15**, 460–63, with permission.

which are reported to show striking synergy, has yet to be thoroughly explored. Some of the more widely used experimental systems are summarized in Table 41.3. There is undoubtedly a valuable place for IFNα in the management of hairy cell leukaemia and of metastatic carcinoid, while IL-2 is effective in about 20% of renal cell carcinomas and has been licensed for use in this condition. In the main, however, single or combined agent systemic cytokine therapy in humans has been unacceptably toxic in relation to its modest clinical benefits and has proved an expensive disappointment.

The principal value of cytokines may well prove to be in augmentation of a suboptimal T-cell response. IFNγ, for example, can induce MHC antigen expression on either antigen-presenting or target cells while IL-2, IL-4, TNF, and granulocyte-macrophage colony-stimulating factor (GM-CSF), among others, will enhance the activation of monocytes, NK cells, and T lymphocytes. Local production of one or more of these peptides within, or close to a tumour, may increase the

concentration of activated tumour-infiltrating 'lymphocytes' which, in turn, could generate further cytokine release and so lead to a cascade process of immunological activation. This is the rationale that underlies several current therapeutic protocols. Systemic use of IL-2, TNF, or IFN, as noted above, has limited value and their toxicity in high dose is often unacceptable. More effective antitumour activity, in some but by no means all, situations seems to be achieved by selective cytokine stimulation of TIL, for example by intratumour injection or by the introduction of a cytokine gene into tumour cells which are then re-implanted. Specific examples of such approaches are discussed below in relation to melanoma.

The use of 'immune stimulants' such as bacille Calmette-Guérin (BCG) or *Corynebacterium parvum*, which have a long history in tumour immunology, probably exploited much the same phenomenon as multiple cytokine therapy. The most striking effects were generally recorded when the injections were

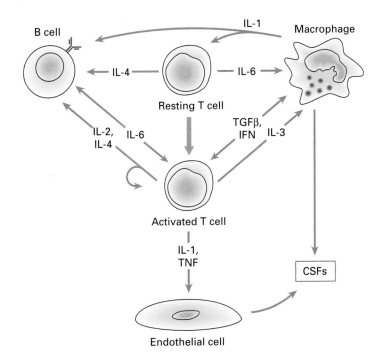

∎ **Fig. 41.5** Examples of the cytokine network that can augment a suboptimal T-cell response to tumour specific antigens. TNF, tumour necrosis factor; TGF, transforming growth factor.

given directly into tumour deposits, e.g. of bladder cancer. Similarly, a number of pharmacological agents have been found to influence *in vitro* assays of immune function and have subsequently been used as enhancers of antitumour immunity. They include muramyl dipeptide, a monocyte activator, lithium, the antihelminthic levamisole, and diethyldithiocarbamate. Despite many accounts of their clinical effectiveness, none has stood the test of time. Non-steroidal anti-inflammatory drugs such as aspirin and indomethacin, which block cyclooxygenase, may be useful adjuvants where an immune response is inhibited by soluble factors elaborated via this pathway. Local release of histamine, as part of an inflammatory response, has also been shown to reduce the effectiveness of specific immune reactivity and the histamine receptor antagonist, cimetidine, may have a place in countering this effect.

Melanoma

Throughout the long history of experimental immunotherapy for cancer, melanoma has stood out as one of the most promising target tumours. Furthermore, conventional therapy has very little to offer in this condition. Although melanoma deposits may regress in response to chemotherapy or radiotherapy, survival is scarcely prolonged and more aggressive combination regimens, which may be more effective, are extremely toxic.

Assessment of clinical trials of immunotherapy, or indeed of any new treatment for melanoma, can be difficult unless a truly randomized protocol is followed as the prognosis in individual cases is notoriously unpredictable. Among the most relevant factors are the depth of the original lesion (Breslow's thickness and Clark's level), the completeness of excision of involved lymph nodes or metastatic deposits and the site of any residual disease. Long experience also warns that it is unwise to extrapolate the often dramatic results of experiments in mice directly to humans. Nevertheless, there are reasons for cautious optimism concerning new developments in immunological approaches to the management of malignant melanoma in humans. As discussed above, tumour-specific and tumour-associated antigens are becoming more clearly defined; several, indeed have been cloned. We have a much better understanding of

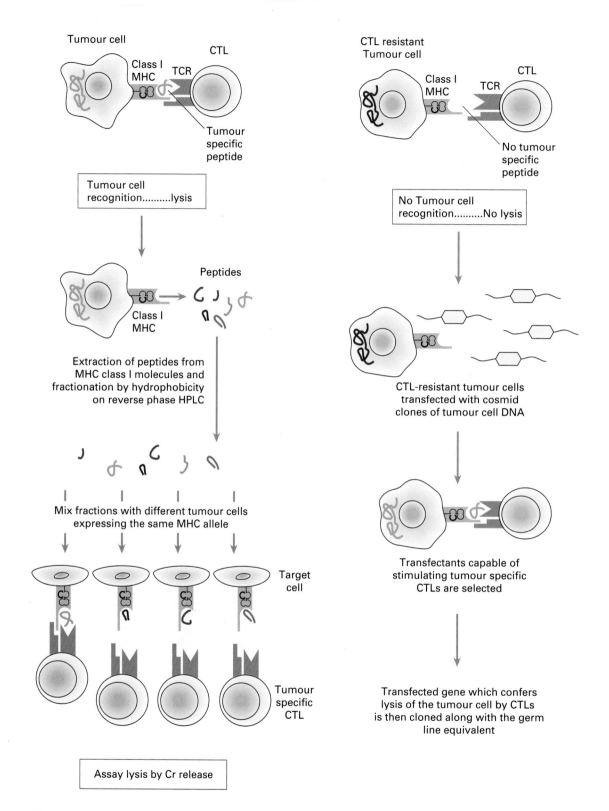

Fig. 41.6 Identification of tumour specific peptide antigens recognised by T cells. (Adapted from Pardoll, *Current opinion in Immunology* (1993) pp. 721).

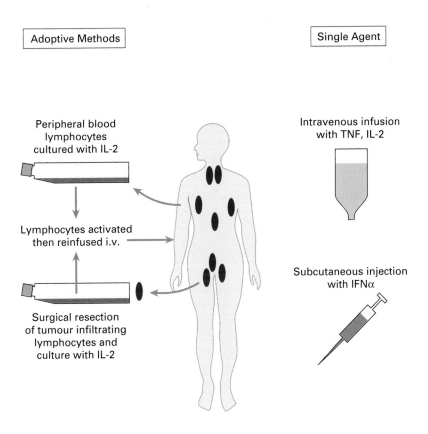

∎ Fig. 41.7a Immunotherapeutic strategies.

antigen presentation, MHC restriction, the role of cell adhesion molecules, and the effects of cytokines. All of these factors have particular relevance to melanoma.

Melanoma antigen

Complex, but rewarding, techniques for characterization of tumour-specific antigens have been applied particularly to melanoma. In essence, a melanoma cell cDNA library is prepared and the cloned products transfected into a cultured mammalian cell line, together with a human MHC class I gene. When a transfected cell is found to stimulate antimelanoma-specific T-cell clones, the cDNA it carries is analysed to identify the precise epitope recognized by the responder population. Alternatively, the antigenic peptide can be eluted from the antigen-presenting fold of MHC class I and sequenced. Confirmation of the identify of the functional epitope can be achieved by

adding defined peptides to APCs with empty MHC I molecules on their surface and testing their sensitivity to lysis by tumour-specific cytotoxic T-cell clones. Table 41.4 lists the principal melanoma antigens identified to date.

Clinical strategies for enhancement of immune responses to melanoma

Adjuvants and cytokines

Intra-or perilesional injection of BCG and of crude cytokine preparations has been practised for many decades but more sophisticated approaches to enhancement of tumour immunogenicity have become popular in recent years. Based on a substantial body of animal data, reviewed by Colombo *et al.* (1994), over 60

▌ **Table 41.4** Melanoma-associated antigens

Antigen	Biochemical	Distribution	Function
Tyrosinase	Protein	Melanosomes	Differentiation antigen, also target for HLA class I-restricted CTL
gp 75	Glycoprotein, tyrosinase-related	Melanosomes	Differentiation antigen
S 100	Ca binding protein 21 kDa, highly acidic	Neural crest-derived tissues, chondrocytes adipocytes, dendritic cells, T lymphocytes	Differentiation antigen, useful marker for amelanotic metastases
GD2, GD3 GM2, GM3.	Gangliosides	Neural crest-derived tumours	Cell adhesion, melanoma differentiation
HMW-MAA	High MW proteoglycan	Melanocye lineage	Differentiation
MAGE-1 MAGE-3	Peptide	Testis, neuroblastoma	?Developmental Targets for HLA class I-restricted CTL
MART 1/Aa	Peptide	Melanocytes	Differentiation marker Target for HLA class I-restricted CTL (as below)
gp 100	Glycoprotein	Melanocytes	Differentiation marker Target for HLA class I-restricted CTL (as below)

CTL, cytotoxic T lymphocyte; HLA, human leucocyte antigen.

protocols have now been approved for transfection of autologous tumour cells with cytokine genes (usually IL-2 but also including IL-4, IL-7, TNF, IFNγ and GM-CSF), the majority for trials in melanoma.

Expansion of tumour infiltrating lymphocytes

The lymphocytes extracted from melanoma deposits differ from those in the peripheral blood, not only in showing higher levels of antitumour activity *in vitro* but commonly also in being oligoclonal, confirming that they are a selected subpopulation. Mere expansion, by culturing with IL-2 does not seem to be effective in clinical practice, possibly because it is difficult to generate substantial numbers for re-infusion into the autologous host, so that current protocols almost all rely upon transfection of cultured TILs with IL-2, IL-4, or TNF.

Vaccines

The earliest human melanoma vaccines, of Coca *et al.* (1912), consisted simply of viable autologous and allogenic tumour cells injected repeatedly over prolonged periods. Many variations on that theme have been tried since. Very often BCG or Freund's adjuvant has been used to enhance the effect of the primary immunogen which may have been viable, irradiated or lysed melanoma cells.

Following anecdotal accounts of tumour regression apparently related to viral infection or antiviral immunization, studies were undertaken on the use of rabies, or vaccinia virus vaccines to stimulate antimelanoma immunity with some evidence of benefit. Thereafter, several groups developed vaccines based on autologous or allogenic melanoma cells infected *in vitro* with Newcastle disease, vesicular stomatitis, vaccinia or other viruses which were usually injected intradermally, commonly with BCG, Freund's, or other adjuvant. With Newcastle disease virus in particular, infection lyses the tumour cells and it was argued that chemical purification of antigen might lead to the development of more concentrated, specific and hence more potent vaccines. In fact soluble shed melanoma membrane components, depleted of MHC antigens and injected with alum as adjuvant, proved moderately successful in clinical trials, although others have reported evidence for the superior immunogenicity of intact viable melanoma cells.

Gangliosides, which are integral components of the cell membrane, are among the most distinctive potential targets for immune attack and several melanoma-derived ganglioside preparations have been developed as antitumour vaccines. Combinations of several gangliosides to produce a polyvalent vaccine may reduce the problem of tumour cell 'escape' through modulation of a single surface antigen and some encouraging

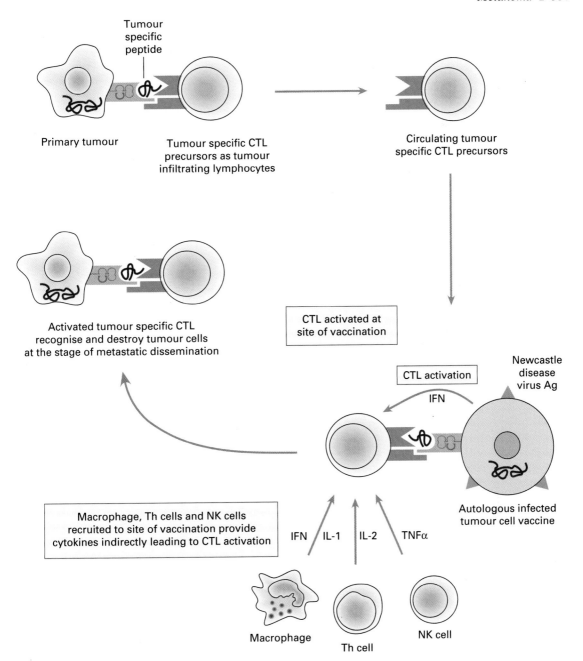

∎ Fig. 41.7b Mechanism of action of virus-modified autologous tumour vaccine. CTL, cytotoxic T lymphocyte; IFN, interferon; Ag, antigen; NK, natural killer (cell); TNF, tumour necrosis factor.

results have been obtained in preliminary trials of this material in patients with advanced melanoma.

The anti-idiotype approach already in use for colorectal cancer, as described above, is also undergoing phase 1 trials in melanoma. The primary antigen is a high molecular weight extract of melanoma cell membranes.

The largest experience of melanoma vaccines in the treatment of human disease is that of Morton's Group (1993) at the John Wayne Cancer Institute, Santa

Monica. After many modifications, they have selected a set of three cultured melanoma cell lines which express, between them, most of the major melanoma-specific antigens that appear to have a role in tumour rejection. Pooled irradiated viable cells from these cultures are injected intradermally with BCG and other adjuvants and with GM-CSF. Patients also take cimetidine in varying doses and the treatment continues for 2 years or more. Responses are measured in terms of antibody titre against melanoma cell membrane antigens, delayed-type hypersensitivity reactions to allogenic melanoma and *in vitro* lymphocyte activation on co-culture with autologous or allogenic tumour cells. Compared with historical controls, increased survival has been demonstrated and benefit appears to correlate with immune reactivity as judged by the above measures.

In an approach that exploits new developments in gene therapy, Nabel *et al.* (1993) have transfected the MHC class I antigen HLA-B7 (not to be confused with the B7 adhesion molecule) into melanoma cells from HLA-B7-negative patients. Tumour-specific cytotoxic T cells are generated by this procedure and there is evidence that, in general, it may not be necessary to alter the antigenicity of 100% of tumour cells in order to achieve complete or near-complete eradication of a cancer by immunological mechanisms. An ill-understood 'bystander effect' means that unaltered cells in the vicinity of those successfully transfected are also killed.

Gene immunotherapy of cancer

The last word has certainly not been spoken on the vexed question of melanoma immunotherapy. At present no regimen is so dramatically effective that it supersedes all others and most incorporate so many components that it is difficult to identify the critical ones. Modification of immunogenicity by gene transfection is an attractive proposition but questions remain as to the most appropriate antigen to introduce or alter and whether adjuvants, cytokines, or immunomodulatory drugs will still have a place. A high proportion of all the cancer gene therapy experimental protocols approved so far in the USA and Britain refer specifically to melanoma (RAC Report, December 1994; GTAC First Annual Report, December 1994) for the obvious reasons that the tumour, when disseminated, responds very poorly to conventional therapy, that metastatic deposits are commonly accessible (e.g. in the skin) for manipulation and assessment of response and that there is already convincing evidence of actual or potential immunogenicity. The approaches being explored are essentially those discussed above, namely transfection

of cytokine genes and of co-stimulatory signal molecules. If they can be shown to have some effect in melanoma, this will undoubtedly be taken as encouragement for further development and wider application of these principles.

Further reading

Baldwin, R. W. (1955). Immunity to methylcholanthrene-induced tumour in inbred rats following atrophy and regression of the implanted tumours. *British Journal of Cancer*, **9**, 652–7.

Bishop, J. M. (1991). Molecuar themes in oncogenesis. *Cell*, **64**, 235–48.

Bodenham, D. C. (1968). A study of 650 observed malignant melanomas in the South West region. *Annals of Royal College of Surgeons*, **43**, 218–39.

Boon, T., De Plaen, E., Lurquin, C. *et al.* (1992). Identification of tumour rejection antigens recognised by T lymphocytes. *Cancer Surveys*, **13**, 23–38.

Browning, M. J. and Bodmer, W. (1992). MHC antigens and cancer: implications for T cell surveillance. *Current Opinion in Immunology*, **4**, 613–18.

Browning, M. F. (1995). In *Cancer metastases: from mechanisms to therapies* (ed. R. G. Vile), pp. 99–122 John Wiley, Chichester.

Challis, G. B. and Stam, H. J. (1990). The spontaneous regression of cancer: a review of cases 1900–1987. *Acta Oncologica*, **29**, 545–50.

Chen, L. Ashe, L., and Brady, W. A. (1992). costimulation of anti-tumour immunity by the B7 counterreceptor for the T lymphocyte molecules CD28 and CTLA-4. *Cell*, **71**, 523–31.

Coca, A. F., Dorrance, G. M., and Lebredo, M. G. (1912). Vaccination in cancer: a report of the results of vaccination therapy as applied to seventy-nine cases of human cancer. *Zeitschrift für Immunitaetsforschung und Experimentelle Therapie*, **13**, 543–8.

Coley, W. B. (1893). The treatment of malignant tumours by repeated inoculation of erysipelas: with a report of 10 original cases. *American Journal of Medical Science*, **5**, 487–511 Form. G.

Colombo, M. P. (1994). Cytokine gene gransfer in tumour inhibition and tumour therapy: where are we now? *Immunology Today*, **15**, 48–51.

Dalgleish, A. G. (1994). Cancer vaccines. *European Journal of Cancer*, **30**(A7), 1029–35.

Esteban, F., Concha, A., Huelin, C., *et al.* (1989). Histocompatibility antigens in primary and metastatic squamous cell carcinoma of the larynx. *International Journal of Cancer*, **43**, 436–42.

Germain, R. N. (1994). MHC-dependent antigen processing and peptide presentation: providing ligands T lymphocyte activation. *Cell*, **76**, 287–99.

Gross, L. (1943). Intradermal immunisation of C3H mice against a sarcoma that originated in an animal of the same line. *Cancer Research*, **3**, 326–33.

Hanto, D. W., Gajl-Peczalska, K. J., Frizzera, G., *et al.* (1983). Epstein–Barr virus (EBV) induced polyclonal and monoclonal B-cell proliferative diseases occurring after renal transplantation. *Annals of Surgery*, **198**, 366–69.

Harawi, S. J. and Hara C. J. (1989). Pathology and pathophysiology of AIDS and HIV-related diseases. Chapman & Hall, London.

Herlyn, M. and Koprowski, H. (1988). Melanoma antigens: immunological and biological characterisation and clinical significance. *Annual Review of Immunology*, **6**, 283–308.

Klein, E., Klein, G., Nadkarni, J. S. *et al.* (1967). Surface IgM specificity on cells derived from a Burkitt's lymphoma. *Lancet*, **ii**, 1068–70.

Klein, G., Vanky, F., Galili, B., and Vose, B. M. (1980). Separation and characteristics of tumour-infiltrating lymphocytes in man. *Contemporary Topics in Immunology*, **10**, 79–107.

Kripke, M. L. (1974). Antigenicity of murine skin tumours induced by ultraviolet light. *Journal of the National Cancer Institute*, **53**, 1333–6.

Lancet (Editorial) (1988). Human papillomavirus and cervical cancer. *Lancet*, **i**, 756–7.

Livingston, P. O. (1989). The basis for ganglioside vaccines in melanoma. In *Human tumour antigens and specific tumour therapy*, pp. 287–96. Alan Liss, New York.

McMichael, A. J. (1992). Cytotoxic T lymphocytes and immune surveillance. *Cancer Surveys*, **13**, 5–21.

Möller, P. and Hämmerling, G. J. (1992). The role of surface HLA-A, B, C molecules in tumour immunity. *Cancer Surveys*, **13**, 101–19.

Morton D. L., *et al.* (1993). Polyvalent melanoma vaccine prolongs survival of patients with metastatic melanoma. *Annals of the New York Academy of Science*, **690**, 120–34.

Nabel, G., Nabel, E., Yang, Z., *et al.* (1993). Direct gene transfer with DNA liposome complexes in melanoma. *Proceedings of the National Academy of Sciences, USA*. **90**, 11307–11.

Old, L. J. (1981). Cancer immunology: the search for specificity. *Cancer Research*, **41**, 361–75.

Oliver, R. T. D. and Nouri, A. M. E. (1992). T cell immune responses to cancer in humans and its relevance for immunodiagnosis and therapy. *Cancer Surveys*, **13**, 173–204.

Penn, I. (1988). Tumours of the immunocompromised patient. *Annual Review of Medicine*, **39**, 63–73.

Prehn, R. T. (1976). Tumor progression and homeostatis. *Advances in Cancer Research*, **23**, 203–37.

Quinn, T. C. (1987). Gastrointestinal manifestations of human immunodeficiency virus. *Current Topics AIDS*, **1**, 155–84.

Rabbitts, T. H. (1994). Chromosomal translocations in human cancer. *Nature*, **372**, 143–5.

Ravindranath, M. H. and Morton, D. L. (1991). Role of gangliosides in active specific immunotherapy with melanoma vaccine. *International Review of Immunology*, **7**, 303–29.

Rege, A. A., Huang, K., and Aggarwal, B. B. (1992). Tumour necrosis factor. In *Cytokine therapy* (ed. D. W. Galvani and J. C. Cawley), pp. 152–76. Cambridge University Press. Cambridge

Rickinson, A. B., Murray, R. J., Brooks, J., Moss, D. J., and Masucci, M. H. (1992). T cell recognition of Epstein–Barr virus associated lymphomas. *Cancer Surveys*, **13**, 53–77.

Rooney, C. M., Smith, C. A., Ng, C. Y. C., *et al.* (1995). Use of gene-modified virus-specific T lymphocytes to control Epstein–Barr virus-related lymphoproliferation. *Lancet*, **345**, 9–13.

Rosenberg, S. A., Lotze, M. T., Yang, J. C., *et al.* (1989). Experience with the use of high dose interleukin-2 in the treatment of 652 cancer patients. *Annals of Surgery*, **210**, 474–84.

Ruiz-Caballo, F., Perez-Ayala, M., Redodndo, M., *et al.* (1991). Molecular analysis of MHC class I alterations in human tumour cell lines. *International Journal of Cancer*, (Suppl) **6**, 123–30.

Slamon, D., Godolphin, W., Jones, L., *et al.* (1989). Studies of the HER-2/neu proto-oncogenein human breast and ovarian cancer. *Science*, **244**, 707–12.

Tyzzer, E. E. (1916). Tumour immunity. *Journal of Cancer Research*, **1**, 125–55.

Urban, J. L. and Schreiber, H. (1992). Tumor antigens. *Annual Review of Immunology*, **10**, 617–44.

Section VIII

Immune interventions

42 Immune interventions

J. Bradley

Introduction

The aim of immune intervention is to manipulate the immune response that causes a disease so that the process is changed, reduced, or abolished. In doing this it is recognized that T cells are pivotal in the development of immune responses, and therefore they have become the target of much intervention therapy.

Animal models

While animal models have some limitations in giving information relevant to human disease processes they have provided much useful information. For example, it was animal models that first illustrated the importance of CD4+ T subsets in determining the pattern of disease; that cytokines and cells in the micro-environment were important in directing T-cell subset differentiation; and showed that immune response can be manipulated. Some illuminating work revealed that in C57/Bl mice infected with *Leishmania* there is a Th1 type of T-cell response to the infection, which leads to effective control and eradication of the infection; but in *Leishmania* infected Balb/c mice the T-cell response is of the Th2 type and severe, chronic and generalized disease develops.

These immune responses to *Leishmania* can be manipulated in various ways:

(1) in susceptible mice (e.g. Balb/c) interferon (IFN)γ can induce a healing Th1 response;

(2) treatment of resistant mice (e.g. C57/Bl) with a single injection of anti-IFNγ monoclonal antibody ablates Th1 cell development and promotes Th2 cell expansion thus making them susceptible to severe generalized disease;

(3) administering anti-interleukin (IL) 4 antibody can convert susceptible mice to resistant mice;

(4) conversely, introduction of a stable transgene of IL-4 into a resistant mouse produces prolonged susceptibility to the organism.

Cytokines in the micro-environment are critical in directing T-cell subset differentiation, and response to infection.

Evidence is now accumulating in animal models of autoimmune disease that Th1 cells are involved in pathogenesis of these diseases, and the use of transgenic animals has demonstrated that IL-2, IFNγ and tumour necrosis factor (TNF) α are important in the pathogenesis of some autoimmune diseases.

CD4+ T cells

CD4+ T cells, also known as helper/inducer cells, see processed antigen peptide in association with MHC class II molecules. Evidence for existence of human CD4+ Th1 and Th2 subsets was first provided by establishing T-cell clones to specific antigens: Th1 clones to *Mycobacterium tuberculosis*, which produced IL-2, IFNγ and TNFβ; and Th2 clones to allergens and *Toxocara canis*, which produced IL-4 and IL-5.

It is now clear that in rodents and humans at least three CD4+ subsets exist:

(1) T0 cells which produce all T-cell cytokines;

(2) Th1 cell producing mainly IL-2, IFNγ, and TNF, and which also activate macrophages, produce delayed-type hypersensitivity (DTH) and switch immunoglobulin production; and

(3) Th2 cells producing IL-4, IL-5, IL-6, IL-10, and IL-13, which promote B-cell development and differentiation.

Among human CD4 subsets IL-6 and IL-10 production are less clearly segregated than in rodents. There are also differences between human CD4+ subsets in their response to lymphokines. While

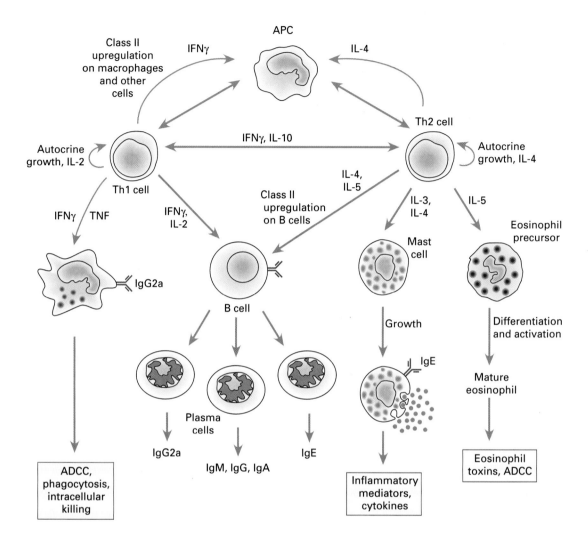

∎ Fig. 42.1 The central role of CD4 T cells in immune responses. TNF, tumour necrosis factor; ADCC, antibody-dependent cellular cytotoxicity; APC, antigen-presenting cell.

human Th1 and Th2 cells proliferate in response to IL-2, Th2 cells are much more responsive to IL-4 than Th1 cells, are not usually cytolytic and provide help to B cells in widely different ratios. In contrast, Th1 cells provide help only at low T:B ratios and in higher ratios may be cytolytic.

IL-1 and IL-4 are needed at the site of antigen-presenting cells (APC)/antigen T-cell interaction for Th2 cell development, whereas the presence of IFNγ, IFNα, TGFβ and IL-12 favour Th1 cell development (see Fig. 42.2). APC influence the pattern of cytokines produced by T cells in two ways. They produce cytokines which determine the T-cell subset. A key

cytokine that converts T0 cells to Th1 cells is IL-12 produced by dendritic cells, macrophages, and activated B cells. This augments production of IFNγ by T cells; causes natural killer (NK) cells to produce IFNγ; and inhibits the development of IL-4 producing cells. IFNγ promotes differentiation of T cells into Th1 cells *in vitro* and *in vivo*. The capacity of intracellular bacteria and some viruses to induce Th1 cells depends on their ability to stimulate IFNγ and IL-12 production by macrophages.

In contrast, early production of IL-4 with little or no IFNγ favours Th2 cell development. Mast cells and basophils can produce IL-4, which pushes T cells to

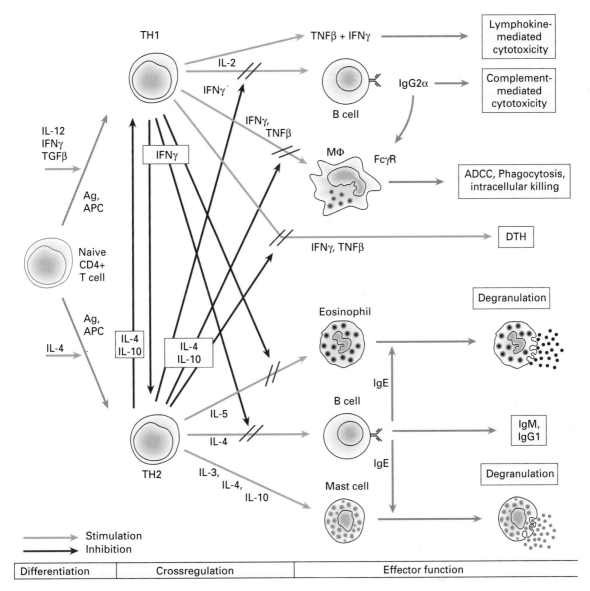

∎ Fig. 42.2 Factors influencing the development of Th1 and Th2 CD4 T cells and the effects of cytokines secreted by them on differentiation, cross-regulation, and effector function. APC, antigen-presenting cell; Ag, antigen; ADCC, antibody-dependent cellular cytotoxicity; DTH, delayed type hypersensitivity; MΦ, macrophage.

the Th2 cell development. IL-4, IL-10 and IL-13 produced by Th2 cells inhibit Th1 cell proliferation and have a strong inhibitory effect on macrophages. Each subset can downregulate activity by the other subset.

CD8+ T cells

CD8+ T cells, also known as the cytotoxic T cell (CTL) — suppressor cell subset, see synthesized antigenic peptide in association with major histocompatibility complex (MHC) class I molecules. The second stimulatory signal is usually provided by the cytokines secreted by activated Th1 cells: IL-2 is the principal cytokine but other cytokines, IL-4, IL-6, IFNγ, have been shown to have some effect. Resting precursor CTL do not express IL-2 receptor (IL-2R). After antigen stimulation the CD4+ and CD8+ CTL respond to production of IL-2 and are dependent on it for proliferation. Activation by antigen causes the precursor CTL to express IL-2R, and undergo differentiation into CTL. A number of

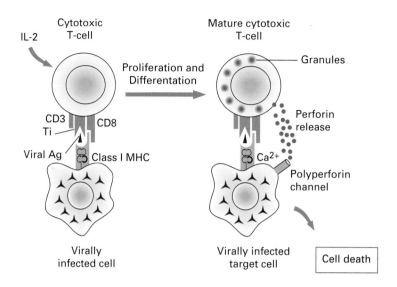

▌Fig. 42.3 The direct effects of CD8 cytotoxic T cells (CTL) on target cells. Ag, antigen; MHC, major histocompatibility complex.

cytokines are produced by CD8+ cells: IL-4, IL-6, IFNγ and TNFβ, but the levels do not appear to be sufficient for a continuing response and cytokines secreted by activated CD4+ cells are, in general, necessary. When levels of IL-2 decline CD4+ and CD8+ CTL undergo programmed cell death by apoptosis.

The means by which CD8+ cells might exert suppressive activity remains controversial. It has been possible to show that CD4+ T cells can be controlled by CD8+ T cells. Immunization with peptides derived from the T-cell receptor (TCR) variable region is capable of inducing CD8+ T cells which recognized these peptides and kill the CD4+ T cells expressing a TCR displaying the relevant peptide.

Apart from killing target cells CD8+ cells may suppress or regulate by cytokine production. Regulatory CD8+ cells have been found in low numbers in experimental animals, e.g. 50–500 in a rat. Initially identified as α–β– they were subsequently found to be γ+δ+ CD8+ cells.

Activation

Antigen is presented to CD4+ T cells in association with MHC class II and to CD8+ T with MHC class I. After engagement of the TCR CD4+ cells begin to synthesize proteins including surface activation markers, e.g. CD69, CD25 (IL-2R), MHC class II DR, and VLA-1. This is accompanied by transcription, translation and secretion of cytokines. The understanding of the fine tuning of events which lead to these

responses is of basic importance to manipulation of immunopathological reactions. Identification of the factors responsible for induction of cytokines which inhibit both release of proinflammatory cytokines and Th1 differentiation may lead to their use in immunotherapy of autoimmune disease.

Human disease

There is much evidence to suggest that human T-cell responses are polarized in a similar way to those of the mouse. Human Th1-like CD4+ cells develop during infections by viruses, intracellular bacteria and protozoa. Th2-like CD4+ cells develop in response to allergens and worm infestations. The activity of T subsets is similar in animal experimental autoimmune disease and human organ-specific autoimmune disease: human CD4+ T cells in autoimmune thyroid disease, Hashimoto's, and in retro-orbital infiltrates of Graves' disease, have a clear-cut Th1 profile with high levels of TNFα and IFNγ production and a cytolytic potential. Similarly most clones isolated from human peripheral blood and cerebrospinal fluid in multiple sclerosis (MS) have a Th1 profile of cytokine production, and TNFα and β are present in the lesions.

In human systemic autoimmune disease there is evidence that a Th1 response is predominant. Rheumatoid synovial fluid contains abundant amounts of 'inflammatory cytokines': IL-1, IL-6, IL-8, TNFα and granulocyte–macrophage colony-stimulating factor (GM-CSF), and lesser amounts of IL-2, IL-3, and IFNγ. It appears that TNFα is important in pathogenesis of rheumatoid arthritis (RA) and antibody to it, but not TNFβ, abrogates the persistent IL-1 production and produces clinical improvement. In rheumatoid synovial fragment culture IL-4 has been shown to depress production of the 'inflammatory cytokines' — IL-6, IL-1β and TNFα. There is evidence for the existence of the same cytokine profile in other systemic diseases, e.g. systemic lupus erythematosus (SLE), Sjögrens syndrome, and primary systemic vasculitis.

Points of intervention

T cells may be unresponsive to antigen due to:

(1) ignorance of the existence of the antigen;

(2) deletion of potentially antigen-reactive T cells

(3) anergy through 'non-professional' antigen presentation;

(4) suppression by other cells including other T cells.

Antigen presentation

Most of the therapies currently being investigated, mainly in animals, revolve around manipulating some component of the complex of MHC, digested peptide lying in the MHC cleft, and the TCR on the T cell as seen in Fig. 42.4. These include:

(1) use of modified epitope;

(2) effects on TCR (T cells vaccination, or use of anti-TCR antibody); and on T cells.

(3) blocking co-stimulatory molecules which are important as second signals.

Epitope modification

All immune responses are initiated by recognition of a specific antigenic (epitope) peptide in association with MHC. Therefore interference with this display may prevent the response developing or continuing. Various ways of blocking the response are possible:

(1) other peptides may bind to MHC molecules and prevent the antigenic peptide from doing so;

(2) identification of the antigenic peptide may allow synthesis of large amounts of the peptide, which could be used to produce high-dose tolerance;

(3) modification of the antigenic peptide to convert the peptide from an agonist to an antagonist.

Recent studies have suggested that subtle changes in the peptide with which TCRs react may change the

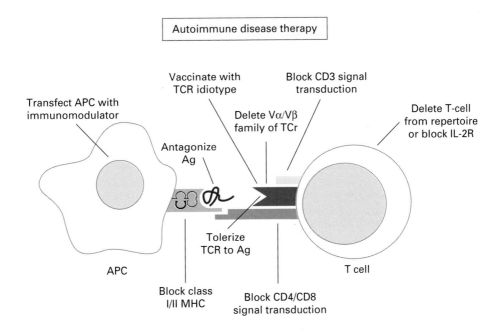

▌Fig. 42.4 Antigen (Ag) presentation. The principal participants in antigen presentation and the sites of immune intervention. APC, antigen-presenting cell; MHC, major histocompatibility complex; TCR, T-cell receptor.

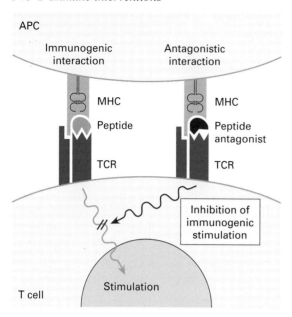

∎ **Fig. 42.5** The effects of antigenic peptide and peptide antagonists. APC, antigen-presenting cell; MHC, major histocompatibility complex.

nature of the signal transmitted to the T cell and that antigen (epitope) analogues can act as powerful and specific inhibitors of T-cell activation.

Antigen analogues which differ by one amino acid in the T-cell epitope site can act as antagonists of the TCR. In TCR antagonism the antigen analogue does not initiate signalling events in its own right and also competitively inhibits antigen initiated signalling. Various groups using single or double amino acid substitution in antigens *in vivo* have shown that it is possible to interfere with autoantigenic recognition by T cells, and that the effects appear to be long-lasting. This effect appears to be associated with engagement of the TCR at other than at the crucial affinity (lower or higher) threshold. For example, Smilek *et al.* (1991) found in experimental allergic encephalomyelitis (EAE) a peptide analogue with a higher affinity for MHC than the the wild-type peptide of major basic protein (MBP) was a potent tolerance inducing agent. This may be because the proper membrane-related events do not take place.

It is possible that engagement of the TCR can be associated with either no activation, partial or full activation. In a DR-1 restricted T-cell clone reactive to haemagglutinin (HA) it has been shown that modification of any of the five major T-cell contact residues of HA 307–319 recognized by the clone could

yield antagonists. When a series of analogues were used in which crucial T-cell contact residues were inserted in to a polyalanine backbone analogues with a single TCR contact residue were neither antagonistic nor antigenic; those with two TCR contact residues were weakly antagonistic; three or four TCR contact residues were strongly antagonistic, and those with all five TCR contact residues were strongly antigenic. These antagonistic effects may be prolonged. Pretreatment of animals with an analogue of encephalitogenic peptide has a long-acting effect and inhibits development of EAE when the encephalitogenic peptide is subsequently given.

HA antigen analogues can inhibit HA antigen prepulsed assays, but not other specific antigen prepulsed assays. Analogues have been used in other antigens systems: proteolipid (PLP), ovalbumin (OVA), haemoglobin, and cytochrome *c*, with similar results. It is therefore likely that this is a general phenomenom.

In contrast to T-cell antagonism there is also the phenomenon of partial agonism. In this an analogue elicits some, but not all, signals, for example IL-4 may be synthesized but the T cells are not induced to proliferate. Some cases of T-cell anergy have also been reported.

TCR engagement can result in:

(1) horizontal signalling (the formation of specific APC/T-cell conjugates via upregulation of specific adhesion molecules and other membrane events; and/or

(2) vertical signalling (VCa^{++} influx, IP turnover, and other intracellular activation events).

Antagonists and partial agonists probably act by uncoupling these two events.

T-cell antagonism, agonism, or anergy have great therapeutic potential and are being evaluated as practical ways of dealing with human allergic or autoimmune disease. An obstacle to this work is that in most instances the relevant antigen which occupies the MHC cleft in human diseases is not known. However, new techniques have been developed to characterize the naturally processed peptides which have been eluted from the binding groove of both MHC class I and II molecules. Animal experiments suggest the possibility that a single antigen analogue may antagonize polyclonal responses if there is a common critical TCR contact residue in these responses.

T-cell receptor

If a reactive restricted T-cell population can be identified as pathogenic it can be modified and rendered immunogenic to induce an anti-idiotype (anti-clonotypic) response by T-cell vaccination. By T-cell vaccination in animal models it has been possible to protect against experimental autoimmune disease, inhibit allogeneic responses and delayed-type hypersensitivity. It has also been recently used to prolong cardiac allograft survival in rats.

It is possible to target the specific TCR α and/or β chains. However, this depends on restriction of the antigen-driven T-cell responses to very limited α and β (or γ/δ) chains usage in the TCR if the effects are not to be too widespread. In EAE the T cells responsible for the lesions have Vβ8 chains in their TCR, and administration of an antibody to Vβ8 chain reverses paralytic disease. If there is a restriction of the α or β chains in the TCR of T cells in a disease process then this can be an effective way of modifying the specific immune response and it has been used in experimental models of human disease, e.g. suppression in the rat of antigen-induced arthritis.

EAE has been successfully treated by immunizing the animals with a peptide from one (residues 39–59 of Vβ8) of the TCR molecules.

Antibody to T cells

Unlike the two previous techniques, this method has been used in humans for many years. Initially, T cells were reduced by polyclonal antilymphocyte globulin (ALG), but now monoclonal antibody (MoAb) anti-CD3 provides more focused therapy. Binding of anti-CD3 MoAb to cells leads to T-cell activation and cytokine release. There is initially almost complete removal of CD3 bearing T cells from circulation due to complement mediated lysis and their clearance by the reticuloendothelial system. Subsequently, T cells appear without CD3 but expressing other T-cell markers. When cultured *in vitro* these T cells will produce CD3. The CD3 receptor may be modulated from the surface of immature cells by continuing presence of antibody. In some patients troublesome side-effects occur: fever, rigors, myalgia, and occasionally hypotension about 1 h after administration due to massive release of cytokines especially TNF and IFNγ. Rarely, the leakage of cells and fluid from blood vessels may be so severe as to lead to severe hypotension and death. However, a longer-term problem is that one-third receiving doses of >75 mg of anti-CD3 antibody develop a malignancy. Another problem is that most of the antibodies used are mouse MoAbs, which are immunogenic to humans. These antibodies may be modified, or 'humanized', by genetical or chemical manipulation to make them less immunogenic. Humanization of mouse MoAb can occur through grafting the mouse antigen binding loops on to a human immunoglobulin molecule; cloning human V

regions into a phage library and selecting for the appropriate antibody; and making mice transgenic for human heavy and light immunoglobulin chains before raising the antibody.

It is possible to use MoAb directed at other molecules on the T-cell surface. Several groups have generated specific tolerance for antigen in animals with anti-CD4+ antibody. Spontaneous and experimental autoimmune disease has been prevented, including insulin-dependent diabetes, thyroiditis, systemic lupus, and arthritis. In patients with RA given anti-CD4+ antibody increased mobility was observed. MoAbs under investigation for use in preventing and dealing with transplant rejection are those against CD2, CD4+, CD6, CD7, CD8, CD25.

T-cell stimulatory molecules

T-cell anergy can result from antigen receptor stimulation in absence of co-stimulation. Several co-stimulatory, or 'second', signals have been proposed: LFA-1/ICAM-1, VLA4/VCAM-1, CD2/LFA-3, and unknown/HSA, but most important is CD28/B7/BB1. CD28 is found on virtually all T cells and it is upregulated during activation. B7/BB1 is found on activated macrophages, dendritic cells, Langerhans cells, and activated B cells. This co-stimulation appears to inhibit negative regulators of IL-2 and therefore allows IL-2 production. *In vivo* blockade of CD28/B7 interaction occurs with CTLA4-immunoglobulin, a soluble form of CTLA4, and an alternative B7-binding molecule. There is little CD28/B7 interaction from small resting B cells which may explain why they have poor APC activity. Poor CD28/B7 interaction can induce anergy, *in vivo* and *in vitro*; facilitate transplantation tolerance; and blockade of B7/CD28 interaction inhibits proliferative response to alloantigen. Inhibition of other, i.e. non-CD28/B7, accessory molecules may induce T-cell anergy and also facilitate graft survival.

CD4+ T cells are susceptible to anergy if exposed to MHC–antigen on chemically fixed APCs, fibroblasts and resting B cells. The anergic T cells can regain their activity *in vitro* by addition of IL-2 or by 'resting' in the absence of the antigen.

Tolerance and suppression of T cells

T-cell responses may be modulated by exposure to antigen. Passive exposure of the mucosae of respiratory or gastrointestinal tracts in mice or rats to low levels of soluble protein antigen stimulates antigen-specific T0- or Th2-like cells in the regional lymph

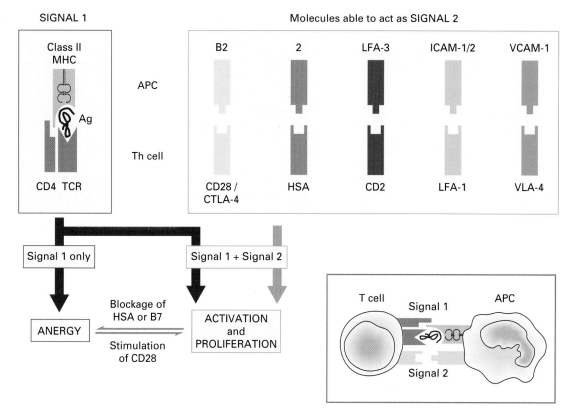

∎**Fig. 42.6** Two signals are required by CD4 T cells for activation and proliferation. Ag, antigen; APC, antigen-presenting cell; TCR, T-cell receptor.

nodes, and brief immunoglobulin (Ig) E antibody production. This is followed on continued exposure by Th1 responses with high IFNγ production and IgE responses cease. This state of 'low zone tolerance' can be transferred by CD8 γ+δ+ cells. Exposure to high doses of antigen leads to T-cell anergy, or may lead to T-cell deletion due to engagement of the TCR by specific antigen while the cell is cycling under the influence of IL-2 which leads to apoptosis.

There are various ways of producing modulation: subcutaneous; intravenous; oral gastrointestinal; intranasal; and tracheobronchial aerosol.

Oral tolerization

It has long been recognized that soluble, deaggregated, antigen in high doses administered orally or intravenously may lead to antigen-specific tolerance. The oral method has been used to induce antigen-specific tolerance/suppression in animal models of MS, uveitis, and diabetes and arthritis induced by type II collagen. In the rodent EAE model oral administration of MBP

before, or during, EAE induction aborted or diminished the disease.

Oral tolerance in animals can be explained by two mechanisms.

1. Large doses produce T-cell anergy to the specific antigen due to presentation of antigen by non-professional APCs i.e. high zone tolerance.

2. Small doses induces generation of MHC class I and II restricted regulatory T cells that release cytokines. For example, the oral effect of MBP is due to inactivation or suppression of proinflammatory cells in the CNS by local production of TGFβ and to a lesser extent IL-4 and prostaglandin (PG) E$_z$ IL-4 by 'regulatory T cells', which migrate from the gut. The production of these inhibitory cytokines correlates with the active suppression of the inflammatory process. The implication of this is that orally administered protein can downregulate immune responses but it is not obligatory for the peptide presented to be the disease inducing peptide. For example in PLP-induced EAE the oral

administration of MBP can suppress the disease; at the site of PLP-induced lesions MBP is also released and activates MBP-specific regulatory T cells which then downregulate the inflammatory activity due to PLP.

The application of this to human disease is being examined.

Suppression

This area has been the topic of much controversy because of the difficulty in identifying suppressor cell and the means of their action. Because of these difficulties the concept of suppressor cells fell into disrepute. However, if Jerne's concept of idiotype is accepted then suppressor cell function would be expected. In any discussion now it is necessary to specify if suppression is specific and non-specific, and in the case of specific suppression if it is idiotypic and antigen specific in nature.

Antigen-specific suppression/Th1–Th2 cell switch

Cells may suppress effector responses through recognition of the same antigen as that recognized by the effector cell. CD8 alloantigen specific suppressor cells have been described in *in vitro* systems. One model proposes that different cells act in a cascade involving Ts1 cells, which are antigen-specific CD4 inducers of suppressor cells.

Suppression of one type of immune response may be due to activation of another type of immune response, for example IL-4 and IL-10 downregulate Th1 cells, and IFNγ may downregulate Th2 cells. Increased IL-4 production has been observed within accepted allogeneic heart allografts in rats, and reduced IL-2 production in renal allografts supports a role for T-cell subset regulation, but caution is needed because this is as yet unproven.

Non-specific suppression

Natural suppressor cells have not been clearly defined but may be CD3+/4–/8–/Thy+/TCR– cells distinct from NK cells present in marrow after lymphoid DXR or CY and in neonatal spleen.

Cytokine and cytokine receptors

The immune response:

(1) may be abolished, changed or increased by cytokine administration, e.g. IL-2, IL-4, IFNγ; transforming growth factor (TGF) β; or IL-4, IL-10;

(2) inhibited by blocking cytokine receptor with antibodies, soluble receptors or receptor antagonists;

(3) may be blocked or inhibited non-specifically, e.g. with corticosteroid or cytotoxic drugs.

Cytokine administration

IL-2 is produced by stimulated C4 T cells. It acts on recently synthesized IL-2R to induce clonal expansion of IL-2 responsive T and B cells, and stimulates activity of NK cells and lymphokine-activating killer (LAK) cells. Intravenous IL-2 provokes massive release of IL-1, IFNγ, and TNF, which are mediators of increased vascular permeability and induce endothelial cell activation. The most serious side-effect is *vascular leak syndrome*, which may produce hypotension, pulmonary oedema, and neuropsychiatric symptoms. IL-2 is produced by three types of cells; CD4 cells; NK cells; and CD8 cells. It make macrophages more microbicidal and tumoricidal, increases the cytotoxic effects of NK cells, and induces B cells to produce antibody.

IL-4 has been shown to depress IL-6, IL-1β, and TNFα in synovial fragments, to downregulate CD5 on B cells and reduces rheumatoid factor (RF) production *in vitro*. The inflammatory cytokine IL-6 is secreted by synovial cells in response to IL-1 and TNF, and is present in inflamed joints and the serum of patients with RA. The serum level correlates with disease activity.

G-CSF and GM-CSF have powerful effects on production of granulocytes, monocytes, and macrophages and enhance the function of mature cells. *IL-3* is a multilineage CSF. These CSFs shorten radiation or drug induced neutropenias. Some malignancies have receptors that could be stimulated before therapy.

IFNs are antiviral glycoproteins which are used to manipulate immune responses. They bind to cell surface receptors and also have antitumour effects due to:

(1) direct antiproliferative effect on some tumour cells;

(2) increased tumour cell antigenicity, MHC and TNF receptors increased;

(3) enhanced antitumour response: enhanced T cell, NK, and macrophage function.

IFNα is produced by B lymphocytes, null lymphocytes, and macrophages. Human IFNα consists of more than 25 structurally similar proteins which consist of 165–166 amino acids. Multiple IFNα genes have been identified. Recombinant IFN-α represent individual subtypes eg IFNα-2a, 2c, etc. Locally IFNα has effects on genital warts, herpes keratoconjunctivitis, laryngeal papillomatosis, and systemically on the course of hepatitis B and (HBV) and C virus (HCV) in chronic carriers, cytomegalouvirus (CMV), and herpes zoster. Its antitumour effect varies with remissions in:

(1) >70% in hairy cell leukaemia, CML, basal and squamous cell cancer;

(2) 30–70% in low or intermediate grade lymphoma and cutaneous T lymphoma;

(3) 10–30% in renal cell Ca Kaposi's, metastatic melanoma, multiple myeloma, and bladder cancer;

(4) <10% in breast, lung, colon, prostatic, hepatocellular cancer, and AML.

In hairy cell leukaemia, renal cancer and cutaneous T-lymphoma IFNα has a major role in treating a condition which responds poorly to other therapy. In HCV hepatitis it induces marked improvement in biochemical and histological in ~50%. The toxic effects are tolerable and include fever, anorexia, flu-like illness, a reversible bone marrow suppression, liver dysfunction, and cardiotoxicity.

IFNβ is produced by fibroblasts, macrophages, and epithelial cells. Human IFNβ has a MW of 22–23 kDa and is 166 amino acids long, and there is only one gene. IFNβ may augment suppressor function, reduce the effects of IFNγ in inducing MHC class II expression, and reduce IFNγ production. In MS a decline in disease progression and lesion activity has been reported after IFNβ.

IFNγ is produced by stimulated T cells and NK cells. There is one gene in humans. Natural IFNγ is a heterogeneous group of molecules of 146 amino acids but of differing MW due to a varying amount of carbohydrate. It binds to a unique receptor, affects many types of cells, and activates macrophages. It is most effective where there is defective cell immune function, e.g. lepromatous leprosy, leishmaniasis, and chronic granulomatous disease (CGD). In CGD after 1 year 70% of those who received IFNγ were free of severe infection, but only 30% of those given placebo. In 1993 reports were published of inactivation and gene knockout of IFNγ. Most striking was vulnerability of mice to intracellular parasites *Listeria* and *Mycobacteria*. IFNγ is critical for activating macrophages and the production of nitric oxide radicals. In vaccinia IFNγ is essential to back up IFNα and β.

Mutated cytokines

These have potential uses in blocking cytokine responses. For example a mutant form of IL-4 in which aspartic acid replaces tyrosine at position 124 amino acids and has a conformation similar to the wild type, blocks IL-13 and IL-4 driven B-cell proliferation,

and IgE and IgG4 synthesis. This may have potential uses in atopic states. Other mutated cytokines, e.g. of GM-CSF are being investigated.

Blocking cytokine/cytokine receptor

At the sites of autoimmune inflammation the presence of IL-2, IFNγ, IFNα, TNFα IL-1α and IL-1β indicates that they may be responsible for disease. From studies with transgenic animals it has been found that the expression of these cytokines may give rise to autoimmune disease. TNFα appears to be of particular importance in RA. Mice that are transgenic for human TNFα developed arthritis which begins 4 weeks after birth, but the disease may be prevented by mab to human TNFα.

Studies in mice on the effect of deficiency of cytokine and cytokine receptors reveal that the effect of the receptor deficiency is more severe than that of cytokine deficiency. In humans this is illustrated by the severe immunodeficiency caused by deficiencies of IL2-Rγ chain and CD40 ligand in the sex-linked combined immunodeficiency (SCID) and hyper-IgM forms of immunodeficiency.

Soluble cytokine receptors are a natural source of cytokine inhibitor. However, soluble cytokine receptors are monomeric, do not exert a prolonged effect, and bind cytokine with less affinity than a dimeric form constructed as a chimeric product with human IgG Fc, e.g. TNF R-Ig. This immunofusion construct does not bind to FcR or activate complement, but does block effects of lipopolysaccharide injection in mice. Similarly, EAE has been blocked by a human fusion protein of truncated IgG1–TNF receptor molecule (IgG1–TNF–Rp55). A soluble IFNγ receptor immunoglobulin (sIFN γR-Ig) construct has been used in animal models of MS and SLE; it delayed the onset of renal damage; reduced and delayed antibodies to ds-DNA; and prevented the onset of membrano-proliferative nephritis. In an IL-4 transgenic mouse model of acute bronchial eosinophilia administration of either sIL-5R or an immunofusion construct inhibited eosinophilic infiltration.

Interference with migration of inflammatory cells

Adhesion molecules

Activated inflammatory cells display adhesion molecules on their surface which facilitate the migration of the cells in tissues. When inflammatory mediators, e.g. thrombin, histamine, and cytokines, are liberated adhesion molecules become expressed; P-selectin within minutes of thrombin, and E-selectin after 3–6 h. The presence of inflammatory cytokines (e.g. IL-1, IL-4 IFNγ, and TNF) also induce ICAM-1 and VCAM-1 after 12–24 h. Leucocytes passing along the blood vessel bind by their selectin ligands to the selectins expressed on the endothelial cells and can come to rest in milliseconds. The next part of the process is activation of leucocyte integrin molecules, e.g. LFA-1 and VLA-4. Chemoattractants binding to receptors on the leucocyte initiate conformational changes in the integrin which then allows it to bind to its ligand.

The activated integrins attach the leucocytes firmly to the endothelium creating bonds, e.g. LFA/ICAM-1 and VLA-4/VCAM-1 (Fig. 42.7(b)). The leucocyte flattens and then moves into the extracellular matrix by moving through the endothelial cell junction. Integrins

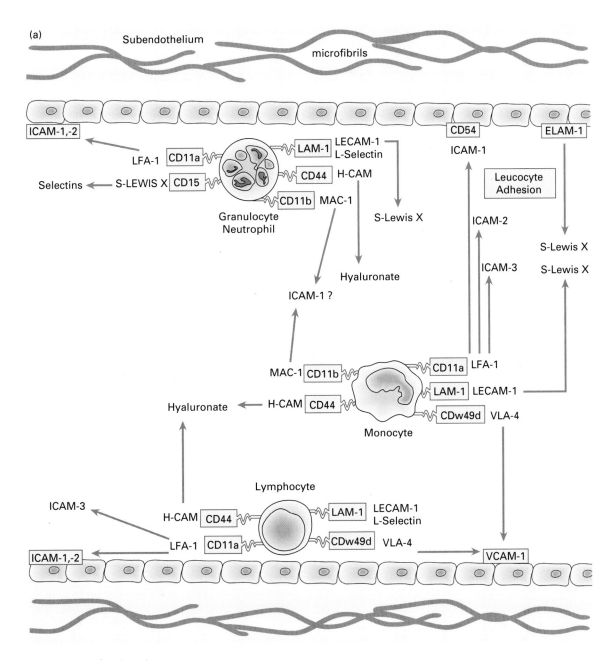

∎ **Fig. 42.7** *Continued*

(b)

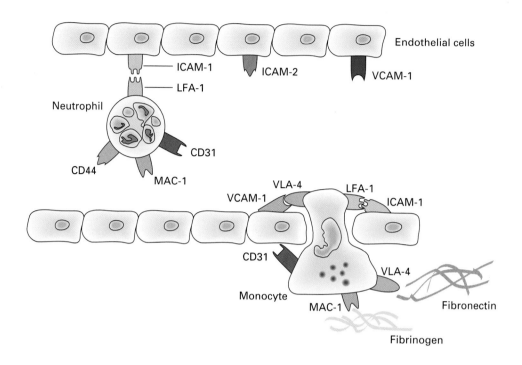

▎ **Fig. 42.7** Inflammatory cell adhesion and migration: the role of selectins and integrins.

are heterodimeric molecules consisting of non-covalently associated α and β units which are involved in cell–cell and cell–substratum adhesion.

Monoclonal antibody to ICAM-1 prevents the induction of collagen-induced arthritis in DBA/1 mice. In mouse EAE antibody to α4 blocks adhesion of lymphocytes and monocytes to inflamed brain endothelium and prevents disease.

Immunosuppression

General suppression of immune responses can be achieved by drugs, radiation, or monoclonal antibodies.

Drugs

Corticosteroids

Immunosuppressive effects

A single dose of corticosteroid causes changes in cell traffic. Within 2 h there is a transient lymphopenia, mainly affecting helper T cells, which disappears within 24 h. The effect depends on dose, method of administration, and timing. In addition reduced macrophage handling of antigen accounts for poor primary antibody responses, and decreased IL-1 production from macrophages affects T-cell proliferation. Because memory cells are more resistant to steroids secondary responses are not affected as much as primary responses. Higher doses of corticosteroid inhibit IL-2 production. In some immunologically mediated conditions the additional anti-inflammatory role and modulation of macrophage function is important, for example in systemic lupus erythematosus (SLE) and idiopathic thrombocytopenic purpura (ITP). In transplantation low doses alone are ineffective in preventing rejection but high doses may do so. A troublesome side-effect of higher doses is the increased susceptibility to infection but this can be reduced by high doses in short courses or giving lower doses combined with another 'steroid sparing' drug, e.g. cyclosporin.

Anti-inflammatory effect

One of the major effects of corticosteroids is due to the inhibition of cytokines produced by lymphocytes and endothelial cells, which in turn leads to less leucocyte adhesion to endothelial cells due to reduced expression of adhesion molecules. Other anti-inflammatory effects are reductions in: oedema; proliferation of fibroblasts and deposition of collagen; neovascularization; and vasodilation. There is less or no fever due to inhibition of cytokine release from macrophages. Corticosteroid induces lipocortin, which inhibits formation of arachidonic acid metabolites — prostaglandins and leukotrienes.

Antimetabolites

Thiopurines

Azathioprine is inactive until it passes through the liver. There it is converted to 6-mercaptopurine (6MP) which inhibits both DNA and RNA synthesis by a negative feedback loop suppressing *de novo* purine synthesis. Because the drug is catabolized by xanthine oxidase the administration of allopurinol can lead to a marked increase in the suppressive and marrow toxic effects of azathioprine. This drug affects all dividing cells by inhibition of DNA synthesis and its main immunosuppressive effect is due to a reduction in NK cells and an effect on T cells. It has little effect on B-cell function. The most important side-effects are neutropenia and thrombocytopenia. It is mainly used in transplantation except when there is liver failure. It is necessary to follow blood counts as long-term effects are seen on granulocyte, platelet, and red cell production.

Methotrexate prevents conversion of folic acid to tetrafolic acid, which is needed for synthesis of thymidylic acid which in turn is needed for DNA synthesis. The major immunosuppressive effect is on lymphocytes, which are inhibited from proliferating.

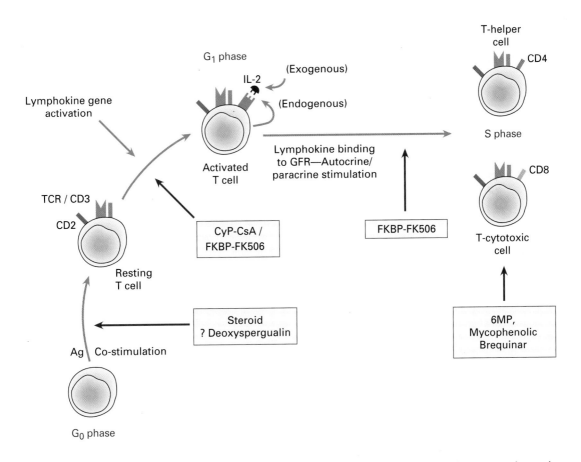

∎ **Fig. 42.8** The cell cycle and the effect of immunosuppressive drugs upon it. TCR, T-cell recetpor; Ag, antigen, GFR, receptor for growth. 6MP, 6-mercaptopurine.

Cytotoxic agents

Alkylating agents affect dividing cells by interfering with DNA at premitotic stage. Tissues vary in their ability to repair DNA damage. These drugs have little direct anti-inflammatory action.

Cyclophosphamide requires to pass through the liver to become active. It impairs specific DTH and antibody production when given before or immediately after antigen. It is clinically useful in aggressive forms of SLE, severe vasculitis, Wegener's granulomatosis, and also in conditioning bone marrow recipients.

Chlorambucil is mainly used for low-grade lymphoma etc. and appears to act on B cells.

Cyclosporin

This is a fungal metabolite which is a strongly hydrophobic cyclic peptide of 11 amino acids. It suppresses humoral and cell-mediated immunity by blocking IL-2 synthesis and preventing clonal expansion of T cells. The immune response relies on production of cytokines to produce its aggressive effects and also to upregulate expression of HLA and adhesion molecules. The principal effect of cyclosporin is to inhibit secretion of cytokines derived from T cells especially the production of IL-2, IL-3, IL-4, IL-5, and IFNγ. It may also effect IL-2R expression. Therefore inhibition of cytokines, especially IFNγ, reduces inflammatory immune responses. Cyclosporin appears to spare suppressor cells and in some animal transplants this leads to tolerance of the graft. For it to exert its activity it must be complexed to the intracellular receptor cyclophilin, a 17 kDa protein. This complex formation inhibits early Ca^{2+}-dependent effects, especially IL-2 and IFNγ production. The immunosuppressive effect may be due to an alteration of folding of transcription factor required for T-cell cytokine expression. However, cyclophilin is present in a number of cells but cyclosporin effects are seen mainly in T cells. This may be due to the cyclosporin–calmodulin complex binding to calcineurin which is the predominant calmodulin binding protein in T cells. The major effects are reduction in IL-2 production, CD4-cell-dependent proliferative responses, and NK activity. The effect on accessory cells is controversial but there is some evidence that IL-1 synthesis may be affected. Cell function returns to normal within a few hours of stopping the drug.

Cyclosporin has a major effect in prolonging graft survival and nearly all transplant protocols now have cyclosporin in them. In animals a short course of cyclosporin may yield long survival of grafts, but in humans this is not so. It has been used in some autoimmune disease, e.g. psoriasis, uveitis and, insulin-dependent diabetes mellitus. There is a quick effect, but a relapse occurs when drug withdrawn, and the clinical course of disease may not be affected. However, it has established a place in the treatment of:

(1) severe psoriasis unresponsive to systemic treatment with methotrexate, PUVA, and topical treatment;

(2) uveitis unresponsive to corticosteroids;

(3) aplastic anaemia, where it is as effective as ALG and prednisone, and in combination with these is even more effective;

(4) severe RA where it has been found to be as effective as azathioprine, penicillamine, and chloroquine.

There has been concern about the nephrotoxic effect of higher doses of cyclosporin. Other side-effects are on renal and liver function, gingival hyperplasia, tremor, hirsutism, lymphoma induction, and increased susceptibility to oncogenic effects of Epstein–Barr virus. Non-Hodgkins lymphoma occurs in 1–10% of transplants, and Kaposi's sarcoma may occur within a few years of transplant.

FK506

This is also derived from a soil fungus. The structure is different from cyclosporin and it binds to a different intracellular protein. It inhibits IL-2, IL-3, IL-4 and IFNγ but is a 10–100 times more potent. Side-effects are similar to cyclosporin.

Mycophenolic acid

Purine synthesis is blocked by this drug, which also inhibits glycosylation of adhesion molecules and the proliferation of smooth muscle.

15-deoxyspergualin

Humoral responses and B cell proliferation are strongly affected.

Rapamycin

Another fungal product which does not inhibit IL-2 but inhibits the signalling pathway used by IL-2R by interfering with protein kinases. This inhibits cell proliferation.

Brequinar sodium

It inhibits pyrimidine synthesis.

Antibodies

Immune responses may be affected by administration of antibodies by:

(1) removing antigen;

(2) removing or inactivating cells that cause damage with antibodies to: TCR, CD3, CD4, CD8, MHC molecules, integrins involved in antigen presentation, vascular endothelium, and B7.1 and B7.2 co-stimulatory molecules;

(3) suppressing antibodies via idiotype-anti-idiotype mechanisms;

(4) neutralizing cytokines or inflammatory agents, and blocking receptors.

Administration of anti-rhesus antibody at the end of pregnancy to rhesus negative women was originally given with the intention of removing rhesus-positive fetal cells (i.e. antigen) rapidly from the circulation before the immune system was activated. It is the most successful form of antibody-mediated immune manipulation, and the widespread use in Caucasians of anti-D has prevented rhesus iso-immunization and dramatically reduced the incidence of rhesus haemolytic disease of the newborn. However, although highly effective clinically, its mechanism of action in inhibiting rhesus iso-immunization is not clearly defined.

Antibodies are also used to deplete populations of cells. Polyclonal antilymphocyte antibody was used in transplantation, but now MoAbs anti-CD3 and anti-CD4 are used. These have been discussed earlier in this section and in the section on renal transplantation. MoAbs are also used *in vitro* to purge bone marrow of immunocompetent and malignant cells prior to marrow transplantation.

Attempts have been made to block the effect of cytokines by administration of MoAbs. In shock-like states and cerebral malaria, TNF levels are very high (two to 10 times controls; the highest in fatal cases), but this partly preventable with administration of MoAb to TNF.

Treatment with intravenous immunoglobulin

Primary antibody deficiency and severe secondary forms of antibody deficiency require replacement treatment with immunoglobulin in order to reduce the infections associated with these conditions. It is also of value in the other condition where it exerts a modulating effect on the immune response. In ITP 1 g immunoglobulin/kg body weight given for 2 days and repeated every 4 weeks helps raise the platelet count, but this rise may be transient.

The means by which intravenous immunoglobulin exerts its effect is not clear and may be due to one or more of the following:

(1) anti-idiotype–idiotype regulation of immune responses;

(2) partial or complete blockade in of the Fc receptors on phagocytic cells by Fc present in the immunoglobulin preparation;

(3) decreased macrophage cytokine production;

(4) reduced production of immunoglobulin by B cells;

(5) suppressor T-cell activation;

(6) alterations in complement-mediated clearance.

The effectiveness of intravenous immunoglobulin has been established in controlled trials in polyneuritis, chronic polyneuropathy, Kawasaki vasculitis. In other conditions it has been tried and benefit claimed, e.g. Wegeners granulomatosis, systemic vasculitits, autoimmune haemolytic anaemia, neutropenia, and polymyositis.

Plasmapheresis

This technique involves separating plasma from cellular components and returning only the cell-enriched fraction to the patient. Lowering the plasma level of IgG, apart from IgG3, slightly reduces the fractional catabolic rate (FCR) of that protein so that the less there is present the less is catabolized (the FCR varies from 18%/day to 2% dependent on the concentration), but the FCR of IgM, IgA, and IgG3 remains constant.

Plasmapheresis may be helpful clinically:

1. Through the removal of pathogenic immunoglobulin in hyperviscosity sydrome due to monoclonal protein (IgM in Waldenström's macroglobulinaemia or IgA myeloma). The symptoms of hyperviscosity: visual problems, abnormal bleeding, neurological symptoms, e.g. headaches, coma, thromboses, and congestive cardiac failure. In Waldenström's macroglobulinaemia as 70–80% of IgM is in the intravascular compartment plasmapheresis rapidly reduces the amount of the hyperviscosity inducing IgM.

2. Through the removal of pathogenic antibody, e.g. in rhesus haemolytic disease, in haemophilia (10% have IgG directed against factor VIII), in

Goodpasture's disease, myasthenia gravis, and Guillain–Barré polyneuritis.

3. Removal of immune complexes and mediators of damage, and relief of the the effects of their clearance by the reticuloendothelial system. In decreasing order of importance this is used in cryoglobulinaemia, Sjögrens syndrome, vasculitis, progressive glomerulonephritis, rheumatoid disease, and SLE.

In plasma exchange the red cell fraction is re-infused in donor plasma and the effect may also be due to the immunomodulating effect of immunoglobulin infused.

Further reading

Cooke A. and Wraith D. C. (1993). Immunotherapy of autoimmune disease. *Current Opinion in Immunology*, **5**, 925–35.

Elliott, M. J., Maini, R. N., Feldmann, M., Long-Fox, A., Charles, P., Katsikis, P., *et al.* (1993). Treatment of rheumatoid arthritis with chimeric monoclonal antibodies to tumour necrosis factor α. *Arthritis and Rheumatism*, **344**, 1105–10.

Khoury, S. J., Hancock, W. W., and Weiner, H. L. (1992). Oral tolerance to myelin basic protein and natural recovery from experimental autoimmune encephalomyelitis are associated with downregulation of inflammatory cytokine and differential upregulation of transforming growth factor β, interleukin 4 and prostaglandin E expression in the brain. *Journal of Experimental Medicine*, **176**, 1355–64.

Norman, P. S. (1993). Modern concepts of immunotherapy. *Current Opinion in Immunology*, **5**, 968–74.

Smilek, D. E., Wraith, D. C., Hodkinson, S., Dwivedy, S., Steinman, L., and McDevitt, H. O. (1991). A single amino acid change in a myelin basic protein peptide confers the capacity to prevent rather than induce experimental autoimmune encephalomyelitis. *Proceedings of the National Academy of Sciences USA*, **88**, 9633–7.

The IFN β Multiple Sclerosis Trial. (1993). Interferon 1β is effective in relapsing–remitting multiple sclerosis: MRI results of a multicentre, randomized, double blind, placebo-controlled trial. *Neurology*, **43**, 662–7.

Index